The Experimental Foundations of Modern Immunology

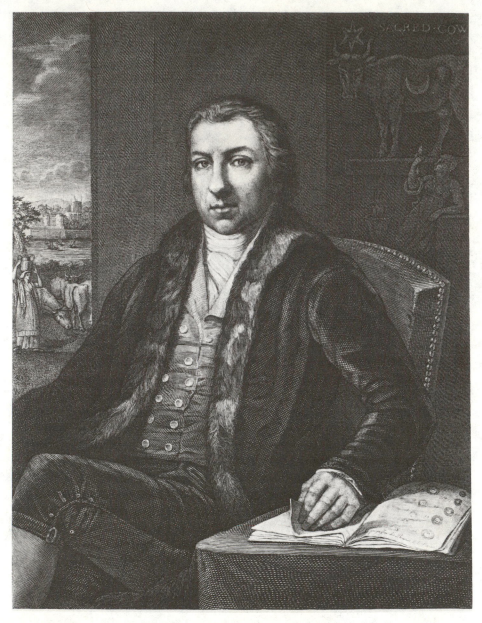

Edward Jenner (1749—1823) discovered that immunization with the relatively innocuous cowpox conferred protection against the more deadly smallpox. This discovery led to the widespread adoption of vaccination and was a major stimulus for the study of the phenomenon of immunity.

Early nineteenth-century line engraving by Antoine Maxime Monsaldi. The original engraving is in the collection of, and is reproduced here with the kind permission of, Dr. Derrick Baxby, Department of Medical Microbiology, Liverpool University. The history of this engraving is discussed in Med. History 22, 335 (1978).

THE EXPERIMENTAL FOUNDATIONS OF MODERN IMMUNOLOGY

THIRD EDITION

William R. Clark

Department of Biology
and the Molecular Biology Institute

University of California, Los Angeles

JOHN WILEY & SONS

New York   Chichester   Brisbane   Toronto   Singapore

Library of Congress Cataloging in Publication Data:

Clark, William R., 1938–
    The experimental foundations of modern immunology.

    Includes index.
    1. Immunology, Experimental—History.   I. Title.
QR182.C53   1986   574.2'9   85-31995
ISBN 0-471-81508-X

Printed in the United States of America

10 9 8 7 6 5 4 3

Preface

The underlying philosophy of this third edition of *The Experimental Foundations of Modern Immunology* remains the same as for the first edition: The best way to learn immunology is to study those landmark experiments that have brought us to our present understanding of how the immune system functions. This is true whether the student is preparing for a career in basic research or in medicine. In either profession, one must always ask not simply *whether* something is so, but *why* it is so and how we *know* it is so.

No textbook for an advanced scientific course can ever be a substitute for reading the primary scientific literature. This text is designed to teach the language of immunology and to describe the most important experiments during the early development of the field, thus preparing the student to begin reading the current primary immunology literature on his or her own as soon as possible.

More recent developments in immunology are also described from an experimental point of view. Some of these were "hot new topics" from the earlier editions of this text. The ones that survive in this edition are beginning to take their place as classic and definitive experiments. Some of the most intriguing new developments described in the present edition will make it to future editions; others won't. That's part of the excitement of being at the leading edge of any field. Many of the most compelling new developments in these chapters are still incomplete, left hanging, as it were, almost in midsentence. If you are curious about the outcome, look up the experimenters or the topic in the most current volumes of *Biological Abstracts* or *Chemical Abstracts,* or thumb through recent issues of the *Journal of Immunology, Nature, Cell,* or *PNAS.*

The present edition represents a major expansion and reorganization of material presented in both previous editions, as well as a comprehensive update. Now that the significance of MHC restriction and Ir genes is better understood, a full discussion of the structure of MHC genes and gene products has been placed earlier in the text (Chapters 8 to 10) and provides a foundation for the discussions of cell–cell interactions that follow (Chapters 11 to 15). Information on clinically related topics has been consolidated into a new section, "Immunology and Human

Health" (Chapters 16 to 20), and has been expanded to include a chapter on "Immunity and Cancer." A number of completely new topics appear with this edition, the most exciting of which is certainly the long-awaited determination of the structure of the T cell receptor (Chapter 12).

I am again indebted to a number of people for direct help in preparing various parts of this text. Eli Sercarz has continued to provide valuable and critical input. Randy Wall once again provided valuable guidance for the section on immunoglobulin genetics. Mayo Yerington undertook the heroic task of getting the entire revised edition onto floppy discs.

William R. Clark

Los Angeles, 1986

Contents

I

Introduction

CHAPTER 1

The Forest before the Trees: An Overview

The Concept of Immunization
What Is the Immune System and What Does It Do?
Fundamental Concepts in Immunobiology
    Antibody Specificity
    Antibody Diversity
    Memory
    Tolerance and Self–Nonself Discrimination
Theories of Antibody Production in Response to Antigen

One of the fascinations of immunology is that it overlaps with, contributes to, and is enriched by such a wide variety of disciplines. Immunology, perhaps to the discomfiture of scientists in less eclectic fields, seems continually to be making contributions to areas as diverse as protein structure, cell differentiation, membrane biology, and eucaryote genetics. Yet at the pedagogical level, immunology has tended to be a rather isolated subject. Most colleges and universities do not have a separate undergraduate course in immunology; even in medical schools immunology is usually buried somewhere in a microbiology course. Although most students of biology are vaguely familiar with at least the concept of an antibody, little of the structure or function of the immune system *per se* is included in lower-division preparatory courses. And because a study of immunology requires the development of a fairly specialized vocabulary, few students develop a casual interest in it on their own.

The requirement for a new scientific vocabulary, or at least the equivalent of a new dialect, also makes immunology somewhat difficult to teach. No matter where one chooses to start, initial progress is bound to be slow until language develops and fundamental concepts become familiar. Thus it is well to spend some time at the beginning of a course or a textbook organizing central concepts and defining fundamental terms. In what remains of this short chapter we do just that. Every idea

3

touched on lightly here will be expanded and expounded on many times over in this text. But it is a good idea to have at least a look at the forest before becoming lost among the trees.

The Concept of Immunization

Most animals are born with virtually no immune protection. A few antibodies cross the placenta from the mother, and in some species antibodies may also be present in the colostrum (milk secreted immediately after birth). Such importation of ready-made immune components from another person or animal is a form of *passive immunization.* The perinatal acquisition of antibodies from the mother is highly variable from species to species, and at best provides protection for only a few months after birth. Another form of passive immunization involves the injection of antibodies (usually against bacterial toxins) produced in animals such as horses or cows. This treatment is given only *after* the development of disease symptoms, and has generally been abandoned now in favor of planned *active immunization.*

Endogenous immune defenses are built up gradually as the newborn is exposed to environmental antigens, principally microbial. This is a natural form of active immunization. Planned active immunization involves the deliberate introduction of foreign matter (*antigen*) into a host animal in order to provoke an immune response prior to natural encounter with the antigen. In the case of smallpox, this process is commonly referred to as vaccination.

References to the efficacy of some form of vaccination in prevention of smallpox have been discovered in ancient Arabic and even earlier Chinese medical manuscripts. The Chinese had developed the practice of inhaling a powder made from smallpox scabs as protection against developing the disease. This method seems to have been sufficiently effective to cause its adoption by various other cultures in the ancient Eastern world. We do not know if the practice was followed in the classical world, but the notion of resistance to a given disease resulting from previous exposure to it seems to have been a common one. Of course, no one had the slightest idea why this should be. The very idea of even asking such a question is a relatively modern development.

The practice of vaccination against smallpox was introduced into Western Europe in the early 1700s by Lady Mary Wortley Montagu, the wife of the British ambassador to Turkey. She had herself been a victim of smallpox, and had observed a form of vaccination against this disease while stationed with her husband in Constantinople. Her daughter was actually the first person in England to receive a smallpox vaccination (1718). Such vaccinations usually consisted of scratching small amounts of dried or powdered scab from healed smallpox lesions into a small wound on the skin. As can be imagined, there was considerable risk associated with this procedure. Nearly everyone became a little ill, and some even died from it. Other diseases could be transmitted with the inoculating material. But most people recovered and were then protected from smallpox for life.

The validity of vaccination in conferring protection against subsequent infection was first put on a firm scientific basis by Edward Jenner at the end of the eighteenth century. Jenner's major contribution was to recognize that persons exposed to cowpox, a relatively mild malady in humans, were protected from smallpox. Specifically, he observed that milkmaids, who often had pockmarks on their hands as a result of cowpox, seemed never to contract the more deadly smallpox even when fully exposed to it. In 1796 he vaccinated an eight-year-old boy with cowpox and then later deliberately exposed him to repeated inoculations of pus from a smallpox lesion. The boy failed to develop smallpox, providing Jenner with a basis for extending his studies to others. Within a few years the validity of vaccination was accepted by most of the medical and scientific community, although its complete acceptance by the general population in England and elsewhere came about only in the middle of the nineteenth century. Inquiry into the means by which vaccination conferred protection against subsequent infection was the beginning of the science of immunology.

Little progress was made in applying the knowledge gained in Jenner's experiments until the second half of the nineteenth century, principally because the biological basis of infectious diseases was completely unknown. Further progress in the field of immunology was thus dependent to a considerable degree on developments in microbiology. By far the most influential figure in the development of both fields was Louis Pasteur. In the course of his studies on the characterization of microbes, he discovered that certain of them could be rendered noninfectious while nevertheless retaining their ability to confer immunological protection. Pasteur found, for example, that anthrax bacilli grown at 42°C (instead of 37°C) could no longer infect sheep, but could confer protection against subsequent exposure to fully active bacilli. Pasteur was thus the first to introduce, in the 1880s, the concept of immunization with attenuated microorganisms. His pioneering work, which also included the development of vaccines for cholera and rabies, opened the way for nothing short of an explosion in the management of infectious diseases. It is difficult to imagine any single contribution, perhaps other than the development of antibiotics, that has had such a profound effect on human health.

Although Louis Pasteur made immunization a highly practical science rather than a vague practitioner's art, the biological basis of the immune response remained unknown for many years. One of the first proposals for a biological mechanism came from Elie Metchnikoff. Working in France and Russia in the 1880s, he observed in several invertebrate species that foreign objects, including microorganisms, were often surrounded by free-living, motile cells that subsequently ingested and destroyed the invading material. This discovery created considerable ferment and quickly led to formation of a school of thought, headed by Metchnikoff, that proposed this phenomenon (called phagocytosis) as the basis for the immune reaction. However, within a few years this proposal was strongly challenged by several scientists, first by an American, George Nuttall (1888), and later, and perhaps more forcefully, by Emil von Boehring and Shibasaburo Kitasato working in Germany (1890). These workers, as well as others, showed that the noncellular, nonclotting elements of blood (serum) from previously immunized animals contained factors that were either directly and specifically lethal to the microorganisms used for the immunization, or capable of neutralizing their toxins. The debate between the advocates of the cellular and humoral theories of the immune response raged vigorously, and rather acrimoniously, until the turn of the century. The English physician, Almroth Wright, showed in 1903 that the immune attack on microorganisms actually involved both humoral and cellular elements. He observed that certain humoral factors, which he called opsonins, in some way rendered bacteria more susceptible to ingestion by phagocytic cells. Opsonins were soon shown to be identical with serum antibodies, which, together with complement, could also directly kill bacteria. In such cases phagocytes ingested the killed microorganisms, as well as damaged host cells, at the site of the infection.

The history of immunology beyond the resolution of the apparent humoral-cellular dichotomy is woven throughout the chapters of this book. The crowning achievement of the immunization process was probably the total eradication of smallpox. In the first half of the twentieth century, two to three million new cases were reported annually. The last case of smallpox in the United States was seen in 1949, and the last verified case in the world was reported in Somalia in 1977. In fact, most Western nations no longer recommend immunization for smallpox; the risk of immunization is considered greater than the possibility of exposure to the disease in its virulent form. It seems fitting that the very problem that stimulated development of the immunological approach of control of infectious diseases has been the first to be totally controlled by this process.

The antibodies that are the basis of the humoral protection conferred by immunization were not to be defined at the molecular level for nearly 50 years after their discovery, although a good deal would be learned about their properties by the early 1900s. Knowledge of the cellular basis of the immune response beyond the phagocytic process has really been developed only in the past 20 years or so. Even today we understand the genetic, molecular, and cellular parameters of immune responsiveness only in broad outline. But enough information has been gathered so that the major questions to be resolved are at least defined, and it is clear that the field of immunology will be an active and exciting one for many years to come.

What Is the Immune System and What Does It Do?

The immune system is actually the body's third line of defense against invasion by foreign substances. The first line of defense is the skin and the various other epithelial linings of those portions of the body in contact with the environment, which present a physical barrier to intrusion by foreign matter. The second line is the battery of nonspecific host mechanisms that compromise the survival and growth of pathogenic microorganisms (pH, cell sloughing, ciliary sweeping, sneezing and swallowing, "genetic" resistance, etc.). These mechanisms are sometimes collectively referred to as innate immunity.

What is meant by "foreign"? In most circumstances, foreign (with respect to the immune system) means anything organic that is not coded for by the host organism's DNA. Although this definition will suffice in nearly all cases in nature, some important exceptions exist or can be created in the laboratory, and these are discussed at various points in this text. It is quite clear that the major selective force behind the evolution of the immune system is the need to combat invasion by pathogenic microorganisms such as parasites, bacteria, yeast (molds), and viruses. As we have already seen, the study of resistance to infectious disease was the major impetus for studying and characterizing the immune system. Such studies, however, now encompass only a very small part of the general field of immunology, the major portion of current efforts being devoted to analyzing the genetic, molecular, and cellular facets that underlie all immune reactions.

There are two ways in which the immune system can deal with invasion by a foreign substance. One way is to produce a globular, circulating glycoprotein called an *antibody*. An antibody molecule recognizes and attaches to the foreign substance in a very specific way. This reaction of the antibody with the foreign substance, or *antigen,* triggers a series of events leading to elimination of the antigen from the system. This type of immune response is called a *humoral immune response* because the active agent (the antibody) is found floating free in the body's "humors" (the blood and lymph systems). Humoral immunity can be directed toward a wide range of foreign substances, both molecular and cellular.

Antibodies (Ab) are produced by a type of white blood cell called a *B lymphocyte*. All antibodies are variations of the basic four polypeptide chain immunoglobulin (Ig) structure shown in Figure 1-1. This structure is composed of two light (L) chains, of molecular weight about 25,000, and two heavy (H) chains of about 50,000 MW. The chains are held together by disulfide bonds. This unit Ig structure has two *antigen-combining sites.* Each site is formed by the NH_2-terminal portions of adjacent H and L chains.

The second way in which the immune system deals with invasion of the body by

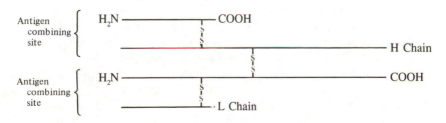

Figure 1-1 A generalized structure for antibody (immunoglobulin) molecules.

foreign material is through a *cell-mediated immune response.* In this case, a specific type of lymphocyte, called a *T cell,* recognizes and binds to the antigen, again leading to the ultimate elimination of the latter from the system. These lymphocytes are distinct in a number of ways from those producing antibodies (B cells). The T-cell reaction is principally, although not exclusively, directed toward antigens associated with the surface of pathologically altered cells such as tumor cells, virally infected cells, etc. The T cell recognizes the aberrant cell by means of a receptor molecule on its surface, which has antibodylike properties but is probably not classical antibody per se. In the case of both humoral and cell-mediated cytotoxic reactions, foreign matter (plus expired host cells) may be removed from the reaction site by *phagocytes,* cells that literally "eat" damaged cells, live or dead bacteria, macromolecular complexes, and even inert inorganic particulate matter.

Fundamental Concepts in Immunobiology

Antibody Specificity

One of the cardinal features of the reaction of antibodies and antigens is the specificity of the reaction. An antibody produced in response to one antigen will cross-react poorly, if at all, with most other antigens.

Antigens are defined as substances, both cellular and molecular, capable of being bound by either an antibody or an immune lymphocyte. Any organic molecule (i.e., with a molecular structure based on carbon) is a potential antigen. It will be obvious from a cursory inspection of the antigen-combining site of an Ig molecule that only a small portion of a macromolecular antigen can actually interact with an antibody molecule. Thus, although an entire macromolecule, cell, or microorganism may be referred to as an antigen, only those discrete portions of the macromolecule that interact with the antigen-combining site, called antigenic *determinants* or *epitopes,* actually trigger the immune response.

A necessary distinction must be made between an antigen and an *immunogen.* An immunogen is defined by its ability to provoke an immune response (either cellular or humoral). Although all immunogens are also antigens, in that they can combine with antibodies, not all antigens are immunogens. The distinction seems to be primarily one of size. Very small molecules (on the order of size of an amino acid, or a single sugar molecule, or a phenol ring, for example) cannot by themselves induce an immune response. However, as Landsteiner showed in the 1920s, if they are coupled to a larger molecule (called a *carrier*), they then become essentially an antigenic determinant or epitope, and can be perceived by and responded to as immunogens by the immune system. Such small molecules, which by themselves are antigens but not immunogens, are often called *haptens.*

The degree to which antibodies are able to distinguish small differences in antigenic structure was demonstrated most forcefully by Landsteiner. He attached small organic haptens to larger carrier molecules and injected these into rabbits. The resulting antiserum contained antibodies that would react with both hapten and carrier. However, by repeatedly reacting the serum with the carrier alone, and removing the resulting precipitate, he could obtain a serum that was specific for the hapten.

Landsteiner then introduced various chemical changes into the hapten, and tested the ability of the antiserum produced against the native hapten to react with altered hapten. Examples of his data are shown in Table 1-1 and Figure 1-2. Serum specific for *meta*-aminobenzene sulfonic acid reacts very well with the same molecule, but hardly at all with molecules in which the sulfonate group is shifted to the ortho or para positions. Moreover, when even a single atom is changed (sulfur to arsenic) in the sulfonate group in the meta position, the antibody barely recognizes the hapten. Equally impressive, antibodies made against one stereoisomer of tartaric acid recognize other stereoisomers either poorly or not at all.

The basis for antibody–antigen reactions is qualitatively similar to the basis for enzyme substrate reactions in that they involve energetically favorable interactions between chemical functional groups in the antigen-combining site, and on the antigenic determinant. Thus, in reality, an antibody produced in response to one antigen could cross-react with any other molecule that had an antigenic determinant of identical or very similar structure. The low degree of cross-reactivity generally observed simply reflects the enormous structural diversity of biological mole-

Table 1-1 The Specificity of Antibodies Made against Various Stereoisomers of Tartaric Acid

	Form of tartaric acid used to induce antibody		
	COOH | HOCH | HCOH | COOH *levo-*	COOH | HCOH | HOCH | COOH *dextro-*	COOH | HCOH | HCOH | COOH *meso-*
Antibody tested against			
l-tartaric acid	+++	0	+½
d-tartaric acid	0	+++½	+½
m-tartaric acid	½	0	+++

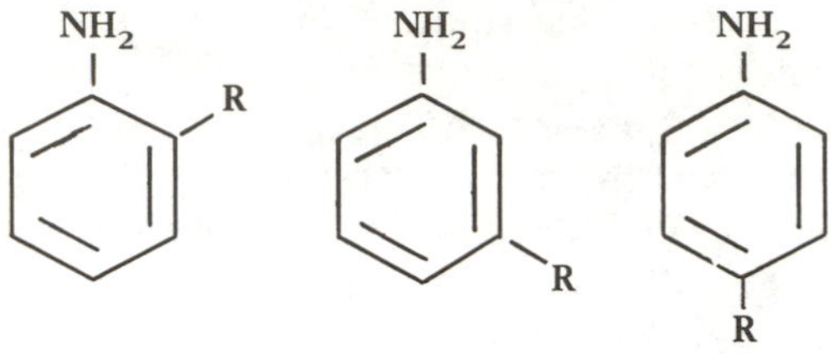

	ortho-R	meta-R	para-R
R = SO$_3$H	$+\frac{1}{2}$	$++\frac{1}{2}$	$\frac{1}{2}$
R = AsO$_3$H	0	$+$	0

Figure 1-2 The reaction of antibodies made against *meta*-aminobenzenesulfonic acid with related molecules.

cules. The important point to keep in mind is that it is not the case that each antibody is made for one—and only one—antigen.

Antibody Diversity

One of the most puzzling features of the immune response, from the point of view of early researchers in the field, was the fact that almost any organic compound known could apparently elicit an antibody that reacted with it in a reasonably specific way. This implied the existence of a very large number of possible antibody molecules. Other organic chemists-turned-immunologists demonstrated that almost any compound they chose to synthesize could elicit the production of a very specific antibody. Thus molecules that had never before existed on earth, and which obviously could not have played any evolutionary role in selecting antibodies, could nevertheless trigger the production of a specific antibody. The basis for this property of immune responses remained a complete mystery until the middle of the present century (see below).

Memory

A characteristic feature of the immune system, with which nearly everyone is familiar, is memory. It is this feature that is referred to when we say someone is "immune" to a particular disease, for example. The first time an individual is exposed to a given pathogen, the resulting disease may progress to the clinically detectable stage or beyond, in some cases even resulting in death. In most instances the immune system will neutralize the pathogen or the microorganism producing it, and symptoms of the associated disease will disappear. On subsequent (secondary) exposure to the same pathogen, the immune response will be mobilized much more rapidly, and will manifest itself much more strongly, than the original (primary) exposure. Very often, the associated disease will not even reach the clinically detectable stage, or at best will cause only mild symptoms. Memory can be generated to virtually any antigen and is characteristic of both the humoral and cell-mediated branches of the immune system. Persistence of the memory state is variable from individual to individual, and also varies among different antigens, but can be quite long—up to 10 years in humans. Any theory attempting to explain the operation of the immune system must be able to account for this feature of immune responsiveness.

Tolerance and Self–Nonself Discrimination

The phenomenon of tolerance can be thought of as an expression of negative immunological memory: As a result of previous exposure to a particular antigen, the subsequent immune response is reduced or totally abrogated. Like memory, tolerance can be demonstrated for both the humoral and cell-mediated branches of the immune system. For the most part, tolerance is an experimental phenomenon, generated in laboratory animals by manipulating the form, dose, or timing of antigen administration. There are, however, examples of tolerance in nature. Among outbred populations such as humans, a skin graft from a child to its mother will usually persist longer than a child-to-father graft, suggesting the induction of limited transplacental tolerance in the mother during embryogenesis to paternal antigens present on the fetus. Experiments with inbred strains of mice have shown that a female mouse repeatedly made pregnant by a male (or males) of a genetically different strain may develop significant tolerance toward skin grafts from mice of the male partner strain. This observation also lends support to the notion that mothers and fetuses may have substantial degrees of histological communication either normally across the intact placenta or briefly at birth at the moment of placental rupture.

The most obvious and important natural expression of tolerance of course is the ability to discriminate self from nonself, and it is likely that all other forms of natural or experimental tolerance are simply expressions of this very central feature of immune responsiveness. The experiments of Landsteiner and others showed that the immune system can respond to almost any conceivable organic molecule—why then does it fail to respond to the organic molecules of which self is composed? Obviously this cannot be allowed to happen, but how is it prevented? Ray Owen reported an observation in 1945 that gives some clue to at least the timing of this event. Genetically distinct cattle twins that share a common blood supply during embryogeny will, as adults, each carry two genetically distinct sets of blood cell elements. The adult uses both sets of blood elements equally well, and neither is immunologically rejected. Were an exchange of blood elements carried out between two normally developed adults of the same two genotypes, rapid, mutual, and vigorous immunological rejection would occur. This was the first suggestion that foreign antigens seen by the immune system during embryological development might be perceived as self, whereas elements encountered for the first time after birth would be considered foreign. In general, this turns out to be true, although as we will see in Chapter 13, the mechanisms by which this occurs are still far from clear.

Theories of Antibody Production in Response to Antigen

We have already pointed out that the great clinical importance of immunology provided much of the early impetus for its development as a field of study. But there were always a few individuals who perceived immunology as a science in its own right, with its own unique challenges and problems to be resolved at the conceptual as well as the practical level. Foremost among the problems requiring a theoretical framework was the question of antibody diversity. How is a specific antibody produced in response to a seemingly infinite variety of molecules, some of which have no natural phylogenetic history of interaction with immune systems? A second but equally important question concerned the immunological distinction between self and nonself. If the immune system can produce antibodies in response to almost any known organic molecule, why does it fail to do so in response to self molecules? Almost any molecule taken from one organism and injected into another will provoke an antibody response, and is thus clearly immunogenic; why then is no antibody made against such molecules in their own immunological environment?

   Paul Ehrlich was the first to propose, in 1894, a theory to account for the cellular origin and diversity of antibody. He suggested that in order for a cell to take up nutrients, it must have specific cell-surface receptors for each type of nutrient molecule. These receptors, he believed, would combine by standard chemical means with defined portions of the nutrient molecules. Thus each receptor would be specific for one or at best a very few closely related nutrients. A mature organism would have a wide range of receptors, capable of combining with almost anything that could potentially serve as a food source. Following a suggestion of Weigert, Ehrlich subsequently proposed that when nutrient materials (antigens) combined with the surface receptors (antibodies), the cell bearing these receptors (or perhaps "sister cells," bearing the same receptors) would overproduce copies of these receptors–antibodies and shed them into the serum. This theory accounted for the existence in serum, and chemical specificity, of antibody in response to antigenic stimulation.

   A key element of Ehrlich's hypothesis was that all possible antibody molecules, in terms of antigenic specificity, preexisted in the host independently of exposure to or contact with antigen. This notion became increasingly difficult to accept as Karl Landsteiner and his colleagues began to publish their work on antibody specificity in the second quarter of the twentieth century. They found that highly specific antibodies could be induced by virtually any chemical, even by molecules that had never existed until manufactured for the very first time in the chemist's laboratory! The dilemma this posed was stated clearly by Stuart Mudd in 1932: "How may it be conceived that the animal body can thus develop substances possessing specific correspondence with the numberless proteins found in nature or capable of preparation in the laboratory?" This was later rephrased by Sir Peter Medawar as the "miracle of immunology . . . a rabbit yet unborn has the ability to make antibodies against a molecule yet unsynthesized." Because there seemed to be no limit to the number of molecules that could serve as antigens, and because antibodies could readily be produced against molecules not found in the natural environment, Ehrlich's hypothesis gradually came to be regarded as untenable. It seemed to require an enormous number of receptors whose primary value to the organism (since their antibody function was considered secondary) was not at all clear.

A conceptual framework for antibody production that appeared to accommodate the difficulties generated by Landsteiner's studies was put forward in the early 1930s independently and almost simultaneously by Breinl and Haurowitz, by Mudd, and by Alexander, and subsequently in a slightly modified and expanded form by Pauling in 1940. This theory, the so-called "instructionalist theory," had great force and influence on the thinking of those immunologists concerned with a rational, scientific interpretation of immunological phenomena. The instructionalists proposed that the immune system contained no a priori information about molecules in the environment, but rather learned about them only as a result of the first direct contact with them. It was postulated that the immune system provided a large number of protein "blanks" or "templates" that, after contact with an antigen, assumed specific and stable conformations that allowed them to interact thereafter in a highly specific manner with only the original antigen. (Nothing was known in the 1940s about the molecular structure of antibodies, or indeed any proteins.) This model engendered widespread enthusiasm principally because it offered relief from the anxiety generated by the experiments of Landsteiner and others with synthetic immunogens. But it ultimately failed for two reasons: one theoretical and one technical. From a theoretical point of view, the instructionalist theory completely failed to account for the ability to distinguish self from nonself. There was nothing in this theory that could explain how a template could be prevented from forming around self-antigens as well as foreign antigens. Furthermore, this theory could not provide a theoretical basis for the phenomenon of *immunological memory.* When an animal is exposed for a second time to a particular antigen, the response is more rapid and the amount of antibody produced is many times greater. When one speaks of being "immune" to a particular substance, one is really referring to immunological memory. Previous exposure to a substance in some ways alters the system so that subsequent responses are dramatically enhanced. Instructional theories could never satisfactorily account for this aspect of the immune response.

As information began to accumulate about protein structure–function relationships, and about the genetic control of protein synthesis, instructional models became technically unfeasible as well. Haber showed that antibody molecules could be denatured, destroying their antigen-binding ability, and then refolded into fully active antibody in the absence of antigen. A real stretch of the imagination would be required to reconcile this finding with instructionalist models for antibody formation. Moreover, it was becoming increasingly clear from genetic experiments with microorganisms that protein structure is determined by information encoded in DNA and cannot be dictated by the environment or be altered in any permanent way by transient intermolecular contacts. It was, in fact, these early experiments in procaryotic molecular biology that directed some immunologists along another pathway of thinking. If every different antibody activity represents a different protein molecule, and if every different protein is coded for by a different gene, then it follows that the genetic information for all possible antibody molecules must preexist in an organism's DNA, independent of knowledge about the types of antigens in the environment. Nils Jerne was the first to propose a selective theory of antibody production, based on this new thinking, in 1955. He hypothesized that all possible forms of antibodies, in terms of antigenic specificity, preexist in the serum, independently of exposure to antigen. The function of antigen was seen as simply selection of one or more of these antibodies for amplified production. He proposed that after combination with an antigen, the antigen–antibody complex was internalized by cells able to make copies of the engulfed antibody. Such a model was able to account for both memory and the ability to distinguish self from nonself. He predicted that as a result of initial exposure to antigen, greater numbers of the initially selected antibody molecules would be present in the serum, leading to a more rapid and enhanced secondary response. Self antibodies, he supposed, would bind tightly to self tissues and could not make their way into the antibody-producing cells for copying and amplification. Although Jerne's "natural selection" theory turned out not to be correct in detail, he nevertheless must be credited with making the intellectual leap from viewing antibody as being *formed* in response to antigen, to postulating that all possible (necessary) antibodies *preexist,* fully formed, independently of exposure to antigen.

Jerne's postulate, although in a sense increasingly demanded by then current developments in molecular biology, was seen as a return to the earlier views of Ehrlich that most immunologists considered impossible in light of Landsteiner's findings. Thus a selective view of antibody production was not at all readily accepted, particularly in view of some minor problems with Jerne's theory, which were seized on and rather vigorously attacked. Nevertheless, the power of Jerne's idea continued to grow and was finally restated in a more biologically sensible form by Burnet in 1957 in his Clonal Selection Theory. This version of the selective theory was overpowering in its simplicity and in its ability to account for all features of the immune response known at the time. In fact, with only slight modification, it still provides the theoretical underpinnings of all of modern immunology. We therefore briefly examine its principal features (in an updated form); it will be referred to many times over throughout this text.

Burnet assumed the existence of a genre of immune system cells, each of which is assumed to be programmed genetically to produce a single antibody with a single type of antigen-combining site. We now know that this cell is the B lymphocyte. Each antigen-combining site will react with only a very limited number of antigenic determinants, or epitopes. The B lymphocyte displays on its surface a copy, in suitable form, of the combining site it is programmed to synthesize and secrete. This combining site acts as a specific antigen receptor through which the cell is activated. Any molecule or cell bearing the antigenic determinant for which this surface receptor is specific (i.e., can chemically combine with) will trigger the B cell to do two things: (1) to proliferate, expanding within the general lymphocyte population, in a clonal fashion, B cells preprogrammed to produce antibodies of this identical specificity, and (2) to initiate the actual mechanics of antibody synthesis and secretion.

This theory was the first to be able to provide a rational explanation for all three major features of immune responses.

1. *Diversity* is accounted for by stipulating that the genetic information to code for the antibodies necessary to combine with all possible antigens exists within an organism's DNA prior to encounter with any antigen. Each B cell may contain a complete set of this information, but will only express the information necessary for coping with a single antigen. Because an antigenic determinant is rather small in size, and of fairly restricted chemical composition (in general only H, C, N, O, P, and S), it is readily apparent that the "universe" of antigenic determinants is by no means infinite. Thus the universe of antibodies needed to deal with possible environmental antigens is also finite. Just how large this universe is, and hence the amount of genetic information that must be carried to deal with it, is still a matter of some debate. The most extravagant estimates, however, do not exceed 1 to 2 percent of the average mammalian genome.

2. *Self–nonself discrimination* is accounted for by assuming that clones capable of reacting with self-antigens are either eliminated during ontogeny or somehow suppressed in their function in the adult. Although specific mechanisms to account for clonal suppression or elimination have not yet been worked out in detail, all available information suggests that this basic premise is correct.

3. *Memory* is explained by the clonal expansion resulting from the initial triggering event (primary reaction). When an antigen is presented to the system a second time, a much larger number of cells bearing a complementary receptor exists in the system, thus giving a greatly enhanced (secondary) response.

The clonal selection theory provides the framework for interpreting all immunological phenomena involving specificity. The challenge now is to understand, within the context of clonal selection, the genetic, molecular, and cellular basis for an immune response at each stage of its development—from first contact with an antigen to its final elimination from the system. The length of this book may suggest to you that this is not a simple process.

Bibliography

Alexander, J., Some intracellular aspects of life and disease. *Protoplasma 14,* 296 (1931).

Breinl, F., and F. Haurowitz, Chemische untersuchung des präzipitats aus hämoglobin und anti-hämoglobin-serum, und bemerkungen uber die natur der antikörper. *Z. Physiol. Chem. 192,* 45 (1930).

Burnet, F. M., A modification of Jerne's theory of antibody production using the concept of clonal selection." *Australian J. Sci. 20,* 67 (1957).

Burnet, F. M., *The Clonal Selection Theory of Acquired Immunity.* Cambridge University Press, London (1959).

Ehrlich, P., On immunity with special reference to cell life. *Proc. Roy. Soc. London (Biol.) 66,* 424 (1900).

Jenner, E., *An Inquiry into the Causes and Effects of the Variolae Vaccinae, a Disease Discovered in Some of the Western Counties of England, Particularly Gloucestershire, and Known by the Name of the Cow Pox.* Sampson Low, Soho, London (1798).

Jerne, N. K., The natural selection theory of antibody formation. *Proc. Natl. Acad. Sci. USA 41,* 849 (1955).

Kolmer, J. A., *A Practical Textbook of Infection, Immunity, and Specific Therapy.* Saunders, Philadelphia (1917).

Landsteiner, K., *The Specificity of Serological Reactions,* Thomas, Springfield, Ill. (1936).

Metchnikoff, E., *Immunity in Infectious Disease,* trans. by F. Binnie, Cambridge University Press, London (1905).

Mudd, S., A hypothetical mechanism of antibody formation. *J. Immunol. 23,* 423 (1932).

Nutall, G., Experimente über die bakterienfeindlichen einflüsse des tierischen körpers. *Z. Hyg. Infekt. Krankh 4,* 353 (1888).

Owen, R. D., Immunogenetic consequences of vascular anastomoses between bovine twins. *Science 102,* 400 (1945).

Parish, H. J., *A History of Immunization,* E. S. Livingstone, Ltd., Edinburgh (1965).

Pasteur: L., De l'attenuation du virus du cholera des poules. *C.R. Acad. Sci. (Paris) 91,* 673 (1880).

Pauling, L., A theory of the structure and process of formation of antibodies. *J. Am. Chem. Soc. 62,* 2643 (1940).

Silverstein, A. M., History of immunology. Cellular versus humoral immunity: Determinants and consequences of an epic 19th century battle. *Cell. Immunol. 48,* 208 (1979).

Wright, A. E., and S. R. Douglas, An experimental investigation of the role of the blood fluids in connection with phagocytosis. *Proc. R. Soc. Lond. (Biol.) 72,* 357 (1903).

CHAPTER 2

Structure of the Immune System

Cells of the Immune System
  The Granulocyte Series
    Neutrophils
    Basophils
    Eosinophils
  The Monocyte Series
  Dendritic Cells
  The Lymphocyte Series
  Mast Cells
  Platelets
Organs of the Immune System
  Bone Marrow
  Thymus
  Bursa of Fabricius
  Spleen
  Lymph Nodes
  Gut-associated Lymphoid Tissue (GALT)
  The Reticuloendothelial System
The Lymphatic Circulatory System

A major portion of the specialized language of immunology stems from what appears at first sight to be a rather bewildering spectrum of organs, tissues, and cells that comprise the immune system itself. Although the medical student who has had a thorough exposure to histology and hematology will, in fact, have much of this terminology at his or her command, the histology and cytology of the immune system are not generally covered in more than a cursory fashion in nonmedical curricula. Therefore, before delving very deeply into the cellular and

17

molecular aspects of immunology, we present, for the unintiated, a reasonably thorough description of the morphological elements of the immune system.

Cells of the Immune System

There are three major groups of blood cells involved in the immune response: granulocytes, monocytes, and lymphocytes. All three arise from one or more stem cells residing principally in the bone marrow, but to some extent in the spleen or liver depending on the age of the animal. Stem cells are primitive, continuously dividing cells that produce more stem cells and, under appropriate conditions, cells that are more highly differentiated along some developmental pathway. The exact number of true stem cells involved in the continuous renewal of blood cells is unknown. The developmental relationship of the various blood elements are shown in Figure 2-1, and the white cell composition of human blood is presented in Table 2-1. In the following sections we examine in some detail the morphology and function of each of the major cell types involved in immune defense mechanisms.

The Granulocyte Series

The granulocyte series is composed of three distinct cell types—neutrophils, basophils, and eosinophils (Figure 2-2)—distinguished by the structure of both nuclear and cytoplasmic components. Although very important in host defenses against microorganisms, granulocytes lack two key attributes we associate with immunity per se: memory and antigenic specificity.

Neutrophils

These are the most numerous and widespread of the granulocytes. They are characterized by highly indented or lobulated nuclei, containing mostly clumped and probably inactive chromatin. The cytoplasm contains numerous granules filled with degradative enzymes and peroxidase. They are generally the first white cells to localize at the site of a foreign invasion, and in the case of microbial infection will actively phagocytize and kill a portion of the invading microbes. Neutrophils are highly mobile and are attracted to the site of an infection by various chemotactic signals, including certain endogenous bacterial products, substances released by damaged tissues, and components of complement (see Chapter 7). Once in the vicinity of the site of an infection, the neutrophils phagocytize invading organisms, plus any damaged host cells. The engulfed material is degraded by substances sequestered in the cytoplasmic granules (see also Chapter 18). In the process, some of the degradative substances used by the neutrophil in intracellular digestion of foreign matter usually leak into surrounding healthy host tissue and cause a local inflammatory reaction.

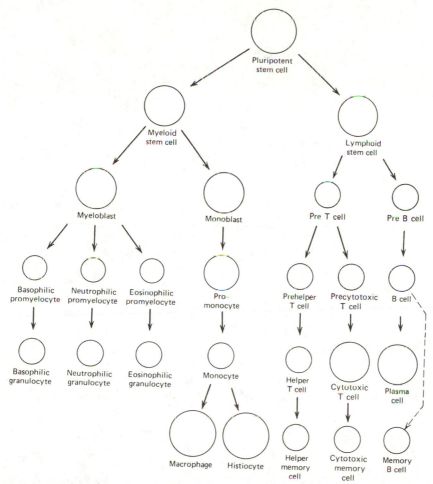

Figure 2-1 Comprehensive maturation scheme for cells involved in the immune response. The nature of the putative pluripotent stem cell is unknown. It may, in fact, be a number of different stem cells. In the bone marrow of the mouse, for example, studies have demonstrated the existence of a common stem cell giving rise to erythrocytes and lymphocytes. In addition, stem cells were identified that gave rise only to myeloid elements or only to lymphoid cells. Ultimately, stem cell activity for all of the blood elements must be accounted for. In the granulocytic series, it is possible that the three end cells may also be distinct at the myeloblast level. The monocyte series as shown in the figure reflects the gradual decrease in cell size with maturation, until the terminal macrophage–histiocyte state is reached, when there is a 3- to 10-fold size increase.

In the lymphocyte series, the pre-T-cell and pre-B-cell forms are almost certainly differentiated within the bone marrow, in spite of the lack of definitive surface markers. The site of maturation of the pre-B cell to the B cell in mammals is uncertain, but probably also occurs in the bone marrow. Differentiation of B cells is antigen driven, and occurs in the lymph tissue. During generation of plasma cells, part of the B-cell population gives rise to memory cells; the antibody-producing plasma cell is a terminal cell type. The pre-T cell matures under thymic influence to several functional forms of immunocompetent T cell (cytotoxic, suppressor, amplifier, see Chapter 13). The final stage of maturation of these forms is also antigen driven. The fully functional cytotoxic effector cell is, like the plasma cell, a large pyrininophilic blastlike cell. Unlike the plasma cell, however, T memory cells are probably generated directly from the mature functional T-cell forms.

Table 2-1 Ranges of Composition of White Cells in Normal Human Blood

Cell type	Percentage range
Neutrophils	40–75
Eosinophils	1–7
Basophils	0–1
Monocytes	2–11
Lymphocytes[a]	15–50

[a]About 70 to 90 percent of normal human blood lymphocytes are thymus dependent (T cells) and the balance are B cells.

Basophils

These are easily distinguished from other granulocytes by their smaller size and by the presence of numerous dark-staining, oval-shaped cytoplasmic granules (Figure 2-2). In this respect they are similar to mast cells, and indeed were originally called blood mast cells. However, true mast cells are confined to peripheral tissues and almost never appear in the blood. On the other hand, blood basophils are

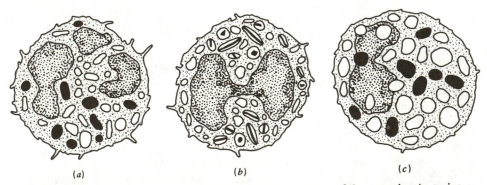

(a)   (b)   (c)

Figure 2-2 Cytological characteristics of the mature members of the granulocyte series. (a) *Neutrophil* (polymorphonuclear leukocyte, or PMN). This, the most common of the granulocyte series, is characterized by a highly lobulated nucleus with densely packed chromatin. When stained with Giemsa stain, the cytoplasm is pale with pink or violet-pink granules. (b) *Eosinophil.* The eosinophil is similar in appearance to the PMN. The nucleus is less lobulated, typically displaying two distinct lobes. The cytoplasm is more granular and, upon ultrastructural analysis, will be found to contain more mitochondria and a more highly developed Golgi than the PMN. (c) *Basophil.* These cells have an irregular nucleus, but it is not usually as lobulated as the other two members of the series. The most distinctive characteristic of basophils is the presence of large, dense ovoid or round granules in the cytoplasm and overlying the nucleus. The granules contain acid mucopolysaccharides and RNA.

often found in tissue, and in fact their presence in blood may be related simply to their transit from bone marrow to peripheral tissue. Because of their low concentration in blood, and diffuse distribution in tissue, definitive studies of basophil function have been difficult to carry out. However, it seems very likely that they do in fact function essentially like mast cells, that is, in the mediation of immediate hypersensitivity reactions (see Chapter 17). The granules in basophil cytoplasm contain pharmacologically active substances such as histamine, serotonin, and heparin and release these into the blood in response to much the same stimuli that cause degranulation of mast cells. There is some evidence that basophils, once degranulated, cannot resynthesize these cell-specific products. They may thus represent a terminally differentiated cell type.

Eosinophils

These granulocytes, first described by Paul Ehrlich in 1879, are present in extremely low concentration in the blood ($300/mm^3$). They are generally similar in overall morphology to neutrophils, but can be distinguished by staining properties and details of nuclear structure.

One of the earliest recognized roles for eosinophils is in the response to infections by helminthic parasites, particularly *S. mansoni* and *T. spiralis* (see Chapter 18). Eosinophils are found in high concentrations during such parasitic infections and can attack and destroy the infecting cells. The overall response to parasites is complex, involving T cells and antibodies as well as eosinophils, but eosinophils appear to be a major factor in the final elimination of the parasites.

The acid-staining cytoplasmic granules of eosinophils contain a number of agents that are toxic to a wide range of cell types, including bacterial and mammalian cells as well as parasites. The principal component of the granules is the so-called major basic protein (MBP), a highly basic peptide of about 10,000 daltons. MBP is released when eosinophils bind to parasitic cells, and both promotes further adhesion of the eosinophil to the target cell, and causes damage to the target cell plasma membrane. Eosinophil granules also contain a family of seven eosinophil cationic proteins (ECP), which are highly toxic to cell membranes, and a peroxidase system.

There is also a considerable body of experimental evidence to suggest that eosinophils may also function to help control inflammatory responses triggered by other components of the immune system. Eosinophils are found in high concentration at sites of inflammatory reactions, including hypersensitivity reactions, usually late in the response. They appear to be attracted by immune complexes and by substances released by mast cells and basophils. Soluble extracts of eosinophils injected into sites of inflammatory reactions can be effective in relieving the effects of histamine and SRS-A on surrounding tissue (see Chapter 17). However, it is not certain that eosinophils carry out such a function *in vivo*.

The Monocyte Series

The mononuclear phagocyte series is composed of a number of functionally and morphologically distinct cell types that form a developmental continuum from the bone marrow monoblast to the tissue macrophage. This series is depicted in Figure 2-1. The *monoblasts* are normally seen only in patients with monocytic leukemia, although their existence in healthy bone marrow can be inferred indirectly from *in vitro* culturing and *in vivo* transfer experiments. The bone marrow *promonocytes*, however, can be isolated and identified. They are glass adherent, 10 to 20 μm in size, rapidly dividing, and only poorly phagocytic. Lysosomes are absent or poorly developed. Some investigators have suggested that it is actually the promonocyte that is the stem cell for the monocyte series. The *blood monocyte* is slightly smaller than the promonocyte, and is the first member of the series to be found in the blood. It is still synthesizing DNA, although not at as high a rate as its bone marrow precursors. Morphologically it is often difficult to distinguish monocytes from the larger members of the lymphocytic series (see below). Monocytes appear considerably more differentiated at the subcellular level than promonocytes; important changes include a distinct increase in the number of lysosomes, a decrease in the nuclear/cytoplsmic ratio, and the acquisition of a characteristically horseshoe-shaped nucleus. The monocytes are intermediate in phagocytic activity between promonocytes and macrophages.

The blood monocytes migrate into peripheral tissues where they enlarge and differentiate into *macrophages* or *histiocytes*. The term macrophage is generally applied to the form found free in the peritoneal, pleural, or alveolar spaces, and to some extent in the blood, whereas the term histiocyte is most often used for those forms found fixed in tissue, particularly attached to the reticulum of the lymph nodes, spleen, and liver. A major histiocyte population is the *Kupffer cells* of the liver, which line the hepatic sinusoids and function to clear antigen from the blood.

The macrophage may grow to be 10 times the size of the blood monocyte and is highly specialized for phagocytosis. There is a marked increase in general metabolism, and the abundant cytoplasm is filled with granules containing hydrolytic enzymes that fuse readily with digestive vacuoles. During active phagocytosis, live macrophages may appear highly granular and irregular in form in an ordinary light microscope, without fixation and staining. The mature macrophage loses the ability to divide and is essentially a terminal cell form. It sticks very readily to most solid surfaces, and advantage can be taken of this fact to deplete lymphoid cell populations of macrophages.

The principal functions of cells of the macrophage series are phagocytosis (Chapter 18), antigen processing and presentation to T cells (Chapter 14), and production of certain monokines (Chapter 13). These functions may or may not be related. Phagocytosis is a rapid and effective means for removing particulate antigens, including bacteria, from the host. During the intracellular degradative process, fragments of the ingested antigen may be transported to and displayed on the macrophage surface, where they may then serve to activate other cells of the immune system (principally T lymphocytes). Other, nonparticulate antigens may be processed and displayed directly on the macrophage surface. In such cases, the phagocytic function of the macrophage may play no role. Apparently all macrophagelike cells, including Kupffer cells and alveolar macrophages, are able to carry out both functions (phagocytosis and antigen presentation). Macrophages that are actively involved in antigen processing and presentation are probably the ones producing monokines, although this is not yet absolutely certain.

Dendritic Cells

The history of dendritic cells is a long and confusing one. Cells with dendritic morphology have been described by many labs over the years, with a variety of often conflicting properties ascribed to them. It is now clear that part of the confusion arises from the fact that there are at least four kinds of dendritic cells. Dendritic cells do have a number of features in common, however. All are characterized by numerous long, slender processes, from which they derive their name, and irregularly shaped nuclei. They display little or no phagocytic or endocytic activity, and bear neither T nor B cell surface markers. It now appears that all dendritic cells display class II MHC antigens (see Chapter 9), and that they function in presenting antigen to T and/or B lymphocytes. Aside from these common features, the various dendritic populations have a number of distinguishing characteristics, reviewed briefly in the following sections.

Lymphoid dendritic cells were first described in mice by Steinman and co-workers in a series of papers between 1973 and 1975. Although their histologic lineage is uncertain, they appear not to be related to lymphocytes, monocytes, or reticular cells. They are derived from bone marrow and are found in both lymph nodes and spleen, but account for less than 1 percent of the total leukocyte population in these organs. Lymphoid dendritic cells were originally identified *in vitro* as part of the population of adherent cells of spleen, and were distinguished by their unique stellate morphology (Figure 2-3), abundant mitochondria, and relative lack of free ribosomes. They display Fc receptors (receptors on cells that allow binding of Ig molecules via the Fc region) and class II antigens, and bind complement fragment C3. They are rather insensitive to γ-irradiation, but are very sensitive to ultraviolet light. Lymphoid dendritic cells are particularly potent in the induction of graft rejection reactions (Chapter 14).

Follicular dendritic cells are seen in sections of lymphoid follicles, and were recently isolated for study by John Tews and his co-workers. These cells have little cytoplasm and few cytoplasmic organelles. One of the distinguishing functional characteristics of these cells is their ability to trap and retain antigen (probably in the form of antigen-antibody complexes) displayed on their surfaces for long periods of time. it has been suggested that they play a key role in the development of memory B cells. When seen in tissue sections *in situ*, it is clear that they are interacting almost exclusively with B lymphocytes.

Like lymphoid dendritic cells, follicular dendritic cells display class II antigens and Fc receptors, and bind C3. Follicular dendritic cells are distinct from lymphoid dendritic cells in that they have many more dendritic processes that are thinner, longer, and may contain beadlike swellings along their length (Figure 2-4). The functional significance of these bead structures is unknown at present.

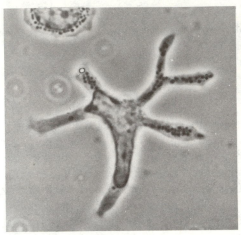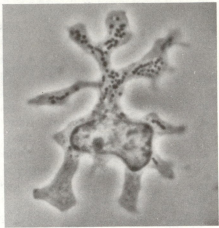

Figure 2-3 Lymphoid dendritic cells. (Photos courtesy of Dr. Ralph M. Steinman, Rockefeller University.)

Interdigitating dendritic cells are found in T-dependent areas of lymphoid tissue, where their processes can be seen to interact intimately with T cell membranes. Numerous mitotic figures can usually be seen in T cells associated with these dendritic cells. It seems possible that the interdigitating dendritic cells may be related to lymphoid dendritic cells; they have many features in common, and the actual tissue localization of lymphoid dendritic cells is unclear because they were defined on the basis of their properties during isolation. However, interdigitating cells have a dense cytoplasmic granule called a Birbeck granule that appears to be absent from the lymphoid dendritic cell. Moreover, the interdigitating cell has no Fc receptor, and does not seem to bind antigen. It is difficult to tell how many of these differences are real and how many are apparent, due to isolation artifacts. Also, much of the work done on interdigitating cells was carried out some years ago, and it is possible that more recently developed techniques would reveal more details about these cells.

Langerhan's cells were described in the 1860s as cells in the epidermis that bind gold tissue stains. More recent techniques have revealed them to be dendritic cells with very long, thin processes that form an extensive network throughout the epidermis. They have the same type of Birbeck granule that is found in the interdigitating cell. The Langerhan's cells are the only ones in the epidermis to bear class II antigens and Fc receptors. Like interdigitating dendritic cells, they appear to interact preferentially with T cells, and their function is almost certainly antigen presentation.

The Lymphocyte Series

Lymphocytes are, by a number of criteria, the most sophisticated of the cells involved in the immune response and possess most of the properties that make the

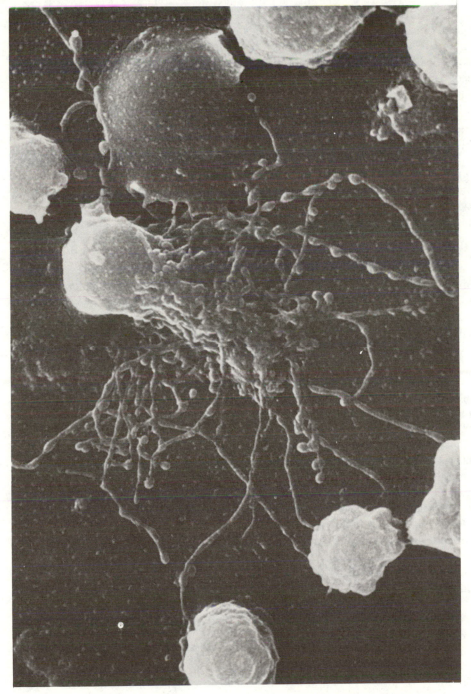

Figure 2-4 Follicular dendritic cells. (Photo courtesy of Drs. Andras Szakal and John Tew, Medical College of Virginia.)

immune mechanism in higher vertebrates unique among biological systems. They are capable of very precise recognition of foreign molecules and cells and have the property of "memory." As a population they are capable of a wide variety of responses to foreignness ranging from the production of antibodies to direct, cell-mediated cytotoxicity. They are also involved in, and subject to, a delicate matrix of cellular regulation.

Lymphocytes are small (7 to 10 μm), free-living cells found in the blood and lymphatic circulatory systems and in all lymphoid organs and tissues. They may also be found singly or in groups in tissues underlying surface epithelium (e.g., the lamnia propria of the gut). The cytoplasm : nucleus ratio is low, and the scant amount of cytoplasm present is relatively devoid of organelles. However, on activation in an immune reaction, lymphocytes undergo blast transformation (i.e., they enlarge) and divide, and the cytoplasm takes on the appearance characteristic of metabolically active cells, accumulating abundant mitochondria and endoplasmic reticulum. After an immune reaction has run its course, at least some of the cells revert to their previous small, apparently undifferentiated form. However, such lymphocytes, called "memory" lymphocytes (as opposed to unstimulated or "virgin" lymphocytes) may be altered in fundamental ways that allow them to respond in a qualitatively different manner on restimulation. The nature of the differences between resting, virgin lymphocytes and memory cells will be discussed more fully in Chapter 13.

Lymphocytes can be broadly divided into three categories on the basis of function and cell surface characteristics. *T cells* are lymphocytes that undergo their maturation in the thymus. They are distinguished by the presence on their membranes of an antigen called *Thy-1*, and the absence of surface immunoglobulin. The Thy-1 antigen is also found on certain cells of the central nervous system; the significance of the presence of this antigen in two such disparate tissues is unclear, but among cells of the immune system only T lymphocytes bear Thy-1, and thus it is a useful surface marker. T cells are important in several types of immune reactions. One subset of T cells are the principal mediators of graft rejection reactions. Another subset helps B cells to mature into plasma cells and secrete antibodies. Yet other T cells may be involved in regulation of the immune response.

B cells are lymphocytes that, on appropriate stimulation by antigen, mature into the antibody-producing *plasma cells.* B cells may be distinguished from other cells of the immune system by the presence on their surfaces of immunoglobulins which, as expected from the Clonal Selection Theory, are copies of the antibody the B cell is preprogrammed to produce. B cells do not display Thy-1.

When both T and B cells have been identified or removed from a pure population of lymphocytes, a small proportion of cells will be left over that express neither Thy-1 nor surface immunoglobulin. This is the so-called "null cell" subset of lymphocytes. The significance of this subset is unclear. It was once thought possibly to be a pool of lymphocytes from which either T or B cells differentiate, but closer examination of these cells (and a fuller knowledge of actual T and B cell differentiation pathways), makes this unlikely. One functional cell type forming at least part of the null cell subset may be the NK (natural killer) cell. These cells are important in the immune response to tumors.

Mast Cells

As seen in Chapter 17, mast cells play an important role in allergic reactions in most species. They were first described by Ehrlich in 1877; he called them "mastzellen" (well-fed cells) because of their appearance and abundance in healthy, well-fed connective tissue. Connective tissue is, in fact, the principal location in which free-living mast cells are found in all species examined. In this sense they are distinct from the other cells involved in immune responses; the latter are found principally in blood or lymph circulation and in the various lymphoid organs. However, during parasitic infections there may be a marked accumulation of mast cells in lymph nodes, principally in the cortical regions, and in gut tissues. The latter accumulation is dependent on T lymphocytes, although by what mechanism is unknown.

The histological origin of mast cells was long a source of debate, but we now know that mast cell precursors exist in bone marrow and are probably similar to the pluripotent stem cells that give rise to most other blood cells. On the other hand, mast cells are phylogenetically much more primitive than blood cells; they can be identified in orders of invertebrates that lack distinct blood cell systems. Mature mast cells do not divide and are quite long-lived.

Mast cells are characterized by numerous large, densely staining basophilic granules in the cytoplasm. In most species the granules contain complexes of histamine, heparin, and zinc, plus a number of hydrolytic enzymes. Although similar to basophils in many respects, mast cells are clearly distinct and the similarities may best be viewed as an example of convergent evolution. Mast cells are triggered to degranulate during the course of immune responses to allergens, and the release into surrounding tissue spaces of histamine and enzymes is largely responsible for the symptoms accompanying an allergic attack (Chapter 17).

Platelets

Platelets are small, anuclear, cell-like bodies found in the plasma fraction of blood. On the basis of histological and biochemical studies of platelet enzymes, principally acetylcholinesterase, Zajicek confirmed the previously held theory that platelets arise from megakaryocytes in the bone marrow, probably by a process of cytoplasmic budding. Platelets contain a number of enzymes and factors important in blood-clotting processes. They are also important in varying degrees, depending on the species, in allergic reactions. Like basophils and mast cells, platelets contain vasoactive amines and enzymes that can lead to damage if released into surrounding tissue spaces. The special situations leading to involvement of platelets in allergic reactions is discussed in detail in Chapter 17.

Organs of the Immune System

Bone Marrow

The bone marrow is more properly a tissue, rather than an organ, and indeed in the medical literature is often referred to as myeloid tissue. It consists of various hematopoietic stem cells and adipocytes embedded in a spongy matrix of reticular cells and blood vessels. It is found in cavities of almost all bones of the body, including skull, ribs, collarbone, and so on, but is most abundant in the long bones such as the femur, and in the sternum and spine. The average adult human volume of bone marrow is on the order of 2 to 3 liters, comprising anywhere from 2 to 5 percent of total body weight.

The major function of the bone marrow in adults is in the generation of all of the cellular elements of the blood, both erythroid and lymphoid, and as such it is the principal repository of hematopoietic stem cells. Although it is not generally possible to identify individual stem cells morphologically, their existence can be inferred by the ability of bone marrow cells to repopulate all of the blood elements of a lethally irradiated animal. In addition to stem cells, the marrow also contains various intermediate developmental forms of erythrocytes, granulocytes, reticular cells, monocytes, lymphocytes, and megakaryocytes. B cells, in various developmental stages, including mature forms, are found in the marrow itself. No cells identifiable as T lymphocytes are found in the marrow per se. However, the blood vessels permeating the marrow contain mature cells of both the erythroid and lymphocytic series. These vessels are usually ruptured when bone marrow cells are collected by flushing the cavities of the various bones, leading to contamination of the resident marrow cell preparation with fully mature cell types from the circulation.

While there are no afferent lymph vessels, bone marrow, like other tissues in the body, is drained by efferent lymphatic vessels.

Thymus

The thymus (so-called because in shape it resembles the leaf of the thyme plant) originates as part of the embryonic pharynx. At a fairly early stage of development (sixth week in humans) the third pharyngeal pouches undergo a rapid enlargement, and very shortly pinch off completely. The two primordia fuse, and migrate into the thorax to a final position just cephalad of the heart. The thymus throughout its existence retains the characteristic appearance of a paired organ. It is the first fetal organ to become lymphoid in character (nine weeks in humans). In late fetal stages and in early postnatal life, the thymus is a relatively large organ, but as body growth continues it becomes progressively smaller in proportion to surrounding structures. The thymus reaches its largest absolute size at about the time of sexual maturation. Beginning in early adult life it gradually involutes, becoming increasingly fibrous and fatty and losing most of its lymphoid character.

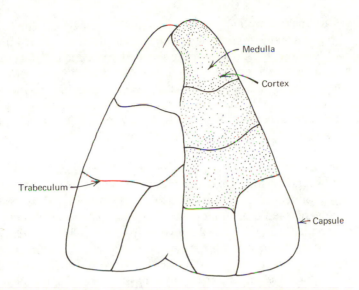

Figure 2-5 The two major lobes of the thymus, like other lymphoid organs, are subdivided into smaller compartments by trabeculae extending in from the capsule. Each "lobule" has a more or less uniform matrix of reticular cells. The periphery or cortex of each lobule is densely filled with rapidly dividing lymphocytes, whereas the central or medullary region is more sparsely populated with mostly nondividing cells. There are no apparent lymphoid follicles or germinal centers in normal individuals, and the thymus proper probably does not have any B lymphocytes. The thymus has only efferent lymph vessels and does not act in any ways as a filter for lymph or blood.

The structure of the thymus is shown schematically in Figure 2-5. Each lobe can be seen to be divided by septa of connective tissue into a series of lobular subcompartments. These septa or *trabeculae* provide the major supporting framework for the thymic tissues. On close histological examination major portions of the thymus can be distinguished—an outer region of densely packed and rapidly dividing lymphocytes called the cortex, and a central area of more loosely arranged lymphoid and epithelial cells called the medulla. The cortical thymocytes are developmentally less mature, and are very sensitive to systemically administered corticosteroids. Medullary thymocytes (about 5 percent of the total) are more mature and relatively corticosteroid resistant. The rapidly dividing cells in the cortex gradually migrate in toward the medulla, where at least some of them enter the bloodstream via the medullary veins. However, careful analysis of the dynamics of the thymic cell populations has led to the conclusion that perhaps as many as 90 percent of the cells dividing and migrating within the thymus die without leaving the organ. The rate of turnover of thymocytes in a young animal or person is such that the equivalent of an entire thymus is generated every two to three days.

Involution of the thymus in humans can begin as early as the late teens (although this is rare), and may not begin until as late at 35 or 40 years of age. The initial stages are marked by a gross reduction in size, principally due to atrophy of the cortical regions and loss of the large, rapidly dividing, relatively immature cell populations. However, the thymus continues to harbor mature T cells for many years after involution, and recent studies have shown that the residual T cells are of the functionally mature subclasses. It is not clear whether the residual mature T cells arise *in situ* after involution, or whether they migrate into the thymus from the periphery. The latter is certainly possible because the involuted thymus is in blood contact with the rest of the immune system, and indeed there is some experimental evidence that this does take place.

The thymus, like any other tissue, is drained by efferent lymph vessels. However, lymph is not brought *to* the thymus by afferent lymph vessels. It is thus normally not a major site of primary immune defense. On the other hand, as we will see in Chapter 13, it is the site of maturation of a major subclass of lymphocytes called T cells. T-cell precursors migrate into the thymus from the yolk sac, in early embryos, and from the bone marrow, at later stages of embryonic development and in the adult, via the bloodstream. Mature T cells also leave the thymus via the blood- stream. The epithelial elements of the thymus produce a hormone, called thy- mosin, that appears to be involved in T-cell maturation and integrity both within the thymus and in other lymphoid organs.

Removal of the thymus in adult animals compromises long-range immune func- tion somewhat, but generally not with fatal results. However, thymectomy at birth has a drastic effect on the subsequent ability of the organism to mount an immune response. The functional consequences of neonatal thymectomy are explored in Chapter 12. Here we simply note the effect of this operation on the structure of other lymphoid organs: neonatally thymectomized animals show severe lympho- cyte depletion in the paracortical and medullary regions of the lymph nodes (Fig- ure 2-8) and around the periphery of germinal centers of both the lymph nodes and the white pulp of the spleen (Figure 2-7). These areas are thus termed thymus dependent or T dependent.

Bursa of Fabricius

The bursa is an epithelial and lymphoid organ that is found only in birds, although possible structural analogs have been suggested in some reptiles. The bursa arises from the epithelium of the gut in the proctodeal region of the cloaca. The structure of the bursa is very similar to the thymus. It is composed of numerous lobes each of which has a cortical and medullary area. The cortex contains mostly large, un- differentiated lymphoid cells, whereas the medulla contains small, apparently ma- ture cells (Figure 2-6). However, in the bursa the cortical and medullary regions are separated by a layer of epithelial cells. Like the thymus, the bursa gradually involutes and atrophies after the onset of sexual maturity.

The functional characterization of the bursa played a key role in the identifica- tion of lymphocyte subpopulations (Chapter 12). The bursa in birds is important for the proper functioning of "B" lymphocytes, which are the lymphocytes that

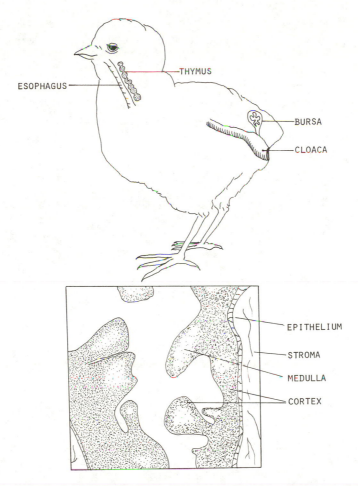

Figure 2-6 The bursa of Fabricius in birds. The bursa develops as an outgrowth of the hindgut epithelium very early in ontogeny. The fingerlike epithelial buds become lymphoid in character much later in development. Each bud or lobe then has a dense outer cortex of rapidly dividing large lymphocytes and a more thinly populated medulla of mostly small, resting lymphoid cells. The overall embryology of the bursa is similar in timing, morphology, and histology to the thymus. (Drawn with the helpful advice of Dr. Joseph A. Price.)

become plasma cells and synthesize and secrete antibody. Removal of the bursa at or before hatching results in a failure of germinal centers to develop in the lymph nodes and spleen in response to immunization, and in a total inability of the bursectomized bird to produce antibodies. However, bursectomy even before hatching does not interfere with normal development of the B cells per se of the chicken immune system. Bursectomized birds have Ig$^+$ B cells, and normal B-dependent regions of lymph tissues. These B cells are able to respond to a variety of signals *in vitro* by secreting antibody. But, for some reason, they are unable to do so *in vivo*. The defect in bursectomized birds is thus not as clear cut as once thought.

A direct analog of the bursa has not been identified in mammals. Numerous gut-associated organs have been proposed, but unconvincingly. It seems likely that in adult mammals the bone marrow itself may be the site of B-cell development; in mammalian embryos, the fetal liver appears to play a bursalike role in the maturation of B lymphocytes.

Spleen

The spleen (Figure 2-7) is a bright-red organ lying in the upper left quadrant of the abdominal cavity. Like the thymus, it is encapsulated by a tough coating of connective tissue, from which arise numerous inward projections or trabeculae that form a general structural matrix for the spleen. The spleen has a dual function—it is the major site for removal and destruction of dead red blood cells, and it is an important (although not indispensable) organ of the immune system.

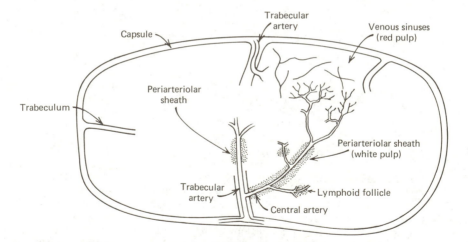

Figure 2-7 Schematic representation of a mammalian spleen. The spleen is surrounded by a tough membranous capsule from which the trabeculae arise and penetrate the inner mass. The splenic artery (not shown) enters and courses along the capsule and into the trabeculae. The major branches of the trabecular arteries, as they leave the trabeculae, are called the central arteries. These are surrounded by thin but densely packed layers of lymphoid cells called the periarteriolar sheath, which are composed principally of T cells. The smaller arterioles branching from the central arteries are often surrounded by B-cell-rich lymphoid follicles, which may contain actively mitotic germinal centers. These lymphoid areas associated with the arterial blood vessels are collectively referred to as the white pulp. Blood from the fine branchings of the arterial system empties into the loosely organized red pulp area, where it is filtered through various venous sinuses and eventually collected into veins that exit via the trabeculae and capsule into the splenic vein.

Like the thymus, the lymphocyte traffic through the spleen is via blood circulation; the spleen has only efferent lymphatics. The splenic artery enters at the hilum, and its branches traverse along the trabeculae gradually breaking up into smaller arteries and arterioles and spreading into the splenic parenchyma. Most of the arteries, at the point where they leave the trabeculae, are surrounded by a pale mass of lymphoid tissue called the "white pulp." This tissue is not well organized, but contains small and large lymphocytes, monocytes, macrophages, reticular cells, and lymphopoietic stem cells. There are also local condensations of lymphocytes called follicles, which often contain "germinal centers" of intense mitotic activity and maturation of B lymphocytes into antibody-producing plasma cells.

The fine branchings of the splenic arterial system empty into a generally unstructured region of venous sinuses called the "red pulp." Although the red and white pulp regions are not clearly segregated, the red pulp is relatively devoid of lymphoid elements, except for phagocytic cells that function in the filtration of foreign elements from the bloodstream. The major function of the red pulp is in the removal and degradation of RBCs that have reached the end of their approximately four-month life span. The sinuses eventually coalesce into defined vessels and unite into the splenic vein, which exits from the spleen near the point of entrance of the splenic artery, and empties into the hepatic portal vein.

Lymph Nodes

The lymph nodes are small (less than 1 cm unless inflamed) bean-shaped structures distributed throughout the entire body and linked together by an equally extensive circulatory system of lymphatic vessels. Each node is surrounded by a dense connective tissue capsule, and is composed principally of lymphocytes embedded in a reticulum cell network (Figure 2-8). The principal functions of the lymph nodes are in the entrapment of foreign matter in the lymph circulation, and as a site for the antigen-driven maturation of lymphocytes. Lymph nodes would appear to be evolutionarily the most recent addition to the immune system.

The lymph nodes are served by both lymph and blood circulation. In fact, it is in the lymph nodes that lymphocytes pass from blood to lymph circulation (p. 39). Afferent and efferent blood vessels enter and leave at the hilus, on the concave side of the node. Afferent lymph vessels enter at various points on the convex surface of the node, whereas the efferent lymph vessel exits at the hilus. The presence of afferent lymph vessels distinguishes lymph nodes from all other lymph organs, and enables them to play their unique role in entrapping and processing foreign antigen from extravascular tissue spaces.

In most species, the lymph node is partially compartmentalized by trabeculae projecting inward from the capsule. The outer region of the node, called the cortex, is rather densely packed with lymphocytes, whereas the inner medullary area, surrounding the hilus, is diffuse with fewer lymphocytes and more open spaces. Immediately under the capsule in the cortical areas are the cortical sinuses, channels of which extend down through the cortex into the medullary region

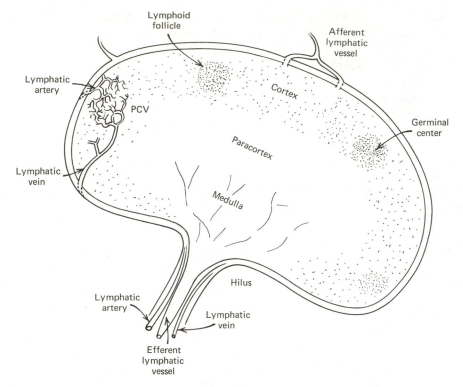

Figure 2-8 Sagittal section of a lymph node. The node can be thought of as containing three principal regions: the outer cortex, containing mostly B lymphocytes embedded in a reticular mesh together with histiocytes; a medial paracortex, containing a high proportion of T lymphocytes plus a few B cells; and a central, sparsely populated medullary region, composed of a reticular network and sinuses populated by various cell types including plasma cells. The cortex contains locally dense aggregates of B lymphocytes called lymphoid follicles, in which can be seen occasional foci of rapid mitotic activity, the germinal centers. The lymphoid artery and vein traverse through the capsule entering and exiting the interior of the node at numerous points. Arterial–venous capillary interchange takes place mainly in the cortical region. Passage of lymphocytes from blood to lymph occurs in the postcapillary venules (PCV).

where they become the medullary sinuses, which then coalesce into the efferent lymph vessel. These sinuses are crisscrossed by networks of reticular cells that are capable of engulfing bacteria or other particulate matter.

Within the cortical region may be found scattered areas of dense lymphocyte aggregations, termed lymphoid follicles. When a particular lymph node is involved in an immune reaction, some of the follicles will have foci of intense mitotic activity called germinal centers. These are created when B lymphocytes within the follicles specific for the infiltrating antigen undergo rapid amplification and maturation to the antibody-producing plasma cells.

The following sequence of events illustrates what might occur in a lymph node during the course of a typical antibody-producing immune response. Lymph carrying the foreign antigen enters the lymph node through the afferent lymph vessels and flows into the cortical sinus. The lymph percolates slowly down through the lymph channels and into and through the lymphocytes populating the cortical region. Reticular cells and fibers trap the antigen and facilitate its interaction with surrounding lymphocytes. T helper cells recognize antigen, divide, and produce factors (lymphokines) needed by B cells in order to develop into antibody-producing cells. Those B lymphocytes that have receptors specific for the antigen in question utilize these T helper factors and undergo a period of rapid proliferation and differentiation to plasma cells. These areas of intense mitotic and metabolic activity are the germinal centers. As noted earlier, during this active period lymphocytes are retarded in their passage out of the lymph node. Finally, the mature plasma cells leave the germinal centers and make their way into the medullary sinuses, where they secrete antibody into the lymph fluid, which leaves the node via the efferent lymphatic vessel, and eventually makes its way into the bloodstream.

Gut-associated Lymphoid Tissue (GALT)

In addition to the major lymphoid organs and tissues described so far, there exist significant concentrations of lymphoid cells and tissues at various points along the gut. These range from loose clusters of a few cells scattered throughout the lamnia propria, through individual but organized lymphoid follicles, up to more complex aggregates of lymph tissue like the tonsils, the appendix, and the Peyer's patches. In combination these gut-associated lymphoid tissues (GALT) may equal or exceed the lymphoid mass of the spleen or the thymus. These structures may represent the phylogenetically most primitive elements of the immune system; they are the only elements to be seen in almost identical form in all vertebrates.

Peyer's patches are compact nodules of lymphoid cells that can be readily seen on the outer wall of the intestine (Figure 2-9). Like the tonsils and the appendix, Peyer's patches show considerable histological organization, with discrete T- and B-dependent areas, lymphoid follicles, and germinal centers during antigenic stimulation. Peyer's patches give rise to B lymphocytes that are committed to making a specialized form of immunoglobulin called IgA. These B cells migrate from the Peyer's patches to epithelial surfaces lining those parts of the body that are open to the outside (the gut itself, tear ducts, salivary glands, mammary ducts, etc.) IgA has a special structure that makes it relatively stable in secretory fluids (Chapter 4) and is an important early line of defense against bacteria trying to penetrate epithelial surfaces.

The tonsils play a role in defense against orally ingested microorganisms. Viruses in particular are trapped in the tonsils, where they induce an immune reaction prior to further penetration into the body. The tonsils contain well-organized lymphoid follicles containing mature B lymphocytes. The exact role of the tonsils is unclear, since there is no evidence that persons who have had their tonsils re-

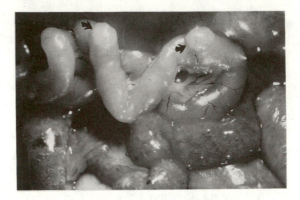

Figure 2-9 Peyer's patches on the small intestine of the mouse.

moved are at higher risk for infections caused by inhaled viruses, or that they experience worse symptoms.

At one time there was considerable interest in GALT as a possible bursal analog in mammals (e.g., a general site of B-cell generation and development). Although this hypothesis still has its defenders, most immunologists consider the bone marrow to be the principal site for B-cell development.

The Reticuloendothelial System

The reticuloendothelial system (RES) is a system of cells and tissues whose functions principally include phagocytosis and degradative metabolism. Antigen and antigen fragments displayed on the surface of RES cells (including fixed macrophages and dendritic cells) are almost certainly the major means of antigen presentation to lymphoid elements of the immune system. Cells of the RES, organized into dense sheets and fibers, form the structural matrix of the spleen, marrow, and lymph nodes. A lymph node, for example, is not just a sac of lymph and free-floating cells. It is, instead, spongelike in construction, with cells and tissues of the RES making up the pliant skeleton of the sponge, and the lymph and free lymphoid cells occupying the interstitial spaces. The RES matrix, is, of course, also infiltrated by trabeculae and blood vessels. The RES cells are all phagocytic, as far as can be determined. Those that remain as part of the fixed tissues within lymphoid organs are often called histiocytes; circulating macrophages are also considered part of the RES. Those histiocytes lining the various sinuses of the lymphoid tissues have a morphology characteristic of endothelial cells. In both lymph nodes and spleen, the RES cells may also be found in germinal centers. In the spleen, RES cells permeate the red pulp as well. It is entirely possible that some cells of the RES are actually stem cells for many elements of the erythroid and lymphoid blood cells.

Fixed cells of the RES filter particulate matter from the blood by processes that are well described morphologically but little understood at the molecular level.

This process is most likely analogous to the phagocytic processes used by macrophages in the elimination of foreign matter and bacteria. RES cells of the spleen can also selectively remove old, dead, or damaged erythrocytes from circulation. These cells are ingested and destroyed, and their hemoglobin metabolized and stored within the RES cells. The iron eventually ends up in the form of ferritin and is refed by the reticulum cells to erythrocyte precursors as they develop in the marrow and elsewhere. There is also some evidence that RES cells may synthesize and secrete bile.

The Lymphatic Circulatory System

Cells of the immune system circulate among lymphoid organs and to other sites in the body via two major circulatory pathways: blood and lymph. Although at any given moment only a minor proportion of the total lymphoid cell pool is found in the circulation, nearly all cells are mobile at some stage in their history and move throughout the system, either in simple transit, or in carrying out immune surveillance.

The system of lymphatic vessels is essentially a complete parallel of the blood system in the sense that wherever blood capillaries and vessels are to be found, so are lymphatic vessels. The lymph drainage system begins as a network of microscopic, single-cell-walled sinuses and vessels embedded in peripheral tissue. Lymph fluid, which is a balanced solution of electrolytes and proteins, plus varying amounts of lipid and carbohydrate, is collected in the lymphatic vessels as it leaks from the blood capillaries. In fact, the principal physiological role of the lymphatic system is to recover the proteins and associated fluids lost in the blood capillary network and return them to the blood system. In humans, the total volume of fluid recovered from interstitial spaces as lymph is between 1 to 2 liters per day. The lymph fluid drains through these vessels into regional lymph nodes, and passes out of the nodes through the efferent lymph vessels that gradually coalesce into the major lymphatics (thoracic duct, right lymph duct), which finally empty into the blood system at the great veins of the neck (Figure 2-10.)

As the lymphatic system returns extravascular plasma proteins from the tissues, extracellular fluids of various sorts may also enter the lymph vessels, together with proteins produced and secreted by cells at various locations in the body. Bacteria and other foreign matter that manage to cross the skin barrier are also collected in the lymph fluid and transported to the nearest lymph node, where an immune reaction is triggered among resident lymphocytes. The lymphatic system is also an efficient route for dissemination of cancerous cells breaking away from a local tumor. Because of the extensiveness of the lymphatic pathway in the body, entry of tumor cells into this system is an extremely serious event, possibly signaling metastasis. Surgical removal of a tumor is usually accompanied by a close examination and possible removal of local nodes in which tumor cells may have lodged.

The circulation of cells of the immune system can be followed starting at a

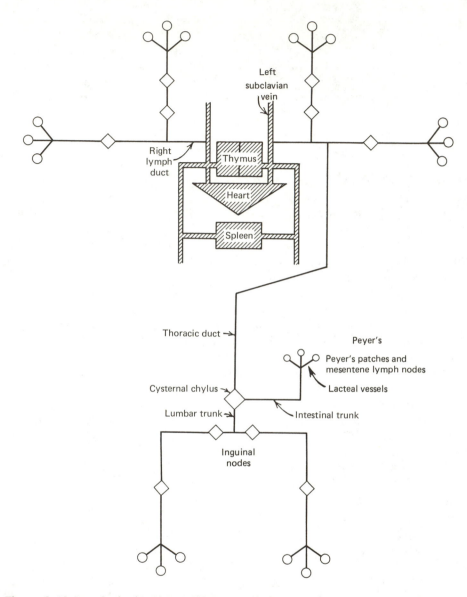

Figure 2-10 Lymphatic circulatory system. Lymph fluid is gathered from the capillary beds in the peripheral tissues and passes through a primary node (○) and various numbers of secondary (◇) lymph nodes, finally emptying into the two major lymphatic trunks: the thoracic duct, which collects lymph from the lower trunk, the left arm and thorax, and the left side of the head and neck, and enters the left innominate (or sometimes, subclavian) vein; and the right lymph duct, which gathers lymph from the right arm and thorax, and the right side of the head and neck and enters the great veins descending through the right side of the neck. The heart and the thymus each have lymphatic drainage to both the left and right side collector systems, while the spleen drains into the thoracic duct. Each lymph node is also in independent communication with

primary lymph node. A primary node is one that receives afferent lymph vessels originating in peripheral tissue rather than an adjacent lymph node. Such vessels do not normally carry white cells, but instead lymph fluid collected from the capillary beds plus miscellaneous proteins and adventitious foreign antigens. Lymph fluid leaving a primary node via an efferent lymph vessel has now entered the closed circuit of the blood-lymphatic system, and contains large numbers of lymphoid cells. Circulating white cells are principally T lymphocytes, with perhaps 15 to 30 percent B lymphocytes. (In normal, healthy individuals red blood cells, granulocytes and monocytes are not found in the lymphatic circulation.) The lymph fluid and lymphocytes carried by the efferent lymphatic vessels may pass through any number of lymph nodes, but, as pointed out earlier, eventually coalesce into the major lymphatic trunks that empty into the bloodstream at the great veins of the neck. The white cells enter the arterial circulation along with other blood elements at the heart, and reach the lymph node once again through the afferent blood vessels. As Gowans showed, it is within the lymph nodes that lymphocytes are able to pass from the blood circulation back into the lymphatic circulation. As blood passes from arterial to venous capillaries located principally in the cortical and paracortical regions of the node, it enters into the postcapillary venules. These vessels are constructed in part of unusual cuboidal epithelial cells (the so-called "high epithelium"), which allow lymphocytes to pass through into adjacent lymphoid sinuses (Figure 2-11). Both T and B lymphocytes cross over from blood to lymph.

Vascular endothelium controls not only the routine passage of lymphocytes from blood to lymph, but traffic of lymphocytes to and from various lymph organs as needed. For example, relatively undifferentiated "pre-T" lymphocytes coming from bone marrow appear to have surface receptors allowing them to identify and cross through thymic vascular endothelium. A similar mechanism is assumed to direct cells leaving the thymus or bone marrow when they arrive at the spleen. The high endothelium of lymph nodes attracts T lymphocytes, whereas at least some B lymphocytes bind specifically to the high endothelium of Peyer's patches.

Endothelial cells themselves produce a number of factors that influence the growth and differentiation of leukocytes *in vitro,* and it is tempting to assume that endothelium plays a similar role *in vivo.* A reciprocal effect, of lymphocytes on endothelium, is readily demonstrable *in vivo:* If T cells are depleted from rats, the high endothelium of the lymph node postcapillary venules will gradually disappear. The study of interactions between cells of the immune system and vascular endothelium is an interesting and very active area of immunological research.

When antigen reaches a lymph node, it can have a number of effects on lymphocyte traffic patterns. There is an initial period of decreased (up to 90 percent)

---

the general arteriovenous network (not shown). The two circulatory systems close by the return of lymph fluid from blood to lymphatic vessels at the capillary beds in the peripheral tissues, and by the return of lymphoid cells to the lymphatic system in the postcapillary venules located in the cortex of the lymph nodes. Hatched areas represent organs connected afferently solely by blood circulation.

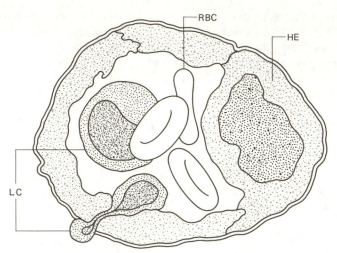

Figure 2-11 Cross-section of a postcapillary venule, showing migration of lymphocytes through the specialized high epithelium. LC: lymphocyte; RBC: red blood cell; HE: high endothelial cell.

egress of lymphocytes (but not of lymph fluid) from the node. The blood vessels within the node dilate considerably, blood flow to the node increases, and this, together with a proliferation of lymphoid cells within the node, cause it to become enlarged. The swelling usually peaks about 5 to 7 days after initial infection and then gradually subsides. Within 24 hours the flow of lymphocytes from the node recommences and will be higher than normal for a period of time. There is good evidence that lymphocytes specific for the antigen in question tend to localize in the node(s) where reaction to the antigen is taking place.

Bibliography

General

Bessis, M., *Living Blood Cells and Their Ultrastructure,* trans. by R. I. Weed, Springer-Verlag, Berlin, Heidelberg, New York (1973).

Butterfield, J. H., D. Maddox, and G. Gleich, The eosinophilic leucocyte: Maturation and function. *Clinical Immunology Reviews 2,* 187 (1983).

Cline, M. J., *The White Cell,* Harvard University Press, Cambridge (1975).

Keller, R., Tissue mast cells in immune reactions. *Monographs in Allergy,* Vol. 2, S. Karger, Basel (1966).

McConnell, I., The lymphoid system. In I. McConnell, A. Munro, and H. Waldmann, eds., *The Immune System, (2nd edition),* Chapter 14, Blackwell Scientific Publications, London (1981).

Tew, J., G. Thorbecke, and R. Steinman, Dendritic cells in the immune response: Characteristics and recommended nomenclature." *J. Reticuloendothelial Soc. 31,* 371 (1982).

Trnka, Z., and R. N. P. Cahill (Eds.), Essays on the anatomy and physiology of lymphoid tissues. *Monographs in Allergy,* Vol. 16, S. Karger, Basel (1980).

Research

Baroni, C. D., et al., The human thymus in aging: Histologic involution paralleled by increased mitogen response and by enrichment of OKT3 + lymphocytes. *Immunology 50,* 519 (1983).

Butcher, E., R. Scolley, and I. Weissman, Organ specificity of lymphocyte migration: Mediation by highly selective lymphocyte interaction with organ-specific determinants on high endothelial venules. *Eur. J. Immunol. 10,* 556 (1980).

Capron, M., H. Bazin, M. Joseph, and A. Capron, Evidence for IgE-dependent cytotoxicity by rat eosinophils. *J. Immunol. 126,* 1764 (1981).

Chin, Y. H., G. D. Carey and J. J. Woodruff, Lymphocyte recognition of lymph node high endothelium. I. Inhibition of in vitro binding by a component of thoracic duct lymph. *J. Immunol. 125,* 1764 (1980).

Drayson, M., M. Smith, and W. Ford, The sequences of changes in blood flow and lymphocyte influx to stimulated rat lymph nodes," *Immunology 44,* 125 (1981).

Eerola, E., S. Jalkanen, K. Granfors, and A. Toivanen, Immune capacity of the chicken bursectomized at 60 hours of incubation: Mitogen-induced cell proliferation and Ig secretion." *J. Immunol. 131,* 120 (1983).

Fossum, S., The architecture of rat lymph nodes. II. Lymph node compartments. *Scand. J. Immunol. 12,* 411 (1980).

Gallatin, W., I. Weissman, and E. Butcher, A cell surface molecule involved in organ-specific homing of lymphocytes. *Nature 304,* 30 (1983).

Glick, B., T. Chang, and R. Jaap, The Bursa of Fabricius and antibody production. *Poultry Science 35,* 224 (1956).

Gowans, J. L., and E. J. Knight, The route of recirculation of lymphocytes in the rat. *Proc. R. Soc. Lond. 159,* 257 (1964).

Guyton, A. C., Interstitial fluid pressure and dynamics of lymph formation. *Fed. Proc. 35,* 1861 (1976).

Hay, J. B., and B. B. Hobbs, The flow of blood to lymph nodes and its relation to lymphocyte traffic and the immune response. *J. Exp. Med. 145,* 31 (1977).

Humphrey, J. H., D. Grennan, and V. Sundaram, The origin of follicular dendritic cells in the mouse, and the mechanism of trapping of immune complexes on them. *Eur. J. Immunol. 14,* 859 (1984).

Kawanishi, H., L. Saltzman, and W. Strober, Mechanisms regulating IgA class-specific Ig production in murine gut-associated lymphoid tissues. II. Terminal differentiation of postswitch sIgA-bearing Peyer's patch B cells. *J. Exp. Med. 158,* 649 (1983).

Kitamura, Y., M. Yokoyama, H. Matsuda, T. Ohno, and K. J. Mori, Spleen colony-forming cell as common precursor for tissue mast cells and granulocytes. *Nature 291,* 159 (1981).

Klaus, G. G. B. et al., The follicular dendritic cell: Its role in antigen presentation in the generation of immunological memory. *Immunol. Rev. 53,* 3 (1980).

Klinkert, W., J. LaBadie, and W. Bowers, Accessory and stimulating properties of dendritic cells and macrophages isolated from various rat tissues. *J. Exp. Med. 156,* 1 (1982).

Lipscomb, M. F. et al., Antigen presentation by guinea pig alveolar macrophages. *J. Immunol. 126,* 286 (1981).

Mandel, T. E. et al., The follicular dendritic cell: Long term antigen retention during immunity. *Immunol. Rev. 53,* 29 (1980).

Mayrhoffer, G., and R. Fisher, Mast cells in severely T cell depleted rats, and the response to infestation with N. brasiliensis. *Immunology 37,* 145 (1979).

McGregor, D. D., and J. L. Gowans, The antibody response of rats depleted of lymphocytes by chronic drainage from the thoracic duct. *J. Exp. Med. 117,* 303 (1963).

Ottaway, C. A., and D. M. V. Parrott, Regional blood flow and its relationship to lymphocyte and lymphoblast traffic during a primary immune reaction. *J. Exp. Med. 150,* 218 (1979).

Parrott, D., and A. Ferguson, Selective Migration of lymphoblasts within the small intestine. *Immunology 26,* 571 (1974).

Rogoff, T. M., and P. E. Lipsky, Antigen presentation by isolated guinea pig Kupffer cells. *J. Immunol. 124,* 1740 (1980).

Steinman, R. M., D. S. Lustig, and Z. A. Cohn, Identification of a novel cell type in peripheral lymphoid organs of mice. III. Functional properties in vivo. *J. Exp. Med. 139,* 1431 (1974).

Szakal, A. et al., Isolated follicular dendritic cells: Cytochemical antigen localization, Nomarski, SEM and TEM morphology. *J. Immunol. 134,* 1349 (1985).

Zajicek, J., Studies on the histogenesis of blood platelets and megakaryocytes. *Acta Physiol. Scand. 40*/Supplement 138 (1957).

II

Antibodies

Until the middle of this century, when lymphocytes were found to be the cells responsible for a wide range of immune phenomena, antibodies *were* immunology. Nearly all of the properties of immune reactions could be accounted for by some defined or inferred property of antibody molecules. Those seemingly immune phenomena that appeared not to involve antibodies (skin graft rejection, for example) tended to be dismissed as not truly immunological in nature. Even the search for cells involved in immune reactions was simply a search for the cellular origin of antibodies, at least in the beginning.

Attempts to isolate and identify the agent or agents in the serum of an immune animal, responsible for the spectrum of reactions that ultimately came to be attributed to a single agent called an antibody, began in the 1890s. Behring and Kitasato showed that serum taken from an animal that had recovered from diphtheria could render a second animal resistant to the disease. The potential health implications of such *antitoxins* were obvious and inspired a literal frenzy of activity over the next several decades as attempts were made to exploit and extend this momentous observation.

As with frenzy generally, these early years of immunology were not very productive or profound. Too many phenomena were being discovered and described all at the same time. No one (except, perhaps, Paul Ehrlich) seems to have had time to sit down and think about how it all might tie together; each set of experimental results was in and of itself just too exciting.

Beginning in the 1920s, some sober-minded scientists in New York and Berlin, who had been trained as chemists, began to take a clearer look at things. They decided to treat the interaction of these mysterious antibodies with their specific antigens just as they would treat the interaction of any two chemical substances. To a surprising degree, antibodies and antigens seemed to play by the same rules as any two chemicals that had an affinity for each other. This finding lent a certain scientific credibility to immunology, and gave rise to the field of immunochemistry. From that point forward, antibodies became one of the prime biochemical models for understanding the structure and function of macromolecules. And once the basic structure of the antibody molecule itself was worked out, understanding how such a complex molecule could be coded for in DNA became one of the major avenues of inquiry in the emerging field of molecular biology. In the next few chapters we examine some of the principal experimental advances that have resulted in our understanding of the structure, function, and molecular genetics of antibody molecules.

CHAPTER 3

Resolution of the Basic Structure of Immunoglobulins

Although the major impetus for the growth of immunology as a science in this century clearly derived from its relevance to understanding and managing infectious diseases, some of its most exciting developments have emerged within the framework of totally nonclinical sciences. And, as we will see time and again in this text, some of these developments, which often read like the best of high-suspense fiction, have had a profound and lasting impact on the sciences that nurtured them. Among such stories, the resolution of the basic structure of monomeric immunoglobulin is perhaps the most important, in terms not only of intellectual excitement, but especially with respect to expanding our appreciation of the scope of eucaryote molecular biology.

At about the beginning of this century, the humoral immune response was defined by the presence in serum (blood, minus cellular elements and clotting factors) of a variety of possible activities directed toward the immunizing substance. In a very scholarly text on infection and immunity published in 1917, Kolmer described several different factors mediating these activities in the serum of an animal immunized with bacteria:

Agglutinins specifically clump or agglutinate just that strain of bacteria used for immunization.

Opsonins facilitate the engulfment of these bacteria by macrophages.

Antitoxins neutralize the toxins associated with the immunizing bacteria, but do not damage the bacterium itself.

Cytolysins, together with complement, lead to lysis and destruction of the bacteria.

Precipitins, which form flocculent precipitates with cell-free culture filtrates of the bacterial growth medium (i.e., with substances shed by the bacteria into the surrounding medium).

All of these activities were found to be highly specific for the immunizing bacterial strain or extracts thereof and were thus grouped under the general heading of antibodies. However, Kolmer, like most immunologists in the first third of this century, had no reason to imagine that all of these activities were mediated by the same entity, and he in fact argued for their distinctness. Zinsser, in an article written in the *Journal of Immunology* in 1921, argued strongly and persuasively in favor of a "unitarian" view of the probable identity of these various immune activities. Today, we know that all of them are, indeed, mediated by the same molecular entity, that is, immunoglobulin.

Immunochemistry: The Early Years

What is the biochemical nature of antibody? How is its structure determined? The biochemical nature of antibody was completely unknown many years into the present century. It was clear that antibody activty was contained in the serum, the two principal protein classes of which are the globulins and the albumins. Fractionation of serum into various protein classes had been carried out as early as the 1850s by selective precipitation with increasing concentrations of salts such as $(NH_4)_2SO_4$. It had been observed already in 1903 that repeated immunizations lead to an increase in the globulin fraction of serum, and that treatments of serum that enrich for the globulin fraction also enrich for antibody. There had also been a suggestion that antibody activity is decreased by treatment with proteolytic enzymes. But the first scientifically based suggestion that antibodies are protein molecules did not come until about 1930, and it was not completely accepted in some segments of the scientific community for many years afterward, mainly because no one was absolutely sure that the active substances precipitated by salt contained *only* globulin protein.

An indirect but key observation that ultimately contributed to the identification of antibodies as proteins was made by Oswald Avery in the 1920s. He showed that certain strains of pneumococci, when grown *in vitro,* shed a substance into the culture medium that react strongly and completely with antipneumococcal antibody. Michael Heidelberger, a chemist working in Avery's group, showed that the shed substance is a polysaccacharide that, importantly, does not contain nitrogen. This was important because the principal method for identifying protein at the time was through its high content of nitrogen. Heidelberger thus had in hand a biochemically well-defined antigen that could precipitate antibody and could unequivocally be distinguished from protein. As a source of antibody, he used antipneumococcal antiserum that had been diluted 20-fold with mild acid solution. This treatment causes a precipitate to form, and Felton had previously shown that all of the antigen-binding capacity of the serum could be recovered from the precipitate, leaving in solution over 90 percent of the serum components. The redissolved precipitate was one of the first sources of enriched antibody.

When the purified pneumococcal polysaccharide was precipitated with enriched pneumococcal antibody, and the resulting immune precipitate recovered and analyzed, it was shown to be composed of a very large amount of protein in addition to the polysaccharide antigen. This experiment confirmed that antigen is indeed a component of immune precipitates (a point that was not entirely clear at the time), and strongly suggested that antibody is protein in nature. By dissociating the antigen–antibody complex with high-salt concentrations, Heidelberger and his colleague, Forrest Kendall, were able to recover the antibody activity from the precipitated protein component, and by re-reacting it with polysaccharide demonstrated that this protein is specific for and essentially 100 percent precipitable by the antigen. Heidelberger went on to use this system to demonstrate that the reaction of antibody and antigen is a bimolecular reaction governed by the same physicochemical laws governing other, simpler chemical reactions. This provided a solid foundation for the branch of immunology that came to be known as immunochemistry.

At this point (about 1935) it was generally accepted that antibody is a serum globulin, although some individuals felt that the possibility that antibodies simply copurified with γ-globulins had not been rigorously excluded. It was also generally accepted that the interaction of antibody with antigen can be understood in terms of the same principles that govern the interaction of simpler chemical moieties. The next major steps in characterization resulted from the application of two recently developed biophysical techniques: analytical ultracentrifugation and electrophoresis. Both of these techniques were developed in Sweden, the former by The Svedberg and the latter by his collaborator, Arne Tiselius. The classic experiment by Tiselius and Elvin Kabat, a student of Michael Heidelberger, is described in Figure 3-1. This definitely established the γ-globulin fraction of serum globulins as the major serum protein class in which antibodies are found. Heidelberger himself went to Sweden and, in collaboration with K. O. Pederson, demonstrated that pure antibody (recovered from a pneumococcal polysaccharide antigen–antibody complex) has a sedimentation coefficient of 7S and a probable molecular weight of about 150,000. More importantly, so does the γ-globulin fraction of serum from an unimmunized animal. Heidelberger and Pederson were the first to make the important suggestion, which later proved to be correct in the most precise detail,

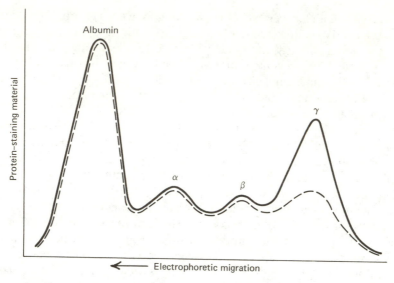

Figure 3-1 The Tiselius–Kabat experiment. In 1939, when this experiment was carried out, it was known that antibodies existed in the serum (blood from which the red cells and clotting factors have been removed). The solid line in the figure shows the electrophoresis pattern of the serum of a rabbit that had been extensively immunized with ovalbumin. The dashed line shows the electrophoresis pattern of the same serum after repeated precipitation with ovalbumin. Note the sharp reduction in the γ-globulin peak of the pattern. This experiment established that the γ-globulin fraction of serum contained the main molecular species of antibodies. [Based on A. Tiselius and E. A. Kabat, An electrophoretic study of immune sera and purified antibody preparations." *J. Exp. Medicine 69,* 119 (1939).]

that there is no major physical difference between purified antibody and the bulk of the proteins comprising the γ-globulin fraction of normal serum. As we now know, virtually all of the proteins present in the γ-globulin fraction of serum are fully functional antibody molecules. Almost identical experiments and conclusions were reported in the same year (1936) by Wykoff at Rockefeller University.

A Second Antibody Species: Macroglobulin (IgM)

Subsequent studies showed the presence in normal serum of another γ-globulin fraction containing antibodies with a sedimentation coefficient of 19S and an approximate molecular weight of 900,000. These were referred to at the time as macroglobulins (now known as IgM). By the early 1940s, it was generally accepted that when the electrophoretically defined γ-globulin fraction of normal or immune serum is isolated and subjected to ultracentrifugal analysis, two distinct size classes are apparent. The major component migrates in the analytical ultracentrifuge with a sedimentation coefficient of about 7S. A minor component of the γ-globulins (about 5 to 10 percent in humans) sediments at 19S. It was shown early on that antibody activity is associated with both size classes, but the relationship between the two, if any, was at first unclear. Some thought that the 19S molecule might be an artifact of the isolation procedure.

In 1955, Franklin and Kunkel and their associates carried out an experiment in which they first separated normal serum into its various components by preparative electrophoresis and then determined the molecular weight of each fraction by ultracentrifugation. They found the 19S species present at the fast end of the γ-globulins, thus establishing it as a normal component of serum γ-globulin. They then used the isolated 7S and 19S proteins as antigens to get anti-7S and anti-19S antibodies and showed that although there is some degree of cross-reactivity, the two are definitely antigenically distinguishable. It seemed quite likely, therefore, that the 7S and 19S γ-globulin molecules would also be structurally distinct.

Deutsch and Morton showed a year or two later that 19S macroglobulin can be dissociated into a 7S γ-globulin by treatment with a sulfhydryl reagent. However, this 7S species retains the antigenic properties of the parent 19S molecule and remains antigenically distinct from the major, originally defined, 7S γ-globulin component. On the other hand, many of the antibody properties of the 19S molecule, particularly agglutination and cytolysis, are greatly decreased on reduction to the 7S species. The reasons for this are clear: the 19S molecule, which is now known to be a pentamer, is a much more efficient cross-linker of antigen and binder of complement (see Chapter 4) than the monomeric, divalent 7S IgM species.

The Discovery of IgA

In 1963, Heremans succeeded in isolating the electrophoretically defined γ_{1A} subfraction of γ-globulin from the serum of two patients recovering from a brucellosis infection and from a volunteer immunized with diphtheria toxoid. All three had active antibodies in their γ_{1A} serum fractions. This was the first suggestion of γ_{1A}-associated antibody activity. Previous studies on the physical properties of proteins in this electrophoretically defined region had shown them to be 7S. Subsequent studies showed them to be antigenically distinct from the 7S and 19S components of serum already known to contain antibody activity, implying the existence of yet a third class of immunoglobulin molecule.

The presence of functional antibodies in various secretions of the body (saliva, mucus, tears, breast milk, etc.) had been described as early as 1917. The presence of γ_{1A} proteins in such secretions was also known. In 1965, Tomasi and his colleagues showed that a wide range of body secretions contain functional antibodies of the γ_{1A} class. However, unlike the γ_{1A} of serum, which is 7S, secretory γ_{1A} was found to be 11S and was concluded to be a polymer of the 7S form. (We now know it to be a dimer.) Thus, the γ_{1A} antibody molecule is unique in that it occurs in two different forms depending on its anatomical location.

In order to bring uniformity to immunoglobulin nomenclature, which continued to be based on the position at which an antibody activity was found on the electrophoretic spectrum (Figure 3-1), an international panel of immunologists was convened by the World Health Organization in Prague in 1964. The three classes of immunoglobulin known at the time were given the formal designations IgG (γ_2, the major 7S antibody class of γ-globulin); IgM (γ_{1M}, also called β_{2M} in the early literature, the "macroglobulin" or 19S component of γ-globulin); and IgA (the previously designated γ_{1A} or β_{2A} component of serum[1]) (see also Figure 6-14).

The Final Resolution of Antibody Structure

In the early 1940s, the question of antibody valence (number of antigen-combining sites per antibody molecule) began to be addressed in a serious fashion. Since antibodies were known to react with antigens as small as 600 to 1000 daltons, a general appreciation of protein structure suggested that antigen-combining sites on proteins would be fairly localized and discrete, and most likely on the surface of the globulin molecules. But the location, shape, or number of such sites was completely unknown. Attempts to analyze the ratio of molecules of antigen per 150,000 MW of antibody in immune precipitates suggested that antibody valence must be very low, on the order of one or two. In a classic early paper on this subject by Hooker and Boyd in 1942, the sites were referred to as "active patches." Considerable insight was evident in their paper, and they were among the first to propose a number of concepts related to the size, shape, and number of antigen combining sites on antibodies that were later firmly established.

The first attempts to determine whether the entire antibody molecule is required for binding antigen involved the use of proteolytic enzymes. Some increase in the amount of antigen binding per gram of antibody, as a result of proteolysis, was noted in experiments carried out in the late 1930s, but in general these experiments were not very informative. Further studies carried out by Petermann and her collaborators in the 1940s showed that antigen-binding activity could indeed be demonstrated in association with enzymatically generated antibody fragments that she estimated by ultracentrifugal analysis to be on the order of quarter molecules. This question was taken up again by Rodney Porter in the mid-1950s, using a much purer preparation of the only enzyme that had given interpretable results in earlier experiments—papain. Limited digestion with papain produced three distinct fragments in equal amounts, each of 50,000 daltons, which could be separated on carboxymethyl-cellulose (CMC) columns (Figure 3-2). Peaks I and II both bound antigen, although they would not precipitate it, whereas peak III did not interact with antigen. On the other hand, peak III material could, under appro-

---

[1]Upon closer analysis of the exact location of the γ_{1A} antibodies in the electrophoretic spectrum of human serum, it was concluded that it was more in the β-globulin peak than the γ. Therefore, it was renamed β_{2A} by some investigators. For a few years, both terms (γ_{1A} and β_{2A}) were used, creating some confusion.

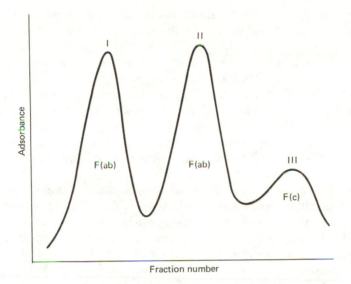

Figure 3-2 Chromatographic profile of γ-globulin digested with papain. After digestion of a sample of γ-globulin with purified papain, the digest was dialyzed and chromatographed on a column packed with carboxymethyl cellulose, which separates molecules on the basis of net electric charge. Peaks I and II later turned out to be essentially identical molecularly. The Fc peak is reduced in relative mass because of crystallization of much of the Fc peptide during dialysis. [Based on R. R. Porter, The hydrolysis of rabbit γ-globulin and antibodies with crystalline papain. *Biochem. J.* **73**, 119 (1959).]

priate conditions, form protein crystals. The ability of fragments generated from heterogeneous, noncrystallizable protein to form protein crystals seemed at the time totally inexplicable, and, indeed, the interpretation of this finding was initially strongly questioned by many scientists. However, this observation was confirmed in several other laboratories and was rapidly accepted as an empirical fact to be accounted for in any model of Ig structure. Peaks I and II, on further analysis, turned out to be essentially identical, their separation on a CMC column being due to slight charge differences brought out during the digestion and isolation procedure.

These data allowed the deduction that the 150,000-dalton Ig molecule is composed of two essentially identical, 50,000-dalton portions, each of which binds antigen (agreeing nicely with the known fact that 7S Ig is bivalent), and another portion of 50,000 daltons, that is apparently exceedingly homogeneous in structure, because it is able to crystallize out of solution. It appeared that each unit is a fairly compact globular structure because, after the initial rapid cleavage by papain liberating the fragments, further digestion is slower. The antigen-binding fragments were subsequently name Fab (for fragment, antigen binding) and the remaining portion was referred to as Fc (fragment, crystallizable). Additional observations Porter noted were that the antigenic determinants that distinguished γ2-globulin

(IgG) from 19S (IgM) and β_{2A} antibody reside on the Fc portion, whereas those determinants cross-reactive among all three known classes reside on the Fab portion.

Additional information about antibody structure was obtained using the protease pepsin. Digestion of the 150,000-dalton γ-globulin molecule resulted in a large fragment of ca. 100,000 daltons, and numerous low molecular weight oligopeptides and free amino acids. The larger fragment was shown to bind two molecules of antigen. Unlike the Fab fragments, the 100,000 dalton piece (called $F(ab)_2$) could also precipitate antigen from solution. Later experiments showed that one $F(ab)_2$ fragment could be converted to two Fab fragments with a disulfide reducing agent such as 2-mercaptoethanol.

A separate approach to looking for subunits of antibody molecules came with the work of Gerald Edelman and his colleagues at Rockefeller University in about 1960. Previous investigators had shown that whereas treatment of γ_{1M} (IgM) antibodies with reducing agents such as mercaptoethanol caused a rapid reduction in both molecular weight and antibody activity, treatment of γ_2 (IgG) antibodies under similar conditions had no effect. However, Edelman demonstrated in 1959

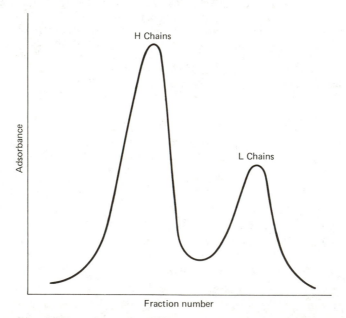

Fraction number

Figure 3-3 Chromatographic profile of reduced and alkylated γ-globulin (IgG). The disulfide bonds of a purified sample of γ-globulin were reacted with a disulfide reducing agent and then alkylated with iodoacetate to prevent reassociation of the bonds. The sample was then chromatographed at low pH on a column that separates molecules on the basis of size. By comparison with standards of known molecular weight, the two observed peaks could be assigned approximate molecular weight values of 50,000 and 25,00 daltons. Because recovery of starting material was essentially quantitative, it was further possible to conclude that γ-globulin must be composed of a total of four chains, two heavy (H) chains of 50,000 daltons each and two light (L) chains of 25,000 daltons.

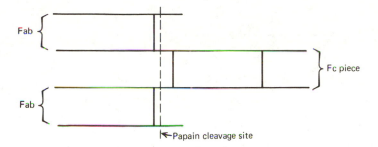

Figure 3-4 The original prototypical structure for γ-globulin (IgG) proposed by Porter on the basis of the proteolytic cleavage data and the disulfide reduction and chain separation data shown in Figures 3-2 and 3-3.

that if IgG is treated with mercaptoethanol in the presence of guanidine hydro-chloride or 6 M urea at pH 3, the 150,000-MW band apparent on starch gel elec-trophoresis is reduced to fragments of lower molecular weight. This provided the first clue that the basic immunoglobulin molecule is composed of more than one peptide chain. Further characterization was difficult because the component frag-ments precipitated out of solution when the reduction medium was dialyzed away. Reduction under such conditions reduces intrachain as well as interchain disulfide bonds, and after dialysis there is a random interaction of all open SH groups, leading to large, nonsensical aggregates. This problem was finally solved by block-ing the exposed sulfhydryl groups either with sodium sulfite or, more routinely, by the use of alkylating reagents such as iodoacetamide, which rendered the dissoci-ated chains soluble in aqueous buffer. When the reduced and alkylated peptides were analyzed by the relatively new technique of Sephadex chromatography, each immunlogublin molecule of 150,000 MW was found to give rise to two heavy (H) chains of 50,000 MW, and two light (L) chains of 25,000 MW (Figure 3-3).

Porter then carried out crucial experiments relating the H_2L_2 structure to the $F(ab)_2Fc$ structure. He found that antibodies prepared to Fab react with both H and L chains, whereas antibodies against Fc react only with H chains. These observa-tions led to his proposal in 1962 of the structure shown in Figure 3-4 as the basic molecular form of immunoglobulin. Over the next several years details of the precise location of inter- and intrachain disulfide bonds, and of enzymatic cleavage sites, were worked out. These studies confirmed Porter's interpretation of Ig struc-ture, and resulted in the refinements shown in Figure 3-5.

Modern Immunochemistry

Myeloma Proteins as Immunoglobulin Analogs

Progress in working out immunoglobulin structure beyond the Porter model was almost entirely dependent on the establishment of myeloma proteins as valid

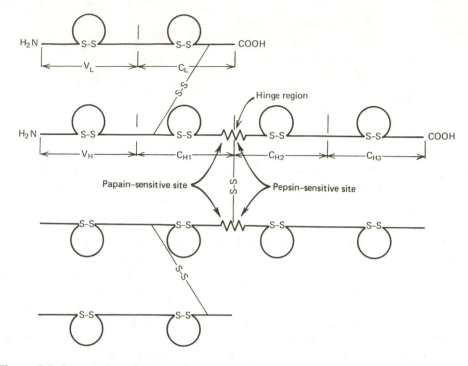

Figure 3-5 Current view of prototypical monomeric Ig structure. Each light and heavy chain is composed of linearly arranged "domains" of about 110 amino acids, each containing an intrachain disulfide loop of about 60 residues. The first domain (from the NH_2-terminal end) of each chain is the variable region (see also Figure 4-12), and the remaining domains comprise the constant region of the chain. The disulfide bonds connecting the L and H chains are always between the C_L and C_{H1} domains, although the precise location of each half cystine within the domain varies from class to class and species to species. The boundary between the C_{H1} and C_{H2} domains is the so-called hinge region, and in all classes of Ig, contains the interheavy chain disulfide bonds. However, the size of the hinge region, and the number of disulfide bonds contained therein, also varies among different species and Ig classes. The papain-sensitive site is in the hinge region, NH_2 terminal of the interheavy chain disulfide bonds. There is a pepsin-sensitive site at the C-terminal end of the hinge region. The Fc fragment generated by this cleavage is then digested further by pepsin, so that an intact Fc fragment is not normally isolated after pepsin treatment.

analogs of normal serum globulin molecules. Myeloma proteins are obtained from the urine and serum of patients with multiple myeloma, a disease in which presumably a single antibody-producing cell or its precursor undergoes oncological transformation. The result is extensive proliferation of the progeny of the transformed cell, which invade and can be found in various body sites, but most prominently the bone marrow. In fact, a serious consequence of this disease is often extensive bone damage. A second concomitant of the disease is greatly elevated levels of serum γ-globulins, which are symthesized and secreted by the antibody-producing (plasma) cells. Any of the classes or subclasses of immunoglobulin may be produced by a particular myeloma, but a given myeloma normally produces only a single type of immunoglobulin molecule. The molecules produced may be intact antibodies (H_2L_2), L chains only (Bence-Jones proteins), or more rarely, H chains only.

As serum globulins began to be characterized in ever greater detail, it became increasingly apparent that myeloma proteins are essentially indistinguishable physically from normal γ-globulins and their component chains. The major difference is an apparent electrophoretic homogeneity of the myeloma proteins in comparison to the highly heterogeneous normal serum γ-globulins. This is due to the fact that myelomas arise in a single antibody-producing cell, and all of the progeny of this cell produce exactly the same species of globulin molecule. Normal serum globulins are made up of a collection of globulin products (antibodies) from many different globulin producing cells, each globulin being slightly different from the others. In multiple myeloma, greater than 95 percent of the total serum globulins may be copies of a single protein molecule. Whereas in electrophoresis γ-globulins as a whole migrate over a fairly broad range, myeloma proteins almost always migrate as a very narrow band. Myelomas from different patients migrate to different points within the γ-globulin mobility range. The advantage of myeloma proteins is thus that they provide a source of protein sufficiently homogeneous for detailed structural analysis.

Although by 1960 the close homology of myeloma proteins with normal γ-globulins was appreciated, there was considerable reservation about their use for studying antibody structure because of the fact that they were produced by a clearly abnormal cell. It was felt that any information thus derived might possibly be misleading or completely erroneous. One major reservation about myeloma proteins expressed by earlier workers was based on their seeming paucity of antigenic markers. An antigenic relatedness of myeloma proteins and antibody molecules was, of course, well established. Nevertheless, if one tested antibodies prepared against γ-globulins with a myeloma protein isolated from a given patient, only a relatively few of the anti-γ-globulin antibodies would react with the myeloma protein. Moreover, myeloma proteins could induce the production of at least some antibodies that did not seem to cross-react with γ-globulins isolated from serum. The resolution of these dilemmas will be apparent when we discuss Ig structure in more detail. Briefly, the former observation is explained by the structural (and thus antigenic) heterogeneity of serum globulins versus the homogeneity of myeloma proteins; the second observation is related to the detectability of idiotypic determinants on myeloma proteins.

A major advance in acceptance of myeloma proteins as analogs of immunoglobulin molecules came about when it was shown that Bence-Jones (B-J) proteins were likely to be identical with the L chain of immunoglobulins. B-J proteins had been known since the 1850s to be present in the urine of multiple myeloma patients. In the early part of this century it was established that they are antigenically related to γ-globulins, but that they are of a very low molecular weight and quite homogeneous in their properties. Exact estimates of the molecular weight were at first confused by the fact that they usually occur as a dimer; the monomer weight was estimated by ultracentrifugal analysis to be about 20,000 to 25,000. The relationship of these proteins to the established γ-globulin proteins was unknown for many years, although it was known that antibodies prepared against B-J proteins cross-reacted with all known antibody classes. With the discovery of distinct H and L chains of the γ-globulins it seemed reasonable to suspect that B-J proteins represented one or the other of the chains of that molecule produced by the malignant cell in the myeloma patient.

The identify of B-J proteins and normal Ig L chains was established in an experiment carried out by Edelman and Gally in 1960. Bence-Jones proteins in urine are characterized by the temperature dependence of their solubility. They are soluble below 60°C, insoluble in the range of about 65 to 75°C, and completely soluble again above 80°C. Edelman and Gally isolated L chains from their own (each other's!) γ-globulins and showed that they had precisely the same solubility characteristics as B-J proteins. This together with previous observations that B-J proteins and L chains are similar in terms of their peptide maps and antigenic cross-reactivity led to acceptance among most immunochemists of the identity of the two molecules, and B-J proteins provided the first source of pure, single peptide chain immunoglobulin protein for detailed structural study. Beginning in about 1967, scanning studies with a wide variety of haptens and antigens allowed determination of the binding specificities of a number of myeloma proteins of H_2L_2 structure, providing definitive evidence for normal antibody function of myeloma proteins.

Antigenic Relationships among L Chains, B-J Proteins, and Immunoglobulins

The identification of separate heavy and light chains as components of the basic structure of immunoglobulins, and the further identification of B-J proteins as L chain analogs, also led to the rapid resolution of a question concerning the antigenic relationships existing among the three known immunoglobulin classes. In 1956, Korngold and Lipari had reported that all B-J proteins isolated from humans were cross-reactive with antibodies made using any of the three known serum globulin classes as the immunizing antigen. Moreover, the B-J proteins fell into two antigenically distinct groups. Members of one group could absorb out a portion of antibodies to, say, IgM. Further absorption with members of the same group of B-J proteins led to no further reduction of anti-IgM antibodies. However, adsorption with members of the other group led to a further pronounced reduction of anti-IgM antibodies. This result suggested that antibody molecules were of two antigenic types: those that cross-react with B-J proteins of type A and another that cross-reacts with B-J proteins of type B. This initial observation was extended by Franklin and Stanworth, who showed in 1961 that antibodies to any one class of Ig cross-react with all other classes of Ig and with B-J proteins. Most importantly, they showed that the antigenic determinants on one class of Ig molecules, that cross-reacted with other Ig classes and with B-J proteins, are localized on the Fab subunit. In 1962, these observations were tied together by Mannik and Kunkel, who reported that all Igs could be classified in two groups based on their antigenic relationship to B-J proteins. For a short time, all Igs were designated as either type I or type II, depending on which antigenic variant of B-J protein they were related to (A or B).

Shortly after the identification of L chains as part of the Ig structure, it was established that there are also two antigenically distinct classes of normal L chains, and that these two classes are identical with the two antigenic groups of B-J proteins originally defined by Korngold and Lipari. In recognition of the importance of this early observation, the two L-chain groups were given the designation K and L, which was soon changed to κ and λ in keeping with the use of Greek letters to identify immunoglobulin chains. All immunoglobulin molecules were found to have either kappa or lambda L chains (but never both). Thus antibodies made against one class of immunoglobulin will always cross-react strongly with all other classes and with B-J proteins, accounting for all of the aforementioned observations. However, antibodies made against the isolated *heavy* chains of one class will cross-react only poorly or not at all with Igs of other classes, or their component H or L chains.

Structural Studies on Immunoglobulins

With the establishment in the early 1960s of myeloma proteins as valid analogs of serum Ig molecules, a number of questions about antibodies that were previously unapproachable could now be addressed. The major question to be resolved was the structural basis for antibody diversity. Electrophoretic examinations of the globulin fractions known to contain antibody activity had revealed considerable electrophoretic heterogeneity of molecules that were otherwise structurally quite similar (molecular weight, hydrodynamic properties, solubility properties, etc.) The γ-globulins were obviously composed of a very large number of related, yet distinct, molecules. Clonal selection theory predicted that this should be the case, because cells were presumed to exist that together produced a wide range of antibodies, each with a distinct antigenic specificity. Comparisons of the amino acid composition of different antibodies with very restricted specificities (recovered from immune precipitates with different antigens) had suggested that the different electrophoretic mobilities were related to variable amino acid compositions of antibodies with different antigenic specificities. Thus an understanding of the detailed structure of antibody (immunoglobulin) molecules became absolutely essential for correlation of structural variability with functional diversity, and ultimately for an understanding of the genetic basis for immunoglobulin structure and diversity.

One of the first approaches to this question, utilizing Bence-Jones proteins, was the comparison of peptide maps of B-J proteins from different sources with one another and with normal L chains. In peptide mapping, the protein to be analyzed is first digested to completion with an enzyme such as trypsin. This will, under ideal conditions, give a collection of smaller peptides that is experimentally reproducible because of the strict site-specificity of the enzyme. The resultant digest is applied to one corner of a square sheet of paper, and electrophoresed along one edge of the paper, separating the peptides on the basis of net charge. The paper is then turned at right angles and subjected to chromatography; the peptides now migrate according to their solubility in the solvent system used. After drying, the paper is sprayed with a peptide-specific reagent such as ninhydrin. The result is a two-dimensional map or "fingerprint" of the peptides generated in the original digestion step. These maps are highly specific for different peptides; differences of only a few amino acids in the overall structure of two closely related proteins will give markedly different peptide maps.

B-J proteins fell into two groups (Figure 3-6). Those belonging to the same group consistently had about one-half of their peptide spots in common, with no obvious relationship among the remaining or "variable" spots. However, proteins from one group had no spots in common with proteins from the other group. These observations were consistent with what was already known about L chains. L

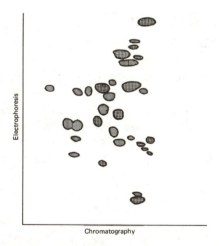

Figure 3-6 Schematic peptide map of a mixture of two type I (κ) Bence-Jones proteins. Two type I B-J proteins were mixed and digested with trypsin. The digest was then chromatographed and followed by electrophoresis at right angles, and the electropherogram was stained with ninhydrin. Spots derived from one of the proteins (as determined by a separate run of that protein alone) are marked by vertical lines; spots associated with the second protein are marked with horizontal lines. Spots common to both B-J proteins are thus marked with cross-hatched lines. [Based on information presented in F. W. Putnam and C. W. Easley, Structural studies of the immunoglobulins. I. The tryptic peptides of Bence-Jones proteins. *J. Biol. Chem.* **240**, 1626–1638 (1965)].

chains belong to either the kappa or lambda groups. All members of one group are antigenically related to one another, although electrophoretically heterogeneous. The kappa and lambda groups are, however, almost totally distinct antigenically.

The next steps involved the arrangement of the peptide fragments into the correct linear order and then the determination of the primary sequence of amino acids throughout the entire peptide chain. This work proceeded rapidly in a number of labs, and in 1965 Hilschmann and Craig published the first completed sequences of two different B-J proteins of the same antigenic type. A comparison of the sequences showed very clearly that all of the variability in amino acid composition occurs in the NH_2-terminal half of the molecule. The sequences in the COOH-terminal 110 or so amino acids were identical in the two proteins. The two halves of the L chain were therefore designated the V (variable) and C (constant) regions; the variable region was assumed to be involved in the antigen-binding function of the Ig molecule. This finding resolved one of the principal questions about the relationship of Ig structure and antibody variability and set the stage for a veritable explosion in accumulation of information about Ig structure–function relationships. Although it was another four years before a complete H-chain sequence was available, it rapidly became apparent that H chains too had a variable region–constant region structure. The first 120 or so amino acids of the H chain contain all of the variability associated with a given subclass of Ig, whereas the remainder of the molecule is essentially identical except for allotypic variations.

As sequence information gradually accumulated on both the H and L chains of myeloma Ig molecules, a great deal of information was learned about Ig secondary and tertiary structure, and about the evolutionary relationships of Ig molecules. The regular spacing of Cys residues along both light and heavy chains, first noticed by Hilschman and Craig and later confirmed by Hill et al. and by Singer and Doolittle, suggested the existence of domains (Figure 3-5) (see also p. 86) which was ultimately confirmed by electron micrograph and X-ray crystallography analysis (p. 132). Each precisely folded domain (or "homology unit") consists of about 110 amino acids and is defined in part by a centrally disposed disulfide loop, the component Cys residues of which are about 60 residues apart. The V domains are concerned with antigen binding. The C_L and C_{H1} domains serve to connect H and L chains and to stabilize V_H-V_L interactions. The remaining C domains are concerned with various biological functions such as complement binding and interactions with cell surface Fc receptors. The amino acid sequences of H-chain domains within a class show from 35 to 50 percent homology. This observation led to the proposal that Ig genes arose from replication of a primordial gene coding for about 100 amino acids. Comparisons of the C region sequences of homologous Ig molecules among various species also disclosed considerable evolutionary conservation of Ig structure, particularly around the Cys residues involved in domain folding. C region domain homology between human and mouse homologous isotypes, for example, is about 30 percent on the average, although it can be as high as 70 percent. As we will see when we study other molecules of the immune system, particularly MHC proteins and the T-cell receptor, there is some evidence to suggest that numerous molecules involved in immune responsiveness may have had a common evolutionary origin.

Detailed comparison of a large number of isotypically identical H and L chains showed that the C regions are not totally invariant. For example, the first κ chains to be sequenced showed a single amino acid difference at position 191. Some κ chains have leucine at this position; the rest have valine. This is true of all κ chains in humans, and represents expression of two different alleles for κ at the population level. The two different forms of κ are thus called allotypes (see also p. 82). Allelic forms for almost all Ig chains have been detected in one species or another. These allelic differences in primary structure usually can be detected as antigenic differences in the chains when they are used to immunize another animal. In fact, antisera capable of distinguishing Ig allotypes had been produced long before identification of allotypes at the level of amino acid sequence.

By the mid-1960s, the basic structure of immunoglobulins was resolved. Two more immunoglobulin classes remained to be defined: IgD, discovered in 1965 by Rowe and Fahey as a rare myeloma protein, and IgE, first described by the Ishizakas in 1967. Both of these immunoglobulins are present in normal serum in very low concentration, and details of their structure would not be worked out for another decade or so. But when their structures were finally derived, they added little to what was already apparent in 1965.

The tremendous burst of excitement and creativity that finally led to the resolution of immunoglobulin structure in the mid-1960s laid the groundwork for a subsequent intellectual challenge: the genetic basis for immunoglobulin structure and diversity. Immunologists could not take up that challenge for another 10 years when molecular biology provided an appropriate technology. We will see what happened in Chapter 5. In the meantime, we will follow developments in the interim period as immunochemists worked out the details of immunoglobulin structure and function at the protein level.

Bibliography

General

Edelman, G. M., Antibody structure and molecular immunology. *Science 180,* 830 (1973).

Natvig, J. B., and H. G. Kunkel, Human immunoglobulins: Classes, subclasses, genetic variants and idiotypes. *Adv. Immunol. 16,* 1 (1973).

Porter, R. R., Structural studies of immunoglobulins. *Science 180,* 713 (1973).

Potter, M., Antigen-binding myeloma proteins of mice. *Adv. Immunol. 25,* 141 (1977).

Putnam, F. W., N. Takahashi, D. Tetaert, Li-C. Lin, and B. Debuire, The last of the immunoglobulins: Complete amino acid sequence of human IgD. In *Immunoglobulin D: Structure and Function,* J. Thorbecke and G. Leslie, eds., *Annals New York Academy of Sciences 399,* 41 (1982).

Research

Heidelberger, M., and O. T. Avery, The soluble specific substance of pneumococcus. *J. Exp. Med. 38,* 73 (1923).

Heidelberger, M., and F. Kendall, A quantitative study of the precipitin reaction between type III pneumococcus polysaccharide and purified homologous antibody. *J. Exp. Med. 50,* 809 (1929).

Nisonoff, A., J. E. Hopper, and S. B. Spring, *The Antibody Molecule,* Academic Press, New York (1975).

Porter, R. R., The hydrolysis of rabbit γ-globulin and antibodies with crystalline papain. *Biochem. J. 73,* 119 (1959).

Putnam, F. W., and C. W. Easley, Structural studies of the immunoglobulins. I. The tryptic peptides of the Bence-Jones proteins. *J. Biol. Chem. 240,* 1626–1638 (1965).

Tiselius, A., and E. A. Kabat, An electrophoretic study of immune sera and purified antibody preparations. *J. Exp. Med. 69,* 119 (1939).

CHAPTER 4

The Properties and Fine Structure of Immunoglobulins

The presently accepted definition of the term *immunoglobulin* contains both a structural and a functional element. Structurally, all immunoglobulins can be related to the prototypical H_2L_2 formula, the derivation of which was described in the preceding chapter. Functionally, immunoglobulins demonstrate an ability to interact in a selective way with the particular antigen used to induce their production.

Despite years of searching, no group of protein molecules meeting either, much less both, of these criteria has been identified in invertebrates. On the other hand, all vertebrates that have been examined, with the possible exception of lampreys, have at least one class of molecules satisfying both of these criteria.

Humans possess a large structural and functional repertoire of immunoglobulins, which for a variety of reasons has been the most intensely studied and most completely characterized among the vertebrates. The properties of other vertebrate immunoglobulins, especially their structural features, are generally defined in relation to the human immunoglobulin classes. The principal features of the classes and subclasses of human immunoglobulin are condensed in Table 4-1; the discussions of the properties of these molecules given below refer only to human Igs.

Immunoglobulin Classes and Subclasses

Before commencing a description of the various classes of human immunoglobulin, let us take a moment to examine the experimental basis for the concept of immunoglobulin classes and subclasses. Immunoglobulins can, of course, themselves serve as immunogens and antigens. They can provoke the production of antibodies directed against structural determinants present in themselves but not present in the animal used to raise the antiserum. However, in a sample of immunoglobulin of a particular structural type taken from normal serum, the effective concentration of individual determinants within the V region will be rather low, being different for each specificity of antibody in the sample. Thus antibodies produced against immunoglobulins tend to be directed against determinants located principally (although not exclusively) in the constant regions of the light and heavy chains.

Classes of immunoglobulins are distinguished solely by structural differences in the heavy chains, because the same two forms of light chain occur in all of the immunoglobulin classes as we have seen. These structural differences are, of course, reflected in distinctive antigenic properties; antibodies made against isolated IgG heavy chains (γ chains), for example, cross-react very poorly with IgM heavy chains (μ chains), and vice versa. The differences in primary sturcture among the H chains of the five classes of human Ig are quite major, most likely reflecting various degrees of evolutionary divergence and modification of a prototypical Ig structure (see following).

Table 4-1 Properties of Human and Murine Immunoglobulins

Ig	H-chain designation	MW (daltons × 10⁻³)	Hinge region residues	Percentage carbohydrate	Number of H-chain domains[a]	Normal serum concentration (mg/ml)	Fixation of guinea pig complement
Human							
IgG1	γ_1	146	15	2–3	4	9	+
IgG2	γ_2	146	12	2–3	4	3	±
IgG3	γ_3	165	62	2–3	4	1	+
IgG4	γ_4	146		2–3	4	0.5	−
IgM	μ	970	0	9–12	5	1.5	+
IgA1	α_1	160	26	7–11	4	3	−
IgA2	α_2	160	13	7–11	4	0.5	−
IgD	δ	~185	64	9–11	4	0.03	−
IgE	ϵ	~190	0	12	5	0.0003	−
Mouse							
IgG1	γ_1	~150	13		4	1–4	−
IgG2a	γ_{2a}	160	16		4		+
IgG2b	γ_{2b}	160	22		4	1–5	+
IgG3	γ_3	~150	17		4	0.1–0.2	−
IgM	μ	~950	0		5		+
IgA1	α_1	~160	14		4		−
IgA2	α_2	~160					−
IgD	δ	~135	32		3	0.008	−
IgE	ϵ		0		5		−

[a]Including V_H domain.

As more and more myeloma proteins became available for study, and were assigned to the various major Ig classes, it was observed that there is also discrete antigenic diversity *within* some of the major H-chain classes. Although it was recognized that such differences probably reflect slight variations in amino acid sequence in the C region of the chains, it was at first thought that these differences might be related to the fact that the proteins are products of aberrant cells. However, it quickly became apparent that the same antigenic variations exist within immunoglobulin classes in the normal population. It is now recognized that these structural variants represent genetically distinct *subclasses* of immunoglobulins and are the products of genes arising fairly recently in evolution by duplication and divergence of prototypical class genes. All of the subclasses of a given Ig class share in common those structural H-chain determinants defining the Ig class, but each of the subclasses differs by minor changes in H-chain amino acid sequence from each of the other subclasses. All of the members of a species carry and express all of the genes for all of the classes and subclasses; the antigenic determinants defining these classes and subclasses are therefore shared by all members of the species, and are called *isotypes*.

IgG

IgG is the principal immunoglobulin of normal human serum. Relatively little IgG is produced during the early portion of a primary immune response, but it is the major form of antibody produced in the secondary reaction (i.e., on rechallenge with the original immunizing antigen). In the adult, because of its preponderance in serum (about 80 percent of total serum Ig), it provides one of the major defenses against bacterial infection. IgG is very important to the human neonate because it is the only immunoglobulin to cross the placenta, thus providing the newborn infant with a supply of ready-made antibodies for protection during the first several months of life. IgG is also found, together with IgM and IgA, in the colostrum (breast milk during the first several days postpartum), which may provide additional protection to the immunologically inexperienced infant. The basic structure of IgG is shown in Figure 4-1.

There are four subclasses of human IgG: IgG_1, IgG_2, IgG_3, and IgG_4. The four subclasses reflect the existence of four antigenically distinct heavy chains, called γ_1, γ_2, γ_3, and γ_4. These chains are similar but not identical in amino acid sequence and general physical properties. For example, they share between 17 and 22 of the 24 peptides generated by trypsin, and they all share identical carbohydrate moieties. One major structural difference is in the number and location of the disulfide bonds. The γ_3 chain, which is somewhat longer than γ_1, γ_2, and γ_4, has an unusually large number of inter-H-chain disulfide bonds. The γ_1 is disulfide bonded to L chains at position 220; the other γ chains form this bond at position 131.

Antisera specific for subclass chains are usually produced by immunization with a subclass-specific myeloma protein and adsorption of the resultant antiserum with myeloma proteins of the other IgG subclasses. IgG as a class is composed of about 65 percent IgG_1, 24 percent IgG_2, 8 percent of IgG_3, and 3 percent IgG_4.

IgG_3 is the most effective binder of complement (see Chapter 8), followed by IgG_1 and IgG_2. IgG_4 in most cases fails to bind complement. All of the subclasses except IgG_2 have been demonstrated to cross the placenta. IgG_1 and IgG_3 bind through their Fc regions to monocytes and may thus be involved in the phenomenon of antibody-dependent, cell-mediated cytotoxicity (Chapter 15). Most antibody responses involve all four subclasses, but some responses seem to be subclass restricted. Antidextran antibodies in humans, for example, tend to be almost exclusively IgG_2. Other properties of the IgG subclasses will be discussed at appropriate points throughout the text.

IgM

The structure of IgM is shown in Figure 4-2. It normally occurs in serum as a 19S pentamer of the basic unit μ_2L_2. Perhaps because of its large size, IgM is not found to any significant extent in tissue spaces; it is essentially confined to the blood circulation. The μ chain has one V_H and four C_H domains; the domains are roughly the same size as those of the γ chain (see section on "Immunoglobulin Fine Structure" later in this chapter for a discussion of domains). The molecular weight of the μ chain is thus about 72,000 daltons, making the monomeric unit molecular

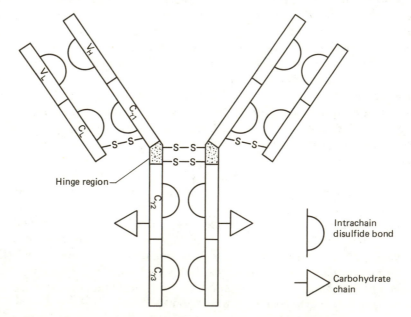

Figure 4-1 Prototypical structure for an IgG molecule. Various subclasses of IgG vary in the number of carbohydrate attachment sites and structure of the hinge region and have minor differences in amino acid sequence.

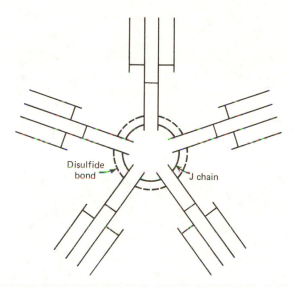

Figure 4-2 The pentameric structure of IgM. The pentameric structure is held together by interchain disulfide bonds linking the C-terminal portions of adjacent monomeric μ chains. The μ chain has a total of four C_H domains and is thus longer than the γ or α chain. The J chain (represented here by a solid line) is a hydrophilic peptide of 15,000 MW. Its precise arrangement in the pentameric structure is not known, but it interacts with disulfide bonds in a short amino acid stretch appended to the end of the C-terminal C_H domain.

weight somewhat over 190,000 daltons. In the pentamer, the five subunits are held together by disulfide bonds linking the C-terminal portions of adjoining μ chains. These intersubunit disulfide bonds are particularly sensitive to mild reduction by thiol reagents at neutral pH, presumably due to their accessibility and to the energetically more favorable state of the monomeric form. The cell agglutinating power of the liberated monomer is 100 to 1000-fold less than the pentamer. Thus, one of the early tests of IgM antibody was based on the reduction of agglutinating capacity on treatment with mild reducing agents.

Each pentamer has associated with it one J chain glycopeptide of approximately ca. 15,000 MW. The J chain (the gene for which is on chromosome 5 of the mouse) is involved in the initial polymerization step of $\mu_2 L_2$ monomers into pentameric IgM. Two μ chains (in different $\mu_2 L_2$ monomers) are joined via their penultimate (cysteine) residues, and the resultant dimer serves as a nucleating unit for assembly of the pentamer (Figure 4-3). These cysteines occur in the C-terminal portion of secreted μ chains, but not of membrane μ, which is probably the main reason that membrane μ is monomeric rather than pentameric. Once the first two μ chains are cross-linked by J chain, it is not clear how the other chains are assembled, or through which cysteine residues they are linked. In virgin B cells, active J-chain synthesis is induced upon antigen stimulation, and may be rate limiting in the production of secreted IgM.

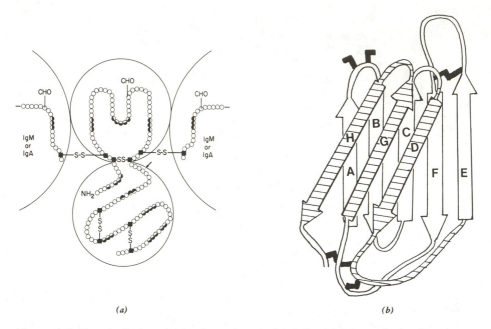

(a)   *(b)*

Figure 4-3 Hypothetical model for the structure of J chain. (a) Schematic drawing of a two-domain model in which half-closed circles (◐) represent hydrophobic amino acids. Closed boxes (■) indicate half-cysteine residues. The arrow indicates a peptide bond sensitive to subtilisin. (b) One domain model showing possible folding pattern of β-pleated sheets. (Photo courtesy Dr. Marian Koshland; reproduced with permission from the *Annual Review of Immunology,* Vol. 3, © 1985 by Annual Reviews Inc., and from the author.)

Koshland has recently worked out the structure for mouse J chain from the sequence of a cloned J gene. Human and mouse J chain share about 77 percent sequence homology. Interestingly, so do the regions of the μ chains to which J chains bind in mouse and humans. This is much higher than the general degree of relatedness of mouse and human Ig chains. (As we will see in the next chapter, the region of the μ chain to which J chains bind is coded for by a genetic element distinct from the μ_4 domains.)

Pentameric IgM has a nominal antigen binding valence of 10. For small antigens, there does seem to be a total of 10 molecules of antigen bound per pentameric IgM; for larger antigens, steric hindrance may be a significant factor in binding, and the number of molecules of antigen bound is often only 5. Steric hindrance seems to be an all-or-none phenomenon in that binding values between 5 and 10 are not usually observed.

IgM does not cross the placenta. It is phylogenetically the most primitive of the immunoglobulins, and variants of the gene for the μ chain appear to have evolved into H-chain genes for the other immunoglobulin classes. IgM is usually the predominant form of antibody found in the serum in the first week after an infection or planned immunization.

IgM is a potent binder of complement. The 7S monomeric IgM subunit binds complement about as well as IgG; however, in the pentameric form, the IgM subunit binds complement at least 15 times as well as IgG. This enhanced affinity of complement for IgM is related to the fact that the first component of complement (see Chapter 8) attaches to several Fc regions simultaneously. 19S IgM has multiple Fc regions in a locally concentrated form and stabilizes the complement molecule almost immediately on attachment. This high efficiency in binding and activating complement, coupled with its early appearance during the course of infection, makes IgM particularly effective in combating bacterial disease.

The monomeric form of IgM is occasionally found in low concentration in normal human serum. Its presence in high concentration is almost always symptomatic of a disease state, such as systemic lupus erythematosus, Waldenstrom's macroglobulinemia, rheumatoid arthritis, etc.

IgA

IgA constitutes about 15 percent of normal human serum immunoglobulins. In serum, it exists primarily as the monomer $\alpha_2 L_2$, but also as various polymers of this basic unit. Serum polymers, containing up to five monomeric $\alpha_2 L_2$ units, are associated with a J chain. Biologically, the most important form of IgA is probably the dimeric form shown in Figure 4-4, known as secretory IgA. This is the predominant (although not exclusive) immunoglobulin component of seromucous secretions such as breast milk, tears, saliva, perspiration, secretions of the lung and gut, etc. Its function is generally to protect the various exposed epithelial elements of the body from invasion by pathogenic microorganisms. IgA in human breast milk is contained in cells, and there has been some suggestion that infants may benefit by the attachment of these cells to the intestinal mucosa where they would release their IgA, providing local protection against potentially pathogenic microorganisms.

IgA is quite resistant to proteolytic digestion, which is an obvious advantage because many of the secretions in which it exists have at least low levels of proteolytic enzymes. It is produced by IgA-specific plasma cells originating in the Peyer's patches. These cells migrate out and are found in association with the epithelial cells producing the primary secretion.

As shown in Figure 4-4, the dimeric secretory form of IgA has associated with it a so-called "secretory component," and a J chain that is identical to the J chain found in IgM. The J chain is synthesized in the plasma cell producing the IgA. It attaches to an α chain at the C-terminal end. Its attachment may be a prerequisite for secretion of the IgA dimer, which is definitely polymerized in the plasma cell prior to secretion.

Secretory component (SC) is a single polypeptide chain of molecular weight about 70,000 that joins the two IgA monomers via disulfide bridges in the Fc regions. Its presumed function is to stabilize the dimeric form, and perhaps protect it from proteolysis. SC is synthesized by epithelial cells lining regions of the body which are in direct or indirect communication with the external environment (lungs, intestine, lacrimal glands, etc.) It is present on the nonlumenal surface of

Secretory component

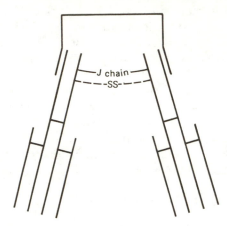

Figure 4-4 The dimeric secretory form of IgA. The two monomers are known to be linked by disulfide bonds in the $C_{\alpha 3}$ domain. The J chain (dashed line) is presumably attached to the C-terminal end of the molecule, similar to IgM (Figures 4-3 and 4-8). However, the precise molecular architecture of these associations has yet to be worked out. Secretory component is a single peptide chain of 70,000 MW and is unrelated in structure to any of the immunoglobulin peptides. The precise nature of its association with IgA is not yet known; the arrangements of both J chain and secretory component shown here are thus only speculative.

these cells as a receptor specific for the Fc regions of dimeric IgA. IgA-producing plasma cells located in or near the epithelial cells secrete dimeric IgA, which then attaches to an epithelial cell surface through interaction of its J chain with the SC receptor. The receptor and (IgA)$_2$ are endocytosed in the form of a membrane vesicle, which migrates to the lumenal side of the cell, where it fuses with the plasma membrane. The extramembranal portion of the SC is then enzymatically cleaved and released as part of the dimeric IgA molecule (Figure 4-5). In addition to epithelial cells of the gut, SC has also been identified as a functional Fc receptor on hepatocytes, where it aids in the transport of IgA from blood to the bile.

There are two subclasses of IgA in humans: IgA$_1$ and IgA$_2$. IgA$_2$ accounts for only about 10 percent of total IgA. Neither subclass binds complement. Both are resistant to proteolysis, especially when complexed with J chain and SC.

IgE

IgE, while very important biologically, is found in extremely low concentration in human serum (30 to 100 ng/ml). It has a half-life in serum of two days. Its discovery was a result of attempts to isolate and identify reaginic antibody, the principal mediator of immediate hypersensitivity (allergic) reactions (see Chapter 17). Reaginic antibody was observed to be neutralized by antisera made against whole

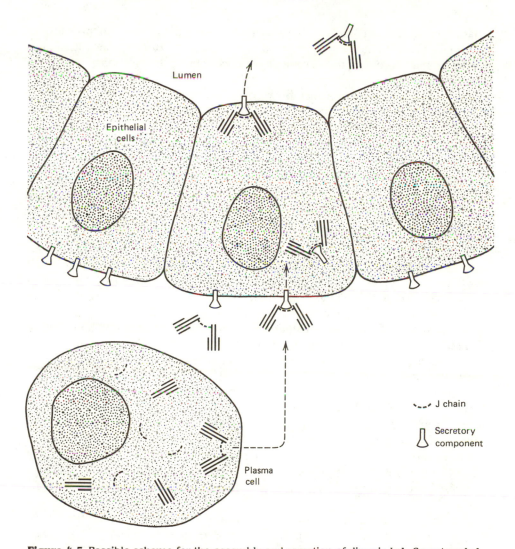

Figure 4-5 Possible scheme for the assembly and secretion of dimeric IgA. Secretory IgA per se is not secreted into external compartments by IgA-producing plasma cells. The IgA monomers and J chain are synthesized and assembled into dimers by plasma cells that lie near the epithelial cells lining secretory structures. Secretory component (SC) is synthesized by and is present on the surface of the epithelial cells. Dimeric IgA attaches to cell surface SC by one or both of its Fc regions, enters the cell, and is secreted (together with firmly attached SC) into the external compartment.

human immunoglobulin but not by antisera against any of the individually purified known immunoglobulins, leading to the suspicion that it might constitute a separate Ig class. Identity of IgE with reaginic antibody was established by the Ishizakas in 1966. The designation E derived from the fact that the allergen most used in the characterization of reaginic antibody was the E antigen of ragweed. IgE may also be important in the humoral immune response to parasitic disease, since it is often found in high levels in the serum of patients with such infections, principally helminthic.

IgE is heat labile and considerably more sensitive to disulfide reducing agents than the monomeric forms of other immunoglobulins. The structure of IgE was worked out only after diagnosis of a patient with an IgE-producing multiple myeloma. The ϵ chain contains one V_H and four C_H domains; the molecular weight of the basic E_2L_2 unit is about 190,000, similar to the monomeric form of IgM. Like μ chains, ϵ chains lack a hinge region. IgE does not cross the placenta, and IgE-antigen complexes do not bind complement.

IgD

The existence of this class of immunoglobulin as a component of normal serum was not suspected until it was discovered in 1964 as a human myeloma protein that could not be typed as IgM, IgG, or IgA (IgE had not yet been defined). Progress in characterization of the IgD molecule has been slow, and only in the past few years has a combination of gene and protein sequencing studies led to a clear picture of IgD structure. Problems that precluded a more rapid resolution of IgD structure included its extremely low concentration in serum, its unusually high sensitivity to protelytic degradation, and the rarity of either spontaneous or induced IgD myelomas.

The protein structure of human secreted IgD was recently worked out by Frank Putnam and his co-workers and is shown in Figure 4-6. Like γ chains, δ chains have three C-region domains. For a time, it was thought that secreted human IgD had four C-region domains, like IgM. However, the slightly larger size of the δ chain (65,000 daltons) turned out to be due to a larger than normal carbohydrate content (about 12 percent) and a relatively long hinge region (64 amino acids). The hinge region is particularly sensitive to proteases, and contains but a single cysteine residue.

The structure of murine IgD was unknown until 1980, when identification of two IgD-expressing plasmacytomas allowed isolation of δ chain mRNA. This was then used to produce cDNA, which was used to isolate the genomic sequences coding for murine δ chain. These were then sequenced, and the surprising structure shown in Figure 4-6 was inferred for murine IgD.

Mice (at least the Balb/c strain, in which these studies were carried out) have lost the coding sequence for the second domain of the δ chain. This is true for both membrane and secreted forms of IgD. That the lost domain is $\delta 2$ was inferred by sequence homology comparisons with human δ chains and by comparison of general properties of C_{H1} domains of other immunoglobulins.

Like human IgD, mouse δ chains have an unusually long hinge region (35 amino acids). The inferred residues would be highly charged and sensitive to proteolysis. There are no cysteine groups, and thus apparently no H-H chain disulfide bonds. It

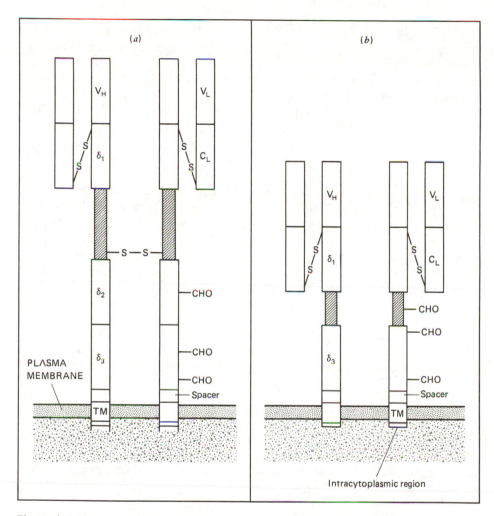

Figure 4-6 Membrane forms of a human and b, mouse IgD. The human structure was determined by amino acid sequencing. The murine structure is inferred from gene sequencing studies. It is possible that murine IgD exists in the membrane only as half-molecules.

is thus possible that murine IgD may exist as half molecules. There is one potential glycosylation site in the hinge region.

IgD does not bind complement, cross the placenta, or bind to cells via its Fc region. It is, however, found on the surface of a high proportion of B lymphocytes, especially in newborns. A discussion of the developmental significance of IgD on cell surfaces, and its possible role in regulating cell activation, is presented in Chapters 13 and 14.

Light Chains

There are two types of light chains in both humans and mice: kappa and lambda. The two types were first distinguished by an immunological comparison of various Bence-Jones proteins: all Bence-Jones proteins fell into two antigenically distinct groups. Subsequent analysis of normal Ig L chains confirmed the existence of the same two antigenic groups. About 60 percent of L chains in humans are of the κ variety, and 40 percent are λ. These two basic types of L chain can also be identified in other vertebrates, although the ratio of κ to λ may vary considerably. (In the mouse, for example, the ratio is about 95 percent κ to 5 percent λ.) In humans, there is about 40 percent sequence homology between the C regions of κ and λ, suggesting a common evolutionary origin. On the other hand, the sequence homology between mouse and human κ C regions is nearly 60 percent, indicating that κ and λ have evolved independently of one another since the initial duplication event. Kappa chains have become more diversified in structure during evolution, compared with the relatively highly conserved lambda sequences. κ and λ occur in association with all Ig classes, although not always in the same proportion. Both L chains of a particular Ig are always either κ or λ.

Monoclonal Antibodies

In Chapter 3, attention was focused on the rapid progress made in understanding immunoglobulin structure once myleoma proteins were recognized as valid immunoglobulin molecules. In the following years, strictly on a trial-and-error basis, antigens that would bind to a number of these proteins with varying affinities were also identified. Thus myeloma proteins could in some cases also be used to study in detail the interaction of antigens with antibody combining sites. The advantage of myeloma proteins for both structural and functional studies of immunoglobulins is the fact that they are monoclonal; that is, all of the myeloma cells in an afflicted individual are descendants of the same clonal precursor and produce identical immunoglobulin products.

Although myeloma proteins provide an excellent source of pure material for studying generalized properties of immunoglobulins, they have, with only a few exceptions, not become a source of antibodies for use as general serological reagents. The immunoglobulin product of a myeloma can be neither predicted nor altered, and individual antigen-binding properties can only be discovered by a costly and time-consuming screening process.

A method for generating continuously growing lines of lymphoid cells that can make and secrete antibody molecules of a *predetermined* specificity became apparent from experiments carried out by Köhler and Milstein in 1975. Using standard techniques developed by somatic cell geneticists, these investigators fused together spleen cells from a mouse immunized with sheep red blood cells, and an Ig-secreting mouse myeloma line. They obtained a double-secreting *hybridoma* line that produced large amounts of monoclonal anti-SRBC antibody (in addition to the Ig produced originally by the myeloma partner) while retaining the perpetual growth characteristics of the myeloma. The selection, propagation and further subcloning of such hybridoma lines, with only minor refinements of Köhler and Milstein's technique, has provided a means of major importance for the production of highly specific monoclonal antibodies (mAbs). These mAbs are now the reagent of choice for the serological detection, identification, and isolation of a wide range of antigens.

A scheme for production of murine mAbs is shown in Figure 4-7. Spleen cells from an immune mouse (taken after four to six days of secondary immunization *in vitro,* to enrich for the desired B cells) are fused with a murine myeloma using an appropriate agent such as polyethylene glycol (PEG). Early experiments had used inactivated Sendai virus, which causes extensive cross-linking and fusion of partner cells. PEG accomplishes the same goal by chemical means. A variety of nonsecreting myeloma cell lines are available for use as the tumor partner; the resultant hybrids with appropriate spleen cells will then secrete antibody only of the spleen cell type. In the initial fusion step, of course, many different types of hybrids will be formed: spleen–spleen, myeloma–myeloma, and a large number of irrelevant spleen–myeloma combinations. Interestingly, the number of hybrids formed between relevant (immune) mouse spleen cells and mouse myeloma cells is much higher than might be expected on the basis of their frequency in the total spleen cell population. Apparently, antibody-producing B cells are particularly susceptible to fusion, perhaps because of their blast cell nature.

Once the hybrids have been formed, the next problem is to distinguish appropriate hybrid cells from nonfused partner cells or irrelevant hybrid cells. The means for doing this were developed some years ago by somatic cell geneticists. The myeloma partner used is selected for absence of the purine metabolizing enzyme hypoxanthine guanine phosphoribosyl transferase (HGPRT). After the fusion step, the entire cell mixture is transferred to a selection medium containing hypoxanthine, aminopterin, and thymidine (HAT) and plated into microwell cultures containing relatively few cells per culture well. The aminopterin blocks the normal nucleotide synthetic pathways, forcing cells into the salvage pathway utilizing hypoxanthine and thymidine. This pathway requires the enzyme HGPRT. Unfused myeloma cells and myeloma–myeloma hybrids thus cannot grow in this medium, but myeloma cells that have hybridized with a spleen cell will survive by utilizing the spleen cell's HGPRT. Unfused murine spleen cells will eventually die out on their own, because unstimulated mouse lymphocytes do not survive more than a few days in culture.

After a week or so of exposure to the HAT medium, viable microwell cultures are identified by microscopic examination. The majority of wells will contain only dead cells. Wells containing viable, proliferating cells are then checked for antibody production. Proliferating cells from individual antibody-positive wells are replated into new wells at a density low enough to ensure that cells derived from the new wells are progeny of single cells (clones). The next step is to determine the

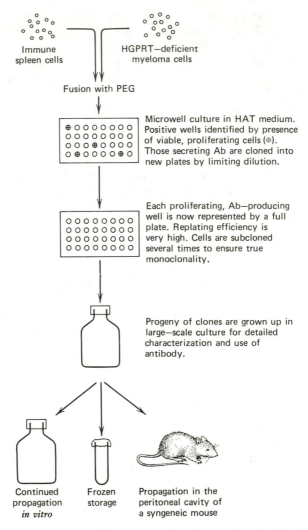

Figure 4-7 Production, selection, and propagation of monoclonal antibodies. (See text for details.)

fine specificity of the various mAbs. As was already known from the study of antibodies present in the serum of immune animals, even relatively simple antigens may induce the appearance of many different types of antibody. These may be of different isotypes, or may react to different epitopes, or may react to the same epitopes with varying degrees of affinity. A similar spectrum of antibody types is represented at the level of Ig-producing cells and in the spectrum of hybridomas rising from the fusion step. These may be identified and selected depending on the needs of the investigator.

Cultures of interest are usually subcloned at least twice to ensure monoclonality. The immunoglobulin produced can be examined by techniques such as isoelectric focusing to ensure that only a single type of immunoglobulin is being produced. Once monoclonality is certain, the cultures can be scaled up to generate large quantities of Ab-producing cells *in vitro,* or cells can be passaged into the peritoneal cavities of animals syngeneic with the cells used for fusion. The mAb can then be harvested from the ascites fluid, usually in concentrations much higher than can be achieved in culture. Hybridoma cells can also be stored frozen, recovered at some future point, and cultured productively either *in vivo* or *in vitro.*

The advantages of large-scale production of monoclonal antibodies of defined specificity are obvious. Less obvious perhaps are some of the disadvantages. Monoclonal antibodies do not precipitate most antigens, because most antigens display the target epitope only once and thus cannot be cross-linked into a precipitin lattice (see p. 146). For similar reasons, mAb will not cap most surface antigens (see p. 156), and, if of the IgG class, may not mediate complement lysis of target cells (p. 168) if target epitopes are spaced too far apart on the target cell surface. Proper identification and characterization of individual mAb is not always trivial, and not all cell hybrids are stable (due to chromosome loss). Most of these problems can be overcome by reasonably simple remedies or precautions. There is no question that the advantages of mAb far outweigh the disadvantages, and the place of mAb in basic and applied research in the future is assured.

Membrane versus Secreted Forms of Immunoglobulin

All of the Ig H-chain isotypes can be synthesized in two forms: membrane bound and secreted. The membrane-bound forms have a stretch of hydrophobic amino acids at the COOH-terminal end of the final C_H domain. One of the first descriptions of this phenomenon involved μ chains in the mouse. In addition to its functions as a circulating antibody, IgM (in the monomeric form) is also found on the surface of virgin B lymphocytes where it functions as an antigen-specific receptor. (As we will see later, IgD may play a similar or related role.) During the 1970s, it was observed by a number of workers that there seemed to be two different IgM molecules associated with B cells. The isolated μ chains from one form of IgM were slghtly larger than the other, and slightly more hydrophobic overall. The two μ chains gave peptide maps that were indistinguishable, except for one or two highly hydrophobic spots associated with the larger μ chain that were estimated to be of a size sufficient to account for the difference in molecular weight.

We now know that these two forms of μ chains are the basis for the difference between the secreted and membrane-bound forms of IgM. Distinct secreted and membrane forms have been identified at either the peptide or the gene level for all of the other H-chain isotypes as well. The structure of the membrane form of the μ

	Secreted form			Membrane form
1	V_H		1	V_H
	μ_1			μ_1
	μ_2			μ_2
	μ_3			μ_3
610	μ_4		610	μ_4
611	P		611	E (−)
	T			V
	L			N
	Y			A
	N			E (−)
	V			E (−)
	S			E (−)
	L			G
	I			F
	M		620	E (−)
	S			N
	D (−)			L
	T			W
	G			T
	G			T
	T			A
J chain —	C			S
628	Y			T
				F
				I
				V
				L
				F
				L
				L
				S
				L
				F
				Y
				S
				T
				T
				V
				T
				L
			646	F
				K (+)
				V
			649	K (+)

Figure 4-8 The C-terminal regions of secreted versus membrane-bound forms of immunoglobulins. The amino acid sequences shown here for the secreted versus membrane forms of murine μ chains (both are from the IgM myeloma MOPC 104E) are typical for essentially all immunoglobulin H chain classes. Both μ chains are identical through position 610, the C terminus of the μ_4 domain. The secreted form of the μ chain has an additional 18 amino acids, the 17th of which (position 627) is the point of attachment for the J chain. The membrane-bound form of MOPC 104E μ chain has an additional 49 amino acids, the majority of which (positions 621 to 646) are hydrophobic, or at least uncharged, amino acids. The stretch of charged amino acids at the beginning (611 to 620) may serve as a "spacer" region, allowing the μ chain a certain degree of rotational freedom on the B cell surface. The charged amino acids at the extreme C-terminal end (647 to 649) may be involved in submembranous interactions.

chain is shown in Figure 4-8. At the end of the μ4 domain is a stretch of a half dozen or so acidic amino acids, which have been postulated to serve as a sort of hinge region, giving the outer portion of the membrane Ig more rotational flexibility. This region is relatively protease sensitive. Immediately following the hinge region is a stretch of 26 relatively hydrophobic amino acids, just sufficient to span a lipid bilayer. Finally, there are several positively charged amino acids at the extreme C terminus of the chain, which may interact with submembranous cytoskeletal elements. These regions bear no homology whatsoever to any of the other Ig domains. The genetic basis for membrane versus secreted forms of Ig heavy chains is presented in Chapter 5.

Biosynthesis and Assembly of Immunoglobulins

Once the structure of immunoglobulin molecules had been determined, the biosynthetic pathways for the component chains was investigated. Biochemists working on this problem, like those who had resolved the structure of immunoglobulins, took advantage of the availability of myeloma cells as a source of homogeneous Ig molecules readily available in large quantities. Up to 30 percent of the protein synthesized by myeloma cells is immunoglobulin.

Myeloma cells were found to have two prominent size classes of membrane-bound polysomes, one of 7 to 8 ribosomes, and one of 16 to 20 ribosomes. These are of the size predicted to translate mRNAs coding for peptides of roughly 25,000 and 55,000 daltons, respectively. It was rapidly established that heavy and light chains are indeed synthesized from separate mRNAs on separate polysomes. N-linked carbohydrates are added cotranslationally, and as far as can be determined both H and L chains fold into their final conformations as they come off the ribosomes.

At the time these studies were carried out, immunologists were rapidly becoming convinced that the V and C regions of Ig chains are encoded separately in the DNA. Such a scheme requires that the V and C portions of the molecule be brought together at some point, either in the DNA prior to transcription, in the RNA prior to translation, or at the peptide level, posttranslationally.

A simple but elegant experiment first reported in 1967 provided strong evidence that both H and L chains are translated from mRNAs that include both V and C region coding information (Figure 4-9). Proteins are always synthesized in the same direction, NH_2 terminal to COOH terminal. If radioactive amino acids are supplied to a peptide synthesizing system for a brief period of time, less than that required for synthesis of a complete peptide molecule (a pulse label), the radioactivity will be present in the highest amount at the NH_2-terminal end of the molecule, because the NH_2-terminal end is the starting point for amino acid incorporation. The researchers reasoned that if a single Ig chain were translated from two

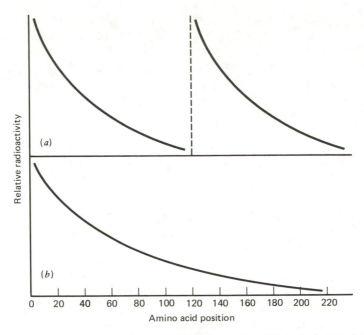

Figure 4-9 Theoretical predictions for two different models of light-chain translation. (a) L chain is translated from two separate mRNAs, one for the V region and one for the C region, and the two peptides are joined posttranslationally. In this case, synthesis starts at two points, position 1 (the NH_2 terminus of the V region) and position 111 (the NH_2 terminus of the C region). Therefore, radioactive amino acids in a brief pulse will be in highest concentration at these two points in the completed L chain. (b) L chain is translated from a single mRNA encoding both V and L regions. In this case, synthesis starts at a single point, position 1, and proceeds without interruption to the COOH terminus. Radioactivity should be highest at the NH_2 terminus, and decrease smoothly toward the COOH terminus. In practice, the results in *b* are observed for both H and L chains.

separate mRNA molecules, and the products of each translation were stitched together posttranslationally, then radioactivity would be present in high levels at two points in the pool of completed peptide chain, reflecting the existence of two starting points. When the experiment was carried out, radioactivity was found to be incorporated into immunoglobulin chains continuously from the NH_2- to the COOH-terminal end. This convinced everyone that both heavy and light Ig chains are translated from single mRNAs containing both V and C region coding information.

The question of coordination of the synthesis of H and L chains intrigued a number of investigators. Because L chains are often found to be synthesized in slight excess by myeloma cells and plasma cells, it was thought that L chains might function to facilitate release of completed H chains from polysomes. However, both H and L chains insert directly into the endoplasmic reticulum, via their hydro-

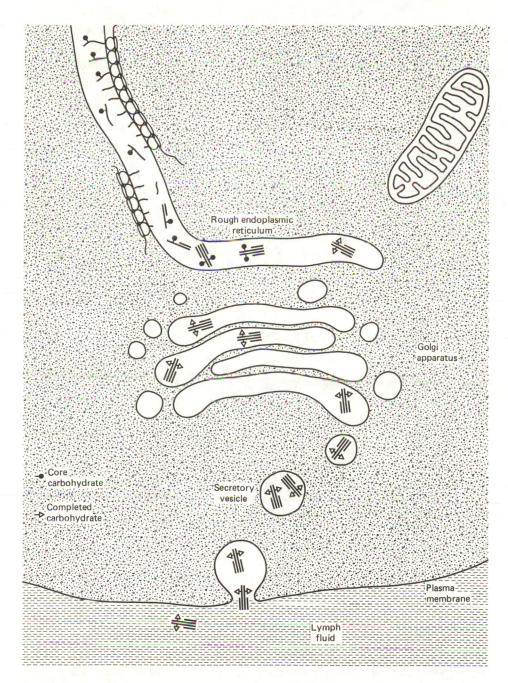

Figure 4-10 Synthesis, assembly, and secretion of immunoglobulin molecules. (See text for details.)

phobic NH_2-terminal leader sequences, and it seems unlikely that they would have much opportunity to interact in the cytoplasm (Figure 4-10). (The leader sequence is cleaved as the completed H or L chain is released from the ribosome.)

After secretion into the cisternal space, the H and L chains assemble into the prototypical H_2L_2 tetramers. Assembly can proceed through H–H dimers or through H–L half molecules. However, only one of these pathways is utilized for a given H-chain isotype. Moreover, in cells that are synthesizing more than one H chain isotype (e.g., $\mu + \delta$) assembly only occurs between homologous H chains. This rule extends also to membrane versus secreted forms of H chain. The initial (core) sugar residues for the carbohydrate structures are transferred from a lipid carrier to the nascent H chains shortly after entry into the ER, and additional buildup of the carbohydrate groups continues during transit to the Golgi apparatus (Figure 4-10). At the Golgi, the completed Ig molecules are packaged into exocytic vesicles for secretion, or into coated pit vesicles for display on the cell surface. The entire process, from synthesis to secretion, requires about 30 minutes. A fully mature plasma cell or myeloma cell will produce about 10^5 immunoglobulin molecules per minute.

Allotypes and Idiotypes

As noted previously, the antigenic determinants defining classes and subclasses of immunoglobulins, which are generated by the primary peptide structure of the heavy chains, are shared by all members of a species and are therefore called *isotypes*. There is at least one separate and distinct gene carried in the germ-line DNA for each immunoglobulin isotype. Some of the genes coding for both the heavy and the light chains, however, occur in allelic form within a species as a whole. These different alleles result in the existence of yet another level of heterogeneity of immunoglobulins, although by definition they do not increase the total number of immunoglobulin genes in the germ-line DNA. The unique antigenic determinants that are the expression at the peptide level of these allelic forms of the same gene are called *allotypes*. They are usually the result of one or two amino acid alterations in a heavy or light chain.

In humans, there are allelic variants of the genes for the γ_{1-4}, μ, α_2, and κ chains. The amino acid changes defining these allotypes in humans are present in the constant region of the H or L chain. Allotype inheritance follows a simple Mendelian pattern and is autosomal. The alleles in a heterozygous individual are codominant, although at the level of single cells only one or the other allele is expressed (allelic exclusion).

The existence of allotypes in humans can be demonstrated in several ways. Serum from patients with rheumatoid arthritis contains antibodies (rheumatoid factor, RF; see Chapter 18) reactive with the IgG of some but not all individuals in the normal population; the target for these alloantibodies turns out to be the Gm allotypes of the IgG class (Table 4-2). Children often have substantial levels of IgG alloan-

Table 4-2 Localization of Gm Factors in Human H Chains

Subclass	C_H1	C_H2	C_H3
		Domain	
IgG1	Gm(4) (Arg 214)		Gm(1) — Arg Asp Glu Leu
			355 — — 358
	Gm(17) (Lys 214)		Gm(-1) — Arg Glu Glu Met[a]
			Gm(2)
IgG2		Gm(23)	
		Gm(-23)	
IgG3		Gm(5)	Gm(6)
		Gm(-5)	Gm(13)
		Gm(15)	Gm(11) (Phe 436)
		Gm(16)	Gm(-11) (Tyr 436)
		Gm(21) (Tyr 292)	Gm(14)
		Gm(-21) (Phe 296)	Gm(b5)[b]
			Gm(c3)[b]
IgG4		Gm(4a) Val Leu His	
		309	
		Gm(4b)[c] Val gap His	

Taken from A. Nisonoff, J. E. Hopper, and S. B. Spring, Localization of Gm factors in H chains, *The Antibody Molecule*, Academic Press, New York (1975), p. 374. Copyright © 1975 by Academic Press, Inc. Reprinted by permission.

[a] In IgG4 the corresponding sequence is Glu Glu Met. In IgG2 and IgG3 the Gm(-1) tetrapeptide is the same as that shown for IgG1; this accounts for the fact that anti(-1) reacts with IgG2 and IgG3 but not IgG4.

[b] Letters are used where WHO numbers have not yet been assigned. However, there is evidence that Gm(c3) is the same as Gm(6).

[c] Gm(4b) lacks the Leu present at position 309 in Gm(4a).

tibodies when the mother has IgG allotypes not expressed in the fetus; maternal IgGs crossing the placenta provide the immunogenic stimulus for production of these antibodies. Alloantibodies may also be found in persons who have received blood transfusions that result in their exposure to allotypic Igs, especially IgA.

Allotypes have also been identified and characterized in the rabbit and in the mouse. The study of allotypy in the rabbit has led to the establishment of some important notions about Ig structure. Allotypy in the rabbit has been identified with both κ and λ light chains, with the C regions of γ, μ, α, and ε chains, and with V_H regions. V-region allotypes are determined by the relatively invariant framework sequences in the V domain (Figure 4-12). A number of laboratories have confirmed the striking observation that the same V_H allotype can be associated with several different classes of heavy chain (the Todd phenomenon). This led to the first serious consideration of the possibility that a single immunoglobulin chain is coded for by two genes—one for the V region, and one for the C region. This idea has since been shown to be true (Chapter 5). Another important concept derived from an analysis of rabbit allotypy is that a given immunoglobulin molecule is composed of identical H chain and idential L chains, a notion subsequently confirmed by amino acid sequence analyses.

Idiotypes are antigenic determinants present on an Ig molecule that are associated with its antigen-binding specificity. These determinants are thus generated as a result of particular amino acid sequences in the hypervariable portion of the V region. Idiotypes may represent the hypervariable sequences themselves or distortions induced elsewhere in the V region as a result of these hypervariable sequences alone or in combination with antigen.

It was observed in the 1950s that antibodies prepared against myeloma proteins could be used to define antigenic specificities unique to the molecule used for immunization. For example, if antibodies to a $(\gamma_1)_2\lambda_2$ myeloma protein from one patient are extensively absorbed with a $(\gamma_1)_2\lambda_2$ myeloma protein from a second patient, it is not possible to absorb out completely all antibodies reacting to the first myeloma protein. It could be argued that the leftover antibodies are directed against allotypic determinants expressed on the first myeloma, not shared by the second myeloma. This is usually true for a small proportion of the leftover antibodies, but it can be shown that the majority do not react with any other immunoglobulin molecule of the same or any other individual. These antibodies thus define antigenic specificities uniquely associated with the immunizing immunoglobulin molecule, and no other. Such specificities are referred to as idiotypic, and the antibodies as antiidiotypic.

It was assumed early on that such determinants are associated with the unique antigen-binding specificity of the immunizing molecule. This assumption was strengthened by the observation that idiotypic determinants could be localized to Fab fragments and even to Fv fragments (see p. 88). Antiidiotypic antibodies have been tested against individual H and L chains derived from the intact immunizing immunoglobulin and shown to react specifically with the V regions. However, idiotypic determinants need not always involve V region amino acids that are in contact with antigen and, in fact, may not always lie within the antigen-combining site. They are simply associated with a particular V_H-V_L combination.

In most cases, idiotypic determinants seem to be associated with H-chain V regions, although L-chain idiotypic determinants are also definitely detectable. In general, isolated H and L chains react less strongly with antiidiotypic antibody than does the intact H_2L_2 displaying the native idiotype. In fact, some idiotypic determinants are lost when the H and L chains are separated and reappear only when the chains are reassociated. Moreover, recombination of an H or L chain taken from an idiotype-bearing Ig molecule, with an L or H chain from a different (heterologous) Ig molecule, may not lead to restoration of the idiotype. These results could be interpreted two ways. Some idiotypes may involve determinants contributed by both H and L chains. Alternatively, an idiotype associated with only one chain may not be expressed in the isolated chain, or when the chain is recombined with a heterologous partner chain, because of incorrect three-dimensional folding.

The detection of idiotypes on normal serum antibodies by immunological techniques is not a simple task. As stated earlier, when serum Igs are used as immunogens, the resultant antibodies are usually directed toward determinants associated with constant regions of H or L chains, because the effective concentration of determinants in the truly variable portion of the V region is quite low. In a few rare cases, however, the serum antibodies produced to a given antigen may be from a relatively restricted number of clones of antibody-producing cells. This means that the number of different V regions represented in the antibody specific for the eliciting antigen is also restricted, and the representation of particular V region determinants is accordingly higher. Such antibodies can be elicited in most rabbits and in some strains of mice by appropriate immunization regimens with pneumococcal or streptococcal polysaccharides and can be used to induce detectable levels of antiidiotype antibody. Occasionally humans will also respond to certain synthetic polysaccharides by producing a restricted number of antibody specificities.

The same idiotype can be associated with more than one class of antibody, as was shown to be the case with V-region allotypes, again presumably reflecting the fact that the V and C regions of immunoglobulin molecules are controlled by separate genes. For example, all of the molecules produced by the progeny of a single clone of cells will have the same idiotype, even though a switchover from IgM to IgG production may occur at some point in the life span of the clone. Idiotypes can also be detected on the surface of lymphocytes involved in the production of antibodies bearing the particular idiotype.

On occasion, the same immunogen administered to different animals will elicit antibodies with cross-reacting idiotypes. If the animals are members of the same inbred strain, such cross-reactivity may well represent expression of identical, probably inherited (germ-line), genes. However, in some cases cross-reacting idiotypes elicited by the same immunogen can be raised in two different strains of animals, and more rarely in animals of two different species. Especially in the latter case, cross-reactivity may be fortuitous, reflecting the existence of similar but not identical V regions that have been elicited in response to the same antigen.

Immunoglobulin Fine Structure

The Concept of Domains

As the primary structure of H and L chains began to be worked out through amino acid sequencing of myeloma proteins, certain features suggesting linear repeats of homologous polypeptide units became apparent. The first of these features to be discerned was the regular spacing of half-cystine residues along the H and L chains. In the native globular state, these residues, about 60 amino acids apart, are known to interact to form intrachain disulfide bonds, with resulting "loops" in the Ig chains (Figure 3-5). In human κ or λ chains, for example, there is a total of four half-cystine residues involved in intrachain disulfide bonding, resulting in one loop each in the variable and constant region. In H chains, there is one such loop in the V_H region, and a total of three or four (depending on the Ig class) loops regularly spaced in the C_H portion of the chain. The V_L and C_L domains line up with the V_H and first C_H domains, and the remaining C_H domains of the two H chains also line up with one another.

   This periodicity of intrachain disulfide bonds led to a closer examination of the amino acid sequences in the C region of H chains; such studies, together with subsequent X-ray crystallographic data (Chapter 6), have confirmed the notion that Ig peptides are composed of consecutive, related sequences of about 110 amino acids ("homology units"). The V_H and V_L regions are, of course, heterogeneous in structure, but their size of about 110 amino acids suggests they they too bear some relation to the basic repeat unit. It is generally thought that the present Ig-chain structure arose by duplication of a primordial structural gene responsible for an approximately 110-amino acid peptide. At some early point, the gene replicate coding for the primitive V region is thought to have split off and come under separate genetic regulation, the various C regions then evolving by a process of gene replication and segregation. In the case of L chains, one V_L and one C_L unit, or "domain," became joined together to form the functional peptide structure. For H chains, the primoridal C_H gene is thought to have undergone additional replication to form a more complex gene coding for three or four domains, which are joined at some point with one V_H domain to complete the heavy chain unit peptide (Figure 4-11). We will see in Chapter 5 that at the molecular level, the DNA sequences coding for C_H region domains are in fact physically separate from one another (although grouped closely together), supporting the idea of coevolution from a domain-sized primitive gene.

   The regions within the disulfide loop of each domain are rather compact,

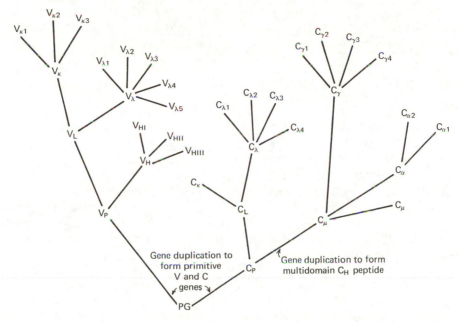

Figure 4-11 Evolution of genes coding for human immunoglobulins. At some point in the distant past, presumably about the time of appearance of the first vertebrates ($4-5 \times 10^8$ years ago) a "precursor gene" (PG) duplicated, and the duplicates diverged to form primitive V and C genes. At this early point of evolution, it is conceivable that a simple VC unit, or a pair of VC units, acted as a primitive sort of antibody molecule. This fairly simple process of gene replication followed by divergent evolution of the new gene copies can easily account for all of the V-region genes, and the various C_L genes. However, at some early point, an important genetic event took place: the "stitching together" of several C_H genes to form coordinately expressed multidomained C_H peptides. The most primitive vertebrates still in existence have multidomained μ-chain-like peptides strikingly similar in overall primary structure to the most recent mammals, suggesting that the "stitching" event must have occurred very early in vertebrate evolution.

globular structures; peptide linkages within each loop are relatively resistant to proteolytic digestion. The intradomain disulfide bonds are much less amenable to reduction by disulfide reagents than are the interchain S–S bonds.

The evolutionary driving force behind development of the multidomained structure for Igs was most likely the addition of useful biological functions with each of the additional domains. The function of the V_H and V_L domains is of course antigen binding. The function of the C_L and C_{H1} domain must certainly be to stabilize the V_L and V_H units so they can interact effectively with antigen. The C_{H2} domain is the site for binding of complement, and either the C_{H3} or the C_{H4} domain (depending on the species and Ig class), appears to be the site for attachment of Ig to cell surfaces (via the so-called Fc receptor). In addition, almost all of the biological functions distinctive of each Ig class (secretability, passage across the placenta) as well as most of the allotypic determinants, are associated with one or more C_H domains.

The Hinge Region

When the distance between the disulfide loops of each of the H chain domains of IgG, IgD, and IgA are compared, it has been observed that the distance between the C_{H1} and C_{H2} loops is substantially greater than between any other domains. This region, composed of from 12 to 60 additional amino acids depending on the species and H-chain isotype, is referred to as the "hinge" region (Figure 3-5). (IgM and IgE do not have hinge regions.) Hinge regions have been identified in electron micrographs of Ig molecules as a locus of flexibility allowing bending between the Fc and the two Fab arms. The amino acid sequence in this region is highly variable among Ig classes, but, in general, is rich in proline and hydrophilic residues, which render it structurally rather flexible as well as accessible to proteases. This is the region preferentially cleaved by mild papain or pepsin treatment. It also contains most of the interchain disulfide bonds holding the two H chains together.

Fv Fragments

In some instances when Fab fragments are treated with pepsin, Fv fragments, which consist of two adjoining V_H and V_L domains, are obtained. The Fv fragments can retain full antigen-binding capacity. The behavior of these fragments and their component chains (half of an L chain and one-quarter of an H chain) have been studied and have provided important insights into the independency as well as the interdependency of immunoglobulin domains. For example, dissociated Fv fragments can spontaneously recombine in solution to give the correctly folded and fully active dimer. This implies that at least these domains contain within themselves complete information for their own three-dimensional structure. Because antigen binding was also restored, we can conclude that not only can the component chains fold into the appropriate tertiary conformations, but the information for appropriate interaction of the two chains into a quaternary structure must also be contained in the primary sequences of the component domains.

V-Region Fine Structure

We have already alluded to the fact that the NH_2-terminal portions of both H and L chains (V_H and V_L domains) are highly variable in amino acid sequence among members of the same V-region family. (As we will see later, each family [κ, λ, and H] is located on a separate chromosome and contains its own V regions.) However, this heterogeneity is not uniformly distributed within the V_H or V_L region, and

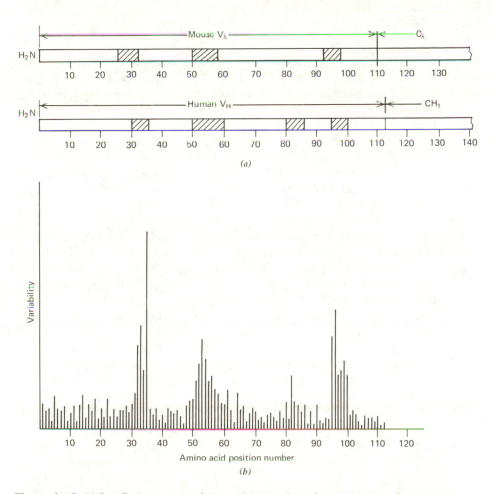

Figure 4-12 (a) Detailed structure of the variable region of Ig chains. The first 110 or so amino acid residues at the NH_2-terminal end of both light and heavy chains comprise the variable region. A combination of one V_L and one V_H forms one antigen-binding site. V_H regions generally tend to be slightly longer than V_L by about 5 to 10 amino acids. Not all portions of the variable region are equally variable. The areas of greatest variability, termed the hypervariable regions (hatched regions), are concentrated in discrete locations along the linear array of V-region amino acids. Light chain V regions have three of these so-called "hot spots," whereas V_H regions have four. It is generally accepted that the variability at these amino acid positions is related to variations in antigen-binding capacity. (b) Graphic representation of variability devised by Wu and Kabat. The variability at any given amino acid position for the known members of a particular family of V regions can be calculated from the following formula:

$$\text{variability} = \frac{\text{number of different amino acids found at position}}{\text{frequency of most common amino acid at that position}}$$

By simple inspection it will be seen that this function will range from 1, for a completely invariant position, to a maximum of 400 for a position in which all 20 amino acids are found with equal frequency. This particular plot is a composite plot representing an "average" human V_H region.

indeed within each family there are regions of fairly constant amino acid sequences common to all members of the family. The function of these constant regions within the V domains appears to be to maintain the correct peptide conformations for appropriate V–V and V–C interactions, and for correct internal folding of the V region itself.

The variability in V-region amino acid sequences is restricted to three sites in V_κ and V_λ regions in both mouse and humans, to three sites in mouse V_H regions, and to possibly four sites within human V_H regions. By comparing the sequences of a great many myeloma protein V regions within the various families, and analyzing the variability of each amino acid position, Wu and Kabat introduced the concept of "hypervariable regions" (Figure 4-12). These regions are not large, consisting of only about 10 or less amino acids each. All of the variability of the V region is restricted to these sites, and affinity labeling studies (see Chapter 7) have shown that the residues in these regions are the ones that interact with antigenic determinants. As such they can be referred to as "complementarity-determining regions." The amino acid sequences outside the hypervariable regions differ very little within different V-region groups (see definition following of family, group, and subgroup). The overall picture of the V region is thus of a series of "framework" regions (FR), which are relatively invariant, among which are interspersed hypervariable or complementarity-determining regions (CDR). The truly variable CDRs may account for no more than 15 to 20% of total V-region amino acids. The framework regions contain the amino acid residues, important for proper folding of the peptide chains, and for interaction with the corresponding V domain in the opposing chain (*trans* interactions) and with the adjacent C domain on the homologous chain (*cis* interactions). The amino acid residues in the hypervariable regions, as just mentioned, contain the information necessary for binding antigen.

Structure of the Antigen-combining Site

Amino Acids in the Hypervariable Regions Interact with Antigen

The antigen-combining site is formed by noncovalent association of the NH_2-terminal domains of adjacent light and heavy chains. Within each of the two contributing domains are regions of high amino acid variability (the hypervariable or complementarity-determining regions) among members of the same V-region family. A great deal of information has been accumulated to show that the amino acids comprising the hypervariable regions are involved in the binding of antigen. Some of this information has come, and continues to come, from applications of a technique known as affinity labeling.

The principal of affinity labeling is illustrated in Figure 4-13. A chemically reactive hapten or hapten analogue is allowed to react with an antibody made against that hapten. After the antibody–hapten reaction occurs, the hapten forms a covalent bond with residues in the antigen-binding site to which it is bound. Subsequently, the precise site of attachment of the hapten can be determined by separation of the chains, and analysis of peptides of the chains generated by enzymatic cleavage.

Examples of haptens used for affinity labeling studies are shown in Figure 4-13. The diazonium derivative of dinitrophenol (*m*-nitrobenzenediazonium fluoroborate, or MNBDF) is typical of chemically activated analogs of specific haptens (in this case, the dinitrophenyl [DNP] group). Antibodies to DNP will bind MNBDF quite readily, and the diazonium group will form a covalent linkage with immediately adjacent tyrosines, histidines, or lysines in the binding site. (in practice, only tyrosines are usually labeled.) The fact that such reagents generally react with a highly restricted spectrum of amino acids has somewhat hampered their usefulness. However, it has been amply documented that, under appropriately controlled conditions, they only react with amino acids within the binding site proper, so that information gathered by this technique is considered solid and definitive.

The reagent ε-(4-azido-2-nitrophenyl)-L-lysine (NAP-lysine) is representative of the class of photoactivated affinity-labeling molecules. NAP-lysine itself can be used to generate antibodies. When NAP-lysine is allowed to equilibrate with its antibody in the dark, and the suspension is then exposed to light, the azide group becomes a highly chemically reactive nitrene and will form a stable covalent bond with *any* adjacent carbon atom. Such reagents are thus not limited to reaction with particular amino acids in the binding site.

Both classes of affinity reagents have been shown to react with residues on both the light and heavy chains of antibody molecules. More precise information on the location of these residues has been derived from recent studies with homogeneous myeloma proteins, which have the ability to bind particular haptens in an immunospecific way. In such cases, because of the purity and high concentration of identical binding sites, it has been possible to show that amino acids that react with affinity-labeling reagents are always associated with the complementarity-determining regions of the light and heavy chains.

Size of the Antigen-combining Site

A great deal of experimentation involving a wide spectrum of techniques has been brought to bear on this question. The approaches used fall into two general categories: ligand competition studies and various forms of direct or indirect physical measurement. In the following sections we examine briefly examples of each type of analysis.

Ligand Competition Studies

Innumerable variations of this type of study have been carried out, using different antigens or modifications of antigens, but they are all basically similar to the

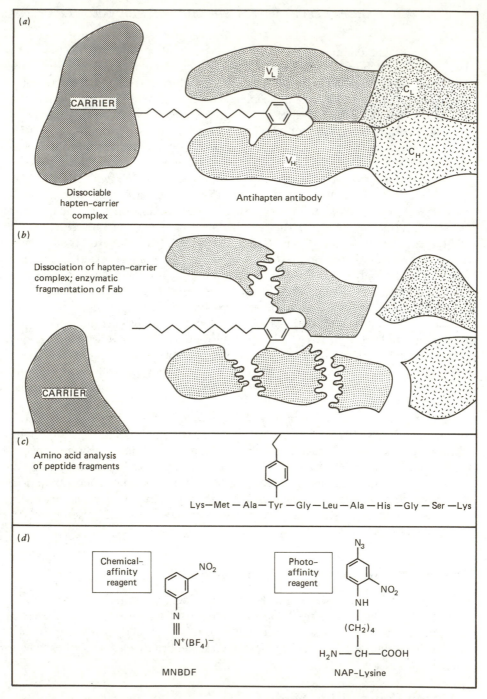

Figure 4-13 Use of affinity-labeling technique to identify sites of antigen–antibody interaction. (a) A form of hapten, identical with that used for immunization except for the presence of a chemical or photoactivatable cross-linking group, is reacted with antibody or its derived Fab. A covalent bond is established between the hapten and an amino acid in

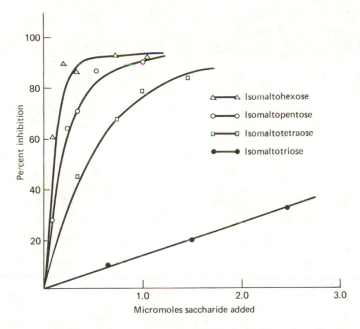

Figure 4-14 Inhibition of dextran–antidextran reaction by various size oligomers of glucose. [From E. Kabat and B. Mayer, *Experimental Immunochemistry*, Charles C Thomas, Springfield, IL (1961). Courtesy of Charles C Thomas, publisher, Springfield, IL.]

classic studies of Elvin Kabat and his co-workers, and have added little to his original conclusions. Kabat's basic approach was to make antibodies to the α-1,6-linked polymer of glucose, dextran, and then to use various glucose oligosaccharides to interfere with the reaction of the antibodies with the native dextran. The results of such an experiment are shown in Figure 4-14. Monomers and dimers of glucose were virtually ineffective. The trimer of glucose had a widely variable effect, depending on the antibody population tested. The tetramer was almost always a good inhibitor of the reaction. Maximum effectiveness was achieved with the hexamer; increasing polymer size over six subunits imparted no additional effectiveness. By chemically modifying each of the first six residues from the reducing end of the oligosaccharides, it was determined that all six were actually involved in binding. Thus, it was concluded that six linearly arranged glucose resi-

its immediate vicinity. (*b*) The hapten is dissociated from its carrier (if carrier is used) and the Fab, enzymatically digested into peptide fragments. The hapten remains covalently attached to that fragment containing the amino acid with which it previously interacted. (*c*) The hapten-binding peptide fragment is sequenced, and its location within the Fab fragment determined by comparison with the amino acid sequences of the H and L chains making up the Fab. (*d*) Representative examples of affinity-labeling reagents.

Table 4-3 Sizes of Various Antigenic Determinants
Reacting with a Homologous Antibody

Antigen	Determinant	Size in most extended form (Å)	Molecular weight
Dextran	Isomaltohexaose	$34 \times 12 \times 7$	990
Silk fibroin	Gly [gly$_3$ala$_3$] Tyr	27	632
	Dodecapeptide mixture	44	1000
G^{60}A^{40}, G^{60}A^{30}T^{10}, and G^{42}L^{28}A^{30}	Hexaglutamic acid	$36 \times 10 \times 6$	792
Poly-γ-D-Glu	Hexaglutamic acid	$36 \times 12 \times 7$	792
Polyalanyl bovine serum albumin	Pentaalanine	$25 \times 11 \times 6.5$	373
Polylysine + phosphoryl bovine serum albumin	Pentalysine	$27 \times 17 \times 6.5$	659
α-DNP heptalysine	α-DNP-heptalysine	$30 \times 17 \times 6.5$	1080

From E. A. Kabat, *Structural Concepts in Immunology and Immunochemistry,* Second Edition, Holt, Rinehart and Winston, New York, p. 127 (1976). Copyright © 1976, 1968 by Holt, Rinehart and Winston. Reprinted by permission of Holt, Rinehart and Winston.

dues defined the upper size limit of an antigen-combining site. Similar studies with synthetic polypeptides suggested an upper limit of five to six linearly arranged amino acids. A summary of such studies is presented in Table 4-3.

Physical Measurements

As with the ligand competition studies, a wide variety of experimental approaches have been used, and again with compatible results. An experiment employing electron spin resonance, carried out by Hsia and Piette in 1969, is illustrated in Figure 4-15. Antibodies to a hapten were reacted with the hapten coupled to an ESR spin label. The hapten and label were separated by a defined number of $-CH_2-$ spacers. Each of the hapten-spacer-label probes was tested separately with the antihapten antibody. As long as the probe is buried within the antigen-combining site, there is a marked rotational restriction of the spin label; outside the binding site, the label can rotate freely in response to the applied magnetic field. Freedom of rotation was observed in those cases where the spin label was greater than 10 Å from its point of attachment to the hapten. The authors concluded from these studies that the depth of the antigen-combining site was on the order of 10 to 12 Å. Direct measurements of other antibody sites suggest this is probably on the low side, the range of values observed being between 10 and 30 Å.

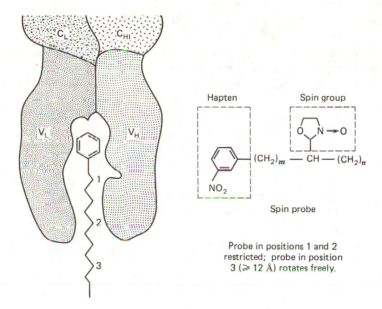

Figure 4-15 Probing the depth of the antigen-combining site using a spin-labeled antigen.

V-Region Groups: Implications for V-Gene Inheritance

During the late 1960s and early 1970s, analysis of the amino acid sequences of a large number of V regions of myeloma proteins belonging to the same *family* (κ, λ, or H) established the existence of distinct *groups* within these families, based principally on sequence similarities in the first (NH_2-terminal) framework portions. V_κ domains of human Igs fall into three obvious groups on this basis ($V_{\kappa I}$, $V_{\kappa II}$, and $V_{\kappa III}$). These three V_κ groups occur together in normal serum of the same individual, and thus are not complex alleles. The degree of sequence homology in the NH_2-terminal portion of V_κ regions of the same group is 70 percent or more, whereas the degree of homology between different human V_κ groups is about 50 percent. Within the same human V_κ group, about 90 percent of the amino acid differences that do occur in the FR1 regions can be related to a single nucleotide change in the codon. Similar patterns appear to hold for human V_λ regions, where at least five groups ($V_{\lambda I-V}$) have been identified. There are three recognized groups of V_H domains in human Igs ($V_{HI-HIII}$). The homology within a V_H group is rather higher than for V_κ and V_λ, being about 90 percent; homology between different V_H groups is usually between 40 to 60 percent. In each case, the V-region genes for different groups within a family are very tightly linked, although occasional segregation has been observed in some animal species.

The situation in the mouse is more complex. Mouse V_κ domains display a great deal of variability even in the framework positions. Although definite mouse V_κ groups can be recognized based on FR1 sequence identities, the number of groups thus defined is very large—perhaps a dozen or more. Lambda light chains in mice, on the other hand, are quite rare, comprising only 3 to 5 percent at most of Ig-associated light chains in the serum, and a correspondingly low frequency of myeloma proteins. Furthermore, the amino acid sequences of mouse λ chains show very little variation. Two groups of λ chains have been identified. Light-chain λ_1 has about a dozen variants, none of which differ by more than a few amino acids; λ_2 is so far defined by a single myeloma protein, which differs substantially from all of the members of λ_1. Lambda chains are very different in amino acid structure from mouse V_κ, and are clearly not a V_κ subgroup. They also are sufficiently similar to human V_λ that little doubt can be entertained about their genetic identity. Variability in mouse heavy-chain V regions lies somewhere between that found in κ and λ chains. V_H sequences in mice fall into seven recognizable homology groups, based on Southern blot (DNA–DNA hybridization) analysis of genomic DNA from 18 inbred strains. There is a total of about 100 different V_H genes. Genes within a group show >80 percent homology; sequence homology between groups is <70 percent.

Amino acid sequence analyses have been important in estimating the minimum number of genes that must be carried in the germ-line DNA. It is generally agreed that each V-region group, and each C-region type or class/subclass must be represented by at least one gene carried in the germ line. However, it appears from direct DNA sequencing studies, both in mice and humans, that a number for V-region genes based on V-region families would be a gross underestimate.

Immunoglobulin Chains Are Coded for by Two Genes

As data from the amino acid sequencing of immunoglobulin chains began to accumulate, speculation arose as to the way in which immunoglobulin genes might be arranged in DNA. At first, it was assumed (since there was no precedent for imagining anything else) that H- and L-chain genes, with continous V and C regions, would simply be lined up end to end in the DNA. The earliest calculations about Ig genes concerned the question of what proportion of the total genome would be required to code for 10^8 or so different antibody molecules. Figures of 1 to 2 percent were generally accepted as reasonable, and because vertebrate genomes were already recognized as having a great deal of extra DNA, this did not seem too large a genetic load to carry.

Before long, however, information began to accumulate that seemed incompatible with the existence of intact V-C coding segments in DNA. For example, several heavy-chain G-region allelic markers are inherited as single-gene Mendelian traits, and these markers (antigenic determinants) are faithfully reproduced in all examples of a given isotype in an animal. If there were hundreds or thousands of copies of that isotypic C region in the genome, one might expect to see some genetic variation around these allelic markers. This is never seen. This observation could be explained, of course, if only a single "master gene" for each H- or L-chain type is carried in the germ line. But then one would have to devise a mechanism whereby a fixed portion (the V region) of a single gene is extensively mutated somatically during ontogeny, without altering a single amino acid specification in the remainder of the gene (the C region).

Another disturbing fact was apparent genetic recombination between V- and C-region coding elements. For example, in the rabbit, the *a* allotype is found within the V_H region (presumably within one of the framework regions), whereas the *d* allotype can be shown to be in one of the C-region domains. Although these two markers are closely linked, occasional crossing over between them has been observed (0.3 percent). When homozygous parents of the genotypes

$$\frac{a1,d11}{a1,d11} \times \frac{a3,d12}{a3,d12}$$

were mated, individual H chains of the heterozygotes were almost always either (*a1, d11*) or (*a3, d12*). However, in a few cases, Ig chains of the (*a1, d12*) or (*a3, d11*) type have been observed, suggesting that crossing over had occurred, and that the two allotypes are coded for by separate but closely linked genes.

In a related study, Todd observed that the same V_H allotypes in rabbits could be found in association with more than one H-chain class. Because allotypes are based on amino acid sequences dictated by nucleotide sequences in structural genes, coding of a complete Ig chain by a single gene would require that nucleotide sequences coding for portions of the V regions of evolutionarily divergent genes (i.e., the H-chain classes) have been rigorously conserved through phylogeny and/or ontogenic somatic mutation.

Similar, and probably related, data has shown that the relatively constant amino acid sequences that help define V-region groups and subgroups also can be found in association with more than one C region.

In a number of cases in rabbits and humans, the same idiotype has also been found in association with different H-chain isotypes. In one particularly striking example, monoclonal IgM and IgG molecules from the same myeloma patient (designated "Til") were shown to share the same idiotype, as defined by cross-reaction with the same antiidiotypic antiserum. Subsequent direct sequencing of the heavy chains of the two Ig molecules showed that they shared identical V_H regions. This finding has since been repeated in several other human patients, and in rabbits. This is the strongest type of evidence that the same V-region gene product can be found in association with different C-gene products.

All of these observations pointed strongly to the notion that individual H and L chains must be coded for by two separate genes, or at least by two separate DNA sequences. Thus as early as 1965, Dreyer and Bennett proposed the "two genes, one polypeptide" theory as a basis for the observed structure of Ig. This proposal, although revolutionary, was accepted almost immediately. It then became important to define the level at which the information in the two genes was joined. There are essentially three possibilities. The genes could be somehow "stiched together" or translocated prior to transcription; mRNA molecules could be combined at some point during or after transcription and processing of HnRNA; or the completed V and C peptides could be covalently linked at some point in the translation or posttranslation stage.

The synthesis of Ig peptide chains has been carefully studied, and it is clear that the Ig chain is translated without interruption from the amino terminus of the V region to the carboxy terminus of the last C domain (Figure 4-9). Furthermore, Ig-chain mRNA has now been isolated from a number of myeloma tumors and can be shown by sequencing and by translation to contain both V and C coding portions. Thus the most likely interpretation seemed to be that the V and C genes were somehow joined or "translocated" in the DNA prior to transcription. However, proof of this had to wait for over 10 years, until the development of the techniques of molecular genetics. What followed is the subject of Chapter 5.

Bibliography

General

Kabat, E. A., *Structural Concepts in Immunology and Immunochemistry,* Second Edition, Holt, Rinehart and Winston, New York (1976).

Möller, G. (Ed.), Immunoglobulin D: Structure, synthesis, membrane representation and function. *Immunol. Rev. 37* (1977).

Möller, G. (Ed.), Immunoglobulin E. *Immunol. Rev. 41* (1978).

Nisonoff, A., J. E. Hopper, and S. B. Spring, *The Antibody Molecule,* Academic Press, New York (1975).

Origins of lymphocyte diversity. *Cold Spring Harbor Symp. Quant. Biol.* Vol. 41/part 2, 627 *et seq.* (1976).

Seidman, J. G., A. Leder, M. Nau, B. Norman, and P. Leder, Antibody diversity. *Science 202,* 11 (1978).

Spielgelberg, H. L., Biological activities of immunoglobulins of different classes and subclasses. *Adv. Immunol. 19,* 259 (1974).

Thorbecke, J., and G. Leslie, Immunoglobulin D: Structure and function. *Ann. N.Y. Acad. Sci. 399* (1982).

Wall, R., and M. Kuehl, Biosynthesis and regulation of immunoglobulins. *Ann. Rev. Immunol. 1,* 343 (1983).

Research

Amzel, L. M., R. Poljak, F. Saul, J. Varga, and F. Richards, The three-dimensional structure of a combining region-ligand complex of immunoglobulin NEW at 3.5-Å resolution. *Proc. Natl. Acad. Sci. USA 71,* 1427 (1974).

Brandtzaeg, P., and H. Prydz, Direct evidence for an integrated function of J chain and secretory component in epithelial transport. *Nature 311,* 71 (1984).

Brodeur, P., and R. Riblet, The Ig H chain V region locus in mice. 100 V Genes comprise seven families of homologous genes. *Eur. J. Immunol. 14,* 922 (1984).

Capra, J. D., and J. M. Kehoe, Hypervariable regions, idiotypy, and the antibody-combining site. *Adv. Immunol. 20,* 1 (1975).

Edelman, G. M., Antibody structure and molecular immunology. *Science 180,* 830 (1973).

Givol, D., Structural analysis of the antibody combining site. *Contemp. Topics Mol. Immunol. 2,* 27 (1973).

Ishizaka, K., and T. Ishizaka, Identification of γE antibodies as a carrier of reaginic activity. *J. Immunol. 99,* 1187 (1967).

Kabat, E. A., E. A. Padlan, and D. R. Davis, Evolutionary and structural influences on light chain constant (C_L) region of human and mouse immunoglobulins. *Proc. Natl. Acad. Sci. USA 72,* 2785 (1975).

Kawanishi, H., L. Saltzman, and W. Strober, Mechanisms regulating IgA class-specific Ig production in murine gut-associated lymphoid tissues. II. Terminal differentiation of post-switch sIgA-bearing Peyer's patch B cells. *J. Exp. Med. 158,* 649 (1983).

Kuan, T. et al., Three monoclonal immunoglobulins; An IgG2, an IgM and an IgM/A hybrid, in one patient. II. Sharing of common variable regions. *Immunology 44,* 265 (1981).

Lamm, M. E., Cellular aspects of immunoglobulin A. *Adv. Immunol. 22,* 233 (1976).

Lennox, E. S. et al., A search for biosynthetic subunits of light and heavy chains of immunoglobulins. *Cold Spring Harbor Symp. Quant. Biol. 32,* 249 (1967).

Mostov, K. E., J.-P. Kraehenbuhl, and G. Blobel, Receptor-mediated transcellular transport of immunoglobulin: Synthesis of secretory component as mutliple and larger transmembrane forms. *Proc. Natl. Acad. Sci. USA 77,* 7257 (1980).

Pollock, R. R., and M. F. Mescher, Murine cell surface immunoglobulin: Two native IgD structures. *J. Immunol. 124,* 1668 (1980).

Porter, M., Antigen-binding myeloma proteins of mice. *Adv. Immunol. 25,* 141 (1977).

Putnam, F. W., N. Takahashi, D. Tetaert, Li-C. Lin, and B. Debuire, The Last of the immunoglobulins: Complete amino acid sequence of human IgD. In J. Thorbecke and G. Leslie, eds., *Immunoglobulin D: Structure and Function, Annals New York Academy Sciences 399,* 41 (1982).

Richards, F., W. Konigsberg, R. Rosenstein, and J. Varga, On the specificity of antibodies. *Science 189,* 130 (1975).

Rowe, D. S., and J. L. Fahey, A new class of human immunoglobulin. I. A unique myeloma protein. *J. Exp. Med. 121,* 171 (1965).

Socken, D. J., K. N., Jeejeebhoy, H. Bazin, and B. J. Underdown, Identification of secretory component as an IgA receptor on rat hepatocytes. *J. Exp. Med. 150,* 1538 (1979).

Weaver, E. et al., Secretion of IgA by human milk leukocytes initiated by surface membrane stimuli. *J. Immunol. 132,* 684 (1984).

Wu, T. T., and E. A. Kabat, An analysis of the sequences of the variable regions of Bence-Jones proteins and myeloma light chains and their implications of antibody complementarity. *J. Exp. Medicine 132,* 211 (1970).

CHAPTER 5

Genetic Basis of Immunoglobulin Structure

In the two preceding chapters, we traced the development of our current under-standing of the structure of immunoglobulin molecules. As we have seen, these studies led to the hypothesis, put forward by Dreyer and Bennett in 1965, that immunoglobulin chains must be coded for by two separate genes—one for the V region and one for the C region. This hypothesis was accepted almost immediately by most immunologists and was validated in the late 1970s by direct sequencing of DNA regions containing immunoglobulin genes.

The "two gene, one polypeptide" hypothesis raised a number of questions that could really only be answered at the level of molecular genetics. (1) How many Ig genes are carried in germline DNA? (2) Where and how are they organized in the genome? (3) How and when are V and C genes joined together; what is the nature of the resulting genetic unit; and how is it transcribed and translated? (4) What is the genetic basis for the tremendous structural diversity of Ig V regions?

Germ-Line Immunoglobulin Genes

There are formally two possibilities for the way in which Ig genes are arranged in DNA. We could imagine that all possible V–C combinations are lined up end to end in the genome; or, the V and C segments could be separated, and recombined when needed to form intact Ig chain-coding genes. In the latter case, we would need very few, perhaps only single, copies of the C-region portions of the final coding unit because this portion of the molecule need not vary within a given isotype.

As discussed at the end of Chapter 4, a variety of experiments—based on C-gene inheritance patterns and on C-gene DNA–RNA hybridization kinetics—had suggested convincingly that individual C-region isotype genes are represented essentially once in the haploid genome. This has now been confirmed by direct DNA sequencing studies.

That left the question of the number of V-region genes. How many V genes must an animal have to deal with the antigenic universe? Are all of these genes carried in the germ line, and transmitted intact from generation to generation, or is some (or all) of this diversity generated somatically after fertilization?

The number of V genes needed to deal with the antigenic universe can only be crudely approximated. We are helped considerably by knowing the approximate size of the antigen-combining site on an antibody molecule, and by the fact that, by and large, only molecules based on the organic elements (C, H, O, N, S, P) comprise the antigenic universe. Clearly the number of truly *different* antigenic determinants that can be constructed given these size and basic composition restrictions is not infinite; most immunologists accept estimates in the range of 10^7 to 10^8. Does this mean then that we need 10^7 to 10^8 V genes? Clearly not. First of all, an antigen-combining site is composed of two separate V regions: V_H and V_L. Thus, if all V_H and V_L could combine randomly, we would immediately be able to lower the number of required genes to 10^3 to 10^4. (However, as we will see later on, there may be some restrictions on V-region pairings.) Another factor that reduces the required number of V genes is the multispecificity of antigen combining sites (p. 144). Virtually all antigenic determinants induce a heterogeneous antibody response; and conversely, an antibody raised in response to one determinant will, if we search long enough, cross-react to some extent with some other antigenic determinant. Moreover, most environmental antigens are multideterminant; if the immune response to one of them were low or absent, survival of the host might not be seriously compromised. Thus, a repertoire of V_L and V_H genes on the order of 10^3 each might well suffice to deal with the antigenic universe.

These are, of course, only guesses, based more on theoretical considerations than on hard data. Ultimately, the only meaningful information must be based on direct quantitation of V-region genes in the DNA. This will likely be accomplished in the not too distant future.

That leaves the question of how many such genes must be carried in the germ-line DNA to be passed on intact from generation to generation. An absolute minimum requirement would be one V gene per immunglobulin *family*, since, as we will see shortly, the three families reside on separate autosomes, and their members never mix (i.e., V_λ associates only with C_λ, V_κ with C_κ, and V_H and C_H). Beyond that, a fairly compelling argument can be made that each identifiable V-region *group* (see p. 95) must also require a separate germ-line gene. These groups are faithfully reproduced in each individual of the species, and it is difficult to imagine how this could occur if only a single V-region gene is inherited for each family. However, as we will see, the number of V genes carried in the germ-line DNA need not be as large as estimates of the total number of V genes needed to deal with the antigenic universe. V-region genes are themselves broken up into segments in the DNA that can be combined in various ways. This combinatorial diversity greatly expands the V-region repertoire that can be generated from a modest number of inherited gene segments. Most molecular immunologists accept estimates on the order of 10^2 to 10^3 total germ-line V-region gene segments as reasonable.

Organization of Ig Genes in the Genome

We have seen that there are three families of immunoglobulin genes: the kappa, lambda, and heavy-chain families. Each of these families is located on a different autosome. In the mouse, the H, κ, and λ families have been assigned to the twelfth, sixth, and sixteenth chromosomes, respectively. In humans, these three families reside on chromosomes 14, 2, and 22, respectively. As we will see in the sections that follow, each of these families is composed of a collection of gene segments that must be spliced together in order to assemble coding information for a continuous immunoglobulin peptide chain.

The general pattern for organization of the gene segments in germ-line DNA for the three Ig families in mice is shown in Figure 5-1. The pattern in humans is virtually identical. In each case, a group of V-gene segments is located some distance away from a cluster of J segments and C-region genes. J segments contain the final 10 to 15 percent or so of the completed V-gene sequence. The J segment groups are located 1 to 3 kilobases (kb) upstream of the C genes. The distance between the V genes and the J segments is not known in most cases. In the case of the H chain genes, an additional gene segment called "D" is required to complete a V_H gene. In germ-line DNA, D segments lie between the V and J segments. Evidence establishing the existence of J and D segments, and possible mechanisms for joining with V segments, are presented in subsequent sections of this chapter; for the present we wish only to obtain an overview of their organization.

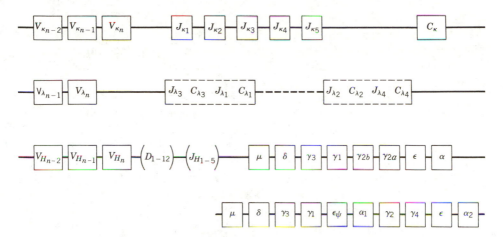

Figure 5-1 The general patterns for organization of the gene segments in germ-line DNA for the three Ig families in mice. In the kappa family, a large number of V gene segments is separated by an as yet undefined distance from a cluster of five J segments and a single C gene segment. So far, the peptide sequence coded for by the $J_{\kappa 3}$ gene segment has not been identified in a κ light chain.

In the lambda family, there are only two V gene segments, separted by some distance from a cluster of interpersed J and C segments. At present, two clusters of two J–C pairs each have been identified directly in the DNA; the order of the two clusters is not yet known. The four C_λ segments are very similar in sequence. In serum Ig, $V_{\lambda 1}$ appears to associate with $C_{\lambda 1}$ and $C_{\lambda 3}$; $V_{\lambda 2}$ associates only with $C_{\lambda 2}$. A $C_{\lambda 4}$ peptide product has not been identified in serum. This pattern for V_λ and C_λ is seen in all inbred strains of mice. In wild mice, the number of V_λ is usually three, and the number of C_λ varies from 2 to 12.

Rearrangement of Light-Chain V and C Regions during Embryogenesis

A major technological advance in molecular biology generally, which has permitted a closer examination of the arrangement of immunoglobulin coding sequences, was the discovery and characterization of restriction nucleases. These enzymes cleave both strands of DNA at the site of enzyme-specific palindromic sequences. For example, the restriction nuclease Eco R1 will cleave double-stranded DNA at any point containing the sequence $\frac{5'\text{GAATTC}}{\text{CTTAAG}5'}$. Using restriction nucleases, one can generate from any source of DNA reproducible collections of small DNA fragments, which can then be used for sequencing or hybridization studies or cloned in an appropriate bacterial vector such as a phage or plasmid. The latter technique can provide the large quantities of homogeneous DNA needed for most sequencing analyses. The advantage of this technique cannot be overestimated; it underlies almost every advance made since 1975 in understanding the structure and organization of genes or gene sequences in DNA. The value of restriction nucleases to science was recognized by award of the 1978 Nobel prize in medicine and physiology to Hamilton Smith, Daniel Nathans, and Werner Arber.

Hybridization analysis of restriction fragments was used by Horumi and Tonegawa to look at the organization and joining of V and C genes in mouse DNA (Figure 5-2). The question asked was whether V and C coding elements are in some way rearranged during the process of differentiation of B cells during ontogeny. DNA from mouse embryos (which was assumed to be representative of germ-line DNA) and from adult myeloma cells was used for hybridization studies with purified λ-chain mRNA. The DNAs in each case were digested to completion with a specific restriction nuclease, and the fragments were hybridized with a specific mRNA coding for the λ light chain. It was found that with digested embryonic DNA, the λ mRNA hybridized by its C-region portion to one DNA fragment and by its V-region portion to a totally separate DNA fragment.

Clearly, the DNA sequences coding for the V_λ and C_λ regions in the embryo are separated by a site for the particular restriction enzymes used. The exact distance

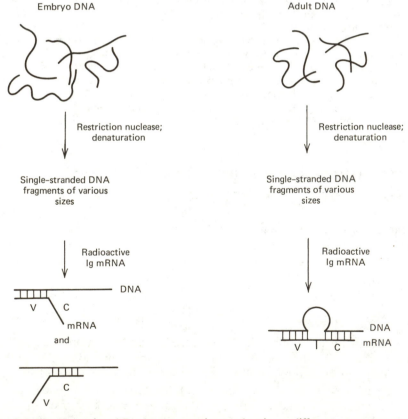

Figure 5-2 The Horumi and Tonegawa experiment showing a different arrangement of V and C genes in embryonic and adult DNA.

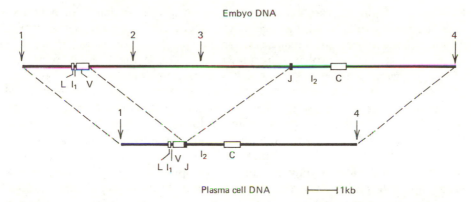

Figure 5-3 Arrangement of mouse λ_1 gene sequences in embryos and in myeloma cells. In embryo DNA, a full λ_1 gene sequence consists of two parts that lie on two separate Eco RI fragments. On one of these fragments (between sites 1 and 2), the coding sequence is split into two parts, one for most of the leader peptides (L) and the other for the rest of the leader peptides plus the variable region peptides (V). These two coding sequences are separated by a 93-nucleotide-long intervening sequence (I_1). On the second Eco RI fragment (between sites 3 and 4), the coding sequence is also split into two parts by a 1250-base-long intervening sequence (I_2). The two parts are for the constant region peptides (C) and approximately 13 residue peptides near the junction of the variable and constant regions (J). In the DNA of a λ_1 chain-producing myeloma (H 2020), the λ_1 gene sequence is rearranged as a result of one (or more) recombination(s) that involves sequences in the two embryonic Eco RI fragments. One recombination takes place at the ends of the V and the J sequences and brings the two sequences into direct contact. The limits of the corresponding sequences in the embryo and the myeloma DNAs are indicated by thin dotted lines. Arrows with numbers indicate Eco RI sites. [Taken from C. Brack et al., A complete immunoglobulin gene is created by somatic recombination. *Cell 15,* 1 (1978). Copyright © 1978 by the MIT Press and the author (S. Tonegawa).]

between them is not known and, in any case, is probably different for different Ig gene systems. On the other hand, in lymphoid system-differentiated (myeloma) DNA, whole λ mRNA hybridized with a single restriction nuclease fragment using the same enzyme. This experiment was taken as the first evidence for a rearrangement of V- and C-region coding elements during differentiation of the immune system. Strictly speaking, however, these experiments only showed the disappearance of a restriction site between V_λ and C_λ elements during differentiation. As it turns out, this is, indeed, associated with a physical rearrangement of V_L and C_L elements.

Further experiments by Tonegawa, and also by Leder at the National Institutes of Health, using cloned fragments of mouse myeloma DNA, showed that after rearrangement the V and C coding sequences for λ and κ light chains are still separated by intervening sequences of about 1 to 4 kilobase pairs (kbp) (Figure 5-3). This appears to be the case in all light-chain systems examined. The conclusion from all of these studies is that V_L and C_L sequences are well separated in mouse embryonic

DNA (although on the same chromosome). During differentiation of lymphoid cells, there is a somatic rearrangement of this DNA such that a particular V_L gene is brought closer to, but still remains separated from, an appropriate C_L gene.

Subsequent studies, involving direct nucleotide sequencing of cloned fragments of DNA containing Ig genes, showed that V–C rearrangement is even more complex. In germ-line DNA coding for L chains, segments containing the nucleotide sequences coding for the last few COOH-terminal amino acids of CDR3, and for all of FR-4, are separated from both the main portion of the V_L gene segment and the C_L gene (Figure 5-3). During B-cell ontogeny, one of the incomplete V segments is somehow selected from the total pool, and transposed to one of these smaller segments (called J for "joining") to make a complete V gene. The completed V segment now lies fairly close to the C-region gene. In the κ and H families, combinatorial permutations of V and J regions obviously increase the possible range of V-region diversity. This diversity may be even more than apparent, since it seems that the precise point at which the V-region segment splices to the J segment during rearrangement can vary by the nucleotide equivalents of one to three amino acids (p. 111).

Assembly of Immunoglobulin V_H Gene Segments

The basic process for assembly of the Ig heavy-chain gene is the same as for κ and λ light chains, with a few additional features. The existence of J_H elements was inferred when it was found that V_H segments per se lack coding information for the carboxy-terminal 15 to 20 amino acids of the completed V-region peptide. Subsequently, several cloned fragments of DNA were found to contain C_H genes with varying numbers (up to five) of J_H segments 5' to the μ gene. All V_H regions end with amino acids coded for by one of these five J_H regions. The other C_H genes are lined up 3' to the C_μ gene, separated by intervening sequences (see Figure 5-4). No J_H sequences are found 5' to any of the other C_H genes; the same set of J_H gene segments serves all C_H isotypes.

However, if one compares the primary sequences of germ-line and rearranged V_H genes with each other and with the corresponding mRNA and protein sequences, there is still a small segment of V region missing. In one case that was studied, the germ-line V_H segment contained information for amino acids 1 to 101; the germ-line J_H segments corresponded to amino acids 107 to 123 of the complete peptide V_H region. When the germ-line V_H and J_H segments are joined in rearranged DNA, they were found to be separated by an additional 13 nucleotides not associated in the germ line with either the V_H or J_H gene segments. The additional nucleotides that appear in the rearranged, complete V_H gene account for amino acids 102 to 106, which fall in the third hypervariable region of the peptide V_H region and thus contribute to antigen-binding diversity.

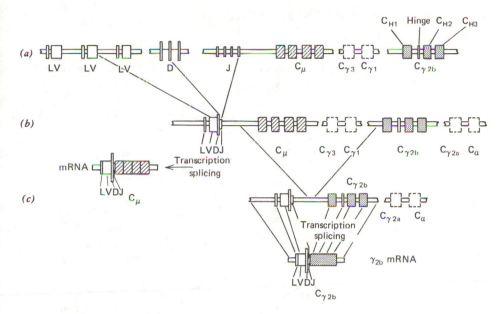

Figure 5-4 Recombination events leading to a complete $_\gamma$2b gene. (a) The germ-line DNA before arrangement. There is a cluster of at least 50 genes (each with a short leader sequence L) coding for part of the variable (V) region, a cluster of D gene segments coding for most of the third hypervariable region, and some distance away there are four J segments that complete the V region coding sequence. The J segments lie about 8 kb from the C_μ gene, which lies at the start of a cluster containing all the C-region genes. The C-region gene sequences are interrupted by noncoding sequences to give a series of exons that coincide with the domains and the hinge region in the C-region amino acid sequence. (b) In the first translocation event one of each of the V, D, and J segments are recombined to give a complete V_H. The V_H, the V_H–C_H intervening sequence, and the C_H segment are transcribed as a single unit. The noncoding sequences (introns) are removed by splicing events during nuclear RNA processing resulting in a continuous coding sequence in the final mRNA. (c) A second translocation event, the heavy chain switch, deletes the C_μ, $C_{\gamma 3}$ and $C_{\gamma 1}$ gene segments and places the VDJ segment and part of the J-C_γ intron near the $C_{\mu 2b}$ gene. Following transcription the introns are removed by splicing leading to a continuous coding sequence in the γ2b mRNA. [From H. V. Molgaard, Assembly of immunoglobulin heavy chain genes. *Nature 286*, 657–659 (1980)].

The approximate location in the germ-line DNA of the gene segments for these additional amino acids is now known, and they have been labeled the "D" (for diversity-generating) segments. So far, 12 D_H segments have been identified in mice. A V_H gene segment is first translocated to a D_H segment, which lies somewhere 3′ to the V gene and 5′ of the J_H gene segment cluster. The joined $V_H D_H$ is then translocated to an appropriate J_H, bringing the completed V_H gene ($V_H D_H J_H$) into proximity to the correct C_H gene. (See also the section, "Isotype Switching.")

The Mechanism of V–D, V–J, and J–D Joining

A detailed study of the nucleotide sequences around the V, D, and J segments of cloned germ-line DNA (Figure 5-5) suggests possible mechanisms for joining them together. There are two types of sequence elements involved: recognition sequences of either 7 or 9 nucleotides, and spacer sequences of either 12 or 23 nucleotides. The recognition sequences, as might be expected, are highly conserved, both within and between genomes (Table 5-1). The 12 and 23 nucleotide sequences are assumed to serve a spacer function because only their length, not their sequence, is conserved. It may be important to note that 12 and 23 nucleotides represent one and two turns of a double helix, respectively.

Note in Figure 5-5 that the recognition sequences have a directional sense to them. That provides one rule for segment joining: only segments with an opposite sense can join. The second rule is that two recognition sequences separated by a 12-nucleotide (12-mer) spacer will only pair with recognition sequences separated by a 23-mer.

How is this information used to join the various components of a V_H or V_L gene? We do not know yet, but two possible models are shown in Figure 5-6. Because the

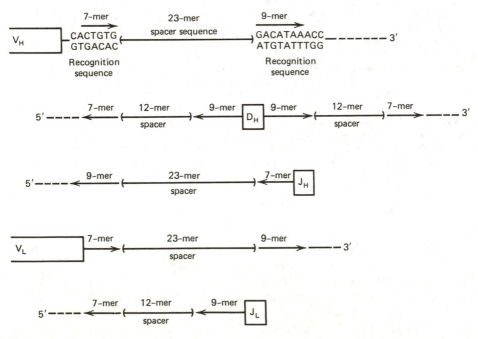

Figure 5-5 Nucleotide organization around the V, D, and J elements of immunoglobulin V genes.

Table 5-1 The Two Conserved Blocks
of Sequences Near the V-J or V-D-J Joining Sites

J DNA segments	Nanomers		Heptamers
$J_{\kappa 1}$	GGTTTTTGT	23	CACTGTG
$J_{\kappa 2}$	AGTTTTTGT	23	CAGTGTG
$J_{\kappa 3}$	GGGTTTTGT	21	CACTGTA
$J_{\kappa 4}$	GGTTTTTGT	24	CACTGTG
$J_{\kappa 5}$	GGTTTTTGT	23	CACTGTG
J_{II}	GGTTTTTGC	12	CACAGTG
J_{H1}	AGTTTTAGT	22	GACTGTG
J_{H2}	GGTTTTTGT	23	TAGTGTG
J_{H3}	ATTTATTGT	21	CACAATG
		23	CAATGTG
J_{H4}	GGTTTTTGT	22	TATTGTG
		21	TACTATG
Basic sequence	GGTTTTTGT		CACTGTG

V DNA segments	Heptamers		Nanomers
$V_{\kappa 21C}$	CACAGTG	11	ACAAAAACC
$V_{\kappa 21B}$	CACAGTG	12	ACAAAAACC
V_{K41}	CACAGTG	12	ACATAAACC
V_{K2}	CACAGTG	12	ACATAAACC
V_{II}	CACAATG	22	TCAAGAACA
$V_{\lambda II}$	CACAATG	23	ACAAGAACA
V_{H141}	CACAGTG	23	ACAAATACC
Basic sequence	CACAGTG		ACAAAAACC

Two blocks of conserved sequences found in the 5'-flanking region of J DNA segments and in the 3'-flanking region of embryonic V DNA segments are compared. The numbers between the two types of sequences indicate the distance between them in base pairs. The bases different from those of the basic sequences in the corresponding positions are underlined. [From H. Sakano, R. Maki, Y. Kurosawa, W. Roeder, and S. Tonegawa, Two types of somatic recombination are necessary for the generation of complete immunoglobulin heavy-chain genes. *Nature 286,* 676–683 (1980).]

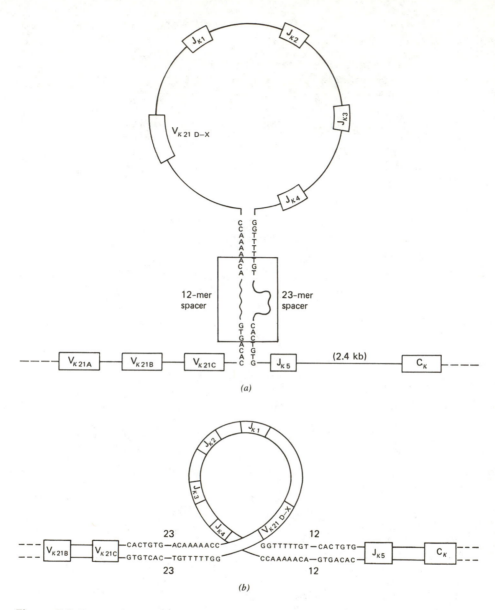

Figure 5-6 Two models for joining of V and J sequences. Both models could apply equally well to joining of V–D or D–J segments. (a) The stem model. The inverted complementary haptamer and nonamer sequences flanking the selected V and J segments ($V_{\kappa21C}$ and $J_{\kappa5}$) on the same strand recombine to form a double-stranded stem structure. This creates a recognition site for an enzyme that excises the stem and loop and joins the V and J segments at the base of the stem. Presumably the same thing happens on the complementary strand. (b) Double-stranded loop model. A protein could bind at one site to the double-stranded haptamer–nonamer 3' of a V segment, and then, either in a directed or random fashion, bind to the inverted complementary structure 5' of a J segment at a second site. Either the same or a different protein could then cut and splice the apposing double strands. In this figure, $V_{\kappa21C}$ would be joined to $J_{\kappa5}$.

V			J		Protein			
DNA								
	3'			5'	95	96	97	98
1.	CCX CCC	— — — — —		TGG ACG	Pro	Trp	Thr	
2.	CCX CCC	— — — — —		TGG ACG	Pro	Arg	Thr	
3.	CCX CCC	— — — — —		TGG ACG	Pro	Pro	Thr	
4.	CCX CCC	— — — — —		TGG ACG	Pro	Pro	Trp	Thr
5.	CCX CCC	— — — — —		TGG ACG	Pro	Pro	Thr	
6.	CCX CCC	— — — — —		TGG ACG	Pro	Thr		

Figure 5-7 Diversity generated as a result of multiple joinings of the same V and J segments. Shown in this hypothetical example are the two 3' codons of a selected V segment, and the two 5' codons of a selected J segment of a light chain. The nucleotides actually joined are underscored with a solid line. Different ways of joining them create different amino acid sequences in the critical third hypervariable region. Similar imprecision of segment joining operates in the assembly of H chains as well.

heptamer and nonamer recognition sequences adjacent to joinable segments are inverted repeats of each other, they could conceivably form a stem structure, which could serve as a signal for deleting the looped out material. A possible problem with this model is that the two spacer sequences are of unequal length, although since they need not interact this may be unimportant. A second model for segment joining would use an enzyme or joining protein that utilizes the nonamer and haptamer sequences to bring the segments to be joined into intimate contact.

Another feature of V–J and V–D joining that will become important when we consider V-region diversity is imprecision at the joining boundary, or *junctional diversity* (Figure 5-7). It turns out that the exact nucleotide at which a V segment is joined to a D or J segment is not precisely fixed. Because the general point at which joining occurs codes for the third hypervariable region, the net result is the creation of several possible hypervariable regions from the same V–D or V–J segments. Of course, if a V segment is joined to a D or J segment out of phase, the resultant frame-shifted gene will likely not be readable. Such rearrangements are termed nonproductive, and indeed most evidence suggests that nonproductive rearrangements outnumber correct or productive rearrangements. If one chromosome rearranges nonproductivity, the cell has the option of rearranging the other chromosomes. If both rearrange nonproductivity, the B cell may be lost.

Isotype Switching

The translocation of the completed V_H gene to a C_H gene involves a level of complexity not seen in the L-chain system. The first H-chain isotype to be selected on antigenic stimulation is always μ. On continued or subsequent stimulation with the same antigen or even with mitogen, some of the clonal progeny will begin to synthesize one of the other H-chain class isotypes. There is good experimental evidence that the initiation of the isotype switch is under T-helper cell control. However, a mechanism must be postulated at the genetic level to account for the phenomenon of H-chain switching pursuant to the T-cell signal.

The details of the mechanism by which a VDJ-C_μ nucleotide sequence is interrupted, and the VDJ gene segment is transposed to a different C_H isotype, are not known. Each C_H gene-segment cluster (C_μ, C_γ, C_α, etc.) is preceded by tandem repeats of homologous nucleotide units of from 20 to 80 base pairs called switch regions. The overall sequence of the switch regions is different for each isotype, and bears no relation to the inverted repeat sequences involved in V–D–J joining. Because each switch region is unique, it seem unlikely that homologous pairing could account for recombination between sequences 3′ to J with different C-region switch signals.

Hood et al. have proposed that a series of class-specific switching proteins may be involved (Figure 5-8). If true, one could then imagine that isotype switching could be regulated by the presence or absence of these proteins. One implication of this model is that after isotype switching, the genes lying between the expressed

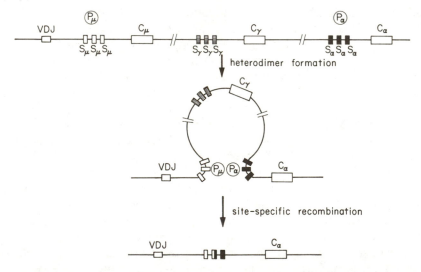

Figure 5-8 Model for class-specific regulation of C_H switching. In this scheme the small boxes represent recognition (S) sequences that bind to switch proteins to mediate C_H switching; the circle represents switching proteins and the large boxes represent coding regions. This model depicts a C_H gene order of C_μ–C_γ–C_α, but this is not a requirement. [From L. Hood, M. Davis, P. Early, K. Calame, S. Kim, S. Crews, and H. Huang, Two types of DNA rearrangements in immunoglobulin genes. *Cold Spring Harbor Symposia on Quantitative Biology, Vol. XLV, Movable Genetic Elements,* Cold Spring Harbor Laboratory, New York (1981).]

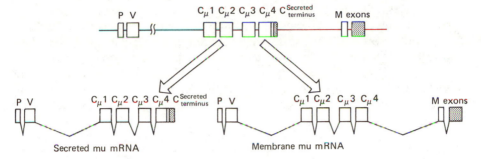

Splicing patterns deduced for μ_m and μ_s mRNAs

Figure 5-9 The μ_m and μ_s mRNAs are assumed to be identical 5′ to $C_\mu 4$. Raised boxes indicate exons; 3′ untranslated sequences are shaded. P refers to the signal peptide exon and V to the rearranged V_H exon. Bent lines indicate RNA splicing between exons. [From P. Early, J. Rogers, M. Davis, K. Calame, M. Bond, R. Wall, and L. Hood, Two mRNAs can be produced from a single immunoglobulin μ gene by alternative RNA processing pathways. *Cell 20,* 313–319 (1980).]

VDJ and the newly selected C gene will be lost, similar to what happens during V–D and VD–J joining (Figure 5-5). In general, this appears to be true. However, in at least one instance, it was found that after switching from IgM to IgG2b production, two copies of the μ gene were still carried in the B-cell DNA. Clearly a "looping out" mechanism did not operate in this case. Current evidence suggests that in this instance a primary transcript was made that extended from VDJ through the γ_{2b} gene—a very long distance indeed (Figure 5-1). The material between VDJ and γ_{2b} is presumed to have been removed in an RNA splicing event as described for the μ-δ choice splice (Figure 5-10) and the membrane-versus-secreted terminus choice splice (Figure 5-9).

Other instances of an extraordinarily long RNA transcript, encompassing several heavy-chain isotypes, have been reported. Usually these are associated with resting memory B cells that have not yet been restimulated by antigen. The possibility has thus been raised that at the end of the initial round of stimulation the B cell's transcription apparatus starts reading through to the H-chain gene selected for secondary expression, but actual rearrangement of the DNA and looping out of intervening genes does not occur until secondary activation of the cell. At present, however, this notion is still controversial.

Organization of Membrane-Form and Secreted-Form Ig Genes

As mentioned in Chapter 4, all Ig H-chain isotypes are synthesized in two forms— membrane and secreted. An obvious question for the immunoglobulin geneticist is whether this is reflected at the genetic level by separate membrane and secreted Ig genes, or whether some posttranscriptional or posttranslational events give rise to distinct peptide products. The first direct solution of this problem involved the μ gene, although it is now known that the same mechanisms hold for the other isotypes as well. Wall and co-workers at UCLA and Hood and his colleagues at the California Institute of Technology showed that the C_μ gene contains both the complete μ_s sequence and an additional, separate coding segment containing the μ_m-specific membrane anchoring sequence (see Figure 5-9). During processing of μ transcripts, either the μ_s sequence is selected to make μ_s mRNA, or the μ_m sequence is selected and spliced to the $C_\mu 4$ domain to make μ_m mRNA. The nucleotides 5′ to the $C_\mu 4$-secreted terminus interface are GT, and the two nucleotides 5′ to the beginning of the M exon are AG. These have been universally found as part of the information required to make an RNA "splice site." The discovery that a cell can use a single gene copy to derive two functionally different proteins through RNA processing is an exciting one and expands the possible interpretation of a number of biological phenomena.

The δ Gene

A special problem arises with respect to the δ gene. In B cells that are developmentally mature and ready to respond to antigen, both μ and δ are expressed on the cell surface, and both have the same V_H region. In lymphomas arising in B cells at this stage of development, both μ and δ are coexpressed over many cell generations, implying continued transcription of both μ and δ genes. It has been absolutely established that the μ gene is the first coding element at the 5′ end of the C_H

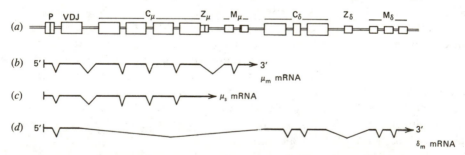

Figure 5-10 Proposed arrangement and transcription of μ and δ gene. (a) Final rearranged form of DNA encoding a μ and δ gene. Z_μ, secreted μ terminus; M_μ, membrane μ termini; Z_δ, secreted terminus; M_δ, membrane δ termini. (b) Primary nuclear RNA transcript for membrane μ. (c) Primary nuclear RNA transcript for secreted μ. (d) Partially processed nuclear RNA transcript for membrane δ (the RNA splice removing the μ sequences has already occurred). In b to d, the heavy lines represent sequences found in cytoplasmic mRNA; thin lines are sequences spliced out during HnRNA processing. (Courtesy Dr. Randolph Wall, UCLA.)

gene cluster; therefore, the δ gene must be 3′ of the μ gene. When the δ gene is expressed, none of the other C_H genes are rearranged or deleted, suggesting that the δ gene is located somewhere between μ and the other C_H genes. But according to the model shown in Figure 5-8, to which few exceptions have been found, expression of a given C_H gene is accompanied by excision and loss of all C_H genes 5′ of the given C_H gene. Thus the continued expression of the same V_{H} in combination with both μ and δ on the B-cell surface seemed somewhat anomalous.

The resolution of this dilemma lies in a rather complex form of RNA processing. The δ gene was cloned and found to be located only 2.5 kbp 3′ of the μ gene. This is much closer than any other two C_H genes, and is even closer than the J_H-μ distance. Several laboratories independently showed that the C gene is not rearranged in cells making both μ and δ; rather, it appears that the VDJ-μ-δ region is transcribed in its entirety, and that splicing to make VDJ-μ or VDJ-δ mRNA, like $μ_m$ versus $μ_s$ mRNA processing, takes place during processing of the resultant complex mRNA precursor (Figure 5-10).

Transcriptional Processing of Ig Genes

In both the kappa and heavy-chain gene families of mice, each of the many V-gene segments is preceded by a set of promoter sequences. This is true in both germ-line DNA and in the rearranged DNA of mature B cells. Yet V-gene transcription begins only after DNA rearrangement. That the germ-line promoter sequences are functional is evidenced by the fact that germ-line V genes can be transcribed in an *in vitro* system, and after transfer into frog oocytes. Yet in B cells they are never transcribed until after rearrangement.

Recent work by a number of laboratories has revealed the existence of so-called enhancer sequences, located in the J–C intron of H and κ genes (but apparently not λ genes), that are necessary for full function of the V-gene promoter. These enhancers appear to facilitate V-region promoter function in a lymphoid cell-specific manner. The cell specificity is presumably imparted by specific enhancer factors found only in the cytoplasm of lymphoid cells. Full and active transcription of the rearranged immunoglobulin gene presumably involves cooperative interactions of the V-region promoter, the enhancer sequence, and the enhancer factor. The details of this interaction are currently under investigation.

Once transcription is initiated, the major task is to clear the transcript of extraneous information contained in the remaining intervening sequences. Although other eucaryotic gene sequences are known to be interrupted by intervening sequences, the mouse Ig gene is unique in two ways. No other gene system has yet been described in which there is a physical rearrangement of nucleotide sequences during embryological development or cell differentiation. Moreover, the way in which Ig coding sequences are interrupted is unique. In other gene systems where the nucleotide sequences coding for the final translation product are interrupted by intervening sequences, the location of the intervening sequences bears

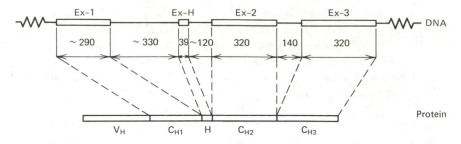

Figure 5-11 Arrangement of DNA sequences coding for components of the mouse γ_1 heavy-chain constant region. Sequences Ex-1, Ex-H, Ex-2, and Ex-3 code for the amino acid sequences of C_{H1}, the hinge region C_{H2}, and C_{H3} of the γ_1 chain, respectively. They are separated in the DNA by intervening sequences ranging in size from 120 to 320 bases. [From H. Sakano et al., Domains and the hinge region of an immunoglobulin heavy chain are encoded in separate DNA segments. *Nature 277*, 627 (1979). Copyright © 1979 by Macmillan Journals, Ltd.]

no discernible relation to structural or functional elements of the translation product. In the Ig gene system (with the exception of J and D segments), intervening sequences separate clearly defined structural, functional, and possibly regulatory elements. It is now established that discrete nucleotide sequences coding for individual mouse H-chain domains, as well as the hinge region, are also separated by intervening sequences (Figure 5-11). On the other hand, none of these intervening sequences shows up in the final Ig product. How and when are they removed?

The laboratories of Wall and of Perry were the first to show that the intervening sequences in mouse myeloma κ-light-chain genes are removed by RNA splicing. For example, the nuclear RNA precursors to κ mRNAs undergo two RNA splicing

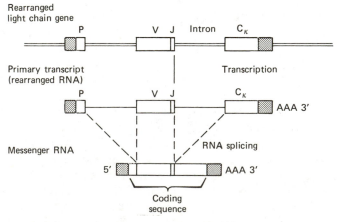

Figure 5-12 Processing of the primary transcript of the mouse kappa light-chain gene. (Courtesy of Dr. Randolph Wall, UCLA.)

events joining the leader peptide-V segments and V–C segments before emerging as the approximately 1250 nucleotide cytoplasmic mRNA (Figure 5-12). The separation of V and C sequences in the κ RNA precursor is the same as the estimated separation in the encoding DNA. The final RNA-splicing step appears to remove the V–C intron and brings the V and C regions into contiguity. Thus, as with other known eucaryote genes, the DNA sequences coding for immunoglobulin chains, including "intervening sequences," are all copied into a single transcript. The sequences not relevant to the final Ig structure are then processed out in a series of RNA splicing steps leading to translatable RNA, which contains information for the V and C regions plus the N-terminal leader peptide.

Allelic Exclusion

In Chapter 4 we encountered the phenomenon of allelic exclusion. This describes the situation in B cells in which the Ig genes of only one parental chromosome are expressed at the level of a surface-displayed or secreted immunoglobulin product. During B-cell differentiation, rearrangement occurs first in the H-chain family, and then in one of the L-chain families. One explanation for allelic exclusion could thus be that rearrangement only takes place on one parental chromosome. But how is one chromosome selected over the other? What would prevent rearrangement from taking place on the other?

In fact, we know that rearrangement quite often *does* occur on both chromosomes. Several studies have shown that in roughly one-third of the cases examined, the nonexpressed (in terms of appearance of membrane or secreted immunoglobulin) genes are, in fact, rearranged. However, in virtually every such case, the rearrangement is defective, usually the result of incorrect splicing. Such "nonproductive" rearrangements are almost never translatable. In the rare instances where two Ig products are translated and present in the cytoplasm, only one is displayed on the surface or secreted. The other could have some defect in structure that prevents glycosylation or other posttranslational processing.

It appears that one of the two chromosomes is randomly selected for rearrangement. If gene rearrangement and processing of the resulting mRNA and protein product proceeds normally, the system switches off. If rearrangement and/or processing is nonproductive, the cell starts to work on the second chromosome. It is likely that a significant number of "double faults" are produced, and indeed cells with two nonproductive rearrangements have been described. The fact that they are more rare than predicted may reflect the fact that they are not usually selected for, or that they are less viable than their normal counterparts.

The molecular mechanisms operating at these various steps are completely unknown. But the level of regulation displayed would seem to indicate rather sophisticated control mechanisms. Somehow, the gene-rearranging apparatus in the nucleus must decide whether or not the Ig chain has reached its appropriate destination: the cytoplasm for pre-B cell H chains; the membrane or exocytotic vesicles for mature B cell H and L chains. It must wait long enough to avoid an unneeded second rearrangement but must remain ready to go if needed. The whole phenomenon of allelic exclusion is one that needs more energy applied to its resolution than it has received in recent years.

V-Region Diversity

In the mid-1960s, when it had become clear that the variability in Ig primary structure resides in the NH_2-terminal portion of H and L chains, and that these V regions are coded for by separate genes, the stage was set for debating one of the most provocative questions in modern immunology: how is this variability generated? Very early in this debate, two opposite points of view emerged. One view (the germ-line theory) held that all of the V regions present in adult lymphoid cells are generated phylogenetically and are transmitted intact in the germ line. A corollary of this view would be that these genes are present in germ-line cells and probably all somatic tissues but are expressed only in differentiated lymphoid cells. The second view held that only a limited number of prototypical V-region genes is transmitted in the germ line, and that expansion and diversification of the inherited information occurs during ontogeny of the immune system (somatic mutation theory). A corollary of this hypothesis would be that the expanded V-region vocabulary is contained only in differentiated lymphoid cells, and not in germ-line or nonlymphoid somatic cells.

Powerful and persuasive arguments were developed in support of each of these theories during the 1960s and 1970s. Because it is now clear that the generation and expression of V-region diversity cannot be adequately explained by a strict application of either theory, we will not spend a great deal of time examining the supporting arguments for each. However, because the two theories fueled some of the more interesting immunological debates over the years, we will examine the stronger points made for each and then assess how each theory has done in light of our recent understanding of V gene coding and expression.

The major arguments for a germ-line model of V-region diversity originated from detailed comparative studies of the amino acid sequences of the NH_2-terminal portions of myeloma H and L chains. These sequences were generated from a number of laboratories, but detailed analysis and comparison of these sequences was carried out principally by Hood at Cal Tech and by Kabat at Columbia University. At first, these analyses focused on the first framework regions (FR-1) of the various chains studied. The assumption implicit in these studies was that V genes identical in FR-1 would be identical in the other framework residues as well. As we saw earlier, this was the rationale for assigning V regions to different groups. The existence of large numbers of V regions with nearly identical framework sequences (members of the same V-region group), found in every member of the species, had been considered by many to be incompatible with a somatic mutation theory. There were basically two arguments. If only a single gene for, say, κ-light-chain V regions is inherited and somatically mutated to produce the adult repertoire of requisite kappa V genes, how is one to account for the fact that the exact same set of V-region subgroups is found in every member of the species? This would imply the existence of a mechanism for closely guiding the somatic mutation process to produce always the same mutant gene products. Such a mechanism, or even a putative basis for it, is totally unknown. Germ-line advocates insisted that as a minimum there would have to be one germ-line gene for every distinct V-region subgroup. In the case of the mouse κ and H gene families, it is clear that identity in FR-1 is no guarantee of identity anywhere else in the molecule (Figure 5-13), and the number of subgroups already identified is approaching the numbers that might be postulated as necessary to deal with the antigenic universe. Thus further expansion by somatic mutation would appear to be of only limited value. The second

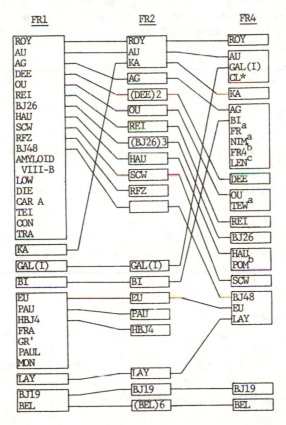

Figure 5-13 Proposed assembly of the frameworks of human V_κI chains from minigene sets. (a) human κ-light-chain subgroup II; (b) human κ-light-chain subgroup III; (c) human κ-light-chain subgroup IV. [Taken from E. A. Kabat, T. T. Wu, and H. Bilofsky, Variable region genes for the immunoglobulin framework are assembled from small segments of DNA—A hypothesis. *Proc. Natl. Acad. Sci. USA* **75**, 2430 (1978). Copyright © 1978 by E. A. Kabat.]

problem with a somatic mutation theory is related to the first. Because the framework regions of V genes appear to be highly conserved within and among individuals, it is clear that somatic mutation would have to be restricted to the hypervariable regions of V genes. Again, no rational genetic basis exists for such a process.

Another observation that gave strong support to a germ-line basis for the V-region diversity has to do with distribution and inheritance of idiotypes. A number of idiotypes in mice are found in virtually every member of an inbred strain, and sometimes even in members of different strains. Furthermore, in breeding experiments, these idiotypes are inherited in a simple Mendelian fashion. It is difficult to imagine that identical idiotypes could be so uniformly and faithfully reproduced by a process of somatic mutation from a single inherited precursor gene. In breeding studies, crossovers can even be observed among V_H-localized idiotypes, allowing a partial ordering of some of them in the genome. There are about 20 such idiotypes at present, but the number keeps increasing. It seems almost certain that they must represent germ-line gene sequences.

In the past few years, enough information about immunoglobulin gene structure, organization, assembly, and processing has been gathered that we can begin directly to assess actual and potential immunoglobulin diversity in the germ-line DNA. In the mouse, it would appear that both the κ and H families contain from 100 to 200 germ-line V-region gene segments. The λ family in mice is very limited in germ-line diversity and certainly contributes little to immunoglobulin diversity in the adult animal. During rearrangement of the germ-line elements necessary for assembly of a complete V gene, additional diversity can be generated in the third complementarity region (CDR-3) of both V_κ and V_H genes. In the κ family, if the 200 or so V_κ gene segments can recombine freely with the four functional J_κ elements, about 800 unique V_κ genes could be generated. Of course, we do not know that all combinations are allowed, and we do not know that all of the CDR3s thus generated would be available for interaction with antigen. On the other hand, the demonstrated and inferred imprecision of joining at the V-J interface is an additional factor for CDR-3 diversity, so the estimate of 800 different V_κ sequences does not seem unrealistic.

Similar arguments hold for germ-line diversity of V_H regions. Two hundred or so V_H segments combining randomly with the estimated 10 D and 4 J_H segments could produce as many as 8000 unique V_H genes. Variability at the site of V–D or D–J joining would expand this number considerably. Thus, assuming random association of H and L chains, there is easily enough information in germ-line DNA to account for 10 million different antibody molecules.

The principal early evidence in support of a somatic mutation mechanism for generation of V-region diversity was derived from hybridization studies using highly radioactive Ig chain mRNA or cDNA. These experiments suggested that nonimmune system DNA (presumed to be representative of germ-line DNA) contained one or at most a very few copies of DNA sequences hybridizing with V-region subgroup-specific probes. Hybridization data are, of course, subject to a number of uncertainties related to sensitivity and specificity, and, indeed, we now know from direct sequencing of germ-line DNA that most Ig families in both humans and mice have very large numbers of V-region sequences. On the other hand, rearrangments of V-region gene segments during lymphocyte maturation could legitimately be considered a form of somatic mutation, because it occurs well after fertilization. Final assembly of the V-region gene involves the splicing together of DNA segments coding for part of the structure of the third complementarily determining region, and as just noted leads to amplification of the possible antigen-combining specificities of the encoded V segments.

A further level of somatic variation has long been inferred from analyses of primary and secondary antibody responses. Many investigators had observed that the variety of V regions produced toward a particular antigen was greater in secondary (IgG) responses than in primary (IgM) responses. Inasmuch as this expansion of the V-region repertoire seemed to occur only after antigen stimulation, it was difficult to relate it to either direct germ-line variability or combinatorial variation.

Direct evidence for such additional somatic mutation in V_H sequences was recently obtained by Lee Hood's group. They compared the amino acid sequences of the first 100 positions of V_H regions of 19 independently derived mouse hybridoma and myeloma proteins capable of binding phosphorylcholine (PC) with mouse germ-line DNA sequences related to V_H regions associated with PC-binding sites. A total of four such genes was identified. However, all 19 V_H amino acid sequences were related to only one of these potential PC V_H gene sequences (T15). Ten of the hybridoma or myeloma proteins were identical with the T15-predicted sequence; nine differed by one to eight residues. Of a total of 24 amino acid differences distributed among the nine variants, about half were in CDRs and half in framework regions (Figure 5-14). The variant V_H sequences were all closer to the T15 germ-line DNA sequence than to any of the other V_H sequences and could not be accounted for by recombination of T15 V_H gene segments with any of the others. Strikingly, the V_H regions (positions 1 to 100) associated with IgM molecules were all identical with the germ-line coding sequence, whereas all of the IgG segments were variants of the germ-line sequence. About half of the IgA V_H segments were also variants.

Similar observations were made by Selsing and Storb in analysis of V regions and gene segments. They were able to show that two myeloma proteins expressing $V_{\kappa 167}$ variable regions could be accounted for by only one known germ-line V_κ segment. Both V_κ regions in the myeloma proteins differed from the germ-line gene sequence by several amino acids, and these could be accounted for by single base changes, involving both framework and complementarity-determining regions. As with the V_H regions studied by Hood's group, Selsing and Storb concluded that the amino acid changes occurred through single point mutations, and not through recombinatorial events in germ-line sequences. More recently, Tonegawa's group has also shown that about 30 known mouse $V_{\kappa 21}$ sequences are derived from about 11 germ-line V_κ genes.

These results provide a clear molecular basis for the observations made at the

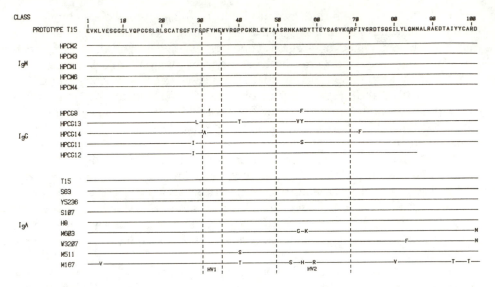

Figure 5-14 The V_H segment protein sequences of myeloma and hybridoma antibodies that bind phosphorylcholine. [From S. Crews, J. Griffin, H. Huang, K. Calame, and L. Hood, A single V_H gene segment encodes the immune response to phosphorylcholine: Somatic mutation is correlated with the class of antibody. *Cell 25,* 59–66 (1981).]

whole animal level on the expansion of the V-region repertoire after isotype switching. Although the consensus among most workers is that somatically generated differences reflect single nucleotide alterations, as opposed to recombinatorial events such as unequal crossing over, the exact mechanism by which the observed changes are introduced is not yet known.

Thus, in the end, both groups of theoreticians can claim at least partial victory. It is clear now from direct sequencing studies carried out with sperm DNA that large numbers of V-gene copies exist in germ-line DNA. These studies are still ongoing, and it is uncertain at present exactly how many copies will be found, but it is obvious that the more extreme forms of a somatic mutation theory, invoking one or at best a few V-region genes per family in germ-line DNA, are untenable. Most of the spectrum of hypervariable regions associated with so-called V-region groups were clearly generated phylogenetically, perhaps by genetic recombination events. On the other hand, it is equally clear that some degree of postconception somatic modification does take place. This can occur prior to antigen stimulation as the result of apparently random assembly of gene segments involving the third hypervariable region. A further, antigen stimulation-dependent generation of V region diversity also plays a role. The genetic basis for this latter mechanism will likely be the subject of considerable research over the next few years. As we noted earlier, direct germ-line diversity plus recombination of germ-line gene segments could provide as many as 10^7 different antibody-combining sites. If the somatic mutation events associated with the T15 family of V_H genes and peptides is at all representative, this capacity could well be increased by an additional factor of 10, for a total of possibly 10^8 different Ig molecules. Such a repertoire is well within the range of binding sites estimated on theoretical grounds to be necessary to deal with the antigenic universe.

Bibliography

General

Honjo, T., Immunoglobulin genes. *Annu. Rev. Immunol. 1,* 499 (1985).

Hood, L., J. Campbell, and S. Elgin, The organization, expression and evolution of antibody genes and other multigene families. *Annu. Rev. Genet. 9,* 305 (1975).

Hood, L., and D. W. Talmage, Mechanisms of antibody diversity: Germ line basis for variability. *Science 168,* 325 (1970).

Seidman, J. G., A. Leder, M. Nau, B. Norman, and P. Leder, Antibody diversity. *Science 202,* 11 (1978).

Valbuena, O., K. B. Marcu, M. Weigert, and R. P. Perry, Multiplicity of germline genes specifying a group of related mouse κ chains with implications for the generation of immunoglobulin diversity. *Nature 276,* 780 (1978).

Weigert, M., L. Gatmaitan, E. Loh, J. Schilling, and L. Hood, Rearrangement of genetic information may produce immunoglobulin diversity. *Nature 276,* 785 (1978).

Research

Alt, F., N. Rosenberg, R. Casanova, E. Thomas, and D. Baltimore, Immunoglobulin H chain expression and class switching in a murine leukemia cell line. *Nature 296,* 325 (1982).

Blomberg, B. et al., Organization of four mouse lambda light chain Ig genes. *Proc. Natl. Acad. Sci. USA 78,* 3765 (1981).

Brack, C., M. Hirama, R. Schuller, and S. Tonegawa, A complete Ig gene is created by somatic recombination. *Cell 15,* 1 (1978).

Capra, J. E., and T. J. Kindt, Antibody diversity: Can more than one gene encode each variable region? *Immunogenetics 1,* 417 (1975).

Cheng, H., F. Blattner, L. Fitzmaurice, J. Mushinski, and P. Tucker, Structures of genes for membrane and secreted murine IgD heavy chains. *Nature 296,* 410 (1982).

Crews, S., J. Griffin, H. Huang, K. Calame, and L. Hood, A single V_H gene segment encodes the immune response to phosphorylcholine: Somatic mutation is correlated with the class of the antibody. *Cell 25,* 59–66 (1981).

D'Eustachio, P. et al., Chromosomal location of structural genes encoding murine Ig λ chains. Genetics of murine λ light chains. *J. Exp. Med. 153* (1981).

Heinrich, G., A. Traunecker, and S. Tonegawa, Somatic mutation creates diversity in the major group of mouse immunoglobulin κ light chains. *J. Exp. Medicine 159,* 417 (1984).

Honjo, T., and T. Kataoka, Organization of immunoglobulin heavy chain genes and allelic deletion model. *Proc. Nat. Acad. Sci. USA 75,* 2140 (1978).

Kabat, E. A., T. T. Wu, and H. Bilofsky, Variable region genes for the immunoglobulin framework are assembled from small segments of DNA—A hypothesis. *Proc. Natl. Acad. Sci. USA 75,* 2429 (1978).

Kurosawa, Y., and S. Tonegawa, Organization, structure and assembly of Ig heavy chain diversity DNA segments. *J. Exp. Med. 155,* 201 (1982).

Kwan, S., E. Max, J. Seidman, P. Leder, and M. Scharff, Two kappa Ig genes are expressed in myeloma S107. *Cell 26,* 57 (1981).

Liu, C.-P., P. W. Tucker, J. F. Mushinski, and F. R. Blattner, Structure of the genes that rearrange in development, mapping of heavy chain genes for mouse immunoglobulins M and D. *Science 209,* 1348–1353 (1980).

Matthyssens, G., and S. Tonegawa, V and C parts of immunoglobulin κ-chain genes are separate in myeloma. *Nature 273,* 763 (1978).

Max, E., J. Battey, R. Ney, I. Kirsch, and P. Leder, Duplication and deletion of human ε genes. *Cell 29,* 691 (1982).

Mercola, M., X. Wang, J. Olsen, and K. Calame, Transcriptional enhancer elements in the mouse immunoglobulin H chain locus. *Science 221,* 663 (1983).

Nikaido, T., S. Nakai, and T. Honjo, Switch region of Ig Cμ gene is composed of simple tandem repetitive sequences. *Nature 292,* 845 (1981).

Sakano, H., R. Maki, Y. Kurosawa, W. Roeder, and S. Tonegawa, Two types of somatic recombination are necessary for the generation of complete immunoglobulin heavy-chain genes. *Nature 286,* 676–683 (1980).

Sakano, H., J. H. Rogers, K. Hüppi, C. Brack, A. Traunecker, R. Maki, R. Wall, and S. Tonegawa, Domains and the hinge region of an immunoglobulin heavy chain are encoded in separate DNA segments. *Nature 277,* 627 (1979).

Seidman, J. G., M. M. Nau, B. Norman, S.-P. Kwan, M. Scharff, and P. Leder, Immunoglobulin V/J recombination is accompanied by deletion of joining site and variable region segments. *Proc. Natl. Acad. Sci. USA 77,* 6022 (1980).

Selsing, E., and U. Storb, Somatic mutation of immunoglobulin light-chain variable-region genes. *Cell 25,* 47–58 (1981).

Tonegawa, S., A. M. Maxim, R. Tizard, O. Bernard, and W. Gilbert, Sequence of a mouse germ-line gene for a variable region of an immunoglobulin light chain. *Proc. Natl. Acad. Sci. USA 75,* 1485 (1978).

Valbuena, O., K. B. Marcu, C. M. Croce, K. Huebner, M. Weigert, and R. P. Perry, Chromosomal locations of mouse immunoglobulin genes. *Proc. Nat. Acad. Sci. USA 75,* 2883 (1978).

CHAPTER 6

Stucture–Function Relationships in Antibody Molecules

125

Immunoglobulins react with antigens through noncovalent interactions of particular amino acids in the antigen-combining site, with various combinations of chemical functional groups on the surface of the antigen called *antigenic determinants*. There is nothing mysterious about this particular reaction—it is governed by the same laws of thermodynamics as any other chemical reaction. A detailed study of antibody–antigen reactions has provided a major focus for immunology research during the past 40 years, both benefiting from and contributing to our evolving knowledge of how macromolecules interact. In this chapter we trace the threads of theory and experimentation that have led to our present understanding of how this most fundamental of immunological processes take place.

The Three-dimensional Structure of Antibody Molecules

The studies leading to the resolution of the structure of the immunoglobulin molecule described in Chapter 3 yielded an essentially linear, two-dimensional representation of what an antibody molecule might look like. Previously obtained hydrodynamic data had already suggested that immunoglobulins were reasonably compact, globular protein structures. Isolated Fab, F(ab)$_2$, Fc, and F$_v$ fragments also behaved as compact globular structures, suggesting conformational independence and integrity of these components of Ig molecules. At any rate, no one expected the actual conformation of Ig molecules in solution to look anything like the stick diagrams shown in Figure 3-5.

Both optical rotatory dispersion and circular dichroism studies, carried out in the early 1960s, suggested that Ig molecules had very little α-helical structure. Isolated Fab and Fc fragments also showed an absence of extensive α-helix, reinforcing the notion that these enzymatically generated subunits of Ig are conformationally independent. The primary amino acid structure of the hinge region made it seem likely, from what was known of protein structure generally, that there would be considerable segmental flexibility between the two Fab fragments and the Fc portion of the molecule. Thus, by the mid-1960s, most immunologists had inferred, from a wide variety of indirect biochemical considerations, that immunoglobulin molecules would be composed of essentially three compact, globular, conformationally independent units, separated by enzymatically labile sites, and essentially identical with the Fab and Fc fragments defined earlier by Porter (see Chapter 3).

These conclusions were confirmed and refined by more direct methods in the late 1960s and early 1970s. In 1967, Valentine and Green published the first electron micrographs of antibody molecules interacting with specific hapten. Since then, numerous EM studies have confirmed their original observations and conclusions, which are summarized in the legend to Figure 6-1.

The availability of crystallizable mouse and human myeloma proteins, and their enzymatically generated fragments, prompted X-ray crystallographers to undertake

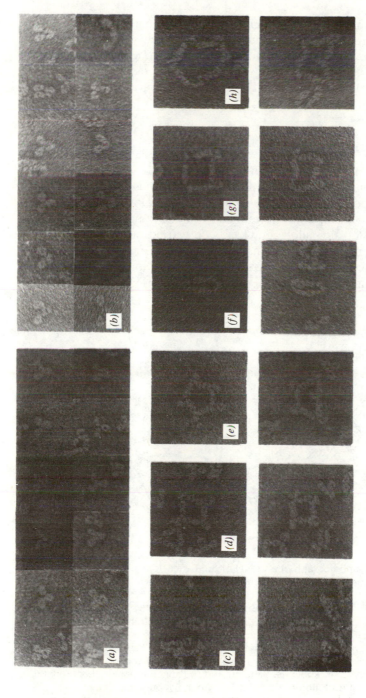

Figure 6-1 Electron micrographs of native and reduced/alkylated antibodies complexed to antigen. Shown are native and reduced monomers (a and b), dimers (c and f), trimers (d and g), and tetramers (e and h) of hapten-linked antibody. The antibodies were reduced under conditons affecting almost exclusively the hinge region interheavy chain disulfide bond. Such treatment has no discernible effect on the kinetics or extent of subsequent antibody–antigen complex formation, although it prevents binding of complement or fixation of the complexes to Fc receptors. In the native monomers, angles between the Fab arms vary from nearly 0° to nearly 180°. The lack of contact between the two C_{H2} domains is readily apparent in the reduced antibodies in all complexes; angles of separation between the C domains is essentially the same as between the Fab arms in native forms. [Electron micrographs courtesy of Drs. George Seegan and Verne Schumaker, Chemistry Department, UCLA ($\times$ 320,000).]

an examination of immunoglobulin structure beginning about 1970. These studies, especially the more recent high resolution (2 to 2.5 Å) analyses, have yielded not only information about the shape of Ig molecules and their fragments, but details of chain folding and domain interactions as well. Studies carried out in various laboratories have revealed different features of Ig structure. We review the more important of these in the following sections.

The Mcg Protein

The Mcg protein is a human $(\gamma_1)_2(\lambda)_2$ myeloma protein. It has been studied in two forms. The intact protein is missing the hinge region, and thus the molecule has no inter-H chain disulfide bonds, nor any H–L disulfide bonds. Interestingly, however, the L chains of the intact myeloma protein are disulfide bonded.

Although some X-ray crystallography has been carried out on the intact Mcg protein, some of the more useful information has come from a study of the Bence-Jones protein obtained from the same patient. In this protein, one of the two light chains assumes a conformation identical with the Fd region (V_H–C_{H1}) of the Mcg H

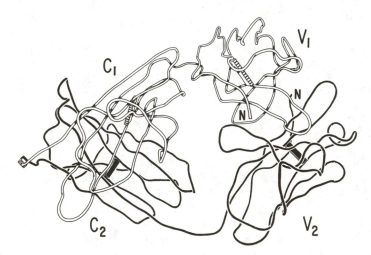

Figure 6-2 Tracing of a photograph of a model of the Bence-Jones dimer, with the polypeptide chains of monomers 1 and 2 shown in white and black, respectively. The solvent channel in which haptenlike molecules can be bound lies between the V domains on the right. The amino–terminal residue in each domain is labeled N, and the interchain disulfide bond between penultimate residues is located on the extreme left. Note the difference between the spatial relations of the V and C domains in the two monomers. Monomer 1 has a conformation similar to that in heavy chains of Fab (antigen-binding) fragments, whereas monomer 2 closely resembles the light-chain components. [From A. B. Edmundson, K. R. Ely, E. E. Abola, M. Schiffer, and N. Panagiotopoulos, Rotational allomerism and divergent evolution of domains in immunoglobulin light chains. *Biochemistry* 14, 3953–3961 (1975). Copyright © by the American Chemical Society, 1975. Reprinted with permission from the American Chemical Society and the author.]

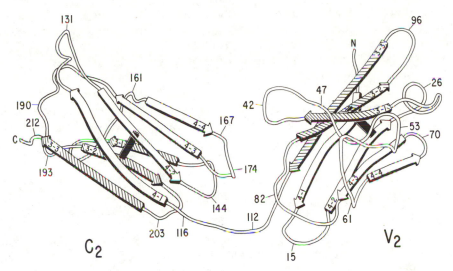

Figure 6-3 Schematic drawing of monomer 2, with directional arrows superimposed on segments participating in antiparellel β sheets. Three-chain layers are indicated by numbered striated arrows and four-chain layers by white arrows. Positions of representative residues are numbered to aid in the correlation of amino acid sequences with the three-dimensional structure. [From A. B. Edmundson, K. R. Ely, E. E. Abola, M. Schiffer, and N. Panagiotopoulos, Rotational allomerism and divergent evolution of domains in immunoglobulin light chains. *Biochemistry 14,* 3952–3961 (1975). Copyright © by the American Chemical Society, 1975. Reprinted with permission from the American Chemical Society and the author.]

chain (Figure 6-2). The interchain disulfide link is located in the COOH-terminal portions of the C regions of each λ chain. The V regions of the two chains lie farther apart from one another than do the C regions. The distance between the intrachain disulfide bonds of V_1 and V_2 is 24 Å, whereas the distance between the C region intrachain disulfides is 18 Å. Thus a well-defined cleft is formed between the two V regions, 15 Å at the mouth and 10 Å deep. The hypervariable regions of each V region are apposed along the lining of the cleft in such a way that binding of a ligand would certainly be possible, although the antigen specificity for protein Mcg is unknown.

Although the two λ chains are identical in sequence, their arrangement in space is significantly different. The distance between the intrachain disulfides in V_1 and C_1 is 25 Å; between V_2 and C_2, 43 Å. By comparison with data on "normal" Fab fragments, this would make the V_1C_1 monomer equivalent to the Fd fragment, and V_2C_2 would correspond to V_LC_L.

The amino acids in each domain are arranged in discrete pleated sheet structures (Figure 6-3). In the C domains, the polypeptide chain is arranged in two layers of antiparallel chain segments of about 12 to 15 amino acids each. The layers are about 9 to 10 Å apart and consist of four chain segments in one layer, and three in the other. The chain segments in the V region follow the same general plan but are more intertwined with one another. In both domains, the middle segment of the three-chain layer is connected by a disulfide bond to a parallel segment of the four-chain layer. The domains along the same chain (*cis* domains) are connected by an obviously exposed stretch of about four to six amino acids called the "switch region."

The C domains face each other at their four-chain surfaces, with the three-chain sheets facing "outside." In the V regions, the situation is reversed, and the three-chain sheets form the interdomain cavity. The hypervariable or complementarity-determining amino acid residues all lie within or very near this cavity.

Protein New

This protein is a Fab fragment of a human IgGl myeloma protein. It has been studied intensively by R. Poljak's laboratory since 1970. It consists of a λ light chain and a V_H-C_{H1} chain (Fd fragment) plus a few amino acids of the hinge region. The λ chain plus Fd fragment are each about $40 \times 25 \times 25$ Å. Within each chain, the V and C domains are separated by a short stretch of unfolded polypeptide chain ("switch region").

The amino acids in each domain are arranged in antiparallel folds of pleated sheet structures (Figure 6-4). Contact between C_{H1} and C_L, as in the Mcg protein, is along the four-strand β-pleated sheet faces. Amino acid residues along these strands tend to be evolutionarily conservative, suggesting that contacts between opposite domains are very critical for overall molecular integrity. This contact is very tight along most of the interface between the two, but loosens up somewhat as they approach the hinge region. The V regions are also arranged in antiparallel pleated sheets but contain one more fold than the C regions. Although the overall structures of each V and C domain within the λ chain and the Fd region are very homologous, the two domains are rotated at nearly right angles to one another along the axis of the chains. In the $V_H C_{H1}$ chain the angle is 80 to 85°, whereas along the λ axis the two domains are rotated about 100 to 110° out of alignment.

More recent analyses of protein New have shown that the interactions between V_H and V_L, and C_{H1} and C_L, are more extensive than those between V_H and C_{H1}, and V_L and C_L. The V_H-V_L domains interact principally through hydrophobic residues that are relatively invariant within V-region groups (and subgroups). The contacts between V_H and V_L are very close, nearly as close as those between C_{H1} and C_L. The cleft between the V_L and V_H domains is, in fact, quite shallow, about 15 Å wide by 6 Å deep. No hapten, antigenic determinant, or even solvent molecule can be accommodated beyond this shallow antigen-combining site, located at the tip of each Fab fragment. The amino acid residues involved in the hypervariable regions are all located on exposure bends of the pleated sheet polypeptide chains in the vicinity of the shallow groove. As far as can be determined, these regions also constitute the idiotypic determinants of protein New.

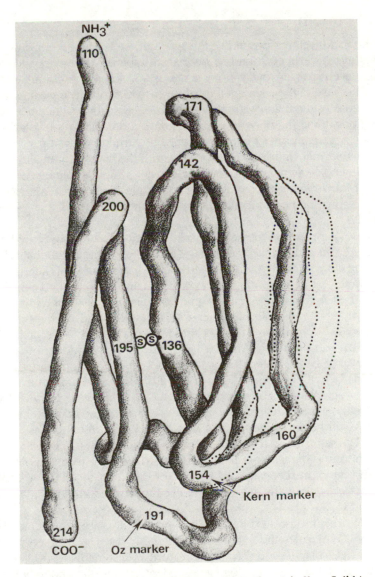

Figure 6-4 Diagram of the basic "immunoglobulin fold" of protein New. Solid trace shows the folding of the polypeptide chain in the constant subunits (C_L and C_{H1}). Numbers designate L (λ)-chain residues, beginning at NH_3^+, which corresponds to residue 110 for the L chain. Broken lines indicate the additional loop of polypeptide chain characteristic of the V_L and V_H subunits. [From R. J. Poljak, L. M. Amzel, H. P. Avey, B. L. Chen, R. P. Phizackerley, and F. Saul, Three-dimensional structure of the Fab fragment of a human immunoglobulin at 2.8-resolution. *Proc. Natl. Acad. Sci. USA 70*, 3305 (1973). Copyright © 1973 by the author (R. J. Poljak).]

The Kol Protein

Kol is a human myeloma protein of the IgG1 subclass. It is one of only a few Ig molecules that have been found to be crystallizable in the intact state. Most Ig molecules, even from a totally homogeneous myeloma source, are difficult to crystallize because of the segmental flexibility associated with the hinge region of the molecule. Most Igs that have been crystallized have subsequently been found to have deletions in the hinge region resulting in a more rigid molecular structure. Kol has an apparently intact hinge region, but turned out to be crystallizable. Nevertheless, segmental flexibility associated with the hinge region allowed the Fc region of the molecule to occupy several different positions in the crystal, making resolution of this region impossible. The enzymatically isolated Fc region of Kol, however, has provided considerable insight into the structure of this region of the Ig molecule.

The two C_{H3} domains of the Fc fragment are very closely apposed in the crystal, whereas the C_{H2} domains make no contact (Figure 6-5). This is rather similar to the usual pairing of V_H-V_L and C_H-C_L domains in Fab fragments. (This similarity is also reflected somewhat in the folding of the two domains. C_{H3} is folded almost exactly like C_{H1} in the Fab fragment. C_{H2} has some of the folding characteristics of a Fab V region.) In the intact Ig molecule, of course, disulfide bonds in the hinge region keep the two C_{H2} domains in a fixed position. The close apposition of the two C_{H3} domains is probably due to fairly extensive hydrophobic bonding of apolar residues; these have largely been replaced by more polar amino acids in the C_{H2} domain. This lack of inherent stable pairing of the C_{H2} domains is obvious in the electron micrographs of IgG molecules in which the hinge region disulfides are reduced (Figure 6-1), leading to a more open structure of the Ig molecule which is, nonetheless, still held together via noncovalent $C_{H3}-C_{H3}$ interactions.

C_{H2} and C_{H3} domains on the same H chain are folded in much the same way as V and C domains in Fab fragments and are separated by a four to six unfolded amino acid switch region. In reconstructed models of the intact molecule, there is very little or no contact along the axis of the molecule between V_H and C_{H1}, V_L and C_L, and C_{H1} and C_{H2}.

The three proteins just described (Mcg, New, and Kol) are representative of the spectrum of Ig molecules and fragments examined to date by X-ray crystallography. Although each displays unique structural features, presumably associated with either its unique function or phylogenetic pedigree, there are nonetheless a fair number of common features that seem to apply to most Ig molecules. The domain structure inferred from studies of the primary amino acid sequences and hydrodynamic properties of Ig molecules is immediately confirmed by even relatively low resolution crystallography. At higher resolutions, the domains come into sharp focus, and one can even see the small linear peptide segments (switch regions) that connect *cis* domains. Individual C-region domains show a highly conserved, nonrandom structural organization of folded polypeptides in the β-pleated sheet conformation (Figure 6-3). This pattern is discernible but somewhat more variable, as might be expected, in the V domains.

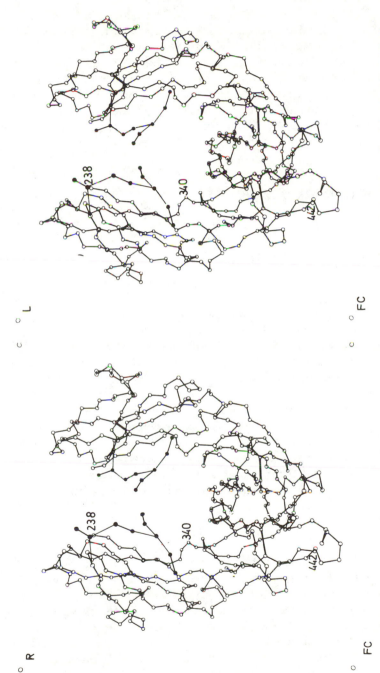

Figure 6-5 Stereo drawing of the C⁴ carbon positions and the centers of the carbohydrate hexose units of the Fc fragment of protein Kol. ●, Approximate centers of carbohydrate hexose units. The carbohydrate attachment site is Asn (297). ○, C⁴ carbon positons. The disulphide linkages are indicated. [From R. Huber, J Deisenhofer, P. M. Colman, M. Matsushima, and W. Palm. Crystallographic structure studies of an IgG molecule and an Fc fragment. *Nature 264,* 415 (1976). Copyright © 1976 by Macmillan Journals, Ltd.]

It is clear that there is no unique structure or shape for the antigen-combining site formed by a V_H-V_L pair. Although the limits of the antigen-binding site are dictated by the limits of the V domains, the site itself can vary from a large, well-defined cleft or groove between the two V regions, to a vaguely defined area at what is more or less the NH_2-terminal end of the antibody molecule. Most of the CD regions within a V domain are displayed on or in the antigen-combining site, but on occasion some CD regions may be buried deep inside the V domains, apparently inaccessible to antigen. (However, it cannot be ruled out that some such conformational aspects of Ig molecules may be related to packing restrictions in the crystalline form, and are thus more apparent than real.)

The Interaction of Antibody with Antigen

Thermodynamic Considerations

The interactions of antibodies and antigens are very similar in many respects to the interactions of enzymes with their substrates, with the important exception, of course, that antibodies do not significantly alter the primary structure of antigens. The binding of antigens by antibodies is effected as a result of interactions between chemical functional groups on the surface of the antigen with amino acid side groups in the antigen-binding site. These amino acids are predominantly associated with the hypervariable regions of the light- and heavy-chain NH_2-terminal domains or V regions.

No covalent bonds are formed or broken in the binding of antigens by antibodies. The types of forces involved in antibody–antigen interactions are essentially those that are important in enzyme substrate interactions: hydrogen bonds, electrostatic interactions, dipole-induced dipole interactions, and, of major importance in Ab–Ag reactions, the formation and disruption of hydrophobic associations. The following paragraphs briefly describe the contribution of these various forces to the overall energetics of the reaction.

Solvation

The ordering and disordering of water molecules around both antigen and antibody is an important factor in the thermodynamics of antigen–antibody interactions. Apolar groups involved in antigenic determinants, and apolar groups in the hypervariable regions that interact with antigenic determinants, can both cause adjacent water molecules to assume a highly ordered structure several layers deep. This results in an energetically unfavorable state, due principally to the decreased entropy of the ordered system. The $\Delta F°$ resulting from the formation or release of such waters of solvation become part of the overall $\Delta F°$ of the interaction of antibody and antigen.

Hydrophobic Bonds

The formation of hydrophobic bonds is a prime example of the importance of solvation in antibody–antigen reactions. The favorable gain of entropy realized by the intimate approximation of apolar groups, deriving from the release of a portion of the ordered water molecules, provides a major driving force for such associations, called hydrophobic bonds. Thus whenever such groups can be brought together within a distance less than the sum of their van der Waal's radii, hydrophobic bonds will form. For the interactions of moderately or highly apolar haptens with their appropriate binding sites, the net change in enthalpy is often insignificant, and the $-\triangle S$ realized constitutes the major element of the free energy change of the reaction.

Hydrogen Bonds

Whenever a hydrogen atom covalently linked to one electronegative atom can interact with the unpaired electron of a second electronegative atom, the system becomes more energetically favorable. The resulting stabilization of such associations are called hydrogen bonds. In antigen–antibody reactions the most important H bonds are O–H–O, N–H–N, and O–H–N. Although the energy of formation of such bonds is significant and can be measured, they do not contribute greatly to the free energy change of most antigen–antibody reactions. The reason for this is that such bonds are formed between antigen and water, and antibody and water, as well as between antigen and antibody. The former two classes of H bond are decreased during the reactions, whereas the latter category is of course formed for the first time. Thus the net energy change realized in the overall reaction is usually very minor when all such changes are algebraically summed.

Ionic Interactions

Coulombic attractions between oppositely charged groups do appear to play some role in the binding of antigens which, under the conditions of the reaction, have highly charged groups within the antigenic determinants. The antigen is presumably partially stabilized in the binding site by interactions with oppositely charged groups. Because both antigen and antibody charge groups will tend to cause some local stacking or ordering of water molecules, opposition of such groups when antigen is bound by antibody causes a modest increase in entropy. However, the decrease in energy thus gained is usually a relatively minor one in the overall thermodynamics of the reaction.

The Physical Chemistry of Antibody Molecules

Antibody Valence

The valence of an antibody refers to the maximum number of molecules of antigen that can be bound per antibody molecule, that is, the number of antigen-

binding sites per molecule. With our present detailed knowledge of immunoglobulin structure, the question of valence may seem academic. However, in
some cases the apparent, functional valence of an antibody may be different from the
actual valence of the immunoglobulin molecule involved. The method classically
used to determine the functional valence of antibody is equilibrium dialysis, illustrated in Figure 6-6. An inner chamber containing antibody is separated from the
outer chamber by a membrane that is impermeable to the antibody but allows free
exchange of smaller molecules between the two chambers. Thus, hapten added to
the system will quickly distribute itself on both sides of the membrane. If the hapten
does not interact with the antibody, the concentration of hapten in the two chambers
will be the same. However, if the antibody is able to bind the hapten, then at
equilibrium the total hapten concentration in the inner chamber will be higher than
in the outer chamber. The concentration of the free species of hapten will be the
same throughout the system, but the inner chamber will contain in addition a certain
amount of bound hapten. The concentration differential will be a function of the
valence and affinity of the antibody for the hapten. The number of molecules of
bound hapten will also be equivalent to the number of antigen-binding sites
occupied at equilibrium. This value will change as the concentration of hapten used
in the system is changed. A careful analysis of the amount of hapten bound at
equilibrium as a function of hapten concentration yields a great deal of information

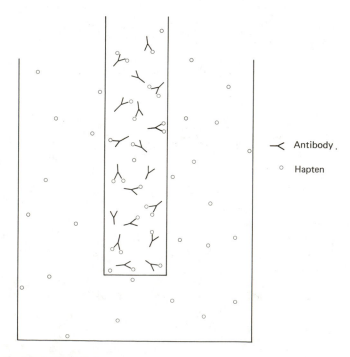

Figure 6-6 Equilibrium dialysis.

in addition to valence, and it is thus worthwhile to examine some of the theoretical aspects of this technique in detail.

The reaction in which a simple, monovalent hapten is bound by antibody can be defined by the equation

$$Ab + H \underset{k_2}{\overset{k_1}{\rightleftharpoons}} Ab \cdot H \tag{1}$$

where k_1 and k_2 are the rate constants for the forward and reverse reactions, respectively. The ratio of these two constants defines the equilibrium constant for the reaction:

$$Keq = \frac{k_1}{k_2} = \frac{[Ab \cdot H]}{[Ab][H]} \tag{2}$$

In order to analyze equilibrium dialysis data in terms of antibody valence, it is useful to alter Equation 2 to the form

$$K = \frac{b}{A_f \cdot c} \tag{3}$$

where K is the equilibrium or association constant from Equation 2 (which also, as we will see later, can be used to define the affinity of the binding site for antigen); b is the equilibrium concentration of bound hapten; c is the equilibrium concentration of free hapten; and A_f is the equilibrium concentration of unoccupied antigen-binding sites. A_f can be related to b by the following substitution:

$$K = \frac{b}{c(nA_t - b)} \tag{4}$$

where n is the number of binding sites per molecule of antibody (i.e., the valence), and A_t is the total concentration of antibody molecules in the system.

If we divide the numerator and denominator of Equation 4 by A_t, we can derive

$$K = \frac{b/A_t}{cnA_t/A_t - cb/A_t} \tag{5}$$

If we now set b/A_t, the ratio of moles hapten bound per mole antibody in the inner chamber, equal to r, Equation 5 becomes

$$K = \frac{r}{cn - cr} \tag{6}$$

which rearranges to

$$\frac{r}{c} = -Kr + Kn \tag{7}$$

Because r and c are variables in the system, and n and K are constants, Equation 7 will be seen to be a form of the slope-intercept formula for a straight line, $y = ax + b$, where a is the slope, and b the intercept on the abscissa. Thus a plot of r/c

versus r will give a line with slope $-K$, an intercept on the abscissa of Kn, and an intercept on the ordinate of n, which defines the valence of the antibody.

In practice, a constant concentration of antibody (A_t) is reacted with various concentrations of hapten, and the equilibrium distribution of hapten in the inner and outer chambers as a function of hapten concentration is determined. The molar concentration of free hapten in the outer compartment is c (Equation 3); r is the bound concentration of hapten in the inner chamber divided by the total antibody concentration (Equations 5 and 6).

Antibody Heterogeneity

A plot of r/c versus r (a form of the Scatchard plot) for the interaction of a single species of antigen-binding site (a monoclonal, monospecific myeloma protein) with a simple hapten is shown in Figure 6-7. In this particular case, the points obtained in the experiment define a straight line. However, when antibody isolated from serum is analyzed by equilibrium dialysis, even if it is specific for a small, monovalent hapten, the Scatchard plot is rarely a straight line function. Examples of plots obtained with samples of serum antibody are shown in Figures 6-8 and 6-9. Although the x-axis intercept is still always 2 (for IgG), the slope is a continuously changing function ranging from a high value for low values of c to lower values for high hapten concentrations. The variation of K values observed is a reflection of the fact that even the simplest hapten interacts with and induces the further production of more than a single species of antibody, each with its own characteristic affinity for the hapten.

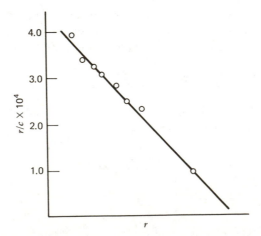

Figure 6-7 Scatchard plot of equilibrium dialysis date for an anti-DNP-specific myeloma protein. [Based on data presented in H. N. Eisen et al., A myeloma protein with antibody activity. *Cold Spring Harbor Symp. Quant. Biol. 32,* 75 (1967).]

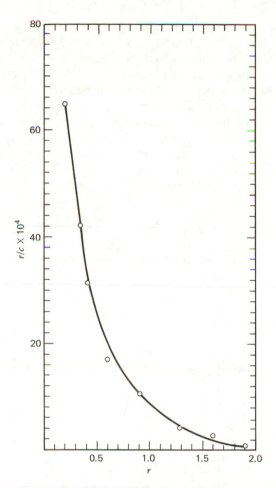

Figure 6-8 Scatchard plot for the binding of whole antiserum with a defined hapten. Calculated and plotted from data represented in J. Marrack and F. C. Smith, Quantitative aspects of immunity reactions. *Br. J. Exp. Pathol. 13*, 394 (1932).]

Affinity and Avidity

Affinity is the term used to describe the tendency of a single antigen-combining site to bind to a particular antigenic determinant. The term most often used to define affinity is simply the equilibrium constant K described in Equation 2 above. From Equation 7 we see that for divalent antibody such as IgG, $r/c = 2K - rK$. Thus, in addition to obtaining a value for K from the slope of the line in a Scatchard plot (Figure 6-7), K can also be obtained by reading the value of r/c on the ordinate when $r = 1$. In other words, for the interaction of a divalent antibody with a soluble, monovalent hapten or antigen, an "average affinity" value can be defined as the reciprocal of the free hapten concentration required to occupy half of the total antigen-binding sites. The range of values observed for K is shown in Table 6-1.

Some complex antigens, such as certain macromolecules, bacterial cell walls, or virus protein coats, are composed of closely packed, repeating antigenic determinants. Animal cell plasma membranes may also have closely packed, cross-reactive antigenic determinants. In such cases, both of the antigen-binding sites of the same antibody molecule are likely to interact with the same or adjoining structures. Once one site has attached to one determinant on the structure, in accordance with the parameter K, the probability of the second site interacting with an antigenic determinant is much higher than for the first. Furthermore, the probability of the anti-

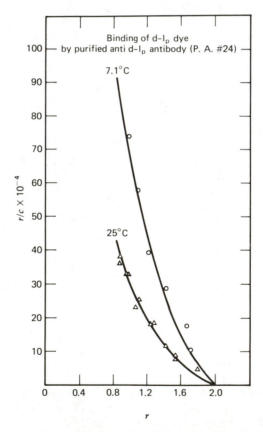

Figure 6-9 Scatchard plot for the binding of purified antibodies with a defined hapten. The solid line represents a theoretical curve based on the assumption of a Gaussian distribution of face energies of binding. Open symbols represent actual data points. [From F. Karush, The interaction of purified antibody with optically isomeric antigens. *J. American Chem. Soc.* **78,** 5519 (1956). Copyright by the American Chemical Society, 1956. Reprinted with permission from the American Chemical Society and the author.]

Table 6-1 Representative Affinities
of Antibodies for Different Types of Antigens

Antigen or ligand	$K_0(M^{-1})$	$T(°C)$
Gastrin	2.7×10^{11}	4
Fluorescein	6×10^{10}	22
Insulin	1.7×10^{10}	37
Digoxin	1.7×10^{10}	24
Vasopressin	4.5×10^{9}	4
Angiotensin	4.3×10^{9}	25
N^ϵ-Dnp-lysine	3×10^{9}	25
Staphylococcal nuclease	8.3×10^{8}	25
Slac-ALME	2.2×10^{8}	25
Ovalbumin	2×10^{8}	1.5
Hexasaccharide	3.2×10^{5}	4
Octasaccharide	1.25×10^{5}	25
Lactose	0.97×10^{5}	25

Adapted from F. Karush, The affinity of antibody: Range, variability, and the role of multivalence. In G. W. Litman and R. A. Goods, eds., *Immunoglobulins* Plenum Publishing Corp., New York (1978). The affinity values shown are defined for the indicated temperatures.

body as a whole dissociating from the structure is much less than the probability of one site dissociating from a single determinant—on the order of 10^{-4}. This increased combining power of a multisite antibody with a multideterminant antigen is generally referred to as avidity. It has recently been suggested, however, that "avidity" has been used in such a large variety of contexts, not always related to thermodynamic parameters, that its precise meaning has been obscured. The term "functional affinity" has been suggested to distinguish the overall preference of a multivalent antibody for its antigen, from that of a single combining site for a particular hapten or determinants (intrinsic affinity).

Free Energy of Antibody–Antigen Reactions

We have seen how the technique of equilibrium dialysis can be used to determine the valence of an antibody molecule. Another value that results from a typical Scatchard plot (Figure 6-7) is K, the equilibrium constant. K can be related to the standard free energy change, $\Delta G°$, resulting from an antibody–antigen interaction by the equation.

$$\Delta G° = -RT \ln K \tag{8}$$

where R is the gas constant and T, the absolute temperature. If K is measured at two different temperatures for a fixed concentration of antibody and antigen, the standard free enthalpy change can be obtained from the van't Hoff equation

$$\frac{d \ln K}{dT} = \frac{\Delta H^\circ}{RT^2} \qquad (9)$$

which can be altered and integrated to the more useful form

$$\log_{10} \frac{K_2}{K_1} = \frac{H^\circ (T_2 - T_1)}{2.303 R T_2 \cdot T_1} \qquad (10)$$

K_1 and K_2 are the equilibrium constants measured at temperatures of T_2 and T_1, respectively. It is preferable in practice to obtain K at a number of different T values. A plot of K versus $1/T$ will then give a line of slope $-\Delta H^\circ/R$. (For important exceptions to this simple relationship, see the previous section "Antibody Heterogeneity.")

Using the value for ΔG° obtained from Equation 8, and for ΔH° as just described, a value for the standard entropy change, ΔS°, can be derived from the relationship

$$\Delta G^\circ = \Delta H^\circ - T \Delta S^\circ$$

Theoretically, therefore, by determining the value of K at several different values for T, and applying this information to Equations 9 and 10, one can obtain the free energy differential driving the association of antibody and antigen. In fact, however, the situation is not quite so simple and ideal in real situations, because only in rare instances is the antibody population one is dealing with homogeneous.

Antibody Specificity

One of the most remarkable features of antibody–antigen reactions, especially to early workers in the field of immunology, is the high degree of specificity observed in many binding reactions. Landsteiner, in the early part of this century, demonstrated that relatively slight modifications of haptens (the term hapten was actually coined by Landsteiner) could dramatically alter their ability to be bound by antibody. Such experiments helped to create a general notion that there are specific antibodies whose exclusive function is to interact with a particular antigen. Indeed, Pauling promoted the rather short-lived notion that individual antibodies are formed in response to a specific antigen by molding themselves around it, essentially using the antigen as a sort of template. This adaptive theory of antibody formation was soon abandoned when it became clear that antibodies, as protein molecules, are assembled *de novo* on ribosomes in response to strict genetic control.

If antigen-antibody reactions are to be understood, it is necessary to abandon any and all teleologic notions about one-to-one relationships of the two molecules. The interaction of an antigen with an antibody will occur if and only if such an interaction is energetically favorable. One of the cardinal dogmas of immunology is that the genetic information coding for the structure of antigen-binding sites is generated completely independently of antigen, at least in the sense that antigen is in any way specifically instructive. At the time an antigen enters the body, a fixed repertoire of potential antigen-combining sites is present on the surface of lymphocytes able to produce antibody. Each lymphocyte is able to produce only that single antibody represented on its surface. If a particular antigen can combine with an existing surface antibody molecule, a reaction will occur (which, as we will see in Chapter 13, leads to further production of that species of antibody).

A particular antigenic determinant may interact with a number of representative combining sites, some more strongly than others, depending on the precise arrangement of amino acid residues within the site. This point is best illustrated from studies in which immunologists screened myeloma proteins for antigen-binding capacity. In analyzing the ability of nearly 350 myeloma proteins for the ability to bind the hapten DNP, Herman Eisen and his co-workers derived the information shown in Figure 6-10. They plotted the proportion of myeloma proteins binding DNP as a function of the affinity with which DNP was bound. A few of the myeloma proteins bound DNP with an affinity within the range of values seen in conventionally induced antibody ($K \geq 10^6$). However, at lower affinity values, the number of myeloma proteins binding DNP increases dramatically. When all affinity values are considered, the proportion of myeloma proteins binding DNP is in the range of 10 to 20%.

These data raise an interesting point. Clonal selection theory predicts that the

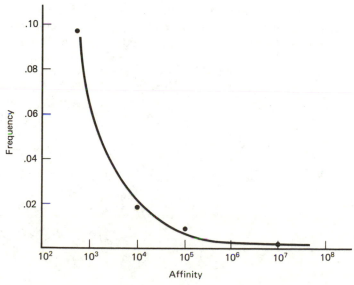

Figure 6-10 The frequency of human myeloma proteins binding DNP as a function of the affinity with which they bind it. [Based on data presented in H. Eisen et al., *Federation Proceedings*, **29**, 78 (1970).]

frequency of antibody specificity for any given antigen, within the repertoire of total antigenic specificities, should be at least approximately inversely proportional to the size of the antigenic universe. Clearly, DNP is not 10 or even 1 percent of the antigenic universe. On the other hand, an affinity of $K = 10^3$ or 10^4 for any antigen is probably not physiologically relevant. The problem is similar to the one molecular biologists face in deciding the stringency conditions for nucleic acid hybridization reactions. How strictly does one nucleic acid sequence have to bind to another in order to infer sequence homology? Here we must ask: At what point in the affinity spectrum is an antibody an antibody? An antibody that binds DNP with an affinity of $K = 10^4$ or so would very probably interact with a different antigen (antigen X) with a higher affinity. Should we then call that antibody "anti-X," "anti-DNP," or both or neither? This gets at the very heart of the definition of antibody specificity. (When an antibody produced in response to one antigen binds a second antigen with a higher affinity, immunologists refer to the second reaction as "heteroclitic.")

Can a single antibody combining site bind more than one antigen? There is ample experimental evidence to support a positive answer. Eisen's lab studied a myeloma protein called MOPC 315, and found that it bound ε-DNP-lysine with a value of $K = 10^7$, a moderately good affinity (Figure 6-11). The same myeloma bound menadione (2-methyl-1,4 naphthoquinone) with an affinity about 15-fold lower, which would be at the very low but probably real end of affinity values for physiologically relevant antibody–antigen reactions.

Because menadione blocked the ability of DNP-lysine to bind to MOPC 315, Eisen postulated that the two molecules, although chemically dissimilar, competed for the same amino acid residues within the binding site. Rosenstein studied another myeloma protein that also bound both of these haptens and presented evidence that they bound to separate parts of the binding site. Whichever view is

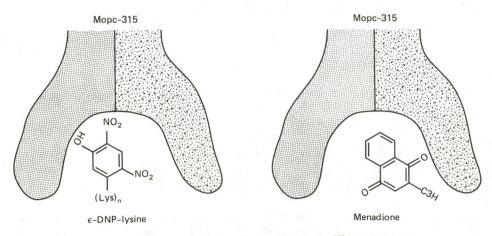

Figure 6-11 The same antigen combining site can bind two different haptens.

correct (perhaps both are, because two different myeloma proteins were studied), these and other studies suggest strongly that more than one biochemical moiety may interact in an energetically favorable manner with the amino acids in a single antigen-binding site. This can really only be seen in a monoclonal antibody population. In an antiserum, composed of many different antibodies binding to the various parts of a given antigen, the different secondary cross-reactivities of each individual antibody are generally not measurable.

Types of Antibody Reactions

The Precipitin Reaction

In many cases, the interaction of antibody and antigen will lead to the formation of an insoluble complex. This happens when antibody and antigen form a cross-linked network or "lattice," which subsequently comes out of solution. Thus a minimal requirement for precipitation is that the antigen molecule involved be at least bivalent, with the individual antigenic determinants sufficiently separated as to accommodate interaction with binding sites on two different antibody molecules. In reality, precipitation usually occurs when large, multivalent antigens interact with a corresponding collection of specific (but heterogeneous) antibodies.

The precipitin reaction is a way of quantitating the amount of antibody present in the serum of an immunized animal. The principal of the precipitin reaction, which essentially involves a titration of antibody by antigen (or vice versa), is shown in Figure 6-12 for the reaction of antibody with a multivalent protein antigen. In the case shown, a fixed amount of antiserum is added to a series of reaction tubes, and to each is added a varying amount of antigen. In the excess antibody zone (prozone), the amount of antigen–antibody precipitate increases with increasing antigen up to some maximum value that defines an equivalence zone. Addition of more antigen actually leads to a decrease in the amount of precipitate formed (excess antigen zone).

An explanation of the zone differences in precipitation is provided by Marrack's lattice theory. When antibody is in excess in the experiment shown in Figure 6-12, complete saturation of each antigen molecule with an antibody is assured. Because most common protein antigens do not have repeats of the same determinant on an individual molecule, an antibody molecule will usually cross-link two different antigen molecules, rather than attach both binding sites to the same molecule. Depending on the concentration of antigen and antibody, complex three-dimensional cross-linked structures will build up with time. The molar ratio of antibody to antigen in the precipitate will vary, depending on the valence of the antigen, but will usually be about 3:1. There will be free antibodies but no free antigens in the supernate of the reaction in this zone.

As more antigens are added, leading up to the equivalence zone, it continues to react with the excess antibodies, and to form lattices. However, as the equivalence

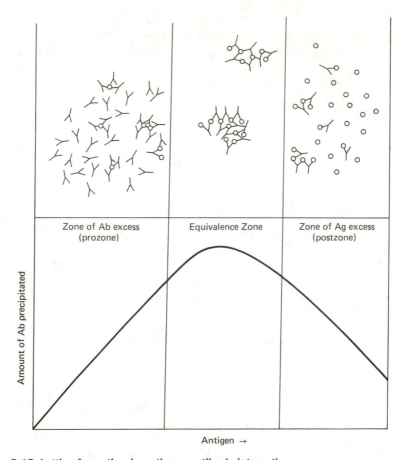

Zone of Ab excess
(prozone)

Equivalence Zone

Zone of Ag excess
(postzone)

Amount of Ab precipitated

Antigen →

Figure 6-12 Lattice formation in antigen–antibody interactions.

zone is approached, the likelihood of each antigen molecule being completely saturated by antibody decreases, due to the competition of antigen determinants for the fixed number of antigen-combining sites. When equivalence is finally reached, by definition there is neither free antibody nor free antigen detectable in the supernates (except for equilibrium dissociation quantities).

As still more antigens are added, the ratio of antibodies to antigens in the precipitates continues to decrease. This is represented in the lattice by individual antigen molecules interacting with fewer and fewer antibody molecules. Nevertheless, for a time, all antigen molecules continue to be cross-linked by antibodies, and a precipitate still forms. However, when the antibody:antigen molar ratio nears unity, the lattice fails to form as individual antigen molecules fail to interact with more than one combining site. This results in the formation of soluble complexes, and both antibody and antigen appear in the supernatant solution (in complexes). In the region of further antigen excess, the theoretical limit of 0.5 is reached in antibody:antigen ratio, beyond which all antigens added remains free in the supernatant. In practice, free antigens may appear in the supernates much earlier, since statistically some antigen molecules will be in higher-order complexes and others will be unreacted.

There are two probable factors contributing to the formation of a physically distinct solid phase (precipitate) during antibody—antigen reactions. First of all, as antibodies (and, in the case of many globular protein antigens, antigens as well) are brought into close intimate contact with one another in a lattice network, hydrophobic protein—protein interactions are fostered. This can lead to reduced interaction with solvent and decreasing solubility. Second, as the size of the complexes increases, they begin to sediment by gravity to the bottom of the tube. This occurs independently of the formation of a physically separate phase, and is accounted for by the volume term in the expression for sedimentation rate $[V(\rho - \rho_0)g]$. Both of these processes (size and hydrophobicity) may be enhanced by the binding of complement to the Ab · Ag complex.

Not all interactions of antibodies and antigens lead to precipitation. Very small, unideterminant antigens form single antibody plus single or double antigen complexes, and can only be precipitated using a second antibody directed against the first. Some antigens may have more than one antigenic determinant but are still too small in size to be easily cross-linked. Larger, more complex antigens that are highly charged may also not be precipitated by antibody, presumably because electrostatic repulsion overcomes the tendency to form hydrophobic complexes. Finally, complexes may not be formed with low affinity antibody, because the concentration of antigen required to drive the binding reaction places the system in the excess antigen zone.

Immunodiffusion

One very useful application of the precipitin rection is in the immunodiffusion technique, based on a method originated by Jacques Oudin but developed by Ouchterlony and often named after him. In this method, the precipitin reaction is carried out essentially in two dimensions rather than three, and in a semisolid medium rather than in solution. As a result, additional information about both antigen and antibody can be obtained.

The basic ideas underlying Ouchterlony immunodiffusion are shown in Figure 6-13. A shallow layer of agar is placed in the bottom of a Petri dish. A well to hold a small volume of antiserum is cut in the center of the dish, and varying numbers of wells to hold samples of antigens are arranged radially around the center well. Depending on concentration and, to some extent, molecular size, antigens and antibodies begin diffusing toward one another at varying rates. At any given moment in time, there will be a concentration gradient extending from each well out to the leading edge of its diffusing component. When two gradients cross, a precipitate will form as a zone for equivalence is established. When both antibodies and antigens are fairly homogeneous, this results in the formation of a visibly observ-

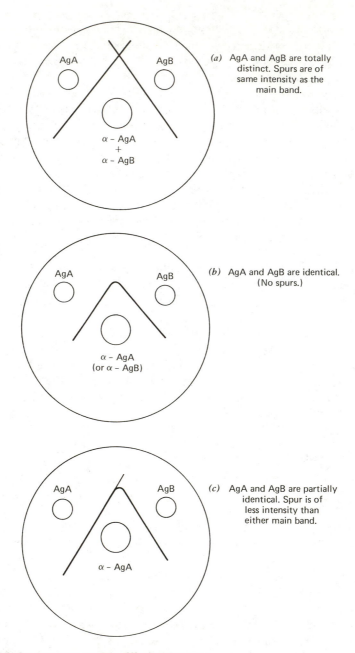

(a) AgA and AgB are totally distinct. Spurs are of same intensity as the main band.

(b) AgA and AgB are identical. (No spurs.)

(c) AgA and AgB are partially identical. Spur is of less intensity than either main band.

Figure 6-13 Ouchterlony double diffusion patterns.

able precipitin line at some point between the two wells. The position of the line between the two wells depends on the relative concentrations of the two reactants in the wells.

A number of kinds of specialized information can be obtained by this type of immunodiffusion analysis. If exactly the same antigen sample is placed in two adjoining wells, the pattern obtained in Figure 6-13*b* is seen. The reason that a portion of the line has disappeared in each case is that the concentration of antigen at the point of intersection of the lines is double that at the front of each line, because of the overlapping radii of diffusion. This region is thus like the zone of antigen excess of a standard precipitin curve. The situation becomes considerably more interesting if the antigen in one well is only partially identical to the antigen in the other well. For example, two phylogenetically related proteins may share some antigenic determinants but have others that are unique. Figure 6-13*c* shows what happens when two such antigens are run against an antibody made against only one of them. The precipitin line formed by the antibody and its specific antigen (A) crosses beyond the line formed by the antibody and the related antigen (B). The reason for this is that all the determinants on B, that are recognized by the antibody, are also on A. At the point of intersection of the two lines, these common determinants go into antigen excess, and the precipitate will not form. However, there are some determinants on A that are not present on B. These determinants are at equivalence all the way along the precipitin line formed between A and anti-A, and thus the anti-A versus A line crosses beyond the anti-A versus B line. This small spur is usually less dense than the main precipitin line, because the amount of antibodies in the anti-A population that react only with these determinants is small compared to the whole anti-A population.

Immunoelectrophoresis

Another analytical application of the precipitin reaction, which combines immunodiffusion with electrophoresis, is immunoelectrophoresis. This method, developed by Curtis Williams and Pierre Grabar in the 1950s, is particularly useful for analyzing samples containing mixtures of many different antigens, because the antigens are first physically separated on the basis of charge before analysis by immunodiffusion. The most common application of this technique has been in the identification of serum components (Figure 6-14). The sample is placed in a round well cut in agar (usually plated on a microscope slide) and subjected to electrophoresis. The various serum components spread out along the axis of the applied current. Immediately after the electrophoresis step is finished, the sample is developed by filling the trough with an appropriate antiserum. As in standard immunodiffusion, the antigens and antibody(ies) diffuse toward one another and form precipitin lines at the respective equivalence zones. The curvature of the lines does not so much reflect differences in molecular weight, but the fact that the various antigens moved through the current as more or less elongated spots.

Standard immunoelectrophoresis, as developed by Williams and Grabar and others, was a major breakthrough in the analytical separation and identification of serum proteins, as well as proteins in the urine, ascites, and various other body fluids. It is still routinely used in the analysis of fluids associated with specific disease states. However, the results obtained with this method are essentially only qualitative. An attempt at quantitating immunoelectrophoresis, as well as improving the resolution of individual components, was introduced by Clarke and Freeman in 1968 (Figure 6-15). This technique involves simple electrophoresis in agarose in one direction, as in the Grabar method, followed by electrophoresis at right angles through agar impregnated with the developing serum. The gel is then stained either with a nonspecific protein stain, or with staining reagents specific for selected proteins. The area under a particular peak is proportional to the concentration of that protein in the fluid studied, and inversely proportional to the concentration of specific antibody in the antiserum used for the second-dimensional electrophoresis. Although absolute quantitation is not usually practical with this technique, very good relative quantitation can be achieved by comparison of the test sample with a standard reference sample.

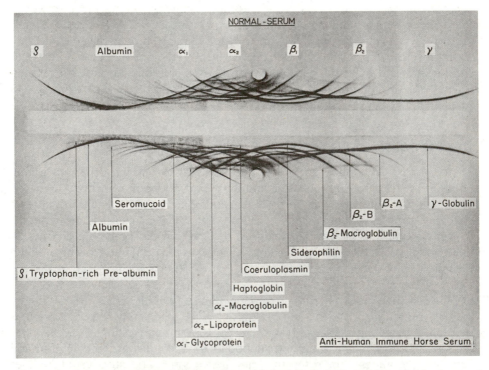

Figure 6-14 Immunoelectrophoretic pattern obtained by first electrophoresing human serum, and then developing with antihuman immune horse serum. [From Philip L. Carpenter, *Immunology and Serology,* Third Edition (1975). Copyright © 1975 by the W. B. Saunders Company, Philadelphia, PA]

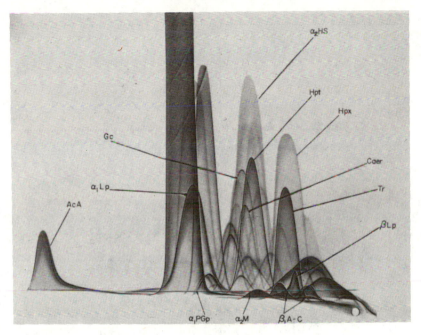

Figure 6-15 Two-dimensional immunoelectrophoresis. [From H. G. Minchin Clarke and T. Freeman, Quantitative immunoelectrophoresis of human serum proteins. *Clinical Science* 35 (1968). Copyright © 1968 by H. G. Minchin Clarke.]

ELISA Assays

A recently introduced immunoassay technique that has rapidly been adapted to a wide range of applications is the *enzyme-linked immunosorbent assay* (ELISA). One very common use of this technique, to screen B-cell hybridomas for antibody production (see pp. 74–77), is illustrated in Figure 6-16 (Scheme 1).

The antigen for which the desired monoclonal antibody should be specific is coupled to the bottom and walls of a microtiter well. In many cases, the antigen will spontaneously adhere to the plastic used to fabricate the microtiter plates. In other cases, the antigen may need to be coupled to the plastic by chemical means. Each antigen-coated assay well is then filled with the supernate from a hybridoma well previously scored as "positive," based on microscopic detection of cell proliferation (Figure 4-7). If the hybridoma supernate contains a monoclonal antibody specific for the bound antigen, the antibody will adhere to the bottom and sides of the microtiter well. The wells are then washed several times with buffer to remove unbound antibody, and each well is filled with a buffer containing a second antibody that is specific for the first antibody. This second antibody has attached to it an enzyme that catalyzes a colorimetric reaction. For example, if, as is usually the case, the hybridomas being screened are murine, then the monoclonal antibody pro-

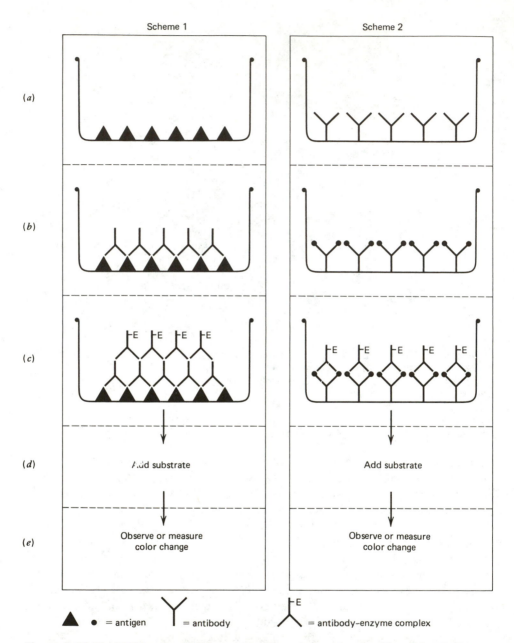

Figure 6-16 The ELISA assay. ELISAs are usually carried out in microtiter plates. Each plate, about 3 $\frac{1}{2}''$ × 5′, contains 96 wells, each of which holds about 0.2 ml. Scheme 1 illustrates the sequence of steps in one of these wells during an assay to detect the presence of a particular *antibody*. Scheme 2 is an ELISA designed to detect the presence of a particular *antigen*.

duced (which binds to the antigen in the microtiter well) would be murine, and so a good second antibody would be goat or rabbit anti-mouse immunoglobulin. The enzyme coupled to this second antibody is usually either horseradish peroxidase, alkaline phosphatase, or β-galactosidase. The only requirements for this enzyme are that it still functions when coupled to the antibody and that it converts a colorless substrate to a colored product. After washing away unbound second antibody, the wells are filled with a reaction buffer containing colorless substrate for the enzyme, plus any necessary cofactors. Those wells in which the specific monoclonal antibody was present in the added supernate will accumulate the colored product of the enzymatic reaction. An entire plate of 96 wells can be scanned visually, or read on an automated plate scanner connected to a computer, in a matter of minutes. As a refinement of this particular assay, the enzyme-linked second antibody can be selected on the basis of reactivity with specific classes or subclasses of murine immunoglobulin. The assay will then not only tell which hybridomas are synthesizing and secreting Ig, but which class or subclass of Ig.

The basic principle of the ELISA, illustrated by this example for detecting mono-clonal antibody production, has been used in a wide range of assays. In another version of the ELISA (Figure 6-16, Scheme 2), one can couple a specific antibody to the microtiter wells, and use this to scan samples for the presence of a particular antigen (e.g., in blood or urine). Samples are incubated in the antibody-coated wells for a period of time, after which unbound sample is removed by washing. A second antibody is then added which also reacts with the antigen.[1] This second antibody is coupled to an appropriate enzyme. As before, substrate for the coupled enzyme is then added to each well. If the sample originally added to a given well contained the specific antigen, then the second antibody will bind to that well, leading ultimately to a positive colorimetric reaction.

ELISA microtiter plates precoated with either antigens or antibodies used in many common assays are now available commercially. Machines are available that can read and record data from 100 or more plates per hour. The ease of use of the ELISA, combined with its extraordinary capacity for processing large numbers of samples, has made this one of the most commonly used immunoassay systems, particularly in clinical laboratories.

Radioimmunoassay (RIA)

The most precisely quantitative application of the precipitin reaction is the RIA. This technique was first developed by Yalow and Berson in the late 1950s, and led

---

[1]This is a good example of when a monoclonal antibody system may *not* be advantageous. Since most antigenic determinants are present only once per antigen molecule, the first and second antibodies must *not* be identical. Although it is certainly possible to have two different monoclonal antibodies for the first and second antibodies, each recognizing a different determinant, the simplest thing to do is to use the same pool of antibodies from whole antiserum for both antibody 1 and antibody 2, since whole antiserum contains a spectrum of antibodies.

to a Nobel prize in medicine in 1977. The methodology is now fairly simple and straightforward (Figure 6-17) but requires that a sample of the material to be tested be available in a highly pure form, and that it can be labeled either synthetically or by secondary derivatization with a radioactive isotope. The amount of radioactive antigen required to just saturate a standard amount of specific antiserum is first determined. To these standard amounts of reactant are added (concomitantly) varying amounts of unlabeled, highly purified antigen. Because the antibodies do not distinguish between radioactive and nonradioactive antigen, the two compete on an equal basis for available antibody-combining sites. In practice, the antibody–antigen complexes formed in the reaction are usually brought down with a second antibody, for which the first antibody is the specific antigen (double antibody method). The amount of radioactivity in the precipitate plotted versus the amount of unlabeled antigen yields a standard curve (Figure 6-16). In an actual experiment, a volume of unknown is added to the reaction system in place of the volume of unlabeled standard antigen. From the degree of displacement of radioactivity from the final RIA precipitate, the amount of antigen in the unknown can be determined by reference to the standard curve.

Reactions of Antibodies with Cells

Antibodies have several types of reaction with cells bearing antigenic determinants that are of practical or theoretical interest. Antibodies may be used to cross-link and clump (agglutinate) cells in suspension, causing them to settle out very rapidly; they may be used to sensitize cells for subsequent lysis by complement or lymphoid cells; or they may be used to induce redistribution of cell surface antigenic molecules (patching and capping).

Agglutination Reactions

Almost any free-living cell type, whether microbial or animal (i.e., red blood cell, lymphocytes, etc.), can be agglutinated by antibodies directed against surface antigens. If clumping is caused by the cell-specific antibody itself, the process is called direct agglutination. If a second antibody, directed against the first, is used to cause agglutination, it is called indirect or passive agglutination.

As with the precipitin reactin, lattice formation accounts in a general way for the formation of complexes between antibody and the obviously multivalent cells. Clumps do not form in regions of antigen excess, probably because not enough bridges are formed to stabilize individual cell–cell associations. Like precipitation of many soluble antigens, agglutination of whole cells is also usually inhibited in regions of antibody excess. The basis of this phenomenon, called the prozone effect, is not clear. It is probably due to the fact that as an antigen-combining site dissociates from the cell or bacterium, it it more likely to be replaced by a free antibody molecule, rather than one already bound to another cell. Another possible explanation is the presence of low affinity "blocking antibody" in serum, which

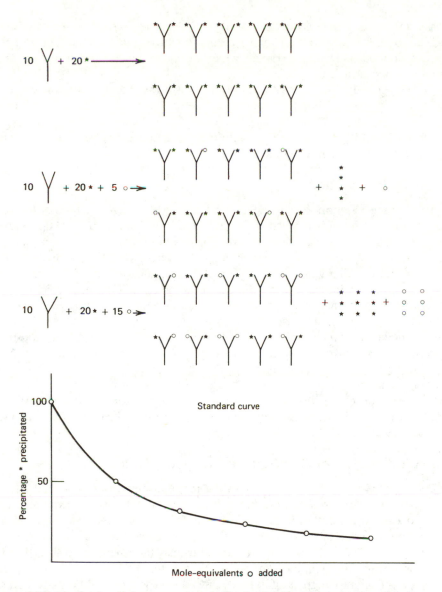

Figure 6-17 Idealized radioimmunoassay. Antibody (Y) is first titrated with radioactive antigen (*) such that essentially 100 percent of * is brought down in the absence of cold antigen (o). In many assays, precipitation is accomplished by a second antibody directed against the first antibody. In practice, less than 100 percent of * may actually be precipitated; this presents no problem, as long as the amount precipitated is fairly reproducible between assays. When o is added together with Y and *, o competes with * for available binding sites on Y, leading to displacement of * from the final precipitate. A plot of known amounts of o added to the reaction leads to a standard curve, which can be used to determine the amount of o in an unknown sample.

masks cell surface antigens but does not cross-link cells effectively. The presence of such antibodies is suggested by experiments in which cells incubated in prozone levels of antibody fail to clump rapidly when washed and incubated in agglutinating antibody concentrations.

Passive agglutination reactions can be used as a rapid test for the presence in serum of antibodies to a wide range of antigens. The antigen to be tested for is coupled to the surface of red blood cells; the ability of the test serum to agglutinate the derivatized RBC can be detected with the unaided eye, bypassing the need for sophisticated equipment or chemicals.

Cytolytic Reactions

The binding of antibodies to living cells can set the stage for lysis of the sensitized cells by one of two mechanisms. IgM antibodies, and most IgG antibodies, can, when complexed with antigen (including cell-bound antigen) fix complement (for a detailed discussion of complement, see Chapter 8). The terminal components of the complement cascade can cause disruption of the cell membrane, leading to osmotic imbalance and cell death. In the case of bacteria, coating (sensitization) by antibody may lead to cytolysis (gram negative bacteria), or may make the bacteria susceptible to phagocytosis (gram positive bacteria) (Chapter 16). The second method by which antibody bound to the surface of cells can lead to destruction of those cells involves not complement but cells as the cytolytic agent. Certain lymphoid cells possessing a receptor for the Fc region of Ig molecules can bind to antibody-sensitized cells through the Fc region of the sensitizing antibody, and lyse the cell by a process called antibody-dependent cell-mediated cytolysis (ADCC). This process may be important in tumor and transplant rejection reactions (see Chapters 19 and 20).

Redistribution of Cell Surface Antigenic Molecules

The interaction of antibodies with a wide range of membrane-associated molecules can lead to the cross-linking and redistribution of the latter. Various stages in this process are illustrated in Figure 6-18. Antibodies directed against a specific membrane molecule are conjugated with a fluorescent label such as fluorescein isothiocyanate (FITC). These labeled antibodies may then be reacted directly with the cells bearing the antigen (*direct staining reaction*). If the density of surface antigen is sufficiently high, a diffuse pattern of fluorescence will be discerned on the cell membrane immediately after staining. Immunoglobulin on spleen B cells is an example of a surface molecule that can be analyzed by direct staining. If the temperature is kept low during observation in the microscope, or if the initial pattern of fluorescence is fixed with a substance such as glutaralydehyde, this diffuse pattern will remain. By focusing down onto the periphery of the cell, the fluorescence is seen as an intense, uninterrupted *ring,* because depth of field of the microscope objective allows a sizable vertical portion of the membrane at the sides of the cell to be viewed. In unfixed cells, the smooth, diffuse pattern of fluores-

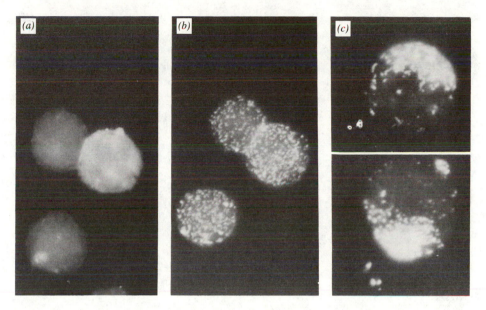

Figure 6-18 Antibody-induced redistribution of the H-2K (histocompatibility) protein antigen of EL4 tumor cells. (a) The native distribution of the H-2K protein was assessed by fixing the cells first with glutaralydehyde, then staining with fluoresceinated mouse anti-H-2K^b IgG. (b) The H-2K proteins were patched by reacting the cells first without mouse anti-H-2K^b, then with fluoresceinated rabbit antimouse IgG, all steps in the presence of sodium azide. (c) The H-2K proteins can be capped at 37°C by omitting the sodium azide in the procedure described in b.

cence breaks up with time to form *patches,* which eventually coalesce at one point on the cell to form a *cap.*

The details of the cellular and molecular mechanisms underlying the patching and capping phenomenon have been extensively reviewed and are beyond the intended scope of this book. However, some aspects of this phenomenon can be mentioned here. The process of patching is relatively energy independent, and is affected principally by the fluid state of the membrane lipids. It requires for its initiation that the membrane molecule be multivalent (i.e., cross-linkable), and probably represents a form of localized precipitin reaction in the plane of the membrane. The aggregation of patches into caps is energy dependent, and, in most cases, dependent on submembranous cytoskeletal elements. The cap is either shed from the surface of the cell or endocytosed.

Most membrane proteins are present in too low a concentration to be susceptible to analysis by direct staining methods. Problems arise because the intensity of fluorescence is too low to permit adaquate observation, and because the greater average distance between individual identical proteins may inhibit cross-linking and aggregation of antibody. In these cases the double-antibody or *indirect stain-*

ing reaction is used. The cells are reacted first with an unlabeled antibody specific for the membrane protein in question. A second antibody, conjugated with FITC and specific for the first antibody, is then reacted with the antibody-cell complex. The pattern of fluorescence seen in such cases is usually somewhat different from that seen in the direct staining method. The initial distribution of fluorescence seen is often patched rather than diffuse. This could be due to any or a combination of several causes: a truly patched distribution of the protein in the native membrane; patching induced by the first antibody, detected only upon application of the second (labeled) antibody; or, rapid patching induced by the second antibody itself. At least in the case of mouse histocompatiblity (H-2) proteins, the initial patchy distribution of fluorescence observed in the double antibody technique is produced as a result of either the first or second antibody and does not represent the true distribution of this protein in the membrane (Figure 6-18).

Bibliography

General

Kabat, E. A., *Structural Concepts in Immunology and Immunochemistry,* Second Edition, Holt, Rinehart and Winston, New York (1978).

Karush, F., The affinity of antibody: Range, variability, and the role of multivalence." In G. W. Litman and R. A. Good, eds., *Immunoglobulins* Plenum Publishing Corp., New York (1978).

Marrack, J. R., *The Chemistry of Antigens and Antibodies,* H. M. Stationery Office, London (1934).

Origins of Lymphocyte Diversity. *Cold Spring Harbor Symp. Quant. Biol. 41* (1976).

Richards, F. F., W. H. Konigsberg, R. W. Rosenstein, and J. M. Varga, On the specificity of antibodies. *Science 187,* 130 (1975).

Yalow, R. S. Radioimmunoassay: A probe for fine structure of biologic systems. *Science 200,* 1236 (1978).

Research

Amzel, L. M., R. Poljak, F. Saul, J. Varga, and F. Richards, The three-dimensional structure of a combining region-ligand complex of immunoglobulin NEW at 3.5 Å resolution. *Proc. Nat. Acad. Sci. USA 71,* 1427 (1974).

Clarke, H. G. M., and T. Freeman, Quantitative immunoelectrophoresis of human serum proteins. *Clin. Sci. 35,* 403 (1968).

Eisen, H., M. Michaelides, B. Underdown, E. Shulenberg, and E. Simms, Myeloma proteins with antihapten antibody activity. *Federation Proceedings 29,* 78 (1970).

Grabar, P., and C. A. Williams, Methode immunoelectrophoretique d'analyse de melanges de substances antigeniques. *Biochim. Biophys. Acta 17,* 67 (1955).

Huber, R., J. Deisenhofer, P. M. Colman, M. Matsushima, and W. Palm, Crystallographic structure studies of an IgG molecule and an Fc fragment. *Nature 264,* 415 (1976).

Landsteiner, K., *The Specificity of Serological Reactions,* Harvard University Press, Cambridge (1945).

Poljak, R. J., X-ray diffraction studies of immunoglobulins, *Adv. Immunol. 21,* 1 (1975).

Poljak, R. J., L. M. Amzel, H. P. Avey, L. N. Becka, D. J. Goldstein, and R. L. Humphrey, X-ray crystallographic studies of the Fab and Fc fragments of human myeloma immunoglobulins. *Cold Spring Harbor Symp. Quant. Biol. 36,* 421 (1971).

Poljak, R. J., L. M. Amzel, H. P. Avey, B. L. Chen, R. P. Phizackerley, and F. Saul, Three-dimensional structure of the Fab[1] fragment of a human immunoglobulin at 2.8-Å resolution. *Proc. Natl. Acad. Sci. USA 70,* 3305 (1973).

Pollock, R. R., and M. F. Mescher, Murine cell surface immunoglobulin: Two native IgD structures. *J. Immunol. 124,* 1668 (1980).

Rajan, S. S. *et al.,* Three-dimensional structure of the Mcg IgGl immunoglobulin. *Molecular Immunology 20,* 787 (1983).

Richards, F., W. Konigsberg, R. Rosenstein, and J. Varga, On the specificity of antibodies. *Science 189,* 130 (1975).

Rosenstein, R., R. Musson, M. Armstrong, W. Konigsberg, and F. Richards, Contact regions for DNP and menadione haptens in an immunoglobulin binding more than one antigen *Proc. Natl. Acad. Sci. USA 69,* 877 (1972).

Saul, F. A., L. M. Amzel, and R. Poljak, Preliminary refinement and structural analysis of the Fab fragment from human Ig New at 2.0 Z. *J. Biol. Chem. 253,* 585 (1978).

Schiffer, M., R. L. Girling, K. R. Ely, and A. B. Edmundson, Structure of a λ-type Bence-Jones protein at 3.5 Å resolution. *Biochemistry 12,* 4620 (1973).

Seegan, G. W., C. A. Smith, and V. N. Schumaker, Changes in quaternary structure of IgG upon reduction of the interheavy-chain disulfide bond. *Proc. Natl. Acad. Sci. USA 76,* 907 (1979).

Valentine, R. C., and N. M. Green, Electron microscopy of an antibody-hapten complex. *J. Mol. Biol. 27,* 615 (1967).

CHAPTER **7**

Complement

The humoral branch of the immune response, as we have described it so far in terms of antibodies and antigens, would at best be only partially effective in protecting the host from disease and harmful substances in the environment. Antibody alone cannot destroy a bacterium, although it can opsonize it for more efficient phagocytosis (Chapter 16). Although an antibody can combine with soluble foreign molecules, it is not in itself very efficient in triggering the elimination of foreign matter from the bloodstream. Many of the biological functions of antibodies require the participation of a group of 11 proteins known collectively as complement.

History

The study of complement began in the earliest years of the study of immune reactions generally. In 1889, Buchner reported that certain bacteriolytic properties of immune serum were lost by heating to 55°C. He called this heat-labile activity alexin. This phenomenon was described more precisely by Pfeiffer in 1894. He showed that the loss of bacteriolytic activity in immune serum could be restored by the addition of nonimmune serum, even though the nonimmune serum by itself had no bacteriolytic properties. The activity of the reconstituting component in nonimmune serum was found to be destroyed by heating to 55°C. Thus the process of bacteriolysis was shown early on to require two components: a heat-stable factor found only in immune serum and a heat-labile factor found in both immune and nonimmune serum. Pfeiffer suggested that only the heat-labile component be called alexin. Pfeiffer later showed that the heat-stable component of immune serum, although unable by itself to lyse bacteria *in vitro,* could be used passively to transfer bacterial immunity to other animals.

Jules Bordet extended Pfeiffer's observations to red blood cells (Figure 7-1), and also reached the conclusion that immune serum contains two components involved in bacteriolysis. The first, a heat-stable substance from immune serum which he termed the "substance sensibilatrice," sensitized cells in some way for the action of the heat sensitive alexin, which he felt was analogous to a "ferment," or enzyme. Ehrlich showed a short time later that it was, indeed, the sensitizing substance (immune body, or antibody) that had specificity for the target cell,

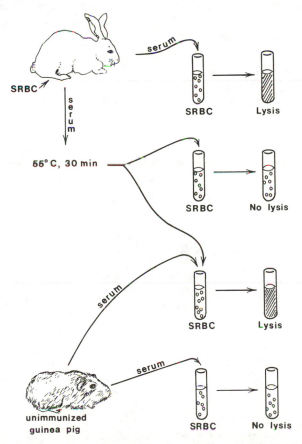

Figure 7-1 Bordet's experiment demonstrating the requirement for complement (alexin) in immune lysis of SRBC. Serum from a rabbit immunized with SRBC will, by itself, lyse target SRBC and release hemoglobin. However, if the serum is first heated to 55°C for 30 minutes, the hemolytic capacity is lost. Lysis can be restored by the addition to the reaction of serum from a nonimmune guinea pig, which by itself has no hemolytic activity.

whereas alexin (which Ehrlich suggested be called complement) had no target specificity but could bind to almost any antibody complexed with an antigen. Thus it was also established early on that antigen-antibody complexes had two kinds of binding sites: one for antigen and one for complement (Figure 7-2).

Bordet's work with red blood cells, their antibodies (hemolysins), and complement led in 1901 to his description of the complement fixation assay, one of the earliest and for many years one of the most useful immunological assay techniques (Figure 7-3). This assay, in addition to its usefulness as a research tool for the detection of antibody, is also the basis of a number of commonly used clinical diagnostic techniques. A standard aliquot of complement is established which contains just enough complement to lyse a set number of red blood cells previously coated with antibody (sensitized red blood cells). An antibody–antigen reaction is then carried out in this complement aliquot. As Ab · Ag complexes form, they bind complement. On centrifugation of the resultant precipitate, the bound complement sediments with the Ab · Ag complexes. When the complement remaining in the supernate is tested in the standard complement assay against sensitized red blood cells, its capacity to mediate lysis is reduced in proportion to the amount of Ab · Ag complex formed in the test reaction.

An interesting aspect of complement, related to its ability to lyse red blood cells,

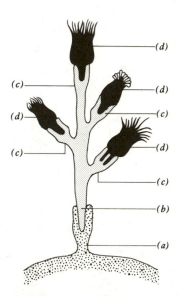

Figure 7-2 Ehrlich's view in 1906 of the relationship between antibody, antigen, and complement. (a) Cell surface receptor, which he equated with antibody. (b) The antigen molecule. (c) Antigen-localized receptors for complement. (d) Complement molecules of various types. This very early view wrongly ascribed the complement binding sites to the antigen portion of the antibody–antigen complex but correctly inferred the existence of more than component of complement.

CONTROL   **EXPERIMENTAL**

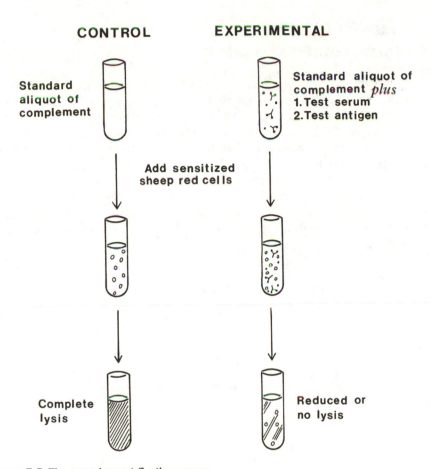

Standard
aliquot of
complement

Standard aliquot of
complement *plus*
1. Test serum
2. Test antigen

Add sensitized
sheep red cells

Complete
lysis

Reduced or
no lysis

Figure 7-3 The complement fixation assay.

is that complement from one species always lyses red cells of another species better than its own. For example, guinea pig complement works much better than rabbit complement in facilitating lysis of antibody-sensitized rabbit erythrocytes. Similarly, rabbit complement works better than mouse complement in facilitating lysis of mouse red blood cells. The reason for this is not well understood but may represent an adaptive-protective mechanism to escape from nonspecific autolysis of red cells by endogenous complement.

The major site for synthesis of the various components of complement is in the liver, although significant amounts are also produced by macrophages. The latter may be important in the progress of local inflammatory reactions involving macrophages (Chapter 17). The synthesis of complement components, particularly C3–C9, is assumed to be under the influence of sex hormones. Serum concentrations of these components is about 10 times higher in males than in females, and the levels can be manipulated by hormone therapy in both mice and humans.

The Classical Pathway of Complement Activation

We now know that complement is actually 11 different proteins in the serum, and not a single factor as earlier workers assumed. The first six components of the classical pathway (Figure 7-4) form a cascade system of zymogens; each component, when activated, becomes an enzyme (a serine protease) that modifies the next component in the pathway. The final five components (C5b–C9) assemble in stoichiometric fashion to form the membrane attack complex. It is this complex that is responsible for the lytic activity initially associated with complement. However, some of the intermediate products of activation, at various points in the activation sequence, have important biological functions. We will look briefly at each of the components of this pathway in terms of biochemistry and, where appropriate, biological function.

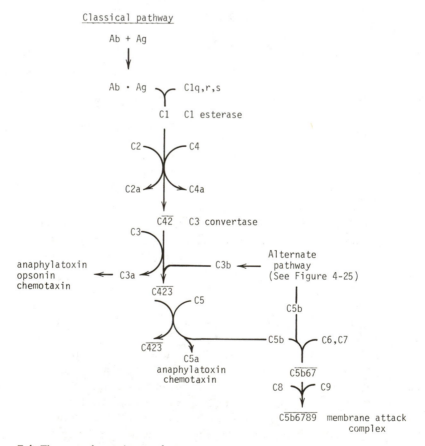

Figure 7-4 The complement cascade.

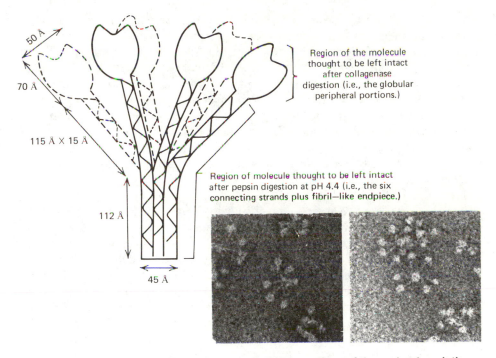

50 Å

70 Å

115 Å × 15 Å

Region of the molecule thought to be left intact after collagenase digestion (i.e., the globular peripheral portions.)

Region of molecule thought to be left intact after pepsin digestion at pH 4.4 (i.e., the six connecting strands plus fibril—like endpiece.)

112 Å

45 Å

Figure 7-5 Proposed model of human C1q. —indicates portions of the molecule pointing toward reader; ———indicates portions of the molecule pointing inward, away from the reader. ~ and ~ indicate collagenlike regions of the molecule proposed to be in triple helix. From the dimensions given, the following comparison can be made: length of collagenlike fiber + fibril-like end piece = 115 + 112 = 227 Å. Length of triple helix proposed from sequence studies = 78 × 2.9 = 226 Å. [Taken from K. B. M. Reid and R. R. Porter, The structure and mechanism of activation of the first component of complement. *Contemp. Topics Mol. Immunol.* 4, 1–22 (1975). Copyright by the Plenum Publishing Corporation, 1975. Electron micrograph of purified C1q molecules (×240,000), courtesy Drs. George Seegan and V. Schumaker, Chemistry Department UCLA.]

C1

C1 is actually composed of three distinct molecules, called, respectively C1q, C1r, and C1s. For a brief time it was believed that a fourth component, C1t, also existed, but this is now known not to be the case. The three component molecules are held together by a Ca^{2+}-dependent bond, and under normal physiological conditions exist only as the complex. The assembled complex exists as a pentamer of the composition $C1qr_2s_2$, which has an average diameter of 300 Å and a molecular weight of 750,000.

C1q is the subcomponent that interacts directly with the Fc portion of μ and γ chains (Figure 7-5). C1q is composed of 18 polypeptide chains arranged into six subunits. Each subunit is composed of a collagenlike stalk, and a globular, 105 residue head. Although the individual peptides that form the approximately 80 amino acid trimeric stalk structure are very similar to the peptides in true collagen trimers, there is sufficient difference to suggest they are coded for by different genes. The globular head structures contain the Fc binding sites. Each subunit is capable of binding to one Fc region. The mechanism by which C1q is activated through binding to a site in the C_{H2} domain of an Fc region of IgM or IgG is unknown. Although C1 complexes will bind to free Ig molecules, activation in such cases is extremely low. Activation is very efficient when C1 binds to IgM or IgG complexed to particulate antigen (usually cell bound). Activation will also occur, although with somewhat less efficiency, when C1 binds to heat-aggregated Ig or Ig that has been chemically cross-linked.

It has been proposed that the crucial event in C1q activation is the binding of C1q at more than one Fc site on a fixed surface or in a precipitin complex. Such multifocus binding would be more avid than binding to single (uncomplexed) Ig molecules and could induce conformational changes in C1q resulting in its activation. This could explain the observation that one molecule of antigen-complexed IgM can form a stable complex with one molecule of C1, whereas more than one molecule of IgG is required. IgM, having five C1q binding sites per molecule, could form a much tighter complex with C1. This can be crucial on the surface of animal cells, where antigenic determinants may be separated somewhat. In such cases the membrane must be sufficiently fluid to allow the determinants to move about and bring two IgG molecules into proximity so that C1q can bind.

C1r and C1s are present in serum as zymogens. As long as Ca^{2+} is present, they spontaneously associate into a $C1r_2C1s_2$ dimer, which in turn associates with one molecule of C1q through sites on C1r. The activation of C1r is rather complex. When $C1r_2s_2$ binds to activated C1q, a conformational change is induced in one of the C1r molecules converting it to an active enzyme. This conformationally activated C1r cleaves the second C1r molecule into two fragments (56K and 27K). The smaller fragment is itself an enzyme that in turn cleaves the first C1r molecule into 56K and 27K pieces. The two C1r 27K subunits then attack and cleave the two C1s chains into similarly sized 58K and 27K chains. The smaller subunits of activated C1s in the activated C1qrs complex ($C\bar{1}$) act on the next component in the pathway, C4.

The autocatalytic step in C1r activation has been observed to occur spontaneously *in vitro*. It occurs in direct proportion to the amount of $C1qr_2s_2$ formed, which is a function of concentration of the individual reactants. However, this only occurs using isolated and purified C1q, r, and s. When normal serum is added to the reaction mixture, association of the C1 complex is inhibited, and no spontaneous activation can be detected.

C4 and C2

C4 and C2 are the next two components activated in the classical pathway. They are considered together because they are both activated by the $C\bar{1}s$ portion of $C\bar{1}$, and act as a complex ($C\overline{42}$) in the activation of the next component, C3.

C4 has a molecular weight of about 2×10^5, and is composed of three subunits: α (93,000 daltons), β (78,000 daltons), and γ (33,000 daltons) that are disulfide bonded. These chains are derived from a single pro-C4 peptide. The α peptide is the substrate for $C\bar{1}s$. A small fragment is released (C4a; MW 8500), which has recently been shown to have moderate levels of anaphylactic activity (see C3a, C5a below). During this process, an internal thioester is cleaved, generating a transiently reactive carboxyl group on the rest of the molecule (C4b) that can become esterfied with hydroxyl groups on a nearby cell surface. Hydrophobic sites may also be exposed on C4b, further stabilizing its interaction with the membrane. The same C4 cleavage step exposes a site on the α chain of C4b for binding of C2. Once C2 is bound to C4b, it is cleaved by $C\bar{1}s$ into two fragments, C2a and C2b. The larger of these, C2a, is the form of C2 that remains with C4b to form $C\overline{42}$.

The activation of C4 by $C\bar{1}$ is one of the principal amplification points in the complement cascade. The molar concentration of C4 in serum is about 5 to 10 times that of C1, and because $C\bar{1}$ is fairly stable, a single molecule of $C\bar{1}$ can activate several hundred, and perhaps several thousand, molecules of C4. About 90 percent of the C4b fragments generated do not bind to either the membrane or C2a fragments and are rapidly degraded in solution. Nevertheless, each Fc region-C1 complex on the membrane may generate up to 100 or 200 $C\overline{42}$ complexes.

In addition to the site of C4b that allows it to bind to the membrane to which antibody and $C\bar{1}$ are attached (the target cell), a second membrane-binding site is also exposed during C4 activation. This second site is recognized by various cell types bearing C4b receptor sites. These sites are present on many different cell types including granulocytes, macrophages, lymphocytes, and erythrocytes. C4b generated either in a soluble immune complex or on the surface of a cell or virus can bind to C4b receptors, leading to the deposition of the entire antibody-antigen-complement complex on the cell surface. In the case of cells with phagocytic activity, this triggers engulfment of the deposited complex. The process of preparation of foreign matter for engulfment by phagocytic cells is called *opsonization*. (See also Chapter 16.) The significance of attachment of these complexes to non-phagocytic cells such as lymphocytes and red blood cells is not clear.

The function of C4 in the $C\overline{42}$ complex is simply to anchor the complex to the cell membrane and to bind C2; it has no enzymatic function. Activated C2 in the $C\overline{42}$ complex acts as an enzyme in the hydrolytic activation of C3 (the complex is thus referred to as C3 convertase). The C2a component of $C\overline{42}$ is rapidly inactivated, making $C\overline{42}$ relatively unstable with time.

C3 and C5

The C3 component of complement is the natural substrate for $C\overline{42}$. C3 is a globular protein synthesized in the liver and also by macrophages and monocytes. It is composed of two peptide chains, α and β, which are disulfide linked and are generated from a single-chain precursor by posttranscriptional cleavage. The α chain has an estimated molecular weight of 110,000: the β chain is approximately

75,000 daltons. $C\overline{42}$ cleaves a small fragment (C3a; MW 9000) from the NH$_2$-terminal portion of the α chain. As in the cleavage of C4, a thioester group is activated on the remaining fragment (C3b) which allows it to interact with cell surfaces. Like the C4b fragment, most of C3b fails to attach to the membrane, and is degraded in solution. C3b also contains a site that allows immune complexes, both soluble and cellular, to bind to cells bearing C3b receptors. The distribution of C3b receptors among cell types is the same as C4b receptors.

C3b attaches to the target cell membrane in the vicinity of $C\overline{42}$, forming a complex $C\overline{423}$. This complex acts as an enzyme that has C5 as its substrate.

C5 is similar in size and structure to C3. It has an α chain of about 115,000 daltons, and a β chain of about 75,000 daltons. Its activation by $C\overline{423}$ also involves liberation of a small peptide (C5a) from the NH$_2$-terminus of the α chain. The larger fragment (C5b) acquires, as a result of the cleavage reaction, a site for attachment to the target cell membrane and sites for the binding of C6 and C7. C5b can bind C6 and C7 either on the target cell membrane or in solution. This trimolecular complex (C5b67) is the foundation for formation of the membrane lytic apparatus (see next section).

The C3a and C5a peptides, although biochemically quite different, have very similar and important biological properties related to inflammation. They can cause histamine release from mast cells, leading to anaphylaxis (see Chapter 6). This property of C3a and C5a led to their being termed anaphylatoxins. Both peptides are also chemotactic for phagocytic cells, attracting both monocytes and neutrophils to the site of an immune reaction. This property is reminiscent of some of the T-cell lymphokines involved in hypersensitivity reactions (Chapter 17). The migrating cells become fixed at the site through surface C3b and C4b receptors. C5a also causes leukocytes to release hydrolytic enzymes into the surrounding space once they arrive at the reaction site. C3a may have properties similar to kinin.

The Membrane Lytic Reaction

As just discussed, C5b can combine either in solution or on the membrane with C6 and C7. This reaction, and subsequent interactions of C8 and C9, does not involve enzymatic modifications of any of the components. However, the components may still be considered activated since the ultimate lytic reaction can only occur if the components interact with one another in the prescribed sequence.

$C\overline{567}$ binds one molecule of C8, and the resultant $C\overline{5678}$ can bind between 8 and 11 molecules of C9. The $C\overline{56789}$ complex can form either on the target cell membrane or in solution (Figure 7-6). $C\overline{567}$ and $C\overline{5678}$ and $C\overline{56789}$ complexes formed in solution can all bind to and ultimately lead to lysis of "innocent bystander" cells of any type. The lytic complex does not acquire significant membrane damaging capabilities until the addition of at least one molecule of C9. Once assembled, this "membrane attack complex" can damage a wide range of membranes, including bacterial (gram negative), mammalian, and synthetic lipid bilayers. In bacteria, complement damages both the inner and outer membranes.

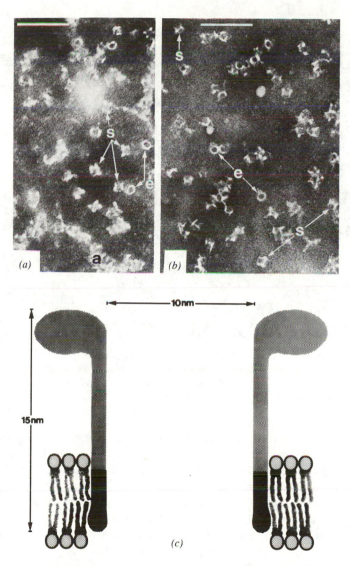

Figure 7-6 Electron micrographs of samples negatively stained with sodium silicotungstate. Scale bars indicate 100 nm. (a) Isolated C5b-9(m). The cylindrical macromolecules are seen in side projections (s) and along the cylindrical axis (e). Some aggregates are seen (a). (b) Isolated, proteolyzed C5b-9(m), showing the unaltered structure of the complex. (c) Schematic illustration of C5b-9(m), anchored in a lipid bilayer by an apolar zone at one terminus of the cylinder (black). [Taken from S. Bhakdi and J. Tranum-Jensen, Molecular nature of the complement lesion. *Proc. Natl. Acad. Sci. U.S.A.* **75**, 5655 (1978).]

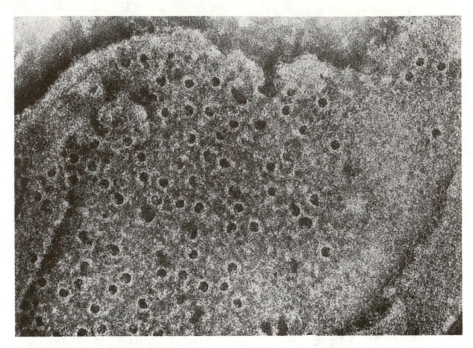

Figure 7-7 Complement-induced lesions in a red blood cell plasma membrane, ×400,000. [From J. Humphrey and R. Dourmashkin, The lesions in cell membranes caused by complement. *Adv. Immunol. 11,* 75 (1969). Copyright by Academic Press, Inc. and the authors.]

The actual mechanisms whereby the terminal components of complement cause cell lysis is still unknown. It has been suggested that the highly hydrophobic lytic complex (C56789) inserts into the membrane, causing disruption of the lipid bilayer. Studies with model membrane systems have shown that complement can lyse liposomes that contain no included protein, suggesting that damage is indeed directed against the lipid bilayer. Although no direct evidence has been obtained for interaction of any complement components with more than the outer surface of plasma membranes, the terminal complement components are known to be rather powerful detergents. What appear to be complement-induced holes have been seen in freeze-fracture electron micrographs of cell membranes (Figure 7-7). Evidence has continued to accumulate to support the notion that these might represent channels formed in the membrane by complement, which would allow exchange of fluids and ions between the intra- and extracellular compartments.

The Alternate Pathway of Complement Activation

The alternate pathway for complement activation can be brought into effect without the participation of antibody or any other element of the immune system. It is not antigen specific and requires no induction period before acting. It thus may be viewed as a form of natural (as opposed to acquired) immunity (see Chapter 16), and it is also not unreasonable to speculate that this pathway may represent an evolutionarily more primitive defense mechanism.

The alternate pathway begins with the apparently random deposition of a molecule of C3b on the surface of a cell or bacterium (Figure 7-8). This surface may be either an "activator" surface, or a "nonactivator" surface. The chemical basis for the distinction between activating and nonactivating surfaces is unclear, although carbohydrate composition appears to be a factor. Many bacterial and some viral and parasitic surfaces are activating, whereas most healthy animal cell surfaces are nonactivating. Attachment of C3b to the surface involves formation of an ester bond between a C3b carbonyl group and a surface hydroxyl group. The C3b carbonyl is made available when an internal thioester bond in the alpha chain of C3 is cleaved during C3 activation. If the available carbonyl group of this "metastable" form of C3 does not interact with a cell surface, it may interact with water to form fluid phase C3b (Figure 7-9).

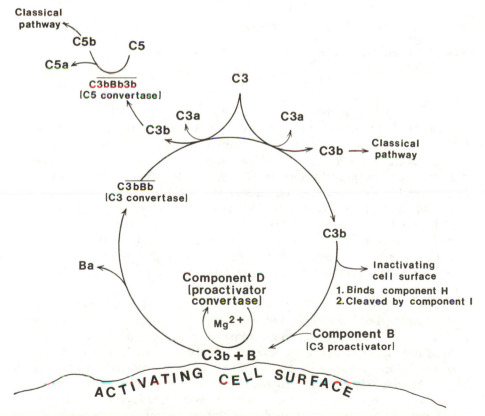

Figure 7-8 The alternate pathway for complement activation. Older nomenclature for some of the components is given in brackets. (See text for details.)

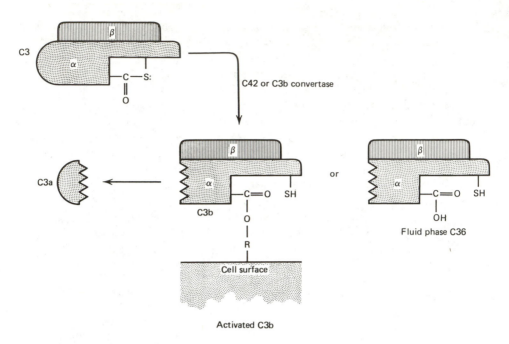

Figure 7-9 Generation of C3b and initiation of the alternate pathway.

If a C3b molecule attaches to a nonactivating cell surface, it will, most likely, bind a molecule of Component H (formerly known as β1H), a glycoprotein of 150,000 MW found in the β-globulin fraction of serum. (*Note*: The nomenclature of the components of the alternate pathway has a long and confusing history. A revised, simplified nomenclature was approved by the Nomenclature Committee of the International Union of Immunological Societies in 1981, and is presented in Table 7-1.) Component H can do two things: it can sensitize C3b for enzymatic cleavage of its α chain by Component I (C3b inactivator), an endopeptidase of 93,000 MW; and, it can block binding of Component B (also known as Factor B) to the C3b molecule. The consequence of binding Component H is thus rapid termination of the alternate pathway. Events regulating the relative levels of Component H in the system are unclear.

If C3b binds to an activating surface, interaction with Component H is disfavored, and C3b will more likely bind Component B. Component B, also known as C3 proactivator, is a single chain β-globulin molecule of 93,000 daltons synthesized by both macrophages and lymphocytes. The C3b·B complex is by itself inactive. However, in the presence of Component D (formerly known as Factor D) and Mg^{2+}, C3b·B is converted to C3b·Bb, also known as C3 convertase. Component D, also known as C3 proactivator convertase, is a 25,000-dalton serine protease found naturally in serum that hydrolyzes Component B into two peptides, Ba and

Bb, with molecular weights of 33,000 and 60,000, respectively. Component Bb when bound to C3b is a potent serine protease with C3 as its natural substrate! However, Component D *only* acts on Component B when the latter is complexed to C3b. The activated C3b·Bb complex (amplification C3 convertase) will now catalyze the hydrolysis of C3 to C3a and C3b. C3a and Component B are functionally (and to some degree even structurally) similar to C4 and C2. C3b generated by this reaction can be used in several ways: it can deposit on the nearby activating surface and interact further with Component B and Component D; it can enter the classical pathway; or it can be utilized to form amplification C5 convertase (see below).

A major feature of the alternate pathway is thus a highly effective positive feedback circuit amplifying an intial, relatively innocuous random event into a major effector mechanism for target cell destruction (Figure 7-8). Component D is not consumed in the reaction, so only C3 and Component B are potentially rate limiting once the cycle begins. C3b molecules will opsonize the involved particle for phagocytosis, and the C3a molecules liberated from the reaction site will attract granulocytes and monocytes to the area, causing further target cell destruction.

As C3b molecules begin to build up in the vicinity of the initial reaction, they may bind to C3b·Bb complexes to form C3b·Bb·3b, or amplification C5 convertase. This will generate additional anaphylactic activity through release of C5a, and can lead to formation of the C5b-9 lytic membrane attack complex.

Properdin, once thought to be a key element of the alternate pathway, is now seen not as a participant in the pathway but rather as a modulator. It can interact directly with C3b·Bb·3b complexes to stabilize them. Properdin, released on dissolution of such complexes ("activated" properdin), can also interact with and stabilize C3b·Bb complexes. Properdin also seems to enhance formation of the membrane attack complex, although the means by which it does so are not known.

The major distinction between the classical and alternate pathways is that in the latter case deposition of C3b on the activating cell surface, and thus initiation of the pathway, is essentially a random event, and does not involve any element of specific target recognition. Initiation is determined solely by the nature of the target cell surface (activating versus nonactivating). In the classical pathway, deposition of C3b on the cell surface is directed by an antigen-specific element of the immune system (antibody) plus five other elements of the complement cascade (C1q-s, C4, and C2). One major result of this difference, especially in an animal not previously exposed to a given pathogen with an activating surface, is in the speed of the response. The alternate pathway can be brought into play immediately on entry of the pathogen into the system, whereas the classical pathway, being dependent on generation of specific antibodies, may not come into play for several days. On the other hand, once the classical pathway begins to function, it is more powerful, due to the ability of antibody to focus higher levels of complement components onto the target cell surface.

An interesting feature of both the classical and alternate pathways is that several of their components map genetically to the major histocompatibility complex. This phenomenon is discussed in more detail in Chapter 10.

Table 7-1 Nomenclature of the Alternate Complement Activating Pathway Components and Intermediates

Component	Former designation	Reaction products	Description
C3	Factor A	C3a	A peptide of relative molecular mass (RMM) 9000 that is hydrolyzed from C3 by a C3 convertase and that possesses anaphylatoxin activity
		C3b	A major fragment, of RMM 180,000, that is derived from C3 by the hydrolytic action of a C3 convertase and that, whether bound to a particle or unbound, may participate in formation of the amplification C3 convertase
		iC3b	C3b that has been inactivated by the peptide hydrolytic action of I in the presence of H without overt fragmentation and that cannot participate in formation of the amplification C3 convertase
B	Heat labile factor; C3 proactivator; glycine-rich β-glycoprotein	Ba	An activation peptide of RMM 30,000 that is hydrolyzed from B by D
		Bb	A major fragment of RMM 63,000 that is derived from B by the hydrolytic action of D and that bears a peptide hydrolase enzymatic site active on C3 and C5
		Bbi	Inactive Bb that has dissociated from C3b and that cannot hydrolyze a peptide bond in C3 and C5
D	GBGase; C3 proactivator convertase		A glycoprotein of RMM 25,000 that is a serine proteinase which hydrolyzes an Arg-Lys bond in B that is complexed to C3b

Table 7-1 *(Continued)*

Component	Former designation	Reaction products	Description
P	Properdin		A glycoprotein of RMM 220,000 that can bind to C3, C3b, and C3b,Bb and that can retard dissociation of Bb from C3b
H	β1H; C3bINA-accelerator		A glycoprotein of RMM 150,000 that can bind to C3b and that can impair binding of B to C3b, accelerate dissociation of Bb from C3b, and facilitate conversion of C3b to iC3b by I
I	C3b inactivator; C4b inactivator; KAF		A glycoprotein of RMM 93,000 that is a peptide hydrolase which converts C3b to iC3b by cleavage of a bond in the α-chain
C3b,B			Magnesium-dependent reversible complex in which B may be hydrolyzed to its Bb and Ba fragments by D
C3b,Bb			Amplification C3 convertase in which Bb can hydrolyze the Arg77-Ser78 bond of the α-chain of C3
C3b,Bb,C3b			Amplification C5 convertase in which Bb can hydrolyze the Arg74-×75 bond of the α-chain of C5
C3b,Bb,P C3b,Bb,C3b,P			P-stabilized amplification C3 and C5 convertases

Reprinted from the *J. Immunol., 127*, 1261 (1981). By permission.

Complement Genes

Genes for several of the complement proteins have now been isolated and their sequence, organization and control are being studied.

The genes for C2 and C4 of the classical pathway, and for component B (Bf) of the alternate pathway, are all closely linked and in both mice and humans are part of the major histocompatibility gene complex (Chapter 9). Different alleles of the C4 gene appear to be transcribed at different rates, resulting in different serum levels of the gene product. The level of expression of C4 is also affected by hormones: males double their levels of C4 after puberty, and the normally lower levels of C4 in prepubescent males and in females can be raised by injecting testosterone. There are two expressed C4 genes in both species, although one of them does not function as a complement component in mice (Slp; see p. 212). At the DNA level there may be three C4 genes in humans, and as many as six in mice. Some of these may be pseudogenes.

C3 is represented by a single gene copy in both mice and humans. The genes show a high degree of homology in these two species. The C3 gene in humans is on chromosome 19.

Bibliography

Research

Bordet, J., and O. Gengou, Sur l'existance des substances sensibilitrices dans la plupart des serums antimicrobiens. *Ann. Inst. Pasteur 15,* 289 (1901).

Houle, J. J., and E. M. Hoffmann, Evidence for restriction of the ability of complement to lyse homologous erythrocytes. *J. Immunol. 133,* 1444 (1984).

Muller-Eberhard, H. J., Complement. *Ann. Rev. Biochem. 44,* 697 (1975).

Porter, R. R., and K. B. M. Reid, Activation of the complement system by antibody-antigen complexes: The classical pathway. *Adv. Protein Chem. 33,* 1 (1979).

Wright, S. D., and R. P. Levine, How complement kills E. coli. *J. Immunol. 127,* 1146 and 1152 (1981).

Zicardi, R. J., Spontaneous activation of the first component of human complement by an intramolecular autocatalytic mechanism. *J. Immunol. 128,* 2500 (1982).

III

Major Histocompatibility Gene Complexes

Nearly 50 years ago, a young British scientist named Peter Gorer was analyzing blood group antigens in mice. During the course of his studies, he identified a rather interesting antigen that he named "antigen II." Antigen II was interesting because it was present on the blood cells of some mice, but not others. Most important, the presence or absence of antigen II turned out to correlate with the ability of mice to reject a particular tumor Gorer was studying.

At first that seemed very exciting, because at least some scientists had suggested that the development of cancer might be under immunological control. But Gorer went on to show that antigen II was present on all cells in the body of the mouse from which the tumor was taken, and so rejection of the tumor was no different (at least in the system he was studying) from tissue transplant rejection generally.

Tumor immunology *per se* thus had to wait another quarter century before getting seriously under way. But Gorer's work led to a veritable explosion in the field of transplantation immunology. His antigen II evolved over the next several decades into the major histocompatibility complex (MHC) of the mouse, which was later renamed H-2. The story of this evolution is recounted in Chapter 9.

MHC complexes in mice and humans, and in all species of birds and mammals analyzed to date, contain genes coding for antigens (called class I antigens) that are expressed on the surface of almost every cell in the body. Class I antigens are recognized by the immune system during rejection of a foreign tissue transplant and are what Gorer was detecting in his earliest studies. But that is only part of the story.

During the 1960s, a second class of genes and antigens was described that turned out to be associated with the MHC. These antigens, called class II antigens, are present principally on the surface of lymphocytes and reticular cells, and were originally defined by their ability to control the antibody response to particular antigens. That is, depending on the type of class II molecules a given mouse might display on its lymphocytes, it might respond well, poorly, or not at all to antigen "X."

Both of these lines of inquiry (transplant rejection and class I MHC gene products; class II gene products and antibody responses) have been pursued vigorously by immunologists over the past two decades. But always in the not-too-distant background lay some troubling questions. Could class I antigens really exist simply to confound transplant surgeons? And what could be the advantage of the class II gene system, which when it did not work exactly right could actually inhibit the response to some foreign antigens?

The answers to these questions have begun to emerge in the past few years, and they display a pleasing unity. Immunologists now believe that the principal role of both class I and class II MHC antigens is in facilitating cell–cell communication among the various components of the immune system involved in antigen recognition and processing. Thus a great deal of information about MHCs that has been treated more or less phenomenologically in recent years can now be integrated into what we knew previously about how immune responses work.

Because an understanding of the MHC at both the genetic and molecular level is crucial to understanding virtually all of immunology beyond the level of immunoglobulin structure, the next several chapters are devoted to describing and analyzing this rather complex subject in considerable detail.

CHAPTER **8**

Historical Development of the Concept of Major Histocompatibility Gene Complexes

Histocompatibility systems of vertebrates, as one might infer from the name, are those systems of genes (histocompatibility genes) and gene products (histocompatibility antigens) that determine whether or not tissues or cells transplanted from one animal to another will be immunologically compatible with and survive in the new host environment. In Chapter 9, which deals specifically with tissue and organ transplantation, we will see that histocompatibility was studied in a number of different ways for a good many years before it was established that survival or rejection of transplanted tissues was an immunological phenomenon. And, in the past 15 years or so, we have become aware that at least portions of these same histocompatibility systems play a crucial role not only in determining whether a graft will be accepted or rejected, but indeed in the facilitation and regulation of a major portion of the known repertoire of immunological responses.

179

Histocompatibility systems have been defined at the genetic level for at least 20 different vertebrate organisms, including humans. By far the best defined of these is the major histocompatibility complex (MHC) of the mouse, designated H-2, which regulates both histocompatibility in the strict sense, and general immune responsiveness as well. There are also several known minor histocompatibility systems in the mouse which, as far as is known at present, seem only to influence graft rejection per se. However, because it is obvious that graft rejection could not have played any recent role in their evolution, the actual biological significance of these minor loci remains a mystery.

The MHC in humans, homologous to H-2 in the mouse, is the HLA system. This complex of genes also influences both graft rejection and general immune responsiveness. Only a major histocompatibility locus has been described for humans, although results of transplantation studies suggest the existence of minor loci as well.

The line of inquiry initiated by Peter Gorer's research on the genetics of mouse blood group antigens in the 1930s evolved into one of the most significant areas of immunological research in the subsequent 50 years. The practical and theoretical implications of this research even now dominate much of our thinking about the immune system. Before summarizing our present state of understanding of the structure and function of MHC genes and gene products, I invite students to familiarize themselves with the background to this fascinating topic. It is an interesting and exciting story. And let us not forget that "those who are ignorant of history are condemned to repeat it." I have no idea who said that, but chances are it was a repentant immunologist.

Early Inquiries into Tissue Compatibility

The transplantation of cells and tissues was studied for many years prior to the demonstration that acceptance or rejection of grafts is an immunological phenomenon. In fact, interest in transplantation as a biological, rather than a surgical, phenomenon was initially directed not toward organ transplantation per se, but to the study of the ability of a tumor derived from one animal to grow in another. It was while studying the *genetics* of this phenomenon, rather than the *immunology* of it, that MHC antigens were first described.

Around the turn of the century, the propagation of tumors through more than one animal was attempted as a means of maintaining a specific tumor for study. The technique of tissue culture was not yet available, so *in vitro* propagation was not possible. Prior to about 1900 the ability of a tumor derived from one mouse to grow in another mouse seemed to biologists to be almost random. Only rarely did a transplanted tumor survive and grow; yet on occasion one would.

Astute observations in a number of quarters gradually led to the realization that groups of animals with restricted breeding patterns had a higher success rate for tumor exchanges than did genetically disparate animals. In a study carried out in Germany in the early 1900s, it was noted that a tumor arising in wild mice captured in a particular neighborhood of Berlin would grow at least transiently in a high proportion of mice trapped in the same neighborhood, with a substantial number of permanent (lethal) takes. However, the same tumor grew less well in mice captured in an adjoining neighborhood, and in only about a quarter of the mice collected in other parts of the city. The tumors did not grow at all in mice obtained from more distant regions.

At this time, various stocks of mice had been maintained around the world in a partially inbred state for many years prior to 1900. These were the so-called "fancy mice," bred to bring out a particular trait such as coat or eye color or peculiar behavioral patterns, considered attractive by mouse fanciers. In 1903, Carl Jensen in Denmark discovered that a tumor arising in a closed-breeding albino mouse stock could be transplanted through nearly 20 generations of mice from the same stock, but was rapidly rejected on transfer to another type of mouse. Loeb in the United States made a similar observation with an Asian strain of mice ("Japanese waltzing mice").

These studies led to the rather vague notion of genetic or "racial" susceptibility to tumors. The first attempt to put the inheritance of tumors on a rational genetic basis came with the work of E. E. Tyzzer at Harvard University, during the first 10 years of this century. He made the seminal observation that the susceptibility of members of a strain of mice to a given tumor could be increased by repeatedly breeding together only those mice within the strain susceptible to that tumor. He was even able to develop sublines of mice within a strain that were not susceptible to tumors growing within other sublines of the same strain.

The Development of Inbred Strains

Analysis and understanding of histocompatibility in the mouse has proceeded much more rapidly than in any other species for one simple reason: the early development of large numbers of *inbred strains*. Members of inbred strains are by some criterion genetically identical. The ultimate criterion, of course, would be direct sequencing of the entire genome of a statistically significant sample of the strain population. The humbler operational criterion used by immunologists is the ability of members of the same sex of an inbred strain to accept permanently transplants of cells and tissues from one another.

In 1912, a mathematical treatment of the genetic consequences of successive generations of brother–sister matings in a single familial line was published. This analysis predicted that by approximately 20 generations, all progeny should be greater than 99 percent identical and homozygous at all genetic loci. Using the already somewhat genetically restricted "fancy mice" as starting stock, a number of truly inbred lines were developed by about 1920. Today, there are literally hundreds of inbred lines of mice, including congenic resistant and recombinant strains (see following), some of which have been maintained by continuous brother–sister matings for more than 200 generations. These provide the working material for a wide range of immunological investigations.

Congenic Resistant (CR) Mouse Strains

The term *congenic* (or coisogenic) in the general sense is applied to two animals (or strains of inbred animals) genetically identical except for some highly restricted genetic region. The ability to thus "isolate" a small genetic segment by comparison of two such animals is highly advantageous for a detailed study of the function(s) encoded in that segment. The term *congenic resistant,* as specifically applied to inbred strains of mice, refers to two inbred strains that are identical throughout their entire genomes, with the exception of some small chromosomal segment containing one or perhaps a few closely linked genetic loci that prevent exchange of tissues between them. These genes are, by definition, histocompatibility genes. However, as noted in Appendix I in the back of the book, one must always bear in mind that the particular gene selected for in the production of the congenic strain may not be the only gene on the chromosomal segment grafted in. An assumption that this is so has led to more than one error in immunogenetics.

The procedures used for producing and characterizing congenic resistant inbred strains of mice are described in detail in Appendix I. The standard notation system used to designate H-2 congenic strains is exemplified by the B10.A strain, which was constructed from the two basic strains B10 (H-2^b) and A (H-2^a). The strain indicated in the left-hand portion of the notation (B10) is the strain providing all of the genetic material *except* H-2. The strain indicated on the right-hand side provides the H-2 locus for the recombinant strain. B10.A mice are thus genetically identical to B10 strain mice, except that they have the H-2 locus of A strain mice. They are therefore of the H-2^a haplotype.

H-2 Recombinant Strains

Recombinant inbred strains of mice used in immunological research are principally those in which a crossing-over event has occurred within a histocompatibility locus. For the H-2 gene complex, which is the only H system in the mouse in which recombination has been produced and selected for, about 1 in 300 F_1 backcrosses will produce a recombinant. Recombinants are also known to occur within the human HLA gene complex. Recombination within the H-2 region occurs during meiosis, and can be detected only by laborious and time-consuming screening of hybrid progeny. For H-2 this is done with serological reagents specific for each of the known loci within the gene complex. Perhaps even more than with CR strains, great care must be taken in the use of recombinant strains to produce specific antisera or to deduce the mapping of genes. It is often difficult to know exactly where, between any two genes, a given crossover occurred. The distance between many genes within H-2, for example, is considerable and may contain other genes whose existence or location is not yet known, but that may nonetheless affect the trait being studied in the recombinant strain.

Gorer's "Antigen II"

The discovery of the major histocompatibility system in mice (H-2) came about as the result of work by Peter Gorer in the 1930s. Gorer was attempting to define blood group antigens in the mouse, so that the genetics and immunology of such antigens could be studied in an animal model. Using recently established inbred strains of mice, he discovered serendipitously that serum from humans with type A red cells would spontaneously react with antigens on RBC from some strains, but not others. The antigen(s) thus defined was heritable in a simple Mendelian fashion. In order to study this in a more reproducible fashion, he injected the RBC of various inbred mouse strains into rabbits and tested the resultant antisera against RBC from each of the immunizing strains. After careful cross-absorption of each antiserum with RBC from each strain, he could demonstrate the existence of strain-specific hemagglutinating antibodies in each antiserum. He was able to define a total of three antigens (Table 8-1).

The next phase of this work, which tied one of these antigens (II) into the acceptance or rejection of tumor allografts, was reported by Gorer in the following year. This paper represents the true foundation of the genetic study of histocompatibility. In it, Gorer demonstrated by backcrossing experiments that the rejection of albino (A) tumors by black (C57) mice correlated with and was dependent upon the existence of antigen II, and that mice that had rejected albino tumors had anti-II antibodies in their serum. Antigens I and III appeared not to be important in this process. He thus suggested that an antigen (II) present on normal tissue (RBC, red blood cells) was also found on tumors, and was in fact the antigen responsible for rejection of the tumor. This was a very important observation, because a major question for many years had been whether tumors transplanted between different animals were rejected because of tumor-specific antigens, or because of antigens present on the tumor that were common to all tissues of the tumor donor. Gorer's work strongly suggested the latter, and moreover suggested that tissue rejection might be immunological phenomenon.

The following year Gorer provided even stronger evidence for the association of antigen II and tumor rejection, and showed that antigen II was present in higher concentration on tumor cells than on RBC.[1] In his last paper before this work was interrupted by the war, he showed that although anti-II antibodies could kill tumor cells *in vitro,* they had no effect on tumor growth when passively injected into tumor-bearing animals. This was a mystery that would not be solved for almost 20

---

[1]It is often assumed that MHC proteins are not present on mouse red blood cells. It is usually forgotten that the initial detection of H-2 antigens was by agglutination of mouse RBC with H-2 antibodies!

Table 8-1 The First Description of H-2 (Antigen II)

Immunizing strain	Antigens		
	I	**II**	**III**
Agouti (CBA)	+++	+	++
Albino (A)	+++	+++	++
Black (C57)	++	−	++

The abbreviations in parentheses are the strain designations later used for these mice which, at the time of this early work, were named only for their coat color.

years, when Mitchison finally demonstrated the cellular, rather than humoral, basis for graft rejection.

The Concept of Histocompatibility and the Discovery of H-2 Alleles

The work on formal transplantation genetics began again after the war, with Gorer's return to the laboratory and the addition of a major new investigator in the United States, George Snell. A series of careful studies of the genetics of skin graft acceptance or rejection in mice had made it clear that although antigen II was a particularly potent inducer of rejection, more than a single gene and gene product was involved in this process. Estimates of the number of additional genes varied from 4 to 15 or more, depending on the strain combinations analyzed.

Snell realized that if either genetic or immunological analyses were to proceed further, the number of genes controlling graft rejection needed to be determined accurately, and each locus individually analyzed. In 1948, he published a classic paper in which he introduced the notion of "histocompatibility" genes, and a method for the production of inbred strains differing by only a single histocompatibility (H) gene. He also described methods for establishing linkage of these genes to other known genetic markers, and for establishing the identity or nonidentity of the various H genes detected in different breeding combinations. He suggested the name "coisogenic" (now commonly called "congenic") for two strains differing at a single H locus. Through the construction and analysis of congenic strains (see Appendix I for details), some 30 to 40 different H genes have been identified and mapped. All code for cell surface antigens that lead ultimately to graft rejection.[2] However, there is considerable difference in the time required for

---

[2]The actual biological functions of the vast majority of these antigens are entirely unclear. However, it is obvious that their ability to provoke graft rejection could have played no role in their evolutionary development or selection.

complete graft rejection across the genetic differences defined by the various H loci. H-2 (renamed from Gorer's antigen II) provokes the stongest reaction, leading to rejection of a skin graft in about 10 to 12 days. Other loci may be nearly as strong, leading to graft rejection in 15 to 20 days, or very weak, sometimes requiring 100 days or more for complete rejection. (Some of these latter loci could not be detected using tumor transplants, because the tumor would prove fatal before rejection could occur.) Because of this difference in "strength," H-2 was called a "major histocompatibility gene," whereas all other H genes were referred to as "minor." As we will see later, the basis for this difference in strength lies in the fact that a very high proportion of host T lymphocytes are capable of directly recognizing MHC products, whereas relatively few T cells can recognize minor H loci. As it turns out, this provides a very important clue to the biological significance of the MHC.

The next major advance in studying the genetics of the H-2 locus also derived from work by Snell and his associates. In 1951, Snell and Higgins published a simple but elegant cross-breeding/transplant method for estimating the number of alleles at the major locus H-2. In this initial study, they identified four; the list has now grown much larger. All of these alleles, at this stage in the study of the H-2 locus, were defined by their ability to provoke strong tissue rejection reactions using strain-specific tumors. These initially described alleles were H-2 (for the A strain, later referred to as H-2^a); H-2^d (strains BALB/c and DBA/2), H-2^b (strains C57BL/6 and C57BL/10), and H-2^p (strain P). At present, nine distinct alleles, based on graft rejection, can be identified in the so-called "foundation strains" of laboratory inbred mice. (The total number of inbred strains is, of course, much larger. Some strains share the identical H-2, or are intra-H-2 recombinants of the basic nine alleles.) A very much larger number of H-2 alleles is being discovered in wild mice by Klein and his associates. This extensive genetic polymorphism of H-2 provides a second very important clue to the biological function of the H-2 system, and a major distinction between H-2 and the minor H loci.

The Definition of H-2 Serological Determinants

A totally separate approach to analyzing H-2 was taken by Gorer, Amos, and Mikulska. They continued the lead established earlier by Gorer in the serological analysis of the antigen II (H-2) system. The serological approach led for awhile to a literal "dark ages" in the study of H-2; the confusion and uncertainty initially generated discouraged all but the most avid H-2 enthusiasts from following its course.

Gorer had shown in 1947 that the antibody response to antigen II was complex, and he suggested that more than a single antigen might be involved. It was soon discovered that the H-2 antigen associated with any given inbred strain (or more properly, with any given H-2 allele) was actually composed of a number of different, serologically distinguishable antigens. The number of such antigens detected grew at an alarming rate. The genetic basis for the existence of so many different antigens associated with a single genetic locus was entirely unclear and was responsible for most of the confusion about H-2 during the 1950s and 1960s. Some of the antigens appeared to be restricted to a single H-2 allele, while others were common to a few or even a majority of strains examined. Tables 8-2 and 8-3 give some indication of the proliferation of antigenic specificities associated with the various known H-2 alleles.

The key questions about the various antigens associated with H-2 were whether they represented different antigenic determinants on a single allelomorphic gene product, or whether they represented separate but tightly linked genes at the H-2 locus that were "turned on" in various combinations in the different alleles. The truth, as we will see later, turned out to be a combination of these two possibilities.

Snell had observed in 1953 that an $H-2^a$-tumor, although rejected by both $H-2^k$ and $H-2^d$ strains of mice, grew in 100 percent of ($H-2^k \times H-2^d$)F$_1$ hybrid mice. The only acceptable explanation for this effect was that the H-2 locus was composed of at least two components (called k and d), and that the $H-2^a$ "allele" arose as a result of a crossing-over (recombinational) event between the *k* and *d* components (Figure 8-1). This experiment was very important because it provided the first evidence that H-2 must consist of at least two genetically distinct loci, providing the groundwork for subsequent development of the two-gene model for H-2. Serological evidence for recombination within the H-2 locus was soon presented by Amos, Gorer, and Mikulska in 1955. In a backcross of ($H-2^d \times H-2^b$)F$_1$ progeny to the homozygous $H-2^d$ parent strain, genetic evidence for a crossover between two of the antigens (B and E of Table 8-2) was obtained. Soon serological evidence for other crossovers within H-2 was obtained, and by 1960 five distinct "regions" controlling the various antigens were defined within H-2 (Figure 8-2). The older

Table 8-2 The Antigenic Structure of Seven H-2 Alleles as Understood in 1956

Strain of mouse	Genotype symbol	Antigens
A	$H-2^a$	CDEFK
BALB/c and others	$H-2^d$	CDEFk
C57BL and others	$H-2^b$	cBEFk
C3H and others	$H-2^k$	CdEfK
ASW	$H-2^s$	CSE? k
P	$H-2^p$	CPE? k
DBA/1	$H-2^q$	CQE? k

From D. B. Amos, P. A. Gorer, and Z. Mikulska, An analysis of an antigenic system in the mouse (the H-2 system). *Royal Society of London, Proceedings (B) 144,* 369 (1955–56).

Table 8-3 Various Antigenic Determinants Associated with H-2 (1960)

Strain	Allele	Antigen															
		A	C	D	E	F	G	H	I	J	K	M	N	Q	S	V	Y
A,AKR.K	a	A	C	D	E	F	—	H	—	J	K	M	N	—	—	—	Y
C57BL,129,LP,STA, etc.	b	—	—	D	E	F	—	—	—	—	K	—	N	—	—	V	—
BALB/c,DBA/2, etc.	d	—	C	D	E¹	F	—	H	—	J	—	M	N	—	—	—	—
A.CA	f	nt²	nt	—	nt	?¹	G	H	I	nt	—	nt	nt	—	—	nt	—
CBA,C3H,C57BR,C58, AKR,101,STB	k	A	C	Dᵏ	E	—	—	H	—	—	K	—	—	—	—	—	Y
DBA/1	q	—	C	—	E	F	—	—	—	—	—	M	—	Q	—	—	nt
RIII	r	nt	?	—	E	nt	—	—	—	nt	K	nt	nt	—	—	nt	Y
A.SW	s	nt	C	—	E	F	G	—	—	nt	—	nt	nt	—	S	nt	—

From P. A. Gorer, The antigenic structure in tumors. *Adv. Immunol. 1*, 345 (1961). As in Table 8-2, each uppercase letter (A through Y) represents a distinct antigenic determinant.

¹ = results of test uncertain.

²nt = no test.

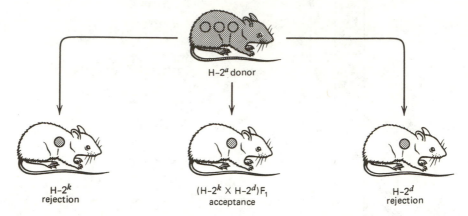

Figure 8-1a When skin from an H-2^a mouse was transplanted to either H-2^k or H-2^d mice, it was rejected. This was no surprise, since it was assumed that the H-2 a, k, and d strains all had different alleles of the H-2 locus. However, when H-2^a skin was transplanted to an (H-2^k × H-2^d)F$_1$ mouse, it was accepted. Such a result was completely unexpected, and incompatible with a single locus model for H-2. The investigators who made this observation suggested the model shown in Figure 8-1b as an explanation.

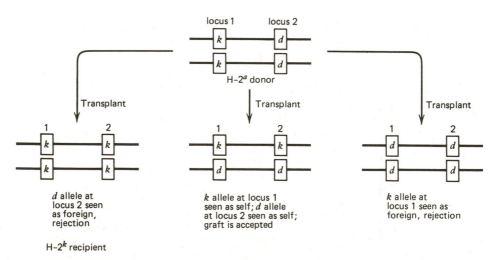

Figure 8-1b If we assume the existence of two (or more) genes at H-2 that code for histocompatibility antigens, we can explain the results in Figure 8-1a. The H-2^k strain would have k alleles at each locus, and the H-2^d strain would have d alleles at each locus. We can then hypothesize that the H-2^a strain H-2 locus arose as a result of a crossover between the two loci when H-2^k and H-2^d strains were mated. The result would be a unique H-2 locus that would have one element foreign to either H-2^k or H-2^d mice, but both elements of which would be recognized as self by an (H-2^k × H-2^d)F$_1$.

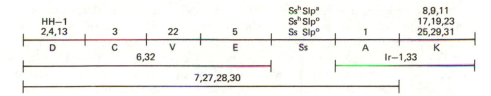

Figure 8-2 A recombination map of the H-2 region. Letters designate subdivisions defined by recombination. Numbers designate genetic determinants of H-2 antigenic specificities. [From D. C. Shreffler, Immunogenetics of the mouse H-2 system. In D. Aminoff, ed., *Blood and Tissue Antigens* Academic Press, New York, pp. 85–99 (1970).]

letter notation for individual antigenic specificities was replaced with a numbering system. The original letters were still retained, at this point, to denote specific regions that were thought to be defined by crossing-over events. Because it was now thought that H-2 represented more than a single gene, or perhaps even more than two genes, it was referred to as a "supergene" or more commonly as the "major histocompatibility gene complex."

Additional evidence that the H-2 gene complex is composed of multiple genes came from studies showing that the loci for two genes unrelated to histocompatibility (as then defined) mapped within the bounds of the H-2 complex. The SS–Slp locus, controlling a serum protein now known to be one of the complement components, was shown to map between the E and A regions of the then current H-2 map (Figure 8-2). The locus for the Ir-1 gene, which controlled the immune response to certain defined polypeptide antigens, was shown to map to H-2 as well, although initially its precise location was unknown.

The problem with the model in Figure 8-2 was that it was inadequate to explain a number of actual experimental observations. For example, specificity H-2.3, which was postulated to be controlled by a gene in the C region, appeared to behave strangely after certain genetic recombination events. In a cross of H-2^a (H-2.3$^+$) by H-2^b (H-2.3$^-$), nine intra-H-2 recombinant offspring (confirmed by distribution of K- and D-region specificities) all were H-2.3$^+$. The model shown in Figure 8-2 would predict that half of the recombinants should be H-2.3$^+$ and half H-2.3$^-$. Similar problems were noted with other H-2 specificities. Shreffler was the first to suggest that the H-2.3 inconsistency could be resolved if this antigen were postulated to be coded for at more than one locus within H-2.

The Two-Gene Model for H-2

The final synthesis of all of the information about the H-2 locus into a coherent model consistent with all of the observed data was made by Jan Klein and Don

Shreffler in a paper published in 1971. The development of this model is similar in both its deductive splendor and its predictive power to the resolution of the four-chain model of Ig structure by Porter and by Edelman in the early 1960s. Klein and Shreffler suggested that the known facts about H-2 could be accounted for by a model in which only two loci (K and D) coded for all of the known H-2-associated antigenic specificities. Most important, they postulated that these two loci arose by duplication of a single primordial gene, and that they coded for proteins with substantial structural (and hence antigenic) relatedness. Thus the same antigenic specificities could be associated with both loci. Moreover, they suggested that the duplicated genes had come to lie on either side of intervening genetic material (Ir and Ss). By studying the recombination of K and D with markers outside of H-2, the order of these two loci, with respect to the centromere, was also changed (Figure 8-3). Because it was now obvious that an H-2 "allele" was actually a collection of alleles of a number of H-2-associated genetic loci, it was suggested that the more definitive term "haplotype" be used.

The reassignment of the various antigenic determinants to two loci also made apparent the existence of private versus public specificities. Further refinement of serology made this distinction even more strict (Table 9-2). Private specificities are restricted to a single locus (K or D) of a single haplotype, whereas public specif-icities can be shared by K- and D-region proteins of the same haplotype, or among either the K- or D-region proteins of any number of natural or recombinant haplotypes. The widely distributed public specificities probably reflect those por-tions of K and D proteins (and, by inference, K and D genes) that have evolved little since the duplication event. The K- or D-restricted public specificities, and the private specificities, presumably reflect accumulated mutational events occuring after gene duplication.

As we will see in Chapter 10, there is evidence from DNA sequencing studies for extensive gene duplication in the D end of H-2, and for at least modest gene duplication at the K end. However, the notion of two distinct and genetically separable regions coding for class I MHC proteins is still valid and fundamental to immunogenetic analyses of a wide range of mammalian species.

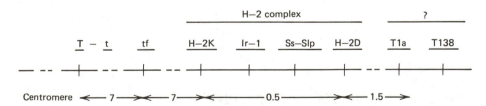

Figure 8-3 A simplified map of linkage group IX of the mouse. From J. Klein and D. C. Shreffler, The H-2 model for the major histocompatibility systems. *Transplant. Rev. 6, 3* (1971).

Discovery and Characterization
of the I Region of H-2

In describing the events leading to the development of the two-gene model for H-2, casual mention was made of a new gene, Ir-1, that appeared to map near or perhaps between the K and D genes. The events that followed from this discovery were far from casual, and indeed a goodly portion of the remainder of this text will deal with attempts to understand the function of genes mapping to this region.

For a number of years prior to the early 1960s, various researchers had tried to determine whether the ability to mount an antibody response was under genetic control, as had been shown for transplantation reactions. A number of studies had suggested this to be the case, although a rigorous genetic proof was lacking. For example, the amount of antibody produced to sheep red blood cells seemed to vary among different genetically defined mouse strains, as did the response to certain bacterial vaccines. But the response to many other antigens, such as large molecular weight proteins, usually elicited a wide range of responses within a given inbred strain, and these ranges overlapped among the different strains in such a way as to make it seem unlikely that any simple, straightforward genetic control was involved.

Such results, in a sense, would not be entirely unexpected because it was already known that large, multideterminant antigens induced the synthesis and secretion of a wide spectrum of distinct antibodies. A protein such as serum albumin, for example, is actually a collection of unique antigenic determinants, each of which is capable of inducing the production of one or more antibodies. The production of each of those antibodies would, in turn, likely be under completely separate genetic control. Thus, while in one strain the ability to respond to one of the component determinants might be genetically determined to be very strong, weak, or even absent, such "fine tuning" would not be apparent when measuring the composite antibody response to the intact, polyvalent antigen.

In the early 1960s, Michael Sela and his co-workers in Israel prepared a series of synthetic polypeptide antigens principally in order to study the afferent (sensitization) phase of the humoral immune response in relation to the molecular structure of the immunogen. In particular, they were concerned with studying discrete molecular alterations that could transform nonimmunogenic molecules into ones capable of provoking antibody production. This approach was conceptually similar to that of Landsteiner, who many years earlier studied the efferent arm of the humoral immune response (the physical interaction of antibodies and antigens), using simple haptens coupled to more complex carriers. Some of the molecules prepared by Sela's group are shown in Figure 8-4.

The development of the simpler, defined polypeptide antigens suggested a way to avoid the problems inherent in analyzing genetic regulation of the antibody response to multideterminant antigens. If the immune response could be entirely

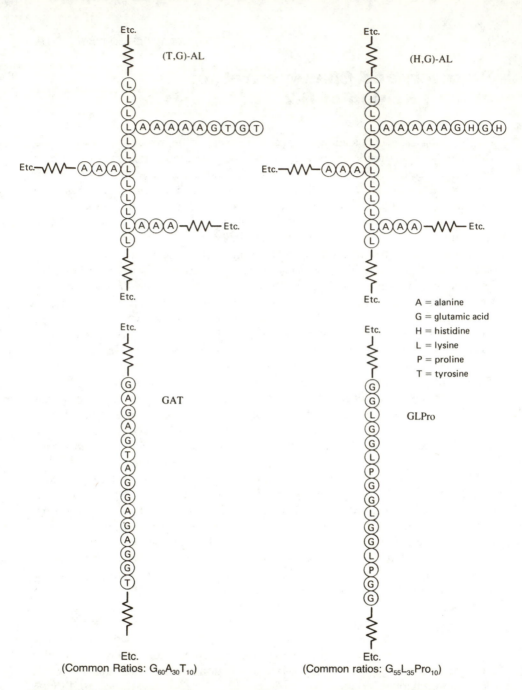

Figure 8-4 Synthetic polypeptides used in Ir gene studies. (T,G)-AL—Poly-l-lysine backbone, with poly-(d,l)-alanine side chains, to the ends of which are appended random linear polymers of tyrosine and glutamic acid; (H,G,)-AL—same as (T,G)-A,L except that tyrosine is replaced by histidine; GAT—random linear terpolymer of glutamic acid, alanine, and tyrosine; GLPro—random linear terpolymer of glutamic acid, lysine, and proline.

restricted to a single type of determinant, genetic analysis would be considerably simplified. With synthetic polypeptides such as (T,G)-AL (Figure 8-4), this is possible since the (G)-AL core of the peptide is nonimmunogenic in mice. The response to (T,G)-AL appears to be restricted to the tyrosine groups in association with glutamic acid.

Studies of this type were begun in Sela's laboratory in collaboration with Hugh McDevitt. They found that when (T,G)-AL and (H,G)-AL were used to immunize CBA (H-2^k) and C57BL (H-2^b) mice, results of the type shown in Figure 8-5 and Table 8-4 were obtained. C57BL mice gave a high response to (T,G)-AL, and a low response to (H,G-AL), while CBA mice gave the reverse pattern. This response was somewhat dose dependent, the difference between the two strains being much less marked at very low ($\leq$ 1 μg) or very high ($\geq$ 100 μg) doses of immunogen. Furthermore, the differential response is observed only in the secondary, primarily IgG, response. The strains give essentially identical primary (IgM) responses to (T,G)-AL. The F_1 hybrids of the two strains gave intermediate (although somewhat to the high side) responses to the immunogens, and backcross analysis (F_1 to either parent) gave a segregation pattern strongly suggestive of alleles of a single dominant gene. The putative gene exercising this control was later designated the Ir1A gene (Ir for immune response, 1 for first reported locus, and A for first reported gene of locus 1). These initial observations paved the way for an intensive investigation, continuing to this day in many laboratories around the world, of the genetic control of immune responses.

It soon became obvious, by comparing the response of a large number of inbred mouse strains to these defined immunogens, that the Ir1A gene(s) most likely mapped very close to H-2. For example, as can be seen from Table 8-4, strains with the H-2^b haplotype are high responders to (T,G)-AL, while all H-2^k haplotypes are low

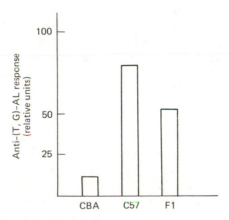

Figure 8-5 Secondary antibody response to (T,G)-AL by CBA and C57 mice and their F_1 progeny. [Based on data presented in H. O. McDevitt, Genetic control of the antibody response. *Hospital Practice 8,* 61 (1973).]

Table 8-4 Response by Representative H-2 Haplotypes to Various Immunogens

Strain	H-2 haplotype	Response to antigen			
		(T,G)-AL	**(H,G)-AL**	**OA**	**GAT**
A; B10.A	*a*	L	H	L	H
C57BL; B10	*b*	H	L	H	H
BALB/C; DBA/2	*d*	H/L	L/M	M/H	H
C3H; CBA; AKR	*k*	L	H	L	H
HTI	*i*	H	L	H	H
B10.A (3R)	*i3*	H	?	?	H
SJL; A.SW	*s*	L	L	?	0
DBA/1	*q*	L	L	H	0

Values shown are for the secondary antibody response only. H = high responder; M = medium responder; L = low responder; 0 = no measurable response; ? = not known. OA = ovalbumin; GAT = glutamic acid–alanine–tyrosine (see Figure 8-4).

responders. Similar H-2 associations are evident for the response to other defined immunogens. In general, strains of the same H-2 haplotype give consistently similar patterns of immune responsiveness to a given defined immunogen.

Analysis of strains congenic for the H-2 complex further substantiated the association of the Ir gene(s) with the MHC of the mouse. For example, strain B10.A, which has only the H-2 complex (plus presumably a few surrounding genes on the transposed chromosomal segment) in common with strain A, responds to (T,G)-AL like strain A, and not like strain B10. The same holds true for other congenic strains (Table 8-4); low-responder strains can be converted to high responders by "breeding in" the H-2 complex from a high-responder strain, and vice versa. Careful analysis of intra-H-2 recombinant strains showed that the Ir gene mapped to a locus between the K and S regions. It thus defined a separate *region* of H-2, the I region. Assignment of this gene to an IA *subregion* came about when a second gene, Ir1B, was also shown to map to the I region of H-2, but was shown to be separate from Ir-1A by crossing over (see next section). Ir-1B thus defines the subregion IB.

The IB subregion of the I region of H-2 was further defined by several genes regulating immune responsiveness, which appeared to be separable from the IA subregion group by crossing over. A gene regulating the antibody response to a homogeneous BALB/c myeloma protein of the IgG$_{2a}$ class was shown by Lieberman in the early 1970s to map in the I region of the H-2 complex. It was originally given the name "Ir-IgG gene." Analysis of the segregation of this gene in H-2 recombinant strains revealed apparent crossing over between the chromosomal region containing Ir-1A and the region containing this immune response gene. Because this gene seemed to be distinct from Ir-1A, it was assigned a formal

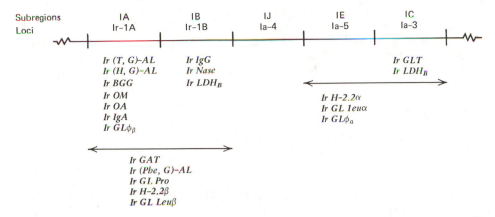

Figure 8-6 Detailed map of the I region as of about 1978, with subregion assignments of representative Ir genes.

designation, Ir-1B. It is the gene that defines the IB subregion of H-2. The IB subregion was also assigned a gene controlling the response to one of the isozymes of porcine LDH. Because it could not be shown that this gene is different from Ir-1B, it was assigned the name Ir-LDH. A third gene, controlling antibody production to an antigenic determinant on staphylococcal nuclease (Ir-Nase), was also mapped to the IB subregion.

During the early 1970s, increasing numbers of synthetic and natural antigens were found to be under Ir gene control (Figure 8-6). Some were thought initally to map to a separately defined IC subregion of H-2, but nearly all of these are now believed to map to IE. As we will see, most antigens are under the control of genes in only *two* subregions of I (IA and IE).

The early map of the I region of H-2, drawn on the basis of gene mapping using intra-H2 recombinants, has been challenged by recent direct gene sequencing studies of the H-2 region. As we will see in the next chapter, firm evidence has been obtained for the existence of the IA and IE subregions, but so far the IB, IJ, and IC subregions have not been detected. Most mouse geneticists now believe that the crossovers within H-2 originally used to distinguish IB from IA and IC from IE may have been misinterpreted. We will also see that the apparent existence of the IJ region may have been due to misinterpretation of congenic strain data. Thus, for the remainder of this text, we will consider the I region of H-2 to be divided into only two subregions: IA and IE.

Bibliography

General

Dausset, J., The major histocompatibility complex in man. *Science 213,* 1469 (1981).
Demant, P., G. D. Snell, M. Hess, F. Lemonnier, C. Neauport-Sautes, and F. Kourilsky, Separate

and polymorphic loci controlling two types of polypeptide chains bearing the H-2 private and public specificities. *J. Immunol. 2,* 263 (1975).

Klein, J., *Biology of the Mouse Histocompatibility-2 Complex,* Springer-Verlag, Berlin, Heidelberg, and New York (1975).

Snell, G. D., J. Dausset, and S. Nathenson, *Histocompatibility,* Academic Press, New York (1976).

Research

Amos, D. B., P. Gorer, and Z. Mikulska, An analysis of an antigenic system in the mouse (H-2 system). *Royal Soc. London Proc. (B) 144,* 369 (1955–56).

Gorer, P. A., The genetic and antigenic basis of tumor transplantation. *J. Pathol. Bacteriol., 44,* 691 (1937).

Gorer, P. A., The detection of a hereditary antigenic difference in the blood of mice by means of human group A serum. *J. Genetics 32,* 17 (1936).

Haaland, M., Beobachtungen über natürlich Geschwultzresistenz bei Mausen. *Berlin Klin. Wochenschr. 44,* 713 (1907).

Klein, J., and D. W. Bailey, Histocompatibility differences in wild mice. Further evidence for the existence of deme structure in natural populations of the house mouse. *Genetics 68,* 287 (1971).

Klein, J., and D. C. Shreffler, The H-2 model for the major histocompatibility systems. *Transplant. Rev. 6,* 3 (1971).

Loeb, L., Uber entstehung einer sarkoms nach transplantation eines adenocarcinoms einer Japanischen mouse. *Zeitschrift f. Krebsforschung 7,* 80 (1908).

Medawar, P. B., The behavior and fate of skin autografts and skin homografts in rabbits. *J. Anat. 78,* 176 (1944).

Mickova, M., and P. Ivanyi, An estimate of the degree of heterozygosity at H loci in wild mouse populations. *Folia Biol. (Praha) 18,* 350 (1972).

Mitchison, N. A., Passive transfer of transplantation immunity. *Proc. Royal Soc. London (Biol.) 142,* 72 (1954).

Snell, G. D., Methods for the study of histocompatibility genes. *J. Genet. 49,* 87 (1948).

Tyzzer, E. E., A study of inheritance in mice with reference to their susceptibility to transplantable tumors. *J. Med. Res. 21,* 519 (1909).

CHAPTER 9

Genetic Organization of the Major Histocompatibility Complexes of Mice and Humans

The Mouse MHC (H-2)

Overview

The major histocompatibility complex of the mouse, commonly known as the H-2 complex, is one of the most intensely studied gene systems in higher organisms. As with all MHC systems, the principal role of molecules coded for by genes within this complex is to facilitate the interaction of T lymphocytes with other cells of the immune system. Coincidentally, the products of the two major gene classes within this complex (class I and class II genes) provide the strongest immunological barrier to transplantation of cells and tissues.

The topography of H-2 is shown in Figure 9-1. The H-2 complex is associated with linkage group IX, which can be assigned to chromosome 17. The H-2 complex has traditionally been considered to be bounded by the K and D/L regions. However, a series of closely related genes lies nearby in the Tla region. As we will see, the structures of most of the Tla region genes, and of their gene products, are homologous with the genes and gene products of the K and D/L regions. Because of their obvious relatedness, some immunologists have suggested they be included as part of the MHC. However, a major definition of the MHC rests in the immune functions associated with its genes. So far, no obligatory immune functions have been assigned to genes in the Tla region, and for that reason we will treat Tla as a distinct, although closely related, region of chromosome 17.

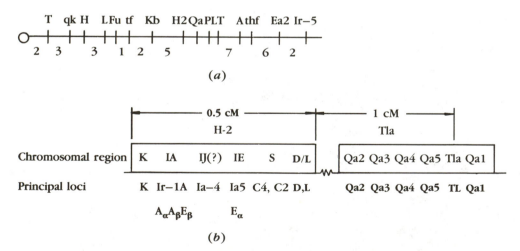

Figure 9-1 (*a*) Genetic map of chromosome 17. Loci from left to right are: T—short tail; qk—quaking; H—hybrid sterility; L—low transmission ratio; Fu—fused; tf—tufted; Kb—knobbly; H-2; Qa—Q region antigens; TL—thymus leukemia antigens; P—phosphoglycerate kinase; A—acid phosphatase (liver); thf—thin fur; Ea2—erythrocyte antigen 2; Ir-5—immune response gene 5. (*b*) The H-2 and Tla regions of chromosome 17.

A *region* within H-2 is defined as a segment of chromosome that serves as the locus for at least one defined gene, *and* that can be distinguished from regions on either side by recombinational (crossing-over) events. A region may actually be the location of a large number of genes, but these genes are tied together by the fact that they have never been observed to segregate independently of one another. The existence of a particular region is inferred from classical gene mapping studies, in which a specific phenotypic trait is associated with the presence or absence of a particular chromosomal segment. However, it is important to remember that when the genes for more than one phenotypic trait map to a given region, there is no way to determine whether these traits are coded for (or controlled) by the same or different genes, until either the DNA containing the genes is directly sequenced and related to distinct gene products responsible for the phenotypic traits, or until the genes can be shown to segregate independently in breeding studies.

The I region of H-2 has at one time or another been divided into as many as five *subregions,* each of which was originally defined by an inferred crossing-over event on both sides. More recently, the I region has been divided into three subregions. The reason for this confusion will be apparent when we discuss the I region in detail later in the chapter. For purposes of drawing a map of H-2 that conforms to molecular genetic evidence, we will consider the I region to be composed of only two subregions—IA and IE.

As we will see in the remaining chapters of this text, the principal function of gene products coded for by known genes in the H-2 complex, with the exception of those in the S region, is in facilitating the interaction of T cells with other cells of the immune system. Thus, in a functional sense, all of these genes are quite similar. However, two major classes of genes that facilitate T-cell reactions can be readily distinguished on the basis of the structure of their products. Genes in the K and D/L regions code for ca. 45,000-dalton peptides involved in the recognition, by cytotoxic T cells, of self cells altered by virus or by oncological transformation. These are referred to as *class I genes and gene products.* Coincidentally, class I gene products are the major target antigens in transplant rejection; we will discuss this topic in detail in Chapter 14.

Genes in the IA and IE subregions code for two peptides associated with each subregion: α (ca. 34,000 daltons), and β (ca. 28,000 daltons). The dimers formed by these peptides facilitate T cell recognition of a wide spectrum of antigens presented on the surface of macrophages, dendritic cells, or B cells. The IA and IE dimers are referred to as *class II gene products.*

Complement and complement-associated genes associated with the S region of H-2 have been referred to as class III genes, although they probably should not be classed as MHC genes at all. We will return to this point later. Monaco and McDevitt have reported a fourth class of genes, mapping to either K or IA, that codes for a family of proteins in the 15,000- to 30,000-dalton size range. These proteins have been identified so far in macrophages, lymphocytes, and fibroblasts. They are not glycosylated and appear not to be expressed at the cell surface. A function for these proteins has not yet been discerned and thus their relationship (if any) to other MHC proteins is unknown.

Class I and class II MHC genes have an extraordinarily large number of alleles distributed throughout a given species. This "polymorphism" of histocompatibility molecules within a species is one of the unique features of both class I and class II MHC products. Various combinations of these alleles occur in different individuals and the different inbred strains that have been produced so far. The particular collection of H-2 alleles assembled on one chromosome of a given individual is referred to as the H-2 *haplotype* for that individual. Each member of an inbred strain is of course identical and homozygous throughout H-2 for the same haplotype. The allele of each gene, locus, or region within the H-2 complex is signified by appending the haplotype designation letter (in lowercase) as a super-script to the designation letter (in uppercase) for the gene, locus, or region. For example, the D gene of strain C3H (H-2^k) is formally identified as D^k. The IA subregion of strain C57BL/6 is written as IA^b.

As we can see from Table 9-1, more than one inbred strain may possess a given H-2 haplotype. By definition, however, such H-2 identical strains differ from one another in at least one (and usually many) other, non H-2 histocompatibility locus (see section on minor H loci below). Also, some haplotypes (H-2^a, for example) clearly arose through an intra-H-2 crossing-over event between two of the "pro-totypical" mouse H-2 complexes. In these cases the individual genes are identified by the haplotype superscript of the strain of origin. H-2^a mice are thus K^{k}I^{k}D^d.

The H-2 complex has been analyzed in great detail, principally by the develop-ment of lines of mice congenic for the H-2 complex. These congenic strains include a large variety of recombinant H-2 haplotypes, and are thus very useful for the production of highly specific H-2 antisera. For example, the A.AL and A.TL strains (Table 9-1) are entirely identical genetically, with the exception of the K region of

Table 9-1 H-2 Haplotypes of Some Representative Mouse Strains

Representative strain	Haplotype designation	Haplotype composition				
		K	IA	IE	S	D/L
Prototypical and H-2 congenic strains						
C57BL/6; C57BL/10; BALB.B; C.SW	*b*	*b*	*b*	*b*	*b*	*b*
C3H; CBA; AKR; B10.BR	*k*	*k*	*k*	*k*	*k*	*k*
BALB/c; DBA/2; B10.D2	*d*	*d*	*d*	*d*	*d*	*d*
DBA/1	*q*	*q*	*q*	*q*	*q*	*q*
H-2 recombinant strains						
A; B10.A	*a*	*k*	*k*	*k*	*d*	*d*
A.AL	*al*	*k*	*k*	*k*	*k*	*d*
A.TL	*tl*	*s*	*k*	*k*	*k*	*d*
B10.AKM; AKR.M	*m*	*k*	*k*	*k*	*k*	*q*

H-2. The B10.BR and B10.AKM strains differ only at the D/L region. Many more such specific combinations are possible.

The K and D/L Regions

As we saw earlier, the existence of products coded for by the gene complex we now call H-2 was first detected by Peter Gorer as a blood group antigen. He and others subsequently showed that, unlike other blood group antigens, H-2 (or antigen II as he originally called it) played an important role in the rejection of nonblood-cell-derived transplantable tumors, and of normal tissues as well. We now know that the antigens Gorer and subsequent workers were detecting are found on the polypeptide products coded for by class I genes of the K and D/L regions of H-2. Class I gene products are ca. 45,000 dalton integral glycoproteins of the plasma membranes of essentially all adult cells, not only in the mouse, but in all vertebrate species examined. They are always found in association with β-2 micro-globulin (ca. 12,000 daltons) at the cell surface. Class I proteins are present in particularly high concentration on leukocytes (ca. 10^5 molecules/cell). Up until a few years ago, it was assumed (in keeping with the two-gene model for H-2) that only two genes (K and D) and two gene products were responsible for the collection of H-2-associated histocompatibility antigens. As we will see shortly, there are

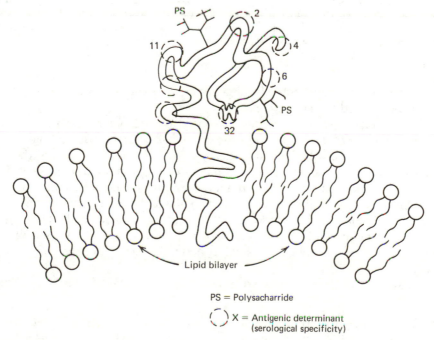

PS = Polysacharride

( ) X = Antigenic determinant
(serological specificity)

Figure 9-2 A schematic view of the orientation of a histocompatibility protein in a lipid bilayer.

Table 9-2 Distribution of Serologically Defined Specificities Among the Major Prototypical Inbred Mouse Strains

	Antigens of the K series																			
H-2 haplotype	**Public**																			**Private**
	1	**3**	**5**	**8**	**11**	**25**	**27**	**28**	**29**	**34**	**35**	**36**	**37**	**38**	**39**	**42**	**45**	**46**	**47**	
b	—	—	5	—	—	—	27	28	29	—	35	36	—	—	39	—	—	46	—	33
d	—	3	—	8	—	—	27	28	29	34	—	—	—	—	—	—	—	46	47	31
f	—	—	—	8	—	—	?	?	?	—	—	—	37	—	39	—	—	46	—	26
j	—	—	c	—	—	—	•	•	•	—	—	—	—	38	—	—	45	?	?	15
k	1	3	5	8	11	25	—	—	—	—	—	—	—	—	—	—	45	—	47	23
p	1	—	5	8	—	—	—	—	—	34?	—	—	37	38	—	—	—	46?	•	16
q	1	3	5	—	11	—	—	—	—	34	—	—	—	—	—	—	45	—	—	17
r	1	3	5	8	11	25	—	—	—	—	—	—	—	—	—	—	45	—	47	•
s	1	—	5	—	—	—	—	28	—	—	—	—	—	—	—	42	45	•	—	19
u	c	—	5	8?	—	—	—	—	—	—	35	36	—	—	—	—	45	•	•	20
v	1	3	—	—	—		•	•	•	—	—	—	—	—	—	—	45	—	•	21
z	—	•	5	—	—	—	27	—	29	—	—	—	—	—	—	—	—	46	47	•

(−) = absence of an antigen; (•) = unknown; (?) = presence or absence of antigen is uncertain; (c) = some antisera cross-react with the indicated H-2 haplotype.

at least two and perhaps more class I genes and peptide products associated with what is now called the D/L region.

The portions of class I molecules exposed on the outer surface of the cell exhibit a number of distinct antigenic determinants or "specificities" (Figure 9-2). These specificities involve only the "heavy chain" of class I molecules; the β_2m chain is relatively invariant among members of the same strain. Each of these specificities is defined by an antiserum monospecific for the determinant in question, that is, one that will not cross-react with any of the other determinants.[1] The rather large number of these seriologically defined specificities, and their irregular distribution among various haplotypes (a reflection of class I polymorphism), made interpretation of the genetic and biochemical nature of H-2 difficult for many years.

The various H-2 specificities are now assigned to one of two fairly distinct

---

[1]The term determinant is used here in the purely operational sense. A determinant could be composed of more than one distinct antigenic structure. If two strains are found which "split" these antigens between themselves, production of a more refined antiserum will be possible, and one determinant will become two. This still happens occasionally in HLA serology.

Antigens of the D series																Antigens of the L series					
Public															Private						
1	3	5	6	13	27	28	29	35	36	41	42	43	44	49		1	27	28	29	64	65
—	—	—	6	—	27	28	29	—	—	—	—	—	—	—	2	—	27	28	29	64	—
—	3	—	6	13	27	28	29	35	36	41	42	43	44	49	4	—	27	28	29	64	65
—	—	—	6	—	27	?	?	—	—	—	—	—	—	—	9	—	27	?	?	•	•
—	—	—	6	—	—	28	29	—	—	—	—	—	44	—	2	—	—	28	29	•	•
1	3	5	—	—	—	—	—	—	—	—	—	—	—	49	32	1	—	—	—	—	—
1	3	5	6	—	—	—	—	35	—	41	—	—	—	49	22	1	—	—	—	•	•
—	3	—	6	13	27	28	29	c	c	—	—	—	—	49	30	—	27	28	29	64	65
1	•	5	6	—	—	—	—	—	—	—	—	—	—	49	18	1	—	—	—	•	•
—	3	—	6	—	—	28	—	•	36	—	42	—	—	49	12	—	—	28	—	•	•
—	3	—	6	?	?	28	29	—	—	41	42	43	—	49	4	—	27?	28	29	•	•
—	•	—	•	—	?	28	•	—	—	—	—	43	—	49	30	—	?	28?	•	•	•
—	—	—	—	—	•	•	•	—	—	—	—	—	—	•	•	—	•	•	•	•	•

although occasionally overlapping categories, public specificities and private specificities (Table 9-2). Public specificities (e.g., H-2.5) are those that occur on K and/or D/L region proteins of a number of different haplotypes, while private specificities (e.g., H-2.2) appear to be both haplotype-specific and restricted to a single K or D/L region gene product.

Serological analysis, as well as direct structural studies of the K and D/L genes and proteins, confirms the notion that the corresponding genes arose through duplications of a common ancestral gene. The widely distributed public specificities may reflect those portions of genes and gene products that are crucial to molecular folding or function, and that have evolved little since the initial duplication event. The more restricted public specificities, and the private specificities, presumably reflect accumulated noncompromising mutational events occurring after gene duplication.

The study of serological specificities associated with class I proteins was for many years a major focus of immunologists trying to understand major histocompatibility complexes. The development of monoclonal antibodies, and the ability to study MHC genes by directly sequencing DNA, has led to a diminished interest in MHC serology per se. The principal value of charts of the type shown in Table 9-2 is to impress on the novice immunologist the tremendous polymorphism of class I MHC genes and gene products.

Evidence for Multiple Class I Gene Loci in the D/L Region of H-2

The two-gene model for the H-2 locus predicted that specificities unique to the K end of H-2 should exist in the membrane independently of specificities assigned only to the D end. This was initially confirmed using monospecific antisera in capping studies. For example, antibodies against specificity 31 (Table 9-2) will cocap the K protein (and associated specificities) of H-2^d haplotype cells, but will not cocap specificities uniquely associated with the D^d region (4, 6, 49, etc.) The same results were obtained when K and D region-associated antigens were independently precipitated from a solution of solubilized H-2 proteins with monospecific antisera. In fact, studies of the latter type provided the first direct biochemical evidence in support of the two-gene model.

However, a more careful application of these two techniques to an analysis of D-region specificities provided evidence for the existence of at least one additional peptide (L) coded for by a gene distinct from the originally defined D gene. The experiments establishing a separate L protein displaying some of the D region specificities (as well as L-unique specificities) were carried out by P. Demant and his colleagues, who pioneered much of the work on isolation and characterization of H-2 and HLA antigens.

In the first series of experiments using cells of H-2^a mice (K^{k}D^d), it was found that antibody against the private D^d specificity, H-2.4, did not cause complete cocapping of the D^d public specificity H-2.28, whereas anti-H-2.4 did induce complete cocapping of the D^d public specificities H-2.3, H-2.35, and H-2.36 (Figure 9-3). This finding taken alone would suggest that H-2.28 was on a surface molecule different from at least some of the molecules containing H-2.4 and H-2.3, H-2.35, and H-2.36. The reverse experiment showed that antibody to H-2.28 always induced complete cocapping of H-2.4. In order to clarify the situation further, these same researchers carried out direct immunoprecipitation of detergent solubilized D^d antigens. In these experiments, antibodies specific for H-2.4 failed to precipitate all of the molecules bearing H-2.28, whereas H-2.28 antibodies precipitated all H-2.4-bearing molecules. The two approaches, surface capping and direct immunoprecipitation, thus gave the same results.

To account for these findings, Demant proposed that the D region of H-2 contains two genes, D and D', each of which codes for a 45,000-dalton surface H-2 protein. The D gene was proposed to code for all of the private and public specificities previously associated with the D region. The D' (now L) gene was proposed to code for at least the specificity H-2.28 (actually the family of antigens H-2.27, H-2.28, and H-2.29, which always occur together), and possibly other specificities. When capping of surface H-2 proteins is carried out with anti-H-2.4, the H-2.28 (and other public specificities) associated with the D-gene product will cap but the

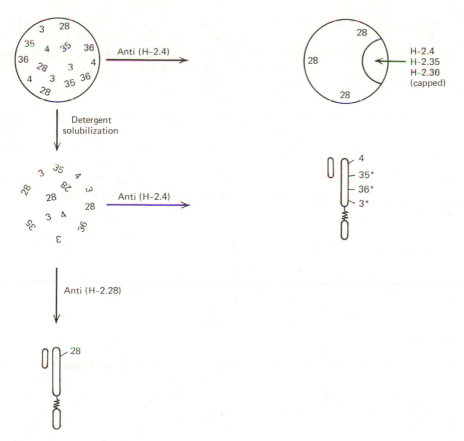

Figure 9-3 Demant's experiment showing that some H-2 specificities cap independently of others.

H-2.28 associated with the L-gene product will remain dispersed on the membrane. On the other hand, when capping is done with antibodies to H-2.28, H-2.4 will obviously be completely capped. A similar interpretation extends to the immunoprecipitation studies.

Demant's findings were rapidly confirmed, and it is now generally accepted that the D region of H-2 is also the locus for the separate gene L. In addition to the specificities H-2.27-29, L proteins may also display H-2.1 and two new specificities, H-2.64 and H-2.65. The L gene has now been cloned and sequenced, and its homology with K and D genes is such that it can be assumed to have arisen from either the K or D gene, or their progenitor, by gene duplication. Just when this may have occurred during evolution relative to formation of the K and D genes is uncertain. So far, the L gene appears to be much less polymorphic than the K and D genes, and in this respect is quite similar to the HLA-C gene in humans (p. 220).

The BALB/c mutant H-2^{dm2} has proved useful in the analysis of the L-gene product, because it does not express an immunologically detectable H-2L protein on its surface membrane. Thus immunization of BALB/c.dm2 mice with BALB/c spleen cells (which do display the L^{d}molecule) provides an antiserum specific for the H-2L^d surface protein. Whether H-2^{dm2} lacks the H-2L gene, or simply fails to express the H-2L surface product, is not known.

More recent work by Demant and by others suggests that the D region may be even more complex. Capping studies with monospecific antibodies have defined two additional molecules, called H-2M and H-2R, that are antigenically distinct from D and L. However, direct DNA sequencing of the D region of several strains shows only a single D region gene, so the additional D-associated molecules must be either RNA-splicing variants of the D transcript, or post-translational modifications of the D-gene product.

Specificities H-2.1 and H-2.28

The public specificities H-2.1 and H-2.28 are deserving of special attention. H-2.28 can probably be considered to be a family, composed of the specificities H-2.27, H-2.28, and H-2.29. These specificities generally occur together in an all-or-none fashion (Table 9-2). Furthermore, expression of the H-2.28 family and H-2.1 seems to be mutually exclusive in that they never occur together on the same K, D, or L molecules. This suggested to some geneticists that these two families might, in fact, be generalized H-2 alleles. That is, the primordial H-2 class I gene (or genes) may have had two allelic forms in the species carrying it: allele 28, and allele 1. All existing variants of class I molecules within an H-2 haplotype (K, D, or L), and all polymorphic variants thereof (e.g., K^b versus K^d versus K^k; D^b versus D^q versus D^s; etc.) would be derivations of one or the other of the two primordial alleles. Resolution of the H-2.1/H-2.28 puzzle should come about in the near future with progress in sequencing class I genes of different haplotypes.

Function of Murine Class I MHC Proteins

The function of the proteins coded for by the H-2K, D, and L genes have been a subject of intense speculation ever since their discoveries. Clearly, they did not evolve simply to prevent organ transplantation. Class I antigens appear on embryonic cells immediately after implantation in the uterine wall. Their existence on virtually every cell in the body and their relative structural conservatism phylogenetically, combined with conservation of an unusual degree of polymorphism within a species, all point to an important biological role for these cell surface proteins.

Various hypotheses have been put forth concerning what this role might be. Among those that have been considered and generally discarded are that these proteins serve as cell surface receptor molecules, as membrane-bound enzymes, as necessary surface markers to guide cell–cell interactions during embryological development, and as recognition determinants in immune surveillance. The latter idea, first formulated in the early 1970s, suggests that these antigens are recognized by immune receptors in the host system. As long as the cell is a healthy self-cell, then its interaction with the host immune system is completely benign. However, if the cell is not self, or if selfness has been altered by disease, then the cell will be attacked by the host's immune system. It was proposed that the location of the receptors for self in this surveillance system would be on some form of T cell.

Although this proposal was intellectually pleasing from a number of points of view, it was initially vague and had virtually no experimental support. In 1974, however, a series of observations made by Doherty and Zinkernagel, concerning the immune response to virally infected self-cells, put the immune surveillance hypothesis on a firm footing. These experiments are discussed in detail in Chapter 14. Briefly, they can be summarized as follows. When a virus infects a cell, the presence of viral antigens on the cell surface is detected by host T cells. However, T cells do not respond to the viral antigen alone, but rather to the viral antigen in the context of self-class I MHC antigens. This phenomenon is known as *MHC restriction*.

The I Region of H-2; Class II MHC Proteins

As we saw in Chapter 8, the existence of the I region was established as the result of mapping of the first immune response gene in mice (Ir-1A). Within a few years, additional Ir genes were detected that mapped to a genetically separable locus, which was called Ir-1B (Figure 8-5). This also defined a new region of H-2. Because of its apparent functional relatedness to the Ir-1A locus, it was decided to make the two Ir loci subregions of the I region, IA and IB, respectively.

By cross-immunizing mice differing in the I region (in an attempt to define an Ir gene product), a series of antigenic specificities was discovered (Table 9-3) that mapped to the IA subregion and to a new, previously undetected subregion of I designated originally as IC. The antigenic specificities were named Ia (for I region associated), and the locus defining IC was designated Ia3. The next splitting occured when an antiserum was found that reacted uniquely with suppressor T cells, defining a determinant not associated with IA or IC. This determinant was found to map to a locus between, and genetically separable from, IB and IC. This locus, called Ia-4, thus defined a new I subregion, IJ. At almost the same time that IJ was described, several laboratories suggested that some and perhaps all of the specificities associated with the IC subregion actually mapped to a separate subregion to the left of IC, but not equivalent to the newly defined IJ. Thus a fifth locus was proposed, Ia-5, which defined the IE subregion.

The composition of the I region is under constant scrutiny by immunogeneticists and molecular biologists and has undergone considerable change in the past few years. It is now generally agreed, for example, that IB is not really a distinct subregion. No new Ir genes have been mapped to the Ir-1B locus, and no Ia-antigenic specificities have ever been uniquely associated with an IB subregion. Moreover, direct gene sequencing of the MHC region provides no evidence for a distinct IB subregion. The genes thought to define IB are almost certainly IA genes.

Table 9-3 Distribution of Ia Antigens
Controlled by Unrelated H-2 Haplotypes

H-2 haplotype	Type strain	Ia antigen 1	2	3	4	5	6	7	8	9	10	11	12	13	14	15
b	C57BL/10	—	—	3	—	—	—	—	8	9	—	—	—	—	—	15
d	B10.D2	—	—	—	—	—	6	7	8	—	—	11	—	—	—	15
f	B10.M	1	—	—	—	5	—	—	—	—	—	—	—	—	14	—
j	B10.WB	—	—	•	—	5	•	7	•	•	10	—	—	—	•	•
k	B10.BR	1	2	3	—	—	—	7	—	—	—	—	—	—	—	15
p	B10.P	—	—	—	—	5	6	7	—	—	—	—	—	13	—	—
q	B10.Q	—	—	3	—	5	—	—	—	9	10	—	—	13	—	—
r	B10.RIII(71NS)	1	—	3	—	5	—	7	—	—	—	—	12	—	—	—
s	B10.S	—	—	—	4	5	—	—	—	9	—	—	12	—	—	—
u	B10.PL(73NS)	1	—	•	—	5	•	7	•	•	—	—	—	—	•	•
v	B10.SM	—	—	•	—	5	•	7	•	•	—	—	—	—	•	•

Taken from J. Klein, L. Flaherty, J. L. VandeBerg, and D. C. Shreffler. H-2 haplotypes, genes, regions, and antigens: First listing. *Immunogenetics 6,* 489 (1978). Copyright by Springer-Verlag, New York (1978).

It is also now generally accepted that the Ia determinants originally assigned to the IC subregion are actually coded for by the IE genes, and there is again no evidence at the DNA level for a distinct IC subregion. It now appears that the inferred existence of the IB and IC subregions was based on misinterpretations of the exact crossover points defining the intra-H2 recombinations of strain pairs used to define these subregions. Thus, by 1982, most immunologists recognized only three subregions of H-2I: IA, IE and IJ.

The I-J Subregion

The history of the so-called I-J subregion is an interesting and instructive one. It was originally defined by antisera made in certain congenic strains of mice such as B10.A (3R) and B10.A (5R) mice. When, for example, lymphoid cells from B10.A (5R) are injected into B10.A (3R) mice, the resulting antiserum detects an antigen present on certain T cells of various H-2^k mouse strains. The IJ antigen is also detected on a "T suppressor factor" (TsF), a molecule produced by T suppressor cells that inhibits T helper cell function. TsF is a dimer; only one of the subunits displays the IJ determinant. Because of the genetic mapping of B10.A (3R) and B10.A (5R), it was assumed that a new subregion, called I-J, must exist between IA and IE. The presence of this antigen correlates well with suppressor T-cell function, so this antigen, called IJ, was assumed to be a differentiation antigen specific for suppressor T cells.

16	17	18	19	20	21	22	23	24	W25	W26	W27	W28	W29	W30	31	32	33
—	—	—	—	20	—	—	—	—	—	—	—	—	W29	W30	—	—	—
16	—	—	—	—	—	—	23	—	—	—	—	—	—	W30	—	—	—
—	17	18	—	—	—	—	—	—	W25	W26	W27	W28	W29	W30	—	—	—
•	•	•	—	•	•	•	•	—	•	•	•	•	•	•	•	—	32	33
—	17	18	19	—	—	22	—	—	W25	W26	—	W28	—	—	31	32	33
—	—	—	—	21	—	—	—	—	•	•	•	•	•	•	—	32	—
16	—	—	—	—	—	—	—	—	—	—	—	—	—	W30	—	—	—
—	17	—	19	—	—	—	—	24	W25	W26	—	W28	W29	—	—	32	33
—	17	18	—	—	—	—	—	24	—	—	W27	—	W29	W30	—	—	33
•	•	•	—	•	•	•	•	24	•	•	•	•	•	•	•	31	32	33
•	•	•	—	•	•	•	•	—	•	•	•	•	•	•	—	32	—

Few immunologists disagree with many of the facts of this story. The 3R anti-5R serum and other sera have been produced in many laboratories. They do, indeed, react with an antigen that correlates with T_S function. But it is quite clear that the gene coding for the antigen detected by the 3R anti-5R serum does not map to the I region of H-2.

The evidence in support of this assertion is now overwhelming. The first direct evidence that a separate IJ region might not exist came from DNA sequencing studies of the H-2 region carried out by Michael Steinmetz and Lee Hood at Cal Tech. They found the A_β, A_α, E_β, and E_α genes—and even a hitherto undetected E_β gene that probably is not expressed—but no IJ gene anywhere in between.

Another line of evidence was provided by Colleen Hayes and her co-workers. She used the 3R anti-5R serum to test a wide range of H-2^k haplotype mice. If an IJ^k gene does exist, then it should be expressed in every nonrecombinant H-2^k strain. As shown in Table 9-4, this turned out not to be true. Although the IJ^k antigen is present in many H-2^k mouse strains, it is not present in all. Certain H-2^k congenic mice are particularly instructive. The AKR mouse is H-2^k, but does not express IJ on its T cells. However, when the H-2^k region of AKR mice is transferred onto a B6 (normally H-2^b) background to form the B6.H-2^k strain, an IJ^k antigen is suddenly detectable! The reciprocal congenic (AKR.H-2^b) is negative, so we can safely infer that *something* in H-2^k is involved. When AKR mice are mated with strain B10, the resultant (B10 × AKR)F$_1$ hybrids display the IJ^k antigen. This looks very much like a two-gene complementation system.

Table 9-4 Distribution of the I-J^k Antigen among Various Mouse Strains

Strain	Haplotype					3R anti-5R reactivity
	K	**IA**	**(IJ)**	**IE**	**D**	
C57BL/6 (B6)	*b*	*b*	(*b*)	*b*	*b*	−
C3H	*k*	*k*	(*k*)	*k*	*k*	+
AKR/J	*k*	*k*	(*k*)	*k*	*k*	−
B6.H-2^k	*k*	*k*	(*k*)	*k*	*k*	+
AKR.H-2^b	*b*	*b*	(*b*)	*b*	*b*	−
C57BL/10 (B10)	*b*	*b*	(*b*)	*b*	*b*	−
B10.A	*k*	*k*	(*k*)	*d*	*d*	+
B10.A (3R)	*b*	*b*	(*b*)	*k*	*d*	−
B10.A (4R)	*k*	*k*	(*b*)	*b*	*b*	−
B10.A (5R)	*b*	*b*	(*k*)	*k*	*d*	+
(AKR × B10)F$_1$	*b/k*	*b/k*	(*b/k*)	*b/k*	*b/k*	+

What is the antigen detected by the 3R anti-5R serum? What sort of genic control is it under? We do not know the complete answers to these questions yet, but an analysis of the origin of the mouse strains used in the original experiments may shed light on some of the confusion surrounding the specificity of the 3R anti-5R serum.

The 3R and 5R strains arose during the "breeding in" of the strain A H-2 region (H-2^a) onto the B10 (H-2^b) background to produce the B10.A (H-2^a) congenic mouse strain. The method for producing such strains is described in Appendix 1. (B10 × A)F$_1$ mice are backcrossed to the B10 parent, and from this mating only progeny retaining the A H-2 region are retained. These are again backcrossed to B10 mating partners, and this basic process is repeated for many generations. As the rounds of backcrossing proceed, the amount of nonselected (non-H-2) material from the original A parent is reduced dramatically. At some point, only A strain genetic material physically linked to H-2^a will be present in the new B10.A strain. With further rounds of backcrossing, the A-strain chromosomal segment containing H-2^a will become smaller and smaller, until it approaches the limits of the H-2^a region itself. This would require many, many rounds of backcrossing.

B10.A (3R) is a spontaneous intra-H-2^a recombinant that arose during the seventh backcross generation, which was isolated and used to establish a separate inbred strain. The B10.A (5R) recombinant arose during the eleventh backcross generation. Both of these represent fairly early points in the establishment of congenicity. The likelihood of having closely linked non-H-2 genetic material from the A strain, on either side of the H-2 locus, is quite substantial. Thus, in retrospect, it is not absolutely certain that the 3R anti-5R serum would be reacting against only H-2-coded antigens.

Another possibility is that a gene within H-2 must interact with a non-H-2 gene to produce the IJ antigenic determinant. This would be consistent with the B6.H-2^k versus AKR.H-2^b data in Table 9-4. Preliminary investigations of this possibility by Hayes and her colleagues suggest a locus on chromosome 4 may be involved, although this has not yet been formally proved. The region of H-2 involved in complementation of the non-H-2 gene is most likely IE. How these two loci interact, and whether either, neither, or both code for structural elements associated with the I-J antigen, remains to be determined.

Function of Class II MHC Proteins

The antigens associated with the IA and IE subregions of H-2 are contained on dimeric glycopeptide molecules (class II MHC proteins). The monomeric subunits are referred to as α (32,000 to 36,000 daltons) and β (26,000 to 29,000 daltons). Alpha chains associated with either subregion display only limited polymorphism among different strains; most of the class II polymorphism is associated with the β chains. As we will see in Chapter 10, the organization of the genes coding for these monomers is somewhat complex. Both of the genes coding for the IA dimer (A_α and $_\beta$) map to IA. However, IA is also the locus for one of the genes (E_β) coding for one of the IE monomers. The gene for the other IE monomer (E_α), which actually controls the expression or nonexpression of the complete IE dimer, maps to the IE subregion. Interestingly, a number of mouse strains do not display class II MHC products associated with the IE region. We will discuss this in more detail in the next chapter.

Class II MHC products have a much more limited distribution than class I MHC products. They are found on all B cells, probably on all dendritic cells of the type described in Chapter 2, and probably on all epidermal Langerhans cells (which may be a form of dendritic cell). Class II antigens are also found on certain subsets of macrophages, possibly on some T-cell subsets, on thymic epithelial cells, and to some extent (depending on the species) on intestinal epithelium and vascular endothelium. In some cases, apparently class II-negative cells may display class II molecules under the inductive influence of lymphokines such as γ-interferon.

As we will discuss in more detail in Chapter 13, class II proteins control the interaction of T helper cells with macrophages and B cells. One of the first steps in the production of antibody is the presentation of antigen on macrophages or dendritic cells to T helper cells. But T_h cells can only respond to foreign antigens presented in the context of self class II antigens coded for the IA or IE subregions. After this initial triggering step, the activated T_h cell must interact with a B cell, and induce it to make antibody. In many cases, this T_h-B cell interaction is also restricted by self class II antigens.

The S Region of the H-2 Complex

The S region of H-2 was originally defined by a gene coding for an allelomorphic protein called simply "serum substance" (Ss). The *b* allele of Ss (Ss*b*) is associated with high levels of this substance in serum, while low levels are found in mice with the *l* allele (Ss*l*). Ss*l* is associated only with the H-2*k* haplotype. Recombinant strains that have acquired *k* alleles of the genes between the I and D regions also have the low serum phenotype (Ss*l*). In males of most inbred strains, the level of Ss protein is partly regulated by sex hormones. After puberty, the amount of this protein in the serum approximately doubles. This increase can be prevented by depriving the male of testosterone. Females have low levels of Ss, like prepubescent males of their strain, throughout life. However, they can be brought up to the adult male level by administration of testosterone.

We now know from work in several laboratories that Ss is component C4 of the complement system. This conclusion was initially based on the observations that Ss has an overall size and subunit composition very similar to C4; that antibody to human C4 cross-reacts strongly with Ss; and that antibody to Ss will agglutinate blood cells with C4 on their surfaces. Recently, the C4 gene has been isolated and sequenced and restriction-mapped to the Ss locus. The C4 gene in humans also maps to the MHC.

A second gene defining the S region of H-2 is the Slp (sex-limited protein) gene. Although the Slp gene is carried by both males and females, it is expressed in (i.e., Slp is found in the serum of) males only. Expression in the various strains is all or none. Positive strains are designated as carrying the Slp*a* alleles, and negative strains are designated Slp*o*. The distribution of Slp alleles seems partially bound up with the Ss system, in that all strains bearing the Slp*o* allele carry the Ss*l* allele. However, both Slp*a* and Slp*o* are found in association with Ss*b*.

Males of Slp*a* strains have no detectable levels of Slp before puberty. Appearance of Slp can be prevented by castration and restored by testosterone. Females of Slp*a* strains develop male levels of Slp when treated with the male hormone. Testosterone has no effect on prepubertal Slp*a* males, or on Slp*o* females.

Slp was known for some years to be structurally and antigenically closely related to the Ss protein (C4). It is now clear from isolation and study of DNA sequences in the S region of H-2 that Slp is a duplication of the C4 gene that has accumulated enough mutations to lose its function as C4, but not enough to prevent its transcription and translation. In the human, where such a duplication is also apparent, both copies of the C4 gene are active.

Genes coding for two other complement proteins are now known to map to the region of H-2 lying between IE and D (Figure 9-4). C2 and B_f, which are closely related both structurally and functionally, lie just upstream from Slp and C4.

From a functional point of view, the complement genes mapping to H-2 are scarcely related to the class I and class II genes, and it may be that their location is purely fortuitous rather than an organizational or functional necessity. Nor are the complement genes mapping to the MHC struturally homologous to class I or class

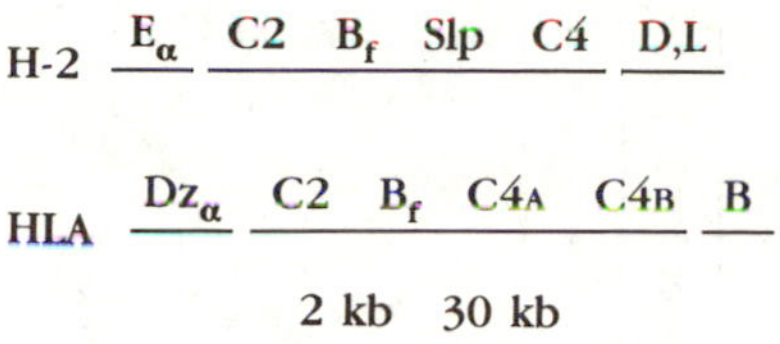

H-2 $\dfrac{E_\alpha \quad C2 \quad B_f \quad Slp \quad C4 \quad D,L}{}$

HLA $\dfrac{Dz_\alpha \quad C2 \quad B_f \quad C4_A \quad C4_B \quad B}{}$

2 kb   30 kb

Figure 9-4 Genetic mapping of complement components associated with the mouse and human MHCs.

II genes. Complement genes seem to be scattered randomly among the various chromosomes, and Jan Klein has made the point that since the other complement genes are not considered MHC genes, neither should C4 and C2. This point of view has some merit.

The "G" Region of H-2

The existence of one or more genetic loci between the S and D regions might be expected on the basis of the large number of S–D crossovers. In 1975, two laboratories proposed that a gene mapping between Ss and D coded for the H-2 specificity H-2.7. This specificity, originally thought to be associated with the K protein, was found to have a different tissue distribution from K/D antigens, being present in high concentration on erythrocytes, but in low concentration or absent on lymphocytes. On the basis of studies with an intra-H-2 recombinant (A.TFRI), it was proposed that the gene controlling H-2.7 mapped to a distinct region of H-2 between Ss and D. This locus was thus given an official designation (H-2G). However, subsequent studies showed that the mapping of the H-2.7 locus using A.TFRI was in error, and that H-2.7 actually maps in the S region. Additional experiments showed that antisera specific for H-2.7 precipitate C4, and in particular react with the C4d fragment. It now seems certain that H-2.7 is passively acquired by erythrocytes from the serum as a result of C4 activation. Both the notion of an H-2.7 specificity, and of a separate H-2G region of the murine MHC containing an H-2.7 gene, have now been dropped.

The Tla Region of Chromosome 17

The chromosomal segment bounded by the H-2K and D regions, which contains the genetic material defined by the early studies of Gorer, Snell, and others, is often thought of as a discrete genetic region, unrelated to adjacent chromosomal regions. It has become clear in recent years that this view is no longer tenable. An increasing number of loci have been defined on the telomeric side of the K-D bounded complex that code for allelic cell surface antigens found principally on lymphoid cells. More importantly, as we will see later, many of the genes and gene products coded for by loci lying to the right of H-2D are also structurally homologous with K and D region genes and gene products.

Table 9-5 Strain Distribution of Tla Region Antigens

Strain	H-2 haplotype	Qa antigens						Allele	Tla[1] Specificities					
		Qa1	Qa2	Qa3	Qa4	Qa5	Qa6		1	2	3	4	5	6
A	a	a	a	a	a?	b	a	a	1	2	3	—	5	6
C57BL/6	b	b	a	a	a	a	a	b	—	—	—	—	—	—
BALB/c	d	b	b/a²	b/a	b/a	b	a/b	c	—	2	—	—	—	—
A.CA	f	c	b	b	b	b	b	d	1	2	3	—	—	—
CBA	k	b	b	b	b	b	b	b	—	—	—	—	—	—
DBA/1	q	b	a	b	a	b	a	b	—	—	—	—	—	—
A.SW	s	b	a	a	a	a	b	b	—	—	—	—	—	—
P/J	p	a	b	b	b	b	b	e	1	2	3	—	5	—

[1]The Tla specificities shown are for the TL antigen on normal thymus cells. Specificity 4 is found only on certain thymus leukemias.
²H-2 identical sublines of BALB/c have been identified that have differences in the Qa2-4 and Qa6 loci.

Boyse first described the Tla locus in the late 1960s. A gene at this locus, which maps 1.5 cM to the right of H-2D, codes for the TL antigen, which is found on immature (cortical) thymocytes and on some T-cell leukemias. A similar gene product has recently been described in humans. There are at least four alleles of Tla in the mouse, and a spectrum of associated antigenic determinants (Table 9-5). On either side of the Tla locus lies a series of loci coding for the Qa antigens, which are also found on the surface of various cells of the immune system (Figure 9-1). Qa antigens as a group have a wide distribution among leukocytes including both T and B lymphocytes and numerous stem cells in the bone marrow. They appear on all of these cells only several weeks after birth, however.

On a purely structural basis, the molecules bearing the Qa and TL antigens could be considered class I MHC gene products. They are approximately 45,000-dalton peptides, found in the membrane in association with β-2 microglobulin. The overall structures of these proteins, and of the genes that encode them, are generally indistinguishable from K- and D-region genes and gene products. However, there are some important distinctions as well. K and D antigens are present on essentially all cells in the body, whereas TL and Qa antigens are found only on immune system-associated cells. On these cells, they are present in much lower concentration than are K-D antigens. Unlike K and D antigens, TL and Qa are not strong transplantation antigens. The degree of polymorphism of the Qa series and of TL is very limited in comparison with K-D antigens. And whereas K and D gene products serve as restricting elements in cell–cell interactions during immune responses (Chapter 14), no such role has been discerned or proposed for TL or Qa antigens. On the other hand, congenic strains differing only at the Tla/Qa loci may reject grafts from each other in a chronic fashion.

It is clear, from structural considerations, that "classical" MHC class I genes and proteins share a common genetic origin with Tla region molecules. There are between 30 and 40 such class I-like molecules (K-D, L + Qa + TL) in the haploid murine genome. The reason why TL and Qa molecules do not share common functions with K-D molecules is unclear at present. Possibly a more detailed study of the structure of these genes and gene products may detect subtle differences that will provide a key to this functional distinction.

Minor Histocompatibility Loci of the Mouse

Although the K and D genes of the H-2 complex code for antigens present the strongest barrier to transplantation, there are many other histocompatibility genes scattered throughout the mouse genome that provide barriers to the exchange of tissues and grafts between mice allogeneic at these various loci. The present estimate of the total number and location of these histocompatibility genes in the mouse is the product of many years of complex genetic experimentation and analysis.

The existence of multiple histocompatibility genes is readily evident when one follows the genetic segregation of loci controlling parental transplant rejection in the F_2 progeny of two allogeneic parents. Consider the illustration in Figure 9-5. The two parental strains, A and B, are allogeneic and will mutually reject skin transplanted from one to the other. Let us assume that such rejection is under control of a single gene, parent A being homozygous for the *a* allele of this gene, and parent B being homozygous for the *b* allele of this same gene. The F_1 progeny of an A × B mating will be uniformly heterozygous (*a/b*) at this locus. Thus, all F_1 progeny will accept a skin graft from either parent. If one examines the allelic composition of the F_2 progeny, then it is quite clear that $(3/4)^1$ of them in a particular experiment will be able to accept a skin graft from either parent.

If we assume two genetic loci controlling mutual rejection of skin grafts, then the same kind of analysis of the allelic constitution of the F_2 generation shows that

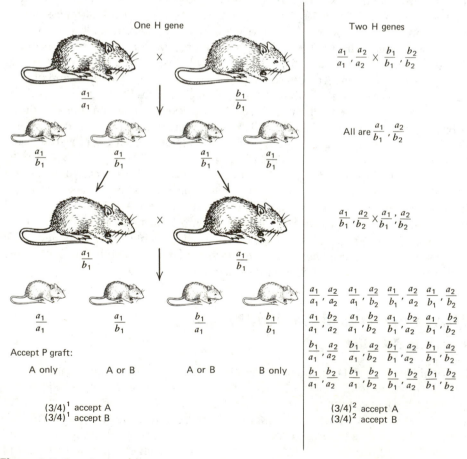

Figure 9-5 Genetic demonstration of multiple H genes in mice.

9/16, or $(3/4)^2$ of the possible combinations should accept a given parental skin graft. Similarly, if three loci control rejection, then $(3/4)^3$ of the F_2 progeny will accept a parental graft. When such analyses are actually carried out, using large numbers of breeding partners, the term n from the expression $(3/4)^n$, which indicates the number of genes involved in histoincompatibility, is quite large, nearly always greater than 10. The number of animals that would be required for a statistically meaningful analysis, if n is of the order of 50, or even 20, is extremely large and thus such studies are not usually practical for the detection of large numbers of genes. Nevertheless, it is quite clear from this type of analysis that graft rejection cannot be controlled by a single genetic locus.

More direct and useful information about minor H loci in the mouse has come from studies with the inbred congenic resistant (CR) lines described earlier in this chapter. Most of these lines were specifically selected for H genes, but some were selected for the presence of other markers and secondarily turned out to carry H loci. So far, nearly 50 H loci have been identified, distributed over most of the 20 mouse chromosomes (including the X and Y). Some of these loci are extremely closely linked to, and may be identical with, other phenotypic marker genes such as Lyt-1 and Lyt-2,3. Three minor loci map on either side of H-2.

H-Y is a particularly interesting minor histocompatibility antigen. It was first described in mice in 1955 by Eichwald and Silmser, who produced an anti-H-Y antibody by injecting male spleen cells into female mice of the same strain. H-Y is thus defined as a male sex antigen. It first appears in mice at the eight-cell stage development and is found on the surface of all cells in the male body. Recent evidence suggests that it is the expression of H-Y on the surface of developing cells, rather than the presence of a Y chromosome per se, that determines testicular versus ovarian development, and thus ultimately maleness. H-Y is apparently highly conserved phylogenetically, at least among vertebrates: anti-H-Y produced in mice reacts very well with male (but not female) cells of frogs and humans.

Similar studies in other species have suggested that the phenomenon of multiple genetic loci affecting graft rejection is a general one. But, again, it should be emphasized that the actual biological significance of these genes is not generally known. They are designated as histocompatibility genes in a purely operational sense. All we can really say about them is that they code for the production of cell surface products detectable by the immune systems of animals allogeneic at these loci in such a way as to lead to graft rejection.

Identification of H loci in the mouse through the generation of CR strains (or by almost any other method) implies the existence of at least two alternative alleles at those loci. The H-2 locus, which has been studied extensively using serological techniques, has at least 15 naturally occurring alleles for each gene, and probably many more if wild populations could be analyzed. The minor H loci in the mouse have not yet been well defined serologically. The F_1 test described earlier in this chapter can be used to detect new alleles at a given H locus, and such studies, where carried out, have confirmed the existence of multiple alleles at some non-H-2 loci. H-1, for example, appears to have over 10 alleles distributed among existing inbred lines. However, such tests are costly and time consuming compared to the value of the information obtained, and few have actually been carried out.

There has been some discussion in recent years about the ability of minor H loci to cause graft rejection in a strictly autonomous fashion. A fair amount of data has been accumulated in support of the notion that minor H antigens are not perceived directly by T cells, but rather can be "seen" only in the context of a class I protein of the MHC. In other words, the T cell responsible for graft rejection does not respond to the minor H antigen alone, but perhaps an "association complex" of the minor antigen plus a K or D protein on the surface of the same cell. We return to this point again when we discuss the phenomenon of MHC restriction in Chapter 13.

The Human MHC (HLA)

Genetics and Serology

The development of our understanding of histocompatibility in humans has proceeded along quite different lines from those just described for the mouse, where immunologists could take advantage of standard inbred and congenic resistant lines of mice and could perform transplant experiments at will. The principal mode of analysis of the human MHC, the HLA system, has been the genetic and serological analysis of families and populations.

The goal of serological analysis of the histocompatibility system of a given species is the development of a collection of individual antisera with specificities for each of the antigens coded for by that system. One can then use these antisera to study the patterns of segregation, within that species, of genes coding for the histocompatibility antigens. Such studies can provide information on the size, location, organization, and polymorphism of histocompatibility systems. Since the mid-1960s, frequent international human histocompatibility testing workshops have met to sort out, by computer and other techniques, the bewildering maze of serological typing data collected on human populations around the world. Sufficient progress has been made to deduce the topography of the HLA gene complex and to define in general terms some of its associated functions.

Crucial to any serological analysis is the production and careful characterization of standard typing sera. Antibodies to the gene products coded for by various components of the HLA complex are obtained from a number of sources. One important source has been from women during or within a few months after a pregnancy, particularly if it is the second pregnancy or beyond from the same father. Antibodies in the sera of multiparous women are directed against the HLA alleles of the father, present in the fetus, which are not shared by the mother. Although some of these antibodies cross the placenta, they appear to be harmless to the fetus.

Another source of anti-HLA antibodies is from patients who have received blood transfusions. A blood transfusion is operationally analogous to a tissue transplant.

However, unlike transplants of solid tissues, rejection of blood cells is principally humoral rather than cellular, and the crucial donor antigens are those of the ABO system rather than those of the HLA complex. As in the mouse, antigens of the human MHC are present in extremely low concentration on mature red blood cells. Nevertheless, antibodies to HLA-coded antigens are produced in the recipient, probably in response to lymphoid elements in the donor blood, and this has proved to be a valuable, although often heterogenous, source (due to the usually high frequency of multiple donors).

A third source of anti-HLA sera is from individuals who have volunteered to undergo planned immunizations (by lymphocyte transfusion) to produce anti-HLA antibodies of a more restricted specificity. This is a particularly useful approach when immunization is between a parent and an offspring. These procedures pose no health problem to the individuals involved and are always and only carried out with the full and informed consent of the volunteers.

Finally, in the past few years monoclonal anti-HLA antibodies have been raised in mice. These antibodies are, of course, extremely specific, and it is occasionally difficult to relate their antigen specificity to the more broadly reactive standard HLA typing sera. However, it seems likely that HLA mABs will become the reagent of choice for HLA typing in the future and will lead to more precise definitions of HLA specificities.

Anti-HLA antibodies can be measured in a number of ways. The method currently used almost exclusively in major HLA typing centers around the world is the lymphocytotoxicity test. In this test, a panel of target cells (usually lymphocytes) is reacted with an antibody source. Antibodies capable of recognizing the HLA antigens on appropriate target cells bind to the cell surface with varying degrees of tightness. When complement is added to these "sensitized" target cells, they will be rapidly lysed; target cells that did not bind the antibody will not. Cytolysis can be detected by release of a radioactive molecule such as ^{51}Cr from the target cell, but in clinical typing procedures is usually measured by uptake into the lysed target cell of a vital dye such as eosin or trypan blue.

Two things are clear from consideration of this type of assay. First of all, by definition we are talking about HLA in terms of molecules present in the plasma membrane of cells, which are capable of provoking an immune response and subsequently binding an antibody. Second, accurate detection of a particular antigenic determinant on a target cell depends upon the specificity (non-cross-reactivity) of the testing antibody, and on its ability to bind complement. These are important factors to bear in mind in interpreting serotyping experiments.

The current view of the structure of the HLA gene complex as derived from such studies is shown in Figure 9-6. The HLA antigens identified by comparative serology in the first few years were shown to fit into two distinct multiallele groups, now defined by the genes called A and B. These are generally accepted as the evolutionary counterparts of the mouse class I MHC products H-2K and H-2D. Because most individuals are heterozygous for these genes, it is possible to follow their distribution among the various offspring. Such distribution is not always totally random—

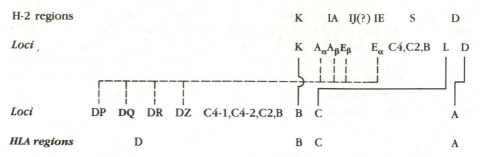

Figure 9-6 Structure of the HLA gene complex, showing probable relationships to H-2 genes and gene products.

some alleles from the A series occur more frequently with certain B alleles than would be predicted on a random basis (see Table 9-6). The reason for this linkage disequilibrium is unknown. Analysis of the occasionally detected crossovers between the two loci established that they were distinct and separate genes.

In the early 1970s, careful work from several different laboratories established the existence of a third gene coding for cell surface alloantigens. This gene, HLA-C, lies between HLA-A and HLA-B, and has so far been assigned eight alleles (Table 9-7). In its more restricted polymorphism, HLA-C appears to be analogous to the class I H-2L gene of mice. In all, there are nearly 10,000 possible haplotypic combinations for human class I surface histocompatibility antigens. The implications of this incredible polymorphism are not presently understood. It should be noted that the specificities listed in Table 9-7 are analogous to the private specificities of the mouse MHC. Because of the manner in which HLA antisera are produced, public specificities are generally not detected in humans although they certainly must exist.

The D Region of HLA

The D region of the HLA complex was originally defined not by serologically detected surface antigens but by the mapping of surface-located gene products that cause stimulation in a mixed lymphocyte reaction (MLR). The MLR is discussed in detail in Chapter 14. Briefly, it is a reaction in which the tendency of lymphocytes to proliferate in response to surface antigens on allogeneic cells is measured. In the early years of HLA analysis, it appeared that human lymphocytes proliferated in direct response to the serologically defined (A + B) antigens that were present on the stimulating cell, but absent on the responding cell. However, in a small but disturbing number of cases, apparently HLA-identical siblings were able to mount vigorous MLR responses. Further analysis showed that siblings differing at the A locus but identical at the B locus occasionally failed to give substantial MLRs. By analogy with the H-2 system of the mouse, it was postulated and subsequently confirmed by extensive population studies that a separate region (HLA-D) exists that is linked more closely to HLA-B than to HLA-A, and which governs the ability to stimulate in the MLR. This region could thus be expected to contain human class II genes.

Although originally detected by its ability to stimulate in the MLR, there have been numerous attempts to define gene products of the HLA-D region serologically as well. In early studies, the ability of the serum of parous women to block MLR activity of their own lymphocytes against a panel of HLA-A, B identical lymphocytes was studied. (HLA-C was not well defined enough at the time to be considered in the study.) Such women may make antisera against antigens present on white blood cells of their offspring; either a few cells leak across the placenta during pregnancy, or there may be a brief comingling of blood elements at the time of rupture of the placenta. Any cell surface antigens contributed by the father, and not present in the mother, will be recognized as foreign and induce production of maternal antibodies. Because the blocking serum and the cells *reacting* in the MLR were autochthonous, it was assumed that any activity of the serum must be directed against *stimulating,* not reacting, lymphocytes. And because reacting and stimulating cells were selected to be HLA-A, B identical, the serum was presumed not to be reacting against determinants on the stimulating cell coded for by these genes.

In these studies, definite patterns of inhibition of MLR activity were observed, suggesting the presence in the sera of these women of antibodies directed against stimulating cell determinants unrelated to HLA-A or B gene products. Further support for this hypothesis came from studies in which the serum antibodies were fluoresceinated, and then reacted with the putative stimulator cells. It was observed that these antibodies react strongly with B cells, to some extent with macrophages, monocytes, sperm, and endothelial cells, but not at all with T cells or platelets. Thus the tissue distribution of the MLR-stimulating gene product is different from the HLA-A, B, and C gene products, which are present on all nucleated cells in the human and is similar to the distribution of class II antigens of the mouse. A similar distribution of target antigens was observed using the test antisera in microcytotoxicity assays. For several years after their discovery, in fact, these determinants were referred to as B-cell antigens. Preliminary biochemical characterization of the membrane proteins precipitated by anti-B-cell antibodies suggested a very strong similarity at the structural level with murine class II molecules. This homology has been supported and strengthened by more recent biochemical studies and by isolation and sequencing of class II genes in the human.

A direct relationship between serologically defined human class II antigens and the MLC-defined HLA-D genes is not yet conclusively proved, and for that reason they are defined by a separate series, HLA-DP, DQ, and DR (Table 9-7; see also p. 248 in Chapter 10). Until just recently, a single region (DR) was usually shown on maps of the type shown in Figure 9-7. However, serological typing data were impossible to reconcile with a single class II locus within HLA. In the past few years, development of more precise monoclonal antibody typing reagents, and, more definitively, direct gene mapping studies at the DNA level, have suggested the segregation of class II genes into three subregions: DP, DQ, and DR. Although the

Table 9-6 Significant HLA Linkage Disequilibria (Δ) and Haplotype Frequencies (HF) of HLA-B Antigens with HLA-A and -C Antigens in European Caucasoids, Blacks, and Japanese

European Caucasoids					Blacks					Japanese				
Haplotype		Δ/1000	HF/1000	Significance	Haplotype		Δ/1000	HF/1000	Significance	Haplotype		Δ/1000	HF/1000	Significance
A1*	B5	13.7	20.6	*						A1	B37	7.6	7.7	***
A1	B8†	57.2	64.1	***						A1	B8†	2.5	2.6	**
A1	B17	16.0	22.4	*										
A2	B12	27.2	64.5	*										
A3	B7	18.5	28.3	*						Aw24	Bw52	30.8	55.6	***
Aw23	B12	17.6	19.3	***						Aw24	B7	34.9	55.1	***
A26	Bw38	5.3	5.5	*	A26	Bw51	9.4	8.1	***	A26	Bw35	16.6	25.8	*
A29	B12	27.3	33.1	***										
Aw30	B18	16.6	17.0	***	Aw30	Bw42	44.6	61.6	***	Aw33	B12	11.5	11.5	***
Aw33	B14	6.4	6.6	***										
B5	Cw1	9.3	12.1	*	B7	Cw4	26.1	33.9	*	B7	Cw2	6.2	6.8	*
B12	Cw5†	40.2	48.2	***						B12	C5†	8.9	9.2	***

B13	Cw6	22.8	25.0	***						B15	Cw3†	30.2	50.9	**
B15	Cw3†	28.3	29.9	***	B15	Cw3†	12.6	13.2	*	B15	Cw4	16.4	19.1	***
B17	Cw6†	35.4	38.7	***	B17	Cw6†	69.8	88.7	***					
B18	Cw5	19.4	23.6	***						Bw22	Cw1†	47.2	51.7	***
Bw22	Cw1†	11.4	12.2	***										
Bw22	Cw3	18.9	20.7	***						Bw35	Cw3	32.2	53.9	**
B27	Cw1	14.6	15.2	***						Bw35	Cw4†	10.5	13.8	*
B27	Cw2	22.6	22.7	***						B37	Cw6†	8.0	8.2	***
Bw35	Cw4†	84.2	89.7	***	Bw35	Cw4†	55.7	61.1	***					
B37	Cw6†	6.1	6.6	*						B40	Cw3†	56.7	106.0	***
B40	Cw2	13.6	14.7	***										
B40	Cw3†	24.5	26.4	***										

Taken from W. F. Bodmer and J. G. Bodmer, Evolution and function of the HLA system. *Brit. med. Bull. 34/3*, 309–316 (1978). Reproduced by permission of the Medical Department, The British Council. $\Delta/1000$ is the difference between the observed and expected haplotype frequency associations. The expected frequency for a given population would simply be the product of the frequencies of the individual haplotypes (see Table 9-8). For example, the frequency of European Caucasoids bearing both the A1 and B8 alleles should, if both alleles are randomly segregating, be $.16 \times .09$, or .014. As shown in this Table, the actual frequency of A1/B8 individuals is .064, more than four times the randomly based prediction.

All analyses are restricted to random healthy individuals.

*, **, *** indicate 5, 1, and 0.1 percent significance levels of χ^2, respectively.

†These haplotypes are found significantly frequently in more than one of the groups.

Table 9-7 1984 Listing of Recognized HLA Specificities

A	B	B	C	D	DR	DQ	DP
A1	Bw4	Bw47	Cw1	Dw1	DR1	DQw1	DPw1
A2	B5	Bw48	Cw2	Dw2	DR2	DQw2	DPw2
A3	Bw6	B49 (21)	Cw3	Dw3	DR3	DQw3	DPw3
A9	B7	Bw50 (21)	Cw4	Dw4	DR4		DPw4
A10	B8	B51 (5)	Cw5	Dw5	DR5		DPw5
A11	B12	Bw52 (5)	Cw6	Dw6	DRw6		DPw6
Aw19	B13	Bw53	Cw7	Dw7	DR7		
A23 (9)	B14	Bw54 (w22)	Cw8	Dw8	DRw8		
A24 (9)	B15	Bw55 (w22)		Dw9	DRw9		
A25 (10)	B16	Bw56 (w22)		Dw10	DRw10		
A26 (10)	B17	Bw57 (17)		Dw11 (w7)	DRw11 (5)		
A28	B18	Bw58 (17)		Dw12	DRw12 (5)		
A29 (w19)	B21	Bw59		Dw13	DRw13 (w6)		
A30 (w19)	Bw22	Bw60 (40)		Dw14	DRw14 (w6)		
A31 (w19)	B27	Bw61 (40)		Dw15	DRw52		
A32 (w19)	B35	Bw62 (15)		Dw16	DRw53		
Aw33 (w19)	B37	Bw63 (15)		Dw17 (w7)			
Aw34 (10)	B38 (16)	Bw64 (14)		Dw18 (w6)			
Aw36	B39 (16)	Bw65 (14)		Dw19 (w6)			
Aw43	B40	Bw67					
Aw66 (10)	Bw41	Bw70					
Aw68 (28)	Bw42	Bw71 (w70)					
Aw69 (28)	B44 (12)	Bw72 (w70)					
	B45 (12)	Bw73					
	Bw46						

The listing of broad specificities in parentheses after a narrow specificity [e.g., HLA-A23 (9)] is optional.

Table 9-8 HLA Gene Frequencies
in Major Populations

Allele	European Caucasoids	Blacks	Japanese
A1	14.9	3.3	0.5
A2	26.0	14.7	24.6
A3	11.6	7.4	0.5
Aw23 } A9	2.3	10.8	0.5
Aw24	9.6	2.9	35.6
A25 } A10	1.9	0.4	0.1
A26	3.7	3.8	9.8
A11	5.9	0.6	9.0
A28	4.0	8.7	0.5
A29	3.8	6.3	0.2
Aw30	2.4	15.4	0.2
Aw31	2.7	2.2	8.0
Aw32	4.5	1.5	0.1
Aw33	1.7	4.6	6.8
Aw34	0.6	6.5	1.0
Aw36	0.3	1.7	0.3
Aw43	0	1.0	0
Blank	4.3	8.4	2.5
B5[a]	5.9	3.0	20.9
B7	8.8	8.9	5.9
B8	8.2	2.9	0.1
B12[a]	16.6	12.7	6.5
B13	2.8	0.7	2.0
B14	3.0	4.1	0.1
B18	5.8	3.9	0
B27	3.9	1.5	0.4
B15[a]	4.8	3.0	9.3
Bw38	2.5	0	0.2
Bw39	2.1	1.8	2.9
B17[a]	5.7	16.1	0.6
Bw21[a]	2.2	1.5	1.5
Bw22[a]	3.6	—	6.5
Bw35	9.5	6.2	7.3
B37	1.5	0.4	0.5

(*continued*)

Table 9-8 (*Continued*)

Allele	European Caucasoids	Blacks	Japanese
B40[a]	8.1	2.0	21.8
Bw41	1.0	1.2	0.4
Bw42	0.3	7.7	0.6
Bw44	11.0	7.1	6.5
Bw45	1.1	3.9	0.2
Bw47	0.4	0.1	0.2
Bw51	7.2	1.4	8.3
Bw54	0	0	7.3
Bw56	0.6	0	1.1
Bw57	3.1	3.9	0
Bw58	1.1	10.7	0.9
Bw62	5.3	1.0	8.8
Blank	6.1	17.1	12.1
Cw1	4.1	0.1	17.6
Cw2	5.1	12.0	0.4
Cw3	10.1	9.2	26.9
Cw4	12.1	15.9	4.7
Cw5	6.0	2.9	0.1
Cw6	7.9	9.0	0.7
Cw7	2.3	2.4	1.1
Cw8	1.9	0.4	0.1
Blank	50.6	47.7	48.5
DR1	6.9	4.9	6.3
DR2	13.4	15.4	20.0
DR3	10.8	17.3	1.6
DR4	9.6	4.9	23.5
DR5	10.3	13.3	2.2
DRw6	2.2	5.3	4.6
DR7	12.5	9.8	0.5
DRw8	2.7	5.6	6.5
DRw9	1.1	2.7	12.2
DRw10	0.7	1.9	0.6
Blank	29.8	19.0	22.0

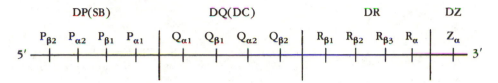

Figure 9-7 Current view of the HLA-D region.

order of these subregions with respect to the centromere is known, the precise order of α and β genes within each subregion is not yet known. The number of α and β genes within each subregion is a consensus of several different laboratories. It is possible that each cell may not express all of the genes shown, but it seems certain now that all humans have multiple α and β genes in each subregion. The overall MLR reactivity associated with the D region appears to be due principally to class II genes in the DR subregion.

Both *cis* and *trans* complementation of α and β genes within a subregion have been observed. Whether all α and β genes within a sub-region can interact freely with one another is unclear, but if they could, it would be possible to generate up to 50 different class II dimers in a completely heterozygous individual. As we will see when we come to consider the function of class II gene products in antigen presentation to T cells, this could be a considerable advantage, and might even be one expression of "hybrid vigor."

Like mouse class II dimers, human class II proteins consist of glycoprotein subunits of 34,000 daltons (α) and 29,000 daltons (β). The α chain associated with a given subregion seems to be almost completely invariant in humans; all of the polymorphism is associated with the β chain.

Other HLA-associated Loci

The genetic fine structure of the human MHC has not been explored in as much detail as that of the mouse because of obvious experimental limitations. The only loci other than A-D that can presently be assigned to HLA with any certainty are related to the complement system. The gene for factor B, a component of the alternate complement pathway, is tightly linked to the HLA-B locus. No crossovers between the two have been reported. Because the gene products are biochemically distinct, however, it is certain that separate genes do exist. Genes coding for complement components C2 and C4 in humans map within HLA. Like the mouse, humans have two genes for C4; however, unlike the mouse, both human C4 genes code for functional proteins. The map position of these various factors is shown in Figure 9-4.

The existence of human minor histocompatibility antigens cannot be demonstrated directly but is inferred from HLA identical sibling transplants that fail.

Bibliography

General

Clement, L. T., and E. M. Shevach, The chemistry of Ia antigens. In F. Inman and W. Mandy, eds. *Contemporary Topics in Molecular Immunology 8,* 149, (1981).

Dausset, J., The major histocompatibility complex in man. *Science 213,* 1469 (1981).

Demant, P. et al., Molecular heterogeneity of H-2 antigens. *Immunological Reviews 60,* 5 (1981).

Demant, P., G. D. Snell, M. Hess, F. Lemonnier, C. Neauport-Sautes, and F. Kourilsky, Separate and polymorphic loci controlling two types of polypeptide chains bearing the H-2 private and public specificities. *J. Immunol. 2,* 263 (1975).

Flaherty, L., Genes of the Tla region: The new Qa system of antigens. In H. C. Morse, ed., *Origins of Inbred Mice,* Academic Press, New York (1978).

Hayes, C., and K. Klyczek, The I-J glycoprotein: Genetic control, biochemistry and function. *Immunological Reviews 3,* 41 (1985).

Klein, J., *Biology of the Mouse Histocompatibility-2 Complex,* Springer-Verlag, Berlin, Heidelberg, and New York (1975).

Klein, J., L. Flaherty, J. L. VandeBerg, and D. C. Shreffler, H-2 Haplotypes, genes, regions and antigens: First listing. *Immunogenetics 6,* 489 (1978).

Origins of lymphocyte diversity, *Cold Spring Harbor Symp. Quant. Biol. 41,* Cold Spring Harbor Laboratory, New York (1976).

Simpson, E., The role of H-Y as a minor transplantation antigen. *Immunol. Today 3,* 97 (1982).

Snell, G. D., J. Dausset, and S. Nathenson, *Histocompatibility,* Academic Press, New York (1976).

Research

Carroll, M. C., H. Passmore, and J. D. Capra, Structural studies on the murine fourth component of complement (C4). IV. Demonstration that C4 and Slp are encoded by separate loci. *J. Immunol. 124,* 1745 (1980).

Carroll, M. C., et al., A molecular map of the human MHC Class III region linking complement genes C4, C2 and factor B. *Nature 307,* 237 (1984).

Cook, R. G., E. S. Vitetta, J. W. Uhr, And J. D. Capra, Structural studies on the murine Ia alloantigens. V. Evidence that the structural gene for the I-E/C beta polypeptide is encoded within the I-A subregion. *J. Exp. Med. 149/4,* 981 (1979).

David, C. S., and S. E. Cullen, Murine Ia Antigens: Identification and mapping of Ia.23 and further definition of the I-E subregion. *J. Immunol. 120/5,* 1659 (1978).

David, C. S., J. Stimpfling, and D. C. Shreffler, Identification of specificity H-2.7 as an erythrocyte antigen: Control by an independent locus, H-2G, between the S and D regions. *Immunogenetics 2,* 131 (1975).

Evans, G. A. et al., Structure and expression of a mouse major histocompatibility gene, H-2L^d. *Proc. Natl. Acad. Sci. U.S.A. 79,* 1994 (1982).

Ferreira, A., C. S. David, and V. Nussenzweig, The murine H-2.7 specificity is an antigenic determinant of C4d, a fragment of the fourth component of the complement system. *J. Exp. Med. 151,* 1424 (1980).

Goding, J., Evidence for linkage of murine β_2 microglobulin to H-3 and Ly-4. *J. Immunol. 126,* 1644 (1981).

Graff, R. J., and D. W. Bailey, The non-H2 histocompatibility loci and their antigens. *Transplant Rev. 15,* 26 (1973).

Hammerling, G., U. Hammerling, and L. Flaherty, Qat-4 and Qat-5: New murine T cell antigens governed by the Tla region and identified by monoclonal antibodies. *J. Exp. Med. 150,* 108 (1979).

Hansen, T. H., S. E. Cullen, R. Melvold, H. Kohn, L. Flaherty, and D. H. Sachs, Mutation in a new H-2-associated histocompatibility gene closely linked to H-2D. *J. Exp. Med., 145,* 1550 (1977).

Hansen, T. H. et al., Immunochemical evidence in two haplotypes for at least three D region-encoded molecules, D, L, and R. *J. Immunol. 126,* 1713 (1981).

Jones, P. P., D. B. Murphy, and H. O. McDevitt, Two-gene control of the expression of a murine Ia antigen. *J. Exp. Med. 148/4,* 925 (1978).

Long, P., W. Lafuse, and C. David, Serologic and biochemical identification of minor histocompatibility antigens. *J. Immunol. 127,* 825 (1981).

Monaco, J. J., and H. McDevitt, "Identification of a fourth class of proteins linked to the murine major histocompatibility complex. *Proc. Natl. Acad. Sci. U.S.A. 79,* 3001 (1982).

Murphy, D. B., L. A. Herzenberg, K. Okamura, L. A. Herzenberg, and H. O. McDevitt, A new I subregion (I-J) marked by a locus (Ia-4) controlling surface determinants on suppressor T lymphocytes. *J. Exp. Med. 144,* 699 (1976).

Natsuume-Sakai, S., T. Kaidoh, K. Sudo, and M. Takahashi, Allotypes of murine factor B controlled by locus within the S region of the H-2 complex. *J. Immunol. 133,* 830 (1984).

Neauport-Sautes, C. M. Joskowicz, and P. Demant, Further evidence for two separate loci (H-2D and H-2L) in the D region of the H-2 complex. *Immunogenetics 6,* 513 (1978).

Neauport-Sautes, C., D. Morello, J. H. Freed, S. G. Nathenson, and P. Demant, The Private Specificity H-2.4 and the Public Specificity H-2.28 of the D Region are Expressed on Two Independent Polypeptide Chains. *Eur. J. Immunol. 8,* 511 (1977).

O'Neill, H., and C. R. Parrish, Monoclonal antibody detection of two classes of H-2K^k molecules. *Mol. Immunol. 18,* 713 (1981).

Ozato, K., H. Takahashi, E. Appella, D. W. Sears, C. Murre, J. G. Seidman, S. Kimura, and N. Tada, Polymorphism of murine major histocompatibility class I antigen: Assignment of putative allodeterminants to disinct positions of the amino acid sequence within the first external domain of the antigen. *J. Immunol. 134,* 1749 (1985).

Roos, M. H., J. P. Atkinson, and D. C. Shreffler, Molecular characterization of the Ss and Slp (C4) proteins of the mouse H-2 complex: Subunit composition, chain size polymorphism, and an intracellular (Pro-Ss) precursor. *J. Immunol. 121,* 3, 1106 (1978).

Shalev, S. et al., β-2 Microglobulin-like molecules in lower vertebrates and invertebrates. *J. Immunol. 127,* 1186 (1981).

Sung, E., and P. P. Jones, The invariant chain of murine Ia antigens: Glycosylation, abundance and subcellular localization. *Molec. Immunol. 18,* 899 (1981).

Taniguchi, M. et al., Functional roles of two polypeptides that compose an antigen-specific suppressor T cell factor. *J. Exp. Medicine 159,* 1096 (1984).

CHAPTER 10

Biochemistry and Molecular Genetics of Major Histocompatibility Gene Complexes

Our knowledge of the structure of MHC genes and gene products, and of the detailed organization of MHC genes in the genome, has increased dramatically in the past several years as a result of the isolation and sequencing of class I and class II genes in mice and humans. A considerable amount of amino acid sequence data for class I proteins had accumulated prior to the beginning of the gene sequencing studies, and this information has been crucial in determining which sequenced genes correspond to which expressed proteins in a given mouse strain, for example. As we will see, this is important because many more class I proteins are encoded in the MHC region than are expressed at the cell surface.

Progress in working out the amino acid sequences of class II proteins had been much slower, for a variety of technical reasons, and the gene sequencing studies have been absolutely essential in developing insights into the detailed structure of the gene products. In the mouse, cloning and analysis of large overlapping segments of MHC DNA has also allowed precise molecular genetic mapping of this region. A comparison of the molecular genetic map of H-2 with the one generated by more classical genetic techniques is, as we will see, both reassuring and surprising.

In the first section of this chapter, we look briefly at the techniques used to analyze MHC genes and gene products. Then we summarize what is currently known about the structure and organization of class I and class II MHC genes and gene products.

Isolation of Class I and Class II MHC Proteins

Class I and class II MHC proteins are transmembrane, meaning that they completely span the lipid bilayer and have at least small portions entering the submembranous cytoplasm. The portion of the MHC protein residing in the lipid bilayer is hydrophobic. Thus, isolation of a complete class I or class II protein presents certain problems of maintaining and working with these proteins in aqueous solution.

There are two basic ways in which MHC-coded proteins may be isolated from the membranes of lymphoid cells (Figure 10-1), and a comparison of the results obtained by the two methods provided important insights into the structural features of these proteins and their arrangement in the membrane.

The first approach involves treatment of whole cells (usually lymphocytes, or cell lines derived from lymphocytes, because of their high density of MHC-coded proteins) with proteases. The rationale behind this approach is straightforward. The antigenic determinants detected serologically are known to be on the outside of the cell surface, and thus at least those portions of the membrane protein bearing these determinants should be accessible to extracellular proteases. And, because the antigenic determinants exist in, and maintain their conformation in direct contact with, an essentially aqueous environment, it seemed likely that antigenic material released by enzyme treatment should be soluble in aqueous buffers and relatively easy to work with.

The protease most commonly used is papain. Fortunately there is a papain-sensitive site on the class I molecule close to the membrane, and limited, non-cytolytic digestion with this enzyme releases an approximately 39,000-dalton glycoprotein containing all of the class I antigenic determinants. This molecule represents the NH_2-terminal 80 percent or so of the class I gene product. It is

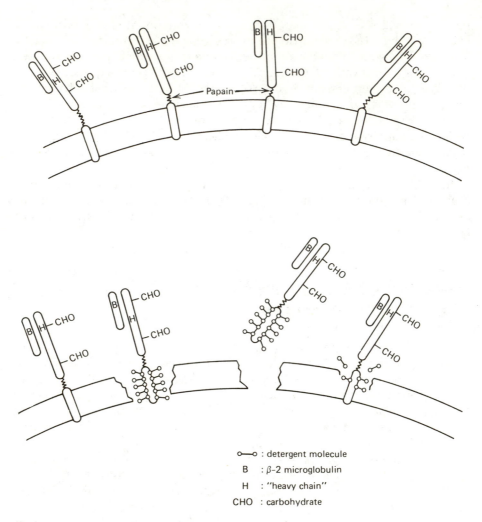

o—o : detergent molecule

B : β-2 microglobulin

H : "heavy chain"

CHO : carbohydrate

Figure 10-1 Enzymatic and detergent solubilization methods for removal of histocompatibility proteins from cell membranes.

always found in association with a molecule of β-2 microglobulin, which bears none of the class I antigenic determinants.

Class II proteins can also be liberated from cell surfaces by treatment with papain, although these proteins are more sensitive to papain and they are extensively degraded if great care is not taken. Class II proteins are thus usually isolated for study by detergent extraction (see following). Both class I and class II antigens reappear on papain-treated cell surfaces within a few hours if the cells are cultured in a nutritive medium at 37°C.

The second method for isolation of MHC proteins from membranes involves detergent extraction (Figure 10-1). This method has the advantage that the entire molecule, not just the extramembranous portion, can be recovered. It has the disadvantage that the molecule thus recovered is not generally soluble in the absence of the extracting detergent. The detergent complexes principally with those portions of the membrane proteins that are hydrophobically bonded to membrane lipids, thereby allowing these regions to associate with the surrounding aqueous medium. If the detergent is removed from the isolated proteins, they will tend to associate with one another through their hydrophobic regions, and precipitate out of solution.

A variety of detergents have been used for extracting membrane proteins from lymphoid cells, but the one most commonly used is Nonidet P-40 (NP-40). NP-40 is a nonionic detergent and, when complexed with MHC-coded proteins, does not interfere with the interaction of antigenic determinants with specific antibodies. This is a useful and important property, as we will see later.

Whole lymphoid cells, or plasma membrane fractions thereof, are incubated for about 1 hour with a 0.3 to 0.5 percent solution of detergent. At the end of this period, the suspension is thoroughly mixed and then centrifuged at 100,000 g for 1 hour. Material not sedimenting under these conditions is considered soluble and, in fact, contains all of the antigenic activity of the original preparation. Under some conditions of isolation, a complex dimer of class I proteins is obtained (two class I chains and the two β-2 microglobulin chains), which is held together by disulfide bonds. However, careful experiments have shown this to be an artifact of isolation. The unit complex in the membrane consists of one chain of each type in non-covalent association.

Purification of MHC Proteins

The MHC-coded proteins account for only a minor fraction of total membrane protein, particularly if one uses whole cells as the starting material. Thus, before any meaningful biochemical experiments can be carried out, it is necessary to achieve a considerable enrichment of the specific protein(s) one is interested in.

A preliminary step often employed in purification involves the use of certain plant lectins bound to a solid substrate (Figure 10-2). When solubilized membrane proteins are passed over an affinity column made from an appropriate lectin bound to Sepharose beads, selective glycoproteins are bound to the column while all other types of molecules pass through. The bound glycoproteins can then be eluted from the column with the free sugar molecules for which the lectin is specific. This procedure leads to a substantial enrichment of MHC-coded proteins in a membrane extract, because all of these molecules are glycoproteins. Interestingly, the lectins that bind to the class I MHC proteins of a given species tend to be T-cell mitogens for that species.

The most important step in purification of serologically detected membrane molecules, however, is immunoprecipitation (Figure 10-2). In this procedure, the antigenic proteins liberated from the membrane are removed from the remaining

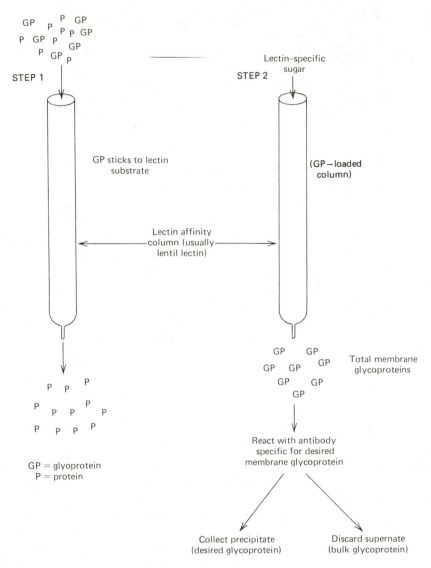

Figure 10-2 Affinity purification and immunoprecipitation steps in isolation of histocompatibility proteins.

molecules by precipitation with a highly restricted antiserum or monoclonal antibody. The specific membrane protein can then be recovered from the antibody–antigen complex for further characterization. Obviously the identity of the antibody used for immunoprecipitation, in terms of its antigenic specificity, must be absolutely beyond question if this technique is to yield meaningful results.

Characterization of MHC Proteins

The biochemical characterization of MHC-coded proteins isolated by the papain digestion technique is nothing more than fairly standard protein chemistry. For large-scale biochemical analyses the products of the enzymatic reaction may be precipitated with $(NH_4)_2SO_4$, redissolved, and analyzed on various sorts of chromatography columns or by electrophoresis.

The characterization of MHC-coded proteins isolated by detergent extraction is complicated by the fact that they are insoluble in water unless complexed to the detergent. Thus analytical systems based on aqueous media, such as column chromatography or standard polyacrylamide gel electrophoresis (PAGE), cannot be used for analysis of the native protein. The analytical technique most often used for detergent-extracted proteins starts with immunoprecipitation of specific proteins, usually after preliminary lectin affinity purification. The precipitated protein is then heated in the presence of sodium dodecyl sulfate (SDS). The SDS molecules replace the larger detergent molecules, and the resultant SDS-proteins can be analyzed directly on SDS–PAGE (Figure 10-3).

Sequencing of MHC Proteins

Because of the difficulty of obtaining large amounts of suitably pure material, standard sequencing techniques have not been practical with many MHC proteins. Instead, a so-called "biolabeling" technique has been used by most laboratories. Lymphocytes are cultured in medium containing a mixture of amino acids, one or more of which is radioactive. The MHC proteins turn over fairly rapidly, particularly in tumor cell lines, such that within a few hours they have incorporated substantial radioactivity. The proteins are isolated from the membrane by one or more of the procedures described earlier, and analyzed one residue at a time, starting at the NH_2-terminal end. The residue from each cycle is mixed with a complete set of appropriately derivatized, nonradioactive carrier amino acids, and the mixture is separated and analyzed by some technique such as high-pressure liquid chromatography. Each amino acid has a characteristic elution profile; the one containing radioactivity is identified as the amino acid at the position just cleaved from the peptide under study. In some instances, corrections must be made for metabolic conversion of one amino acid to others (e.g., glutamine to glutamic acid). Such corrections present no real problem, and the sensitivity of the biolabeling method is at least an order of magnitude greater than standard colorimetric methods.

Isolation and Characterization of MHC Genes and cDNA

Beginning in about 1980, it became possible to study MHC genes directly at the level of DNA. The progress made in the past five years in our understanding of the

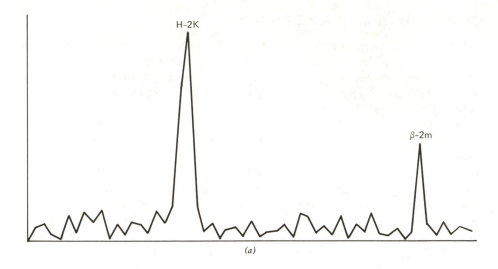

(a)

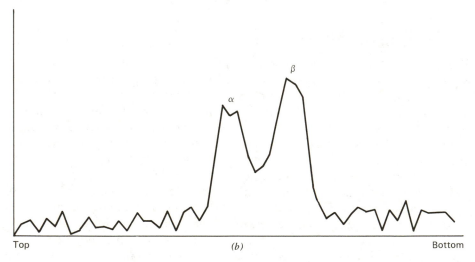

Top   (b)   Bottom

Figure 10-3 Facsimile SDS–PAGE profiles of mouse MHC proteins. Isolated and partially purified membrane proteins coded for by the MHC are loaded onto the tops of SDS gels and migrate through the gel under the influence of electric current. Separation of the proteins is on the basis of size and hydrodynamic properties, smaller and more compact molecules moving more quickly through the gels. The class I and β-2m proteins are quite homogeneous and migrate as single, sharply defined peaks (panel a). The α and β peptides coded for by the IA region, however, may have broader and more irregular peaks on the gel, suggesting multiple proteins with some heterogeneity in size in each peak (panel b). This may reflect varying degrees of glycosylation. The α peak also contains I_i protein (γ chain; see p. 244).

structure and function of major histocompatibility complexes and the gene products they encode has been impressive.

Because class I and class II gene products are not particularly predominant cytoplasmic proteins, it was initially somewhat difficult to get at the related nucleic acid sequences. Several approaches were finally successful. In one instance, a short stretch of DNA corresponding to a small portion of the inferred coding sequence of a class I peptide was synthesized *in vitro*. This short stretch of DNA was then used as a primer: it was mixed with whole mRNA extracted from lymphoid cells (a good source for MHC mRNAs) and incubated with reverse transcriptase and free nucleotides. Because the primer would only hybridize with mRNAs for a class I MHC product, only class I cDNAs should be generated. In fact, a cDNA clone for an HLA-B locus gene product was rapidly generated with this approach and used to isolate and characterize related genomic sequences.

A different approach resulted in the isolation of one of the first H-2 class I cDNA clones. mRNA from the membrane polysomes of lymphoid cells (where one would expect to find the mRNA for membrane proteins like class I antigens) was isolated and size fractionated on a sucrose gradient. The 17S size class (corresponding to the inferred mRNA size for class I proteins) was obtained from the gradient; translation *in vitro* verified the presence of highly enriched class I mRNA. This mRNA fraction was reverse transcribed *en bloc* into cDNA and cloned. Each clone in the resulting library was used to select mRNA from the enriched class I mRNA source. The selected mRNAs were translated one by one *in vitro* until an mRNA coding for a class I protein was found. The cDNA clone corresponding to that mRNA was then grown up and used for further characterization of mouse class I genes.

One additional technique that has proved useful in determining gene organization in the H-2 region is the use of "cosmid" clones. Most cloned fragments of complementary or genomic DNA are in the 1 to 3-kb size range, and are used mostly as probes or for direct sequencing studies. Cosmid clones contain much larger fragments of partially digested genomic DNA (30 to 50 kb) and may contain portions or complete copies of several adjacent genes. Determining the linear arrangement of cosmid fragments from a single genetic region can allow the precise mapping of genes within that region.

These and other related techniques were used by a number of laboratories to isolate in rapid succession probes for all of the human and mouse class I genes, and shortly afterward, all of the class II genes.

Structural Studies on Class I Gene Products

Determination of the primary amino acid sequence of murine class I MHC proteins was begun in earnest in the mid-1970s in the hope that such information would provide insight into the degree of evolutionary relatedness among the various class

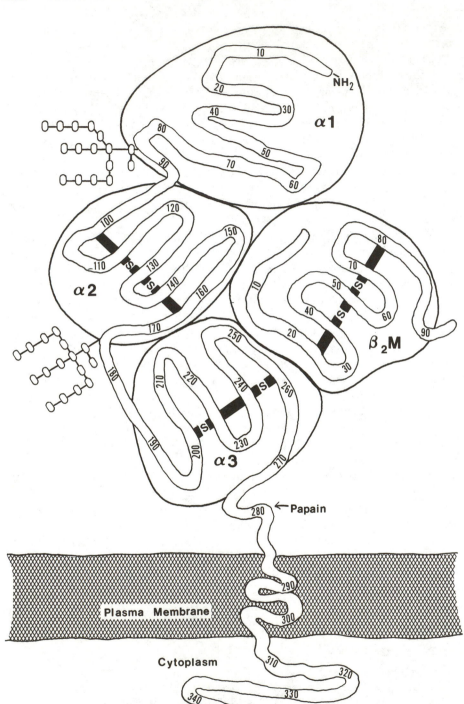

I genes, and the structural basis for both the function of these proteins and for the extensive polymorphism seen among the various MHC haplotypes.

Progress in working out the primary sequences of murine H-2 class I proteins was hampered by difficulty in obtaining sufficiently large quantities of these proteins from mouse lymphoid cells. Early studies were carried out principally on material obtained by papain treatment of spleen or liver cells, or of lymphoid cell lines. Later studies utilized detergent-solubilized class I molecules from lymphoid tumor lines. Nathenson and his colleagues were the first to complete the entire amino acid sequence of a class I H-2 molecule (Figure 10-4). Detergent-solubilized membrane proteins were isolated from cells that had been grown in the presence of radioactive amino acids, and analyzed by peptide mapping and amino acid sequencing. This procedure took several years. More recently, probes have been developed for isolating class I genes from both mice and humans, and inferred amino acid sequences can now be obtained fairly quickly (see below).

The H-2K^b molecule studied by Nathenson et al., which is typical of all class I molecules studied so far, has 346 amino acids, with two intrachain disulfide bonds and two carbohydrate moieties. (The number and location of carbohydrate groups may vary slightly from species to species.) There is a stretch of 25 hydrophobic amino acids (residues 285 to 310) that presumably spans the plasma membrane. The short C-terminal portion of the molecule is hydrophilic, slightly basic, and presumably resides on the cytoplasmic side of the membrane. There is a highly papain-sensitive site at about residue 280, cleavage of which under controlled conditions will result in a high yield of intact extracellular H-2K protein. There is an inferred second papain-sensitive site near residue 185.

The H-2K^b peptide can be arranged into three extracellular domains, in agreement with the structure proposed for human class I molecules, and with the structure of class I genes (see below). Each of these domains is about 90 amino acids long. The α2 and α3 domains contain an internal disulfide bond and should fold in much the same way as an immunoglobulin domain. For reasons to be discussed shortly, it seems most likely that β-2m associates with the α3 domain. The arrangement of coding sequences for the transmembrane portion of the molecule, and for the intracellular portion (see below), also suggests that these can be considered as distinct domains.

Each class I molecule has two or three N-linked carbohydrate groups attached. The structure for the murine carbohydrate groups is shown in Figure 10-5. Each moiety contains about 15 residues, for a total carbohydrate mass of about 3300 daltons per H-2 chain. In the early period of H-2 biochemistry it seemed likely that carbohydrates would be involved in H-2 antigenicity, if for no other reason than by

Figure 10-4 Proposed structure of class I MHC proteins. The structure shown is for the H-2K^b molecule, modified slightly from the structure presented by Coligan et al., but is prototypical for all class I MHC molecules. From J. E. Coligan, T. J. Kindt, H. Uehara, J. Martinko, and S. G. Nathenson, Primary structure of a murine transplantation antigen. *Nature 291*, 35 (1981).]

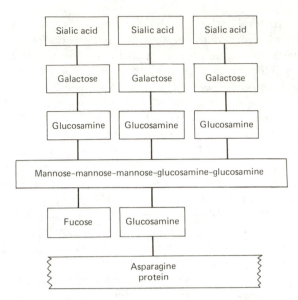

Figure 10-5 Proposed structure for the carbohydrate moiety of mouse H-2K and D chains. [Taken from J. Klein, Biochemical aspects of H-2 antigens in *Biology of the Mouse Histocompatibility-2 Complex*, Chapter 15, Springer-Verlag, New York (1975).]

analogy with known blood group antigens. However, it now seems virtually certain that they are not. The carbohydrate moieties of H-2 proteins of widely varying antigenic makeup are essentially identical. The isolated polypeptide fragment containing the intact carbohydrate structure has no antigenic activity. Enzymatic removal of nearly all the sugar residues has essentially no effect on the antigenicity of solubilized H-2 proteins. Blockage of glycosylation during synthesis does not prevent reexpression of class I on the cell surface, or prevent it from being recognized by either antibody or T cells. Precisely what the role of carbohydrates is in the structure or function of H-2 molecules is still unknown.

Comparison of amino acid sequences among various H-2 and HLA class I proteins (Figure 10-6) reveals a remarkable degree of evolutionary conservation, ranging from 75 to 85 percent when comparing class I proteins within a species, to about 70 percent when comparing such proteins between mice and humans. Many of the amino acid differences are relatively minor and involve single base changes in DNA. Interestingly, variant positions between different allotypes are not randomly distributed along the chain, but occur in clusters or "hot spots." Small clusters of differences are apparent at residues 18 to 24, 30 to 32, 41 to 45, and 95 to 100. A major area of variability is found between positions 61 and 83 in both mice and humans, suggesting this may be a principal locus for allelic variations in both species.

As noted earlier, the D and L genes within the D region of H-2 have not been separated by a crossing-over event. However, a mutant mouse strain (H-2^{dm2}) has

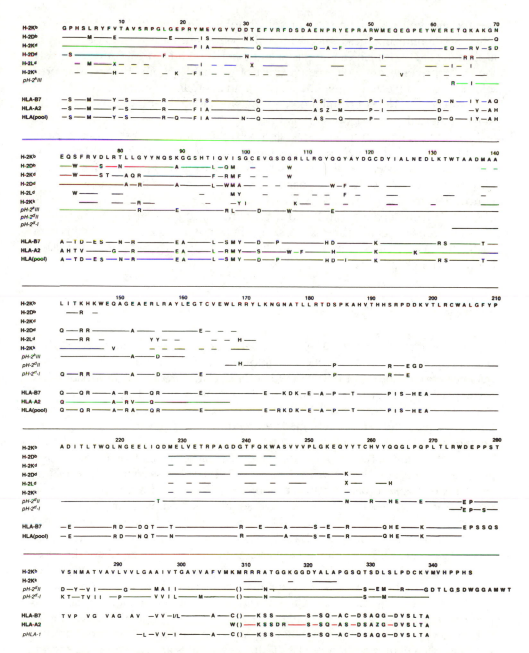

Figure 10-6 Comparison of primary amino acid structures of human and murine class I MHC proteins. [From J. E. Coligan, T. J. Kindt, H. Uehara, J. Martinko, and S. G. Nathenson, Primary structure of a murine transplantation antigen. *Nature* 291, 35 (1981).] Solid line indicates same amino acid at a given position as the H-2K^b molecule at the same position.

been found which lacks the H2L^d protein, but has normal H-2K^d and H-2D^d proteins. By immunizing these mice with cells from a normal H-2^d mouse, antisera against the H-2L^d protein can be raised and used to immunoprecipitate selectively the H-2L^d protein from a detergent extract of normal H-2^d membranes. This protein has been subjected to peptide mapping analysis, and compared to H-2K and H-2D molecules. The structural difference between L and K or L and D is about the same as the difference between K and D.

Increasingly, gene products associated with the Tla region are included, on a structural basis, in the category of class I MHC proteins. The proteins coded for by the Tla and Qa genes are all approximately 45,000-dalton glycoproteins (except Qa2, which may be only 40,000 daltons) and exist in the plasma membrane in noncovalent association with β-2 microglobulin. Recent peptide map comparisons of Qa-2 H chain peptides with K and D proteins suggest a sequence homology of 75–90 percent, about the same as that seen when comparing K and D proteins with each other. As we will see below, the structure of Tla region genes is indistinguishable from H-2 class I genes.

Class I MHC Genes

Restriction nuclease fragments encoding MHC genes were isolated and cloned beginning in 1979–1980, and the first information about gene structure and sequence began to appear in 1981. Since that time, a large amount of information has accumulated about the structure and organization of both class I and class II genes. The relative speed with which DNA fragments can be sequenced, compared to peptide sequencing, has brought the latter technique virtually to a halt as a means of studying MHC gene product structure.

A representative structure for class I genes typical of H-2 and Tla in the mouse, and HLA in humans, is shown in Figure 10-7. The most striking feature of this structure is its concordance with the domain structure inferred for class I gene products from studies of their amino acid sequences. Complete structures of numerous class I genes in both mice and humans have now been determined, and certain features common to all class I genes can be discerned. Of the three gene segments coding for extracellular domains (Figure 10-4), α1 and α2 are the most variable in sequence (70 to 85 percent inferred peptide homology), whereas α3 seems to be highly conserved (greater than 90 percent homology). Overall sequence homology among K, D, L, Qa, and Tla class I genes in the mouse is about 80 percent. The gene segment encoding the transmembrane region of class I molecules shows considerable variation among haplotypes (about 70 percent homology). The intracellular portion of class I MHC molecules are coded for by several gene segments. The region closest to the membrane (IC-1) appears to show the highest degree of conservation (nearly 100 percent), whereas the other segments show the lowest degree of homology of the entire molecule (less than 70 percent). Interestingly, the introns in class I MHC genes appear to be relatively conserved.

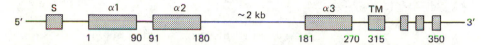

Figure 10-7 Structure of class I genes, based on available data from both mouse and human sequences. The organization scheme shown appears to be a general one. S = signal (leader) peptide. $\alpha 1$, $\alpha 2$, and $\alpha 3$ correspond to the peptide domains of the same designation shown in Figure 10-4. TM codes for the transmembrane portion of the molecule, and the three small segments 3' of TM code for the intracytoplasmic portion of the molecule. The numbers shown below the exons represent amino acid positions in the class I peptide.

The significance of this is unclear at present, but it is unlikely to be biologically meaningless.

The entire MHC, Qa, and Tla regions of the mouse genome have been mapped by Steinmetz and Hood, using class I DNA probes to analyze large cloned DNA restriction fragments (cosmids). A surprisingly large number of class I genes was found in the Qa and Tla regions (Figure 10-8). However, of the 30 or so genes identified using DNA hybridization probes, only about half may actually be expressed. Some have been sequenced, and have internal termination sequences or other abnormalities. Others have been transfected into cells, and do not cause a net increase in surface β-2m, suggesting they are not normally expressed at the cell surface. A number of other genes in the Qa and Tla regions apparently are expressed at the cell surface in association with β-2m, but do not react with any of the typing sera used to define class I molecules. This would suggest that they are not polymorphic in the mouse, and thus do not provoke the production of antibodies when injected into otherwise allogeneic mice. The possible function of these heretofore undetected class I genes is currently being investigated.

Biochemical Characterization of Class II MHC Proteins

Class II MHC proteins are usually obtained by detergent extraction rather than by papain digestion, because the latter treatment tends to degrade these proteins more than class I proteins. The first class II proteins to be analyzed were those

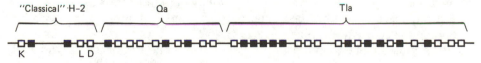

Figure 10-8 Class I genes found in the H-2/Tla region of the BALB mouse chromosome 17. Open boxes represent expressed genes. Products of the genes represented by closed boxes have not yet been detected on the surface of lymphocytes.

controlled by genes in the IA and (in some strains) IE subregions of the mouse MHC. Early studies suggested that each of these proteins is composed of two subunits. Whereas the class I proteins of mice and humans migrate as a single, sharply defined band of approximately 45,000 daltons on SDS–PAGE, the class II gene products of mice migrate as two rather more heterogeneous peaks of 32,000 to 36,000 daltons (α subunit) and 26,000 to 29,000 daltons (β subunit) (see Figure 10-3).

If the gels are run over a greater distance, the heavier peak resolves into two peaks, one of about 31,000 daltons (I_i subunit), and a second peak of 34,000 to 36,000 daltons (the α subunit). The 31,000-dalton peak was first identified by Pat Jones on 2D gels. Detailed analysis of two-dimensional gel patterns showed that immunoprecipitates of both IA- and IE-associated class II proteins from whole cells also contain a third peptide chain, of about 31,000 daltons. This chain does not vary in structure among the different haplotypes, and is thus called the I_i (i for invariant) protein, or the γ chain of class II. An identical arrangement exists in humans, and probably for other species as well. The α, β, and γ chains are all synthesized on rough ER, and pass into the cisternal space together where all three form a trimeric complex. The α and β chains are glycosylated as they traverse the Golgi, and are brought to the cell surface. There the association with the γ chain apparently ends. Some free γ chain may be found on the cell surface (it is a transmembrane protein), but it does not remain associated with the class II α-β dimer. Thus the γ chain may function to transport the α and β chain to the surface, just as the β-2m molecule is thought to transport class I peptides to the cell surface, although in the latter case β-2m remains associated with the molecule it transports. The reason that the γ chain is found associated with α and β chains in immunoprecipitates is that the bulk of class II molecules precipitated are intracellular (mostly in the ER and Golgi) rather than surface-associated.

Analysis of Class II Protein on 2D Gels

A close analysis of the two-dimensional gel patterns of mouse class II MHC proteins led Patricia Jones and her colleagues at Stanford to conclude that although the genes for both subunits of the IA-associated Ia protein are, indeed, located in the IA subregion of H-2, only one of the genes for the IE-associated protein (α) is located in the IE subregion; the gene for the other subunit (β) is actually located in the IA subregion. This conclusion rested on the following kind of evidence. Using an antiserum specific for IE^k-coded gene products, she immunoprecipitated corresponding molecules from spleen cells of various strains carrying the k allele(s) of the IE subregion. She found that the biochemical properties of the IE^k dimer, as revealed by electrophoretic behavior, were different when the IE^k gene was present in a genome carrying an IA^b gene, either by virtue of an intra-MHC recombination (B10.A(3R): *cis* effect), or by formation of an F_1 hybrid with a strain carrying an

IA^b gene (B10 × B10.A: *trans* effect), from those defined when it was present only with an IA^k gene (B10.A) (Figure 10-9, Table 10-1).

If the IE subregion-associated dimer is coded for entirely by genes in the IE subregion, then how could B10.A and B10.A(3R) have different IE^k dimers? The only difference between the two is the presence of *b* alleles in the latter to the left of, and on the same chromosome with, IE^k (*cis* effect). Jones concluded that one of these genes must be in some way influencing the structure of the IE-associated Ia

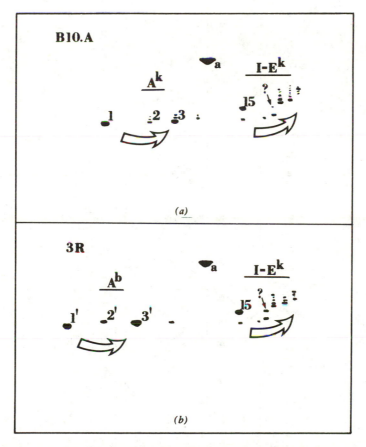

Figure 10-9 Schematic representation of isoelectric focusing gels of molecules precipitated by anti-IE^k antibodies from B10.A and B10.A(3R) spleen cells. Spots 1, 2, and 3, and the spots near them represent carbohydrate-modified forms of an IA^k polypeptide chain. Spots 1′, 2′, and 3′ represent carbohydrate modified forms of an IA^b polypeptide chain. Spot 15 and the spots near it are coded for by the IE subregion. Actin is labeled a. The large arrows indicate the direction of increasing modification of the polypeptide chains. Note the general displacement to the left of the IA^b spots compared to the IA^k spots. [From P. P. Jones, D. B. Murphy, and H. O. McDevitt, Two-gene control of the expression of a murine Ia antigen. *J. Exp. Med.* **148**, 925 (1978).]

Table 10-1 Production of Two Structurally Distinct IE^k Dimers by Mice Possessing the Same IE^k Gene

										IE^k dimer	
Strain	**K**	**IA**	**IB**	**IJ**	**IE**	**IC**	**S**	**G**	**D**	**B10.A-like**	**3R-like**
B10	b	b	b	b	b	b	b	b	b	(no IE^k dimer)	
B10.A	k	k	k	k	k	d	d	d	d	+	−
B10.A(3R)	b	b	b	b	k	d	d	d	d	−	+
B10 × B10.A	b/k	b/k	b/k	b/k	b/k	b/d	b/d	b/d	b/d	+	+

The dimers are distinguished by their location and pattern after two-dimensional gel electrophoresis. Based on information presented in P. P. Jones, D. B. Murphy, and H. O. McDevitt, "Two-Gene Control of the Expression of a Murine Ia Antigen," *J. Exp. Med.*, *148*, 925 (1978).

dimer. If both genes coding for the two IE^k-associated monomers are located in the IE subregion, then one of the "grafted-in" b alleles would be altering the structure of one of the IE^k genes, which seemed unlikely.

The B10 haplotype, of course, has no IE^k dimer; cells of the b haplotype do not express an IE-associated Ia antigen on their surface. (The same is true of the $s, f,$ and q haplotypes.) The B10.A haplotype produces a single type of IE^k dimer—the prototypical B10.A-like IE^k molecule. Yet an F_1 hybrid of these two haplotypes produces two kinds of α-IE^k precipitable molecules—the B10.A-like and the B10.A(3R)-like. Here, the presence of some b allele of a B10 MHC gene is contributing structural information to a molecule thought to be associated with the IE^k gene on the opposite chromosome (*trans* effect; Table 10-1).

How can all of this be explained? Jones and her colleagues put forward the following model. Both of the genes coding for the subunits of the Ia dimer associated with the IA subregion are actually located in the IA subregion. However, the case for the IE subregion-associated Ia dimer is different. The gene coding for one of the monomeric chains is, indeed, located in the IE subregion. The gene coding for the *other* subunit is located in the IA subregion (Figure 9-1). In two of the haplotypes not expressing an IE-associated Ia dimer (b and s), Jones had found that the IA-coded β subunit of the IE dimer was present in the cytoplasm, but not on the cell surface. She thus hypothesized that the presence of the E region-coded α subunit was necessary for expression of the A region-coded β subunit (as part of a dimer) on the cell surface. (As it turns out, the f and q haplotypes do not even have the IA-coded β-subunit for the IE molecule.) This simple and elegant explanation accounts for all of the observations made so far, the most elementary of which are those set forth in Table 10-1. The class II molecule associated with the IE subregion of a B10.A animal will be composed of one subunit coded for by a gene in IA^k, and one subunit coded for by a gene in IE^k. Its composition could be represented thus: $A^k E^k$. In a B10.A(3R) animal, the IE subregion-associated class II molecule would have the composition $A^b E^k$. This is a molecule biochemically distinct from the B10.A class II molecule.

The α and β chains from one I subregion of the mouse can interact with α and β chains from the same subregion in different haplotypes, but not with α and β chains of the other subregion (even though IE_α is actually coded for by a gene in IA). Since the E_α and E_β genes can be separated by crossing over, one can observe the interaction of E_α and E_β subunits from different haplotypes by *cis* as well as *trans* complementation. When α and β subunits from different haplotypes mix, such as in an F_1 by transcomplementation, or in an intra-I region crossover by *cis* complementation, new Ia antigenic determinants may be observed that are not associated with either parental (or prototypical) Ia molecules.

As we will see later, class II proteins play a role in antigen presentation to helper T cells, much like class I proteins are involved in the recognition of virally infected cell surfaces by cytotoxic T cells. T lymphocytes are activated by antigen on the surface of antigen-presenting cells, but only in the context of an appropriate class II protein. Presumably, the class II protein and the foreign antigen together create a structure recognizable by the T cell. It would thus seem advantageous for the antigen-presenting cell to express a wide variety of possible class II structures. Normally heterozygous humans, in fact, may have as many as 60 different class II α–β combinations for use in antigen presentation (see Figure 9-7). On the other hand, homozygous inbred strains of mice may express only two different class II molecules, but would appear quite capable of dealing with their (admittedly restricted) antigenic universe. Moreover, some strains of mice do not even express the IE subregion structure, suggesting that this molecule may not be crucial for survival. It is possible that IE is in the process of being lost from the gene pool. But the bottom line is that some strains of mice get along quite well with only a single type of class II molecule on their surface (IA), suggesting that having a variety of different class II proteins is not necessarily a rigid requirement for processing environmental antigens.

Class II Genes

The general structure of the I region of H-2 and D region of HLA was shown in Figure 9-6. Four HLA class II loci have been identified so far: DP, DQ, DR, and DZ. Each of these loci contains one or more α and β genes. However, how many of the α and β genes mapping to each locus are actually expressed at the cell surface is uncertain. Sequence comparisons suggest that human DQ and DR are the homologs of mouse IA and IE, respectively.

A typical structure for a class II gene, in this case a DC β (light-chain) gene, is shown in Figure 10-10. Five exons are apparent. The first exon includes coding information for a 5′ untranslated sequence, a 32-amino acid leader sequence, and codons for the first 4 amino acids of the first extracellular domain. The second exon codes for the remainder of the first domain, while the third exon contains information for the second extracellular domain (closest to the membrane). The fourth exon codes for a short connecting peptide between the second domain and the membrane, plus the transmembrane region, and the first 6 amino acids of the cytoplasmic tail. Finally, the fifth exon codes for the rest of the cytoplasmic tail and the 3′ untranslated sequence.

There are four cysteine residues located in positions indicating that there are two internal disulfide bonds, suggesting the existence of two folded domains. An asparagine at position 19 probably is the attachment point for an N-linked carbohydrate group. These are common features of all β genes sequenced so far. A comparison of different β-chain sequences suggests that class II polymorphism is mostly in the first (membrane distal) domain. The second domains of different β chains are about 95 percent homologous.

An exon organization pattern similar to the β system can be seen in a typical α (heavy-chain) gene (Figure 10-10). The first exon codes for the 5′ untranslated sequence, a 25-amino acid hydrophobic leader peptide, and 2 amino acids of the first cytoplasmic domain. The second and third exons encode the rest of the first domain and the complete second domain, respectively. The fourth exon codes for

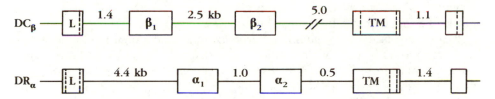

Figure 10-10 Human class II alpha and beta genes. The structures of the corresponding murine genes is very similar. Dashed lines represent peptide domain boundaries.

a 22-amino acid transmembrane region, a 15-amino acid cytoplasmic tail, and the first few amino acids of the 3′ untranslated sequence. The fifth exon codes for the remainder of the 3′ UT sequence. Like the β chain, and unlike class I genes, the gene segments for α chains approximate, but are not exactly congruent with, the discrete peptide domains of the gene product.

The complete peptide coded for by the α chain gene in Figure 10-10 is 229 amino acids long. There is only one potential disulfide loop in this and other α chains, in the second (membrane proximal) domain. On the other hand, there are two likely carbohydrate attachment sites, one in each domain.

The exact number of β genes associated with the three human class II gene loci is not yet clear. There may be as many as three β-chain genes coded for at the DR locus, two at DP, and probably two at DQ. There appear to be six α-chain genes in humans, two each for DP and DQ, and one each for DR and DZ. One of the α genes in DQ is highly polymorphic, the other showing the typically more limited sequence variability typical of α chains. As noted earlier, the α chains of DR and DQ share 50 percent or more sequence homology with E_α and A_α; the DP α chain shows homology to both.

β-2 Microglobulin (β-2m)

β-2m was originally described as a small (12,000 dalton), carbohydrate-free protein found in the serum and urine of various mammals, including humans. The significance of β-2m found in the serum is unclear. In 1973, two groups reported that β-2m was also found in association with HLA antigens isolated from human lymphocytes. These reports were soon followed by others demonstrating β-2m in association with H-2K and H-2D antigens (1974) and with the TL antigen found on mouse thymocytes (1975). In none of these cases does β-2m contribute to the antigenic properties of the serologically defined antigen. β-2m is not associated with Ia proteins, Thy-1 antigen, or surface immunoglobulin. Most evidence suggests that very little free β-2m occurs on the membrane in the mouse, although small amounts may exist on human cells. The gene for β-2m in humans is associated with chromosome 15 in humans, and chromosome 2 in mice. Thus although found in physical association with class I MHC proteins in both species, it is not genetically linked to MHC in either species. In mice there are two known allelic forms of β-2m, differing by a single amino acid.

β-2m is associated with membrane proteins in a noncovalent fashion, whether they are isolated by the papain method or by detergent extraction. The question quite naturally arose whether this association reflected a relationship existing in the membrane, or whether such associations were generated artifactually during isolation procedures. Two types of studies have shed light on this question. First of all, using chemical cross-linking reagents with intact membranes it has been shown that β-2m cross-links only to those cell surface structures defined by the isolation studies already mentioned. Second, it has been shown that β-2m redistributes in capping studies only with these same antigens on the cell surface, whether the antibody used is against β-2m or against the antigen. Antibodies against antigens other than the ones identified in the isolation studies fail to cocap β-2m. Thus all available evidence points to a real association of β-2m with H-2D, H-2K, and TL in mouse membranes, and with HLA-A, HLA-B, and HLA-C in the human cell membranes. β-2m itself is not an integral membrane protein, but rather "floats" on the cell surface in association with these proteins, which are integral.

The most likely function for β-2m is in facilitating the transport of class I peptides to the cell surface. Both mouse and human cell lines with β-2m defects fail to express cell surface class I proteins. This situation may be analogous to immunoglobulins: heavy chains are synthesized in B cells before L chains, but are neither expressed at the cell surface nor secreted until rearrangement and expression of the L-chain gene.

Extensive amino acid sequencing studies have been carried out on β-2m molecules from various sources. The structural homology between β-2m and a single immunoglobulin constant region domain was obvious from the beginning. Human β-2m is about 100 amino acids long and has a single disulfide joining residues 25 and 81. The degree of homology between β-2m and any C_H domain of IgG_1 is about the same as the degree of homology between any two IgG C_H domains. Recently, antibodies made against certain mouse L chains have been shown to cross-react with β-2M, and vice versa. Thus the conclusion that genes for Ig domains and for β-2m are evolutionarily related is tempting, and this relationship is all the more interesting genetically in that so far β-2m does not seem to be linked to any of the Ig gene groups.

Genetic Basis of MHC Polymorphism

As we have pointed out at several points in this and the preceding chapters, both class I and class II (β) genes are highly polymorphic within the same species. Both mice and humans probably have 100 or more alleles of class I and class II proteins. Unlike other allelic eucaryotic genes, which differ in ways that can be traced to fairly simple point mutations, deletions or insertions, the differences among MHC alleles is usually rather extensive. It is not at all unusual for two different H-2K proteins, for example, to differ by 15 to 20 percent of their amino acid sequences.

	150					155					160
K^b	Ala	Gly	Glu	Ala	Glu	Arg	Leu	Arg	Ala	Tyr	Leu
K^{bml}	—	—	Ala	—	—	Tyr	Tyr	—	—	—	—
L^d	—	—	Ala	—	—	Tyr	Tyr	—	—	—	—

Figure 10-11. "—"means same amino acid as the k^b protein.

On the other hand, some amino acid stretches in class I proteins are very highly conserved, not only within the species but between species as diverse as mice and humans. Similar degrees of polymorphism are seen in the β chains of class II proteins. This extensive polymorphism of MHC proteins has been observed in every species in which sufficiently detailed analyses have been carried out, suggesting strong selective pressures for its generation and maintenance.

One striking feature of polymorphism may be seen when any two alleles of the same gene are examined. Sequence differences between them tend to be clustered in short stretches, rather than scattered randomly throughout the gene. A particularly striking example of this can be seen in the case of recently derived MHC mutants of the H-2^b haplotype. A large number of spontaneous MHC mutants have been identified in C57BL6 mice (H-2^b), and a number of them have been characterized at the protein and gene level by Stanley Nathenson and colleagues. Mutant bm-1 has an altered H-2K protein which differs from the normal K^b protein by three amino acids. This change occurred in a single mutational event. Moreover, the three altered amino acids are clustered rather than randomly distributed (Figure 10-11). The K^b and K^{bml} genes are completely identical 5' and 3' to the altered cluster. This suggests that mutant K^{bml} arose by a gene conversion event, in which a short stretch of the K^{bml} gene was "corrected" against a gene sequence somewhere else in the genome. If this were true, one might expect to see similar corrections or "donor" sequences in other class I genes. This, in fact, happens: The K^{bml} altered sequence is seen in the exact same form and at the same location in the L^d gene.

In fact, when alterations in a wide range of both class I and class II genes or proteins are compared we see a similar pattern. Alterations tend to involve small clusters of amino acids at a restricted number of sites, and these clusters are found both in alleles of the same gene or in other isotypes of the same gene class (I or II), suggesting that the correcting mechanism is not isotype specific. In fact, most class I and class II genes are composites of numerous corrections.

The mechanism by which gene conversion occurs is completely unknown, but one possible scheme might involve pairing with short, nearly homologous stretches of DNA, followed by excision–repair of mismatched sequences. In the case of class I genes, it has been suggested that some of the "silent" class I-like genes in the Tla region may serve as a correcting gene pool.

Bibliography

General

Clement, L. T., and E. M. Shevach, The chemistry of Ia antigens. In F. Inman and W. Mandy, eds., *Contemporary Topics in Molecular Immunology 8,* 149 (1981).

Cook, R. M. et al., "Studies on the protein products of murine chromosome 17: A status report." *Transplant. Proc. 10,* 695 (1978).

Hood, L., M. Steinmetz, and B. Malissen, Genes of the major histocompatibility complex of the mouse. *Ann. Rev. Immunol. 1,* 529 (1983).

Möller, G. ed., Molecular genetics of class I and II MHC antigens. *Immunol. Rev. 84* and *85* (1985).

Research

Auffray, C. et al., Isotypic and allotypic variation of human class II histocompatibility antigen α-chain genes. *Nature 308,* 327 (1984).

Benoist, C. et al., The murine Ia α chains, E_α and A_α, show a surprising degree of sequence homology. *Proc. Natl. Acad. Sci. USA 80,* 534 (1983).

Coligan, J. E., T. J. Kindt, H. Uehara, J. Martinko, and S. G. Nathenson, Primary structure of a murine transplantation antigen. *Nature 291,* 35 (1981).

Coligan, J. E., T. J. Kindt, R. Nairn, S. G. Nathenson, D. H. Sachs, and T. H. Hansen, primary structural studies of an H-2L molecule confirm that it is a unique gene product with homology to H-2K and H-2D antigens. *Proc. Natl. Acad. Sci. U.S.A. 77,* 1134 (1980).

Cook, R. G., E. S. Vitetta, J. W. Uhr, and J. D. Capra, Structural studies on the murine Ia alloantigens. V. evidence that the structural gene for the I-E/C beta polypeptide is encoded within the I-A subregion. *J. Exp. Med. 149/4,* 981 (1979).

Das, H., S. Lawrance, and S. Weissman, Structure and nucleotide sequence of the heavy chain gene of HLA-DR. *Proc. Natl. Acad. Sci. USA 80,* 3543 (1983).

Evans, G. A. et al. Structure and expression of a mouse major histocompatibility gene, H-2L^d. *Proc. Natl. Acad. Sci. U.S.A. 79,* 1994 (1982).

Gates, F. T., J. Coligan, and T. Kindt, Complete amino acid sequence of murine β-2 microglobulin. Structural evidence for strain-related polymorphism. *Proc. Natl. Acad. Sci. U.S.A. 78,* 554 (1981).

Hess, M., Immune response region-associated antigens of the mouse—Biochemical properties of detergent and papain solubilized molecules. *Eur. J. Immunol. 6,* 188 (1976).

Koch, N., S. Koch, and G. Hammerling, Ia invariant chain detected on lymphocyte surfaces by monoclonal antibody. *Nature 294,* 644 (1982).

Larhammer, D. et al., Exon-intron organization and complete nucleotide sequence of a human MHC antigen DC$_\beta$ gene. *Proc. Natl. Acad. Sci. USA 80,* 7313 (1983).

Malissen, M., M. Damotte, D. Birnbaum, J. Trucy, and B. Jordan, HLA cosmid clones show complete, widely spaced human Class I genes with occasional clusters. *Gene 20,* 485 (1982).

Mengle-Gaw, L., S. Connor, H. McDevitt, and G. Fathman, Gene conversion between murine class II MHC loci. *J. Exp. Med. 160,* 1184 (1984).

Ramanthan, L. et al., Purification and characterization of mouse β-2 microglobulin: Allelic variants from two different strains. *Mol. Immunol. 19,* 435 (1982).

Shalev, S. et al., β-2 microglobulin-like molecules in lower vertebrates and invertebrates. *J. Immunol. 127,* 1186 (1981).

Steinmetz, M. et al. A pseudogene homologous to mouse transplantation antigens: Transplant antigens are encoded by eight exons that correlate with protein domains. *Cell 25,* 683 (1981).

Winoto, A., M. Steinmetz, and L. Hood, Genetic mapping in the MHC by restriction site polymorphisms: Most mouse class I genes map to the Tla complex. *Proc. Natl. Acad. Sci. USA 80,* 3425 (1983).

IV

The Cellular Basis of Immune Responsiveness

The 1940s and early 1950s were crucial years for immunology; very little happened. The reason that very little happened was that immunology had gone about as far as it could go as a clinical, purely descriptive science. Although there would be further developments in clinical immunology, they would be mostly refinements of existing information and procedures. Progress in working out the structure of immunoglobulins had floundered for technical reasons, and research into cellular parameters of the immune response had not yet recovered from the defeat of Metchnikoff's and Ehrlich's ideas 50 years earlier. The analysis of transplantation genetics and serology was becoming hopelessly Byzantine. The groundwork for the growth of immunology as an independent biological science, able to contribute in a broader way to our understanding of life processes, had not yet been laid down. This building of a foundation for the coming explosion in immunology that would begin in the 1960s is what occurred during most of the 1940s and 1950s. It was an unspectacular time and, as often is the case when blind men try to describe elephants, a confusing time.

In the mid-1950s, everyone believed that immune responses involved antibody, complement, and macrophages. It was also generally agreed that antibody was produced by plasma cells. A few people wondered from which cell type plasma cells were derived, but from a histological rather than an immunological point of view. However, with the acceptance of Burnet's clonal selection theory at the end of the 1950s, the histological origin of the plasma cell became a question of the most fundamental immunological importance, because this would be the cell predicted by clonal selection to display—as a population—the body's complete repertoire of antigen-specific receptors.

What was really missing up until the 1960s was an understanding of the cellular basis of immune responses generally. Blood leukocytes are mostly granulocytes and monocytes, with about 25 percent or so lymphocytes. Lymph nodes were known to be centers of immune reactions, as was the spleen. These organs are also the locations of plasma cells, which actually produce antibodies. Most leukocytes in these organs are lymphocytes, with a few granulocytes and some macrophages or histiocytes. Lymphatic vessels such as the thoracic duct contain almost exclusively lymphocytes. Yet the identification of the small, nondividing lymphocyte as the direct precursor of cells involved in immune responses was not established until the late 1950s and early 1960s.

The first definitive association of an immune function with small lymphocytes came with the studies of Simonsen, Billingham, and others who showed (1957–1960) that graft-versus host disease (Chapter 14) is caused by small, resting lymphocytes. A highly likely association of graft rejection with small lymphocytes was also established in the early 1960s when it was shown that treatments that reduced this type of cell in the circulation (neonatal thymectomy, cortisone treatment, irradiation, thoracic duct drainage) reduced the ability of an animal to reject foreign cells and tissues. Moreover, lymphoid cells from lymph nodes draining a graft site could be demonstrated to attack and destroy graft cells in an antigen-specific fashion *in vitro,* suggesting a possible mechanism underlying graft rejection. A key paper published by Gowans et al. in 1962 also suggested the small lymphocyte as the precursor of the antibody-producing plasma cells. Gowans et al. showed that chronic drainage of the thoracic duct in rats, the principal cellular component of which is the small lymphocyte, severely reduces the antibody response of the rats, just as it reduces the ability to reject grafts. Immune responsiveness could be restored by infusing small lymphocytes into the bloodstream. In a sense, these early results of Gowans may have been somewhat misleading, because as we will see shortly, *two* populations of small lymphocytes are needed to produce an antibody response: a helper cell and the actual antibody-producing cell. It is possible that what Gowans was really detecting was not reduction and reconstitution of antibody-producing cells, but helper cells. However, his conclusion that small lymphocytes are the precursors of the antibody-secreting plasma cells was essentially correct, and to him must go the principal credit for establishing this fact.

Thus a role for the small lymphocyte in immune phenomena was becoming increasingly apparent in the late 1960s. However, it was generally assumed that lymphocytes are homogeneous, and that the same cells are involved in both transplant rejection and antibody production. The rather troubling observation that immunity to soluble and microbial antigens could be passively transferred with immune serum, whereas immunity to grafts of tissues and cells could not, had been around since Gorer's work in the late 1930s. Mitchison confirmed in the 1950s that graft immunity could not be transferred with immune serum but could be transferred with lymphoid cells from an immune animal. However, neither observation led immunologists to suspect that the immune response to tissues was fundamentally different from the immune response to anything else. In the next few chapters we will see, among other things, just how wrong they were!

CHAPTER 11

Lymphocyte Subpopulations

Clinical Observations Leading to the Concept of a Two-Compartment Immune System

At about the same time that Gowans and his colleagues were confirming the small lymphocyte as the key cell of the immune system, an important idea was beginning to develop among clinicians working with patients suffering from a variety of different immunodeficiency diseases. The total spectrum of such diseases is very wide and complex, and includes both primary and secondary deficiencies. Primary immunodeficiencies are present at birth (although they may not be detected for several months to a year or more), and usually represent genetically based lesions in the immune system itself. A rather high proportion of these lesions are linked to the X chromosome. Secondary, or acquired, immune disorders arise somewhat later in life and may represent the delayed expression of a genetically linked immune dysfunction, or may arise as the result of malfunction of some portion of the immune system incident to a nonimmunologically based disease. It was the systematic study and classification of primary immunodeficiency diseases in humans that contributed to the idea of two separate compartments within the immune system.

Many primary immunodeficiency states can now be grouped with one of three general classes (Table 11-1). The first category includes those dysfunctions resulting primarily in the inability to produce normal quantities of serum immunoglobulins. One of the earliest definitive reports of such a disease was made by Bruton in the early 1950s, and concerned a particular congenital, recessive, sex-linked agammaglobulinemia affecting principally males. Diseases of this type are usually only detected toward the end of the first year of life, when maternally supplied antibodies begin to be depleted. The infant is subject to repeated infections by a wide range of microorganisms, primarily pyogenic bacteria, but including fungal and even protozoan infections. There is usually fairly good resistance to viral disease. This category of disorders is characterized by varying degrees and combinations of the following symptoms: low amount of serum immunoglobulins (0 to 25 mg/100 ml serum, compared with over 1000 mg/100 ml in normal serum); absence of the ability to produce specific antibodies; generally atrophic, aplastic, or absent germinal centers within the lymph nodes and spleen; and a virtual absence

Table 11-1 Categorization of Human Primary Immunodeficiency Diseases According to the Type of Dysfunction Manifested

Primary dysfunction	Specific disorders	Other manifestations
Inability to produce specific antibody	Bruton-type agammaglobulinemia; transient infantile hypogammaglobulinemia; selective Ig deficiencies	Susceptible to bacterial infections; low serum Ig; low or absent plasma cells; atrophic germinal centers
Inability to reject homografts	DiGeorge syndrome; Mauer-Sorenson disease	Susceptible to viral infection; low circulating lymphocytes; thymus usually vestigial or atrophic
Inability to produce antibody or to reject homografts	Swiss-type agammaglobulinemia; other combined immunodeficiency diseases	Susceptible to essentially all infectious organisms; almost always fatal within 1 to 2 years

of plasma cells anywhere in the immune system. On the other hand, the total number of circulating small blood lymphocytes is usually within the normal range, if somewhat at the lower end; the thymus is normal; thymus-dependent regions of the lymph nodes and spleen are normal in appearance; skin homografts are rejected, although graft survival time may occasionally be slightly prolonged; and apparently normal delayed hypersensitivity reactions are observed. Although the defenses of these patients against a wide variety of diseases are seriously compromised in early life, some compensation is usually achieved through periodic administration of pooled human serum γ-globulin, which contains antibodies to most of the common infectious microorganisms.

The second important category of primary immunodeficiency diseases encompasses those lesions that primarily affect the ability to mount delayed hypersensitivity and homograft rejection reactions. Included in this category, among others, are the DiGeorge syndrome and the Mauer-Sorenson agammaglobulinemia. In these states, the ability to produce antibodies against common bacteria is relatively unimpaired, although antibody production to a number of other synthetic and natural antigens may be depressed. The level of plasma cells is within the normal range, and germinal centers of lymph nodes and spleen are well developed. On the other hand, the absolute number of small lymphocytes in the blood is drastically reduced, and so-called "thymus-dependent" areas of the lymph nodes (paracortical regions) are seriously depleted of lymphocytes. Susceptibility to viral infections is very high. In fact, these disorders were often detected as the result of development of specific disease symptoms after injection of smallpox vaccine. The thymus is usually vestigial or congenitally atrophic. A limited degree of success in treating this disorder has been achieved by transplantation of neonatal thymus tissue; success is dependent on the ability to control eventual rejection of the grafted tissue.

The third category of immunodeficiencies is somewhat broader, and includes those disorders generally referred to as "combined immunodeficiency diseases." An example of this condition is the Swiss-type agammaglobulinemia. This disease is caused by an autosome-linked recessive genetic defect and combines the symptoms found in the two categories just described. All of the lymphoid organs are rudimentary and aplastic, even in the face of massive local or systemic infection. Infants born with this disease are virtually defenseless, within a few months of birth, against all sorts of infection, and rarely survive beyond a year or two of life. For reasons that are discussed later, current strategies for treatment of this category of disorders center on bone marrow transplantation. To date, only limited successes have been achieved.

Not all primary disorders of the immune system can be placed unequivocally in one of these three categories, although as more data from clinical observation and laboratory analysis are collected and scrutinized, an increasing number of these diseases are being assigned to one or another group. What has clearly emerged from these studies is that a significant number of immunodeficiency diseases involve a primary defect either in the ability to produce antibodies, or in the ability to mount graft-type reactions, or both.

These observations made on human immune disorders by themselves might not have led to the concept of a functionally dual immune system. But as is so often the case when rapid advances are made in scientific understanding, these findings intersected with, and were elegantly complemented by, entirely separate sets of experimental findings from laboratories studying what at first glance would seem to be a relatively unrelated problem: the ontogeny and function of the immune system in lower animals. What began as two rather unrelated scientific endeavors rapidly evolved into a highly productive and synergistic joint field of investigation. Before drawing any further conclusions about immune function based on the analysis of human immunodeficiency diseases, therefore, it will be profitable to review the critical experimental findings in animal models.

Contributions from the Study of Animal Models Toward the Concept of a Functionally Dual Immune System

Some of the most illuminating animal experiments yielding information on the functional organization of the immune system have been performed not on mammals but on birds, especially domestic chickens. Birds have an organ called the "bursa of Fabricius," the exact morphological counterpart of which is not known in other vertebrates. The bursa is an organ with a histological appearance not unlike the thymus, but it is located at the lower end of the gastrointestinal tract. Glick first showed in 1956 that removal of the bursa in newly hatched chicks severely impairs the ability of the adult birds to mount antibody responses. An intensive investigation into the precise role of the bursa over the next decade led to the notion that it plays a crucial role in the development of the humoral immune response in fowl. The effects of bursectomy before or immediately after hatching are summarized in Table 11-2. Adults derived from bursectomized chicks are agammaglobulinemic and cannot mount specific antibody responses. Germinal centers are lacking in the lymph nodes and spleen, even after repeated antigenic stimulation. Plasma cells are greatly reduced. On the other hand, removal of the bursa in adult chickens has no noticeable effect on the immune system either functionally or morphologically. Moreover, removal of the bursa around the time of hatching has no effect on the ability of the adult chicken to reject skin grafts.

At the same time that studies were being carried out on the role of the bursa in the development of immunity in the chicken, other workers were carrying out similar experiments with the thymus. As in the case of the bursa, removal of the thymus in newly hatched chicks was found to have a serious effect on development of immunity in the adult (see Table 11-2). However, the way in which the immune system is affected is quite different. The ability to form antibodies to some antigens, especially those related to bacteria, is relatively unimpaired, although the response to other antigens is, in fact, notably inhibited. Serum immunoglobulin levels gener-

Table 11-2 Effects of Surgical Removal of the Thymus or Bursa in Newly Born/Hatched Animals

Operation	Effects on the adult immune system						
	Specific antibody response	Serum immunoglobulin levels	Plasma cells	Germinal centers	Paracortical regions	Homograft response	Circulating small lymphocytes
Bursectomy (chicks only)	Absent	Low	Absent	Absent	Normal	Normal	Normal
Thymectomy (chicks, newborn mice)	Normal or reduced[a]	Normal	Normal	Normal	Thinly populated	Absent	Very low

[a]Depending upon antigen used in test.

ally are not significantly affected. The formation of germinal centers and the frequency of plasma cells is normal. By contrast, the ability to reject allografts, and to mount delayed hypersensitivity responses, is drastically reduced. The number of small lymphocytes in the circulation is markedly depressed, and the paracortical regions of the lymph nodes and the white pulp of the spleen are only sparsely populated by lymphocytes.

Essentially identical conclusions about the role of the thymus in the immune response were derived from experiments in mammals. Neonatally thymectomized mice were found to have the same immune defects as adults, both morphologically and functionally, as chickens derived from thymectomized newly hatched chicks (Table 11-2). Because no organ has yet been found in mammals that can be conclusively identified as a bursal equivalent, the experiment corresponding to neonatal bursectomy could not be (nor has it yet been) carried out.

Nevertheless, the striking similarities between the patterns emerging from the classification of human immunodeficiency diseases, and the results obtained from ablation experiments in animals, could not be ignored. By the mid-1960s, both clinical and basic research immunologist were convinced that there were indeed two separate arms of the immune system—one dealing almost exclusively with the need to produce circulating antibodies and another that at least in part was involved in the mediation of transplant and delayed hypersensitivity-type reactions. This duality of function was now firmly correlated with specific organs—the bursa or its equivalent, of prime importance in the production of antibodies—and the thymus—playing a key role in delayed-hypersensitivity and graft rejection reactions. However, the means by which these separate organ systems controlled the immune response was not yet clear. The final phase of this story involved the identification of two major populations of lymphocytes controlled by these organs and a definition of their respective roles in providing the complete repertoire of immune responses.

The Discovery of Two Separate and Interacting Populations of Lymphocytes

It is always difficult to point to any given experiment as being the first critical step in the resolution of an important scientific question, because almost every experiment that is done is an extension of some previous investigation. Nevertheless, the experiments of Henry Claman and his collaborators, first published in 1966, seem like an appropriate place to begin tracing the development of the concept of a cellular basis for the apparent dual function of the immune system.

As frequently happens in experimental science, the results of Claman's studies that were most important in triggering what would prove to be a very productive and exciting line of investigation were, in fact, not the original objective of his experiments. He had designed an experiment to test the capacity of lymphocytes from various organs to reconstitute the ability to produce antibody in mice whose immune responsiveness had been suppressed by irradiation (Figure 11-1). After exposing the animals to 650 to 750 R, he introduced cells from the thymus, bone marrow, or spleen of syngeneic animals into each mouse. He then tested the ability of these irradiated, reconstituted mice to produce antibodies against sheep red blood cells (SRBC), as measured in a version of the hemolytic plaque assay (see Appendix 1). The results of these experiments are summarized in Table 11-3. Thymus cells gave a slight, marginally significant restoration of the ability to produce antibodies to SRBC, whereas injection of cells from the bone marrow had no effect at all. Mice reconstituted with spleen cells, as had been observed by others, gave a strong, positive antibody response to SRBC. However, the most significant observation was that although thymus cells or bone marrow cells given alone were of little or no benefit, injection of a mixture of thymus and bone marrow cells gave a response that worked as well or better than spleen cells. Claman's interpretation of this rather startling finding, which turned out to be the correct one, was that one of these two populations probably contained cells capable of making and secreting antibody, but only in the presence of cells from the other population. Although he could not conclude from his experiments which population was which, he predicted on the basis of information known at the time that bone marrow would be the most likely source of antibody-producing cells.

These results were followed rapidly by others. Mosier showed first that macrophages as well as lymphocytes were required for a primary immune response. Using a recently developed system for generating an antibody response entirely *in vitro,* he showed that purified lymphocytes alone could not produce antibodies to sheep red blood cells, nor could macrophages alone. However, a mixture of the two gave a normal response. Mosier also showed that antigen could first be "fed" to the macrophages, noningested antigen washed away, and the resultant antigen-charged macrophages used to mix with purified lymphocytes to elicit a specific antibody response in the absence of free antigen. In subsequent experiments, he looked closely at the reaction order of each cell type (macrophages and lymphocytes) and concluded that although only a single population of macrophages was involved, two populations of lymphocytes seemed to be required for a primary humoral response. His "three cell interaction model" has proved to be correct, as we will see.

The next major advance in understanding the cellular basis of the two arms of the immune response came largely with the work of Mitchell and Miller and their colleagues. They had shown that removal of the thymus in mice during the first 24 hours after birth (neonatal thymectomy), in addition to suppressing delayed hypersensitivity-type responses in the adult, also depressed the ability to make antibodies against SRBC to about 5 to 10 percent of the normal response. This defect could be corrected in the adult (unirradiated) by the injection of either thymus cells or thoracic duct lymphocytes, but not by bone marrow cells. This established in an experimentally useful way the important notions that the antibody response to

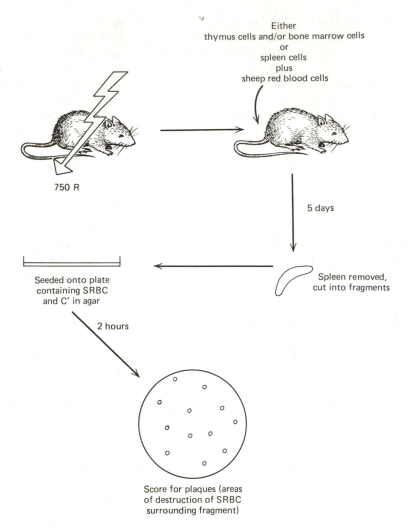

Figure 11-1 The Claman experiment. The assay used was a version of the plaque technique developed principally by Nils Jerne. Those spleen fragments containing cells secreting antisheep red cell antibody are surrounded by clear spots in the otherwise red "lawn" of sheep erythrocytes in agar. These clear spots or plaques arise when the secreted anti-SRBC antibody binds to surrounding erythrocytes and activates the complement included in the agar. This leads to lysis of the SRBC and diffusion of their hemoglobin away from the fragment. [In the more frequently used version of the Jerne assay, the spleen is dissociated further into single cells, so that the actual number of plaque-forming cells (PFC) in the spleen can be determined. A single PFC is equated to a single antibody-secreting cell.] Plaques formed around fragments or cells secreting IgM can be seen after an hour or two of incubation, and are called direct plaques. However, IgG-secreting cells do not usually have readily visible plaques associated with them. The anti-SRBC IgG secreted by these cells binds to surrounding erythrocytes, but because of the relative inefficiency of IgG in activating complement, plaques may not be formed. This problem is

Table 11-3 Synergy of Thymus and Bone Marrow Cells in the Production of Antibodies to Sheep Red Blood Cells

Cells injected		Relative level of response to SRBC
None		7.4
$35-50 \times 10^6$ Thymus	+ SRBC	12.3
10^7 Bone marrow	+ SRBC	1.6
5×10^6 Spleen	+ SRBC	66.1
50×10^6 Thymus plus 10^7 bone marrow	+ SRBC	70.7

From H. N. Claman et al., *Proc. Soc. Exp. Biol. Med. 122,* 1167 (1966).

some antigens was dependent on an intact thymic function, and that thoracic duct cells could work as well as thymus cells in restoring that function.

Mitchell and Miller then turned their attention to an experimental system somewhat similar to the one used by Claman. They observed that in adult thymectomized, irradiated mice, thoracic duct cells could cooperate with bone marrow cells in restoring the antibody response to SRBC. Under appropriate conditions, this could be done using allogeneic combinations of thoracic duct cells and bone marrow cells. This allowed them to construct a crucial experiment designed to determine which cell type actually produced the antibody (Figure 11-2). Adult CBA mice were thymectomized and irradiated with 800 R, and immediately reconstituted with CBA bone marrow cells. Two weeks later, each mouse was given an inoculum of (CBA × C57BL/6)F1 thoracic duct cells, plus SRBC. Five to seven days after that, the spleens of the reconstituted mice were removed and tested for the presence of cells producing antibody against SRBC in the Jerne hemolytic plaque assay. Prior to being tested in the plaque assay, however, the spleen cells were treated with normal serum, or with antiserum specific for CBA antigens, or with antiserum specific for C57BL/6 antigens.

Table 11-4 summarizes the results of these experiments. When these immune spleen cells were first treated with normal serum, before being tested in the Jerne assay, there was, as expected, no effect on the total number of plaque-forming cells (PFCs) observed. When the cells were pretreated with antiserum directed toward

---

circumvented by adding a second antibody (developing antibody), which is specific for antibody secreted by PFC. The plates are prepared exactly as for the determination of direct plaques. This antibody binds to secreted antibodies that have by then bound to surrounding erythrocytes. Because several developing antibodies can bind to each original IgG molecule, the efficiency of complement activation is increased, and plaques develop within a few minutes. By a comparison of these "indirect" plaques with direct plaques, an approximation of the ration of IgG to IgM-secreting PFC can be determined.

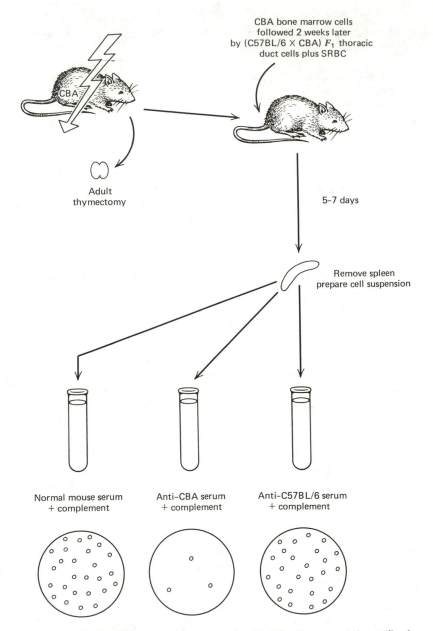

Figure 11-2 The Mitchell-Miller experiment showing that T cells are not the antibody-secreting cells.

Table 11-4 Experimental Evidence That Thoracic Duct Cells Are Not the Antibody-producing Cells

Experiment	Cells injected	Average PFC per spleen	Number of PFC per aliquot remaining after treatment with		
			Normal mouse serum	Anti-CBA serum	Anti-C57BL/6 serum
1	10^7 Thoracic duct cells + SRBC	10,980	80 (100%)	4 (5.0%)	88 (110%)
2	3.5×10^7 Thoracic duct cells + SRBC	69,300	604 (100%)	20 (3.3%)	571 (94.5%)
3	5.0×10^7 Thoracic duct cells + SRBC	85,850	1454 (100%)	70 (4.8%)	1660 (114%)

From G. F. Mitchell and J. F. A. P. Miller, Cell to cell interaction in the immune response. II. The source of hemolysin-forming cells in irradiated mice given bone marrow and thymus or thoracic duct lymphocytes. *J. Exp. Med. 128*, 821 (1968).

CBA antigens, the number of PFCs was reduced to only a few percent of the value obtained with normal serum. This result simply says that the PFCs had CBA antigens on their surfaces. Because both the thoracic duct cells and the bone marrow cells used for reconstitution had CBA surface antigens, such a result would be expected, and does not enable us to conclude anything about the source of the PFCs. However, when the cells were pretreated with antiserum specific for C57BL/6 antigens, no reduction in the number of PFCs was observed. This is clear evidence that the cells producing and secreting the antibody (the PFCs) did not have C57BL/6 antigens on their surfaces and were, therefore, not derived from the thoracic duct cells or their progeny. In a subsequent experiment, the PFCs were actually physically isolated from the hemolytic plaques and identified karyotypically as coming from the donor of the bone marrow cells. These data confirmed in a powerful way the concept of an obligatory collaboration between a "helper" cell influenced by the thymus, and an antibody-producing cell found in bone marrow, in the production of antibody to at least some antigens.

A second elegant proof of the existence of two interacting subsets of lymphocytes involved in antibody production is best exemplified by the experiments of Katz and Benacerraf and their co-workers, and by Rajewsky and his colleagues, on the immune response to haptens and carriers. These investigators made a striking and puzzling observation, which is exemplified by the data in Tables 11-5 and 11-6. As the reader will recall, a hapten is defined operationally as a molecule that is not by itself immunogenic, but which is capable of interacting with antibody molecules. In the experiments shown in Table 11-5, which exemplifies work done by Katz and Benacerraf, it can be seen that preimmunization of the animals with the carrier alone (BGG) is capable of causing an enormous increase in the amount of antibody to hapten produced by subsequent primary immunization with the hapten (DNP)-carrier conjugate. The exposures to hapten in the three experiments shown were

Table 11-5 Effect of Preimmunization with Carrier on the Subsequent Antibody Response to Hapten Coupled to the Carrier

	Immunization protocol		Anti-DNP antibody (μg/ml serum)	
Experiment	Day 0	Day 7	Day 11	Day 14
1	—	DNP_7–OVA	0.40 (1)	0.26 (0.6)
2	—	DNP_{28}–BGG	0.10 (1)	0.22 (2.2)
3	OVA (50 μg)	DNP_7–OVA	1.14 (1)	41.6 (36.5)
4	BGG (1 μg)	DNP_{28}–BGG	0.13 (1)	22.1 (170)
5	BGG (50 μg)	DNP_{28}–BGG	0.17 (1)	139.8 (822)

From D. H. Katz, W. E. Paul, E. A. Goidl, and B. Benacerraf, *J. Exp. Med., 132,* 261 (1970). Numbers in parentheses in the "Day 14" column are the ratio of the antibody value on Day 14 to the antibody value on Day 11.

Table 11-6 Effect of Intermediate Immunization with Carrier on the Secondary Antibody Response to Hapten

Experiment	Immunization protocol				Anti-DNP antibody (μg/ml serum)			
	Day 0	Day 7	Day 28		Day 28	Day 32	Day 35	
1	DNP_7–OVA	—	DNP_7–OVA		3.2 (1)	9.0 (2.8)	73.4 (22.9)	
2	DNP_7–OVA	—	DNP_{28}–BGG		14.7 (1)	6.2 (.42)	14.1 (0.9)	
3	DNP_7–OVA	OVA	DNP_7–OVA		0.82 (1)	31.2 (38.0)	603.4 (736)	
4	DNP_7–OVA	BGG	DNP_{28}–BGG		4.2 (1)	26.7 (6.4)	627.0 (149.3)	

From D. H. Katz, W. E. Paul, E. A. Goidl, and B. Benacerraf, *J. Exp. Med.* *132*, 261 (1970). The numbers in parentheses under the "day 32" and "day 35" columns are the ratio of the antibody values on those days to the antibody value on day 28.

all identical in timing and amount. Simply by preexposing the guinea pigs to the carrier molecule, which is not immunologically cross-reactive with the hapten, the production of antibody specific for hapten could be increased up to 800-fold!

As shown in Table 11-6, similar results could be obtained for the secondary antibody response (reexposure of a primed animal to the same stimulating antigen). Experiments 1 and 2 of this table define the normal secondary response to hapten–carrier conjugates. Note especially that in order to develop a secondary reaction the carrier used in the second immunization must be the same as (homologous to) the carrier used in the priming injection. Thus, even though the animal is seeing DNP for the second time, it displays memory to the hapten only when coupled to the homologous carrier. Experiment 3 shows the effect analogous to that seen in Table 11-5: Animals receiving a boost of carrier alone prior to the secondary challenge with the hapten–carrier complex develop a much higher antibody response to hapten upon subsequent challenge with the complex. Experiment 4 shows an even more striking phenomenon: animals rechallenged with hapten on a heterologous carrier will produce a strong antibody response to hapten if they are given a temporally intermediate exposure to the heterologous carrier alone.

These experiments were carried out in about 1969–1970, and the investigators involved were, of course, aware of the mounting evidence that production of antibody to many antigens seemed to require the interaction of two separate classes of lymphocytes: an antibody-producing cell found in adult bone marrow, and an auxiliary or "helper" cell found in thymus and the thoracic duct. They were therefore able to construct a hypothesis to account for their findings in the hapten–carrier system related to these findings. This hypothesis consisted of essentially the following elements.

1. In response to any immunogen, a result of exposure to the immunogen is the selection and expansion of clones of cells reactive to the various antigenic determinants or epitopes present on the immunogen. In the present case, clones to both hapten and carrier would be expanded after exposure to a carrier–hapten conjugate.

2. In the response to the present immunogens (hapten–carrier conjugates), two cell types are required for the production of antibody; a helper cell and an antibody-producing cell. These two cell types each recognize various small portions of the conjugate, portions not very different in size from an antigenic determinant. Thus, on the average, the two cell types would be interacting with different portions of the molecule at any given time. It is assumed that each cell type is free to interact with all of the various epitopes.

3. If one dissociates a complex immunogen into component parts, and uses one or more parts to immunize an animal, clones of both helper cells and antibody-forming cells reactive to the epitopes thus presented will be activated and expanded. On subsequent challenge with the intact, complex immunogen,

those clones previously expanded in response to particular immunogen components will now be represented in a relatively high frequency in the system.

Does this hypothesis explain the results in Table 11-5 and 11-6?

Let us first analyze the effect of preimmunization with carrier on the primary antibody response to hapten (Table 11-5). As a result of preexposure to BGG, two kinds of clones should be expanded: helper cells for BGG epitopes and antibody-forming cell (AFC) clones for BGG epitopes. Seven days later, the animal sees the DNP–BGG complex for the first time. In order to respond by producing antibodies to the various epitopes present on the complex, two cell types will be needed: helper cells and AFC. As a result of previous exposure to BGG, there should be an expanded set of clones capable of acting as helper cells in the response to BGG determinants. (There are also, of course, expanded clones of AFC for BGG, but these do not enter into our present analysis.) These helper cells can react with the BGG determinants present on the DNP–BGG conjugate and present the conjugate to the spectrum of AFCs specific for the various epitopes on the conjugate, including DNP. The hypothesis thus accounts for the enhanced primary response values seen in experiments 3 to 5.

It is important to note that the initial exposure to BGG did not affect the clones potentially responsive to DNP, either at the helper or the AFC level. When the animal receives DNP–BGG, it is truly seeing DNP for the first time. The clones responsive to DNP therefore need to be activated in a primary fashion, and both the kinetics of the response and the class of antibody produced are characteristic of a primary reaction. This primary response will be quantitatively enhanced, however, because of the expanded clones of helper cells capable of interacting with the BGG determinants on the complex immunogen. Finally, although it cannot be concluded from the present experiments, we should note that under normal circumstances haptens alone (even in an immunogenic form) fail to stimulate significant expansion of helper cell clones specific only for hapten.

How does the proposed hypothesis fit with the data obtained from the experiments of Table 11-6?

Experiment 1. As a result of the primary challenge with DNP–OVA, we would expect to see expanded clones for OVA helper cells, OVA AFC, and DNP AFC. Thus, on secondary challenge with DNP–OVA, we should get a true secondary response in terms of kinetics, magnitude, and antibody class. These data show that at least the magnitude of the response is strongly affected by such a protocol; other independent data have confirmed the secondary nature of the reaction in terms of kinetics and antibody class.

Experiment 2. We should get the same expanded clones as in experiment 1 as a result of the primary challenge with DNP-OVA. However, here the secondary challenge is with DNP–BGG. There are no expanded clones of either type (helper or AFC) for BGG. There is an expanded clone of AFC for DNP, but no helpers for

DNP, because it is a hapten and, as stated before, under normal conditions we do not get easily detectable production of helper cells specific for haptens. Because production of antibody to DNP requires both helpers and AFC, there is neither a secondary nor even an enhanced primary response to DNP. Presumably, there *is* a normal primary response to DNP as part of the DNP–BGG complex, which should result a slight increase in antibody to DNP across the 28- to 35-day period, but this increase, if it occurs, is apparently offset by decay of existing antibody to DNP generated by the original DNP-OVA immunization.

Experiment 3.   This group shows what we might call an enhanced secondary response, due to the additional expansion of helper cell clones caused by the intermediate exposure to carrier.

Experiment 4.   Here, the so-called "carrier effect" seen so dramatically in Table 11-5 is again obvious. Intermediate exposure to the heterologous carrier changes the results seen in experiment 2, because such exposure results in expan-

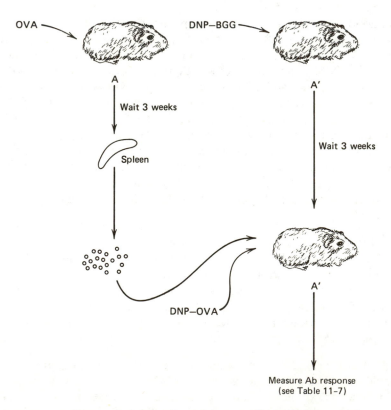

Figure 11-3 Conclusive demonstration that hapten-specific antibody producing cells are physically distinct from carrier-specific helper T cells.

sion of helper cells that can subsequently aid in the immune response to DNP coupled to the heterologous carrier (BGG).

These experiments were repeated many times over in a number of laboratories with the same results. The only model that is consistent with these data is one that postulates two separate populations of cells cooperating in the production of antibody in both the primary and secondary response to antigen.

But consistency between models and data, although comforting for the creators of models, is not quite adequate for general proof of a theory. A chief virtue of a hypothesis, if it is a good one, should be its suggestion of performable experiments, and an accurate prediction of the results. The foregoing hypothesis assumes the existence of separate clones of helper cells and AFC. If this is indeed true, then one ought to be able to raise helper cells independently of AFC and transfer them into a second animal where they can interact with other AFC raised independently of helpers.

An example of an experiment to test this prediction of the hypothesis is shown in Figure 11-3. In this experiment, the carrier ovalbumin (OVA) alone is injected into guinea pig A. On the basis of the foregoing hypothesis, we would predict the expansion of clones for OVA helpers and OVA AFC. Guinea pig A′ is separately primed with DNP–BGG. Three weeks later, spleen cells from the OVA-primed guinea pig are transferred into the DNP–BGG-primed animal, which is then challenged with DNP–OVA. As a control, a separate group of DNP–BGG-primed guinea pigs received no primed cells, followed by a DNP–OVA challenge. A few days afterward, the antibody response to DNP is measured in both groups of animals. The data from such an experiment are shown in Table 11-7. From previous experiments, we know that DNP–BGG-primed mice will not produce anti-DNP antibody in response to DNP–OVA; this is confirmed in the control group in the present

Table 11-7 Passive Transfer of Carrier-primed Helper Cells into Hapten-primed Recipients

Experiment	Number of carrier-primed cells transferred	Anti-DNP antibody (μg/ml serum) Day 0	Day 7
1	None	1.4 (1)	0.74 (.53)
	10^9	0.7 (1)	49.3 (70.4)
2	None	0.99 (1)	0.62 (.63)
	10^9	1.2 (1)	57.1 (47.6)
	2×10^8	2.0 (1)	29.4 (14.7)
	5×10^7	1.0 (1)	13.6 (13.6)

After W. E. Paul, D. H. Katz, E. A. Goidl, and B. Benacerraf, *J. Exp. Med. 132,* 283 (1970). The numbers in parentheses in the Day 7 column are the ratio of the antibody value on Day 7 to the antibody value on Day 0.

experiment. However, cells transferred from an OVA-primed guinea pig into the DNP–BGG-primed animal prior to challenge with DNP–OVA do, as the hypothesis predicts, allow the second mouse to respond to DNP-OVA by producing anti-DNP antibodies.

Cell Surface Markers Used to Distinguish T and B Lymphocytes

Studies defining the functional heterogeneity of lymphocytes were paralleled by investigations in other laboratories aimed at establishing morphological criteria for distinguishing lymphocyte subpopulations. Although some early scanning electron microscope studies had been interpreted as showing physically discernible structural differences between thymus-influenced cell (T cells) and bursal-equivalent cells (B cells), this is no longer accepted. The method most often used to distinguish among lymphoid cell populations takes advantage of the differences in protein antigens present on the cell surface membranes.

There are, as might be expected, a large number of antigens detectable on lymphocyte surfaces, only a few of which are present exclusively on lymphocytes. Nevertheless, various of these antigenic markers are quite useful, not only for distinguishing among various lymphocyte subpopulations, but also among different stages of development, within a single lymphocyte lineage. We present here a brief description of those surface antigens most useful in identifying functionally and developmentally distinct lymphocyte populations in mice and humans.

The Thymus Leukemia (TL) Antigen

This antigen was originally identified on a murine thymus leukemia, but its principal utility is that it is found among normal mouse tissues only on cortical thymocytes. Mature (medullary) thymocytes and peripheral T cells are TL-. The gene for TL maps near H-2 on chromosome 17, and the structure bearing the TL antigen is similar to proteins coded for by class I genes of the H-2 complex (Chapter 9). A similar antigen, called T-6, has been identified in humans (see below).

Thy-1

The Thy-1 antigen, formerly referred to as the theta (θ) antigen, is coded for by a single gene located on chromosome 9 of the mouse. There are two alleles, Thy-1.1 (formerly θ_{AKR}) and Thy-1.2 (formerly θ_{C3H}). The Thy-1 molecule is a 111-amino acid glycoprotein with an overall molecular weight of about 18,000 and a protein molecular weight of 12,500. The complete amino acid sequence is known in the mouse, and nearly complete sequences are available for rat and human analogs of Thy-1. The two mouse alleles of Thy-1 differ by a single amino acid at position 89.

The overall sequence and molecular conformation of Thy-1 shows strong homology with immunoglobulin domains. Thy-1 molecules have extensive β-pleated sheet structure with an inferred folding pattern similar to Ig domains. There is also a potential internal disulfide bond linking positions 19 and 85. Amino acid sequence homologies with Ig domains can be as high as 40 percent. It has been suggested that the Thy-1 genes may be similar to the primordial immune system gene that produced immunoglobulins by repeated duplication and linear association in the DNA.

The principal value of the Thy-1 system is in the identification of murine T lymphocytes, since mouse B cells, macrophages, and granulocytes do not display Thy-1. However, the Thy-1 antigen in mice is found on a variety of cell types other than lymphocytes. It is found in high concentrations on nerve cells and in lower concentrations on epidermal cells and fibroblasts. Thy-1 is present on both thymocytes and peripheral T cells. The amount of Thy-1 present on cortical (immature) thymocytes is about 5 to 10 times greater than that present on medullary thymocytes or peripheral T cells. In fact, it is often difficult to kill mature T cells with Thy-1 antiserum plus complement.

Molecules with antigenic and physical properties similar to murine Thy-1 are found in most other species, although because of differing tissue distributions it is not a generally useful marker. Rat Thy-1 is found on most thymocytes, but not on peripheral T cells, and on 40 percent of bone marrow cells (including B-cell precursors). Humans have a Thy-1-like antigen of MW 30,000, present on fixed (noncirculating) cells in lymph node and spleen, but display no Thy-1 on circulating lymphocytes or on cells readily released by teasing lymphoid tissue. Thy-1 is also found on a small proportion of thymocytes in humans.

Class II MHC Antigens

Class II MHC antigens are coded for by genes in the IA and IE subregions of the H-2 complex of mice, and the HLA-D region of humans. They are found on probably all B cells, on some macrophages, and on dendritic cells. They are not found on resting T cells, although there have been suggestions that they may be found on some mitogen- or antigen-activated T cells. When class II antigens are detected on T cells, they are present in concentrations at least 100-fold less than on B cells. Thus class II antigens are generally useful for distinguishing T cells from B cells.

Surface Immunoglobulin (sIg)

Surface immunoglobulin (sIg) is, in all species examined, the most useful surface marker for the identification of B lymphocytes. An endogenously synthesized, special membrane form of immunoglobulin (see Chapter 4) serves as the B-cell receptor for antigen. The bulk of sIg present on mature circulating B cells is restricted to a single molecular species, corresponding to the H- and L-chain isotypes, allotypes, and V-region idiotypes of the immunoglobulin the cell is programmed to produce upon antigenic stimulation. (See Chapter 12 for discussions of multiple isotypes on virgin B cells.)

The Ly Antigen System in Mice

A system of antigens restricted to lymphocyte surfaces in the mouse has been identified during the past 20 years (Table 11-8). Some (Lyt) are reasonably restricted to T cells, some (Lyb) to B cells, while others (Ly) are found on both T and B cells. It is not the case that each antigen defines a different T or B cell subpopulation; most lymphoid cells have more than one antigen on their surface.

The Ly-1 and Lyt-2,3 Antigens

The Ly-1 and Lyt-2,3 antigens have proved particularly useful in defining functional subpopulations of T cells. These antigens are defined by specific antisera produced by immunization of mice with purified thymocytes or T cells from an appropriate strain, followed by suitable adsorptions to remove antibodies to other cell surface antigenic specificities. The gene coding for Ly-1 resides on mouse chromosome 19; the gene or genes coding for Lyt-2 and Lyt-3 map to chromosome 6. Each gene has two alleles: 1 and 2. The mouse species as a whole thus expresses Ly-1.1, Ly-1.2, Lyt-2.1, Lyt-2.2, Lyt-3.1, and Lyt-3.2. Any given mouse strain expresses some combination of alleles of the three genes.

The distribution of Ly-1 and Lyt-2 and -3 antigens among various lymphoid organs in newborn and adult mice is shown in Table 11-9. At birth, virtually all Thy-1$^+$ cells in the mouse are equally positive for all three antigens, and throughout life cortical thymocytes are always Ly-1$^+$, Lyt-2,3$^+$. As postnatal development proceeds, the proportion of triply positive cells in the medullary regions of the thymus and in peripheral lymph tissues decreases, with the gradual appearance of cells that are either Ly-1$^+$, Lyt-2,3$^-$ (Lyt-2,3$^-$ cells) or Ly-1$^-$, Lyt-2,3$^+$ (Lyt-2,3$^+$ cells). Actually, these latter cells are not really Ly-1$^-$. During T-cell maturation, some Ly-1, Lyt-2,3$^+$ cells lose sensitivity to lysis by Ly-1 antiserum plus complement. Whether this is due to a decrease in surface density of the Ly-1 antigen, or to a change in some other surface property of the cells displaying the antigen, is not clear. Analysis using fluorescent Ly-1 antibodies shows these cells to be definitely positive for Ly-1, displaying perhaps as much as Ly-1, Lyt-2,3$^+$ cells. However, to distinguish them from the anti-Ly-1 sensitive triply positive cells found both in the thymus and in the periphery, these cells are usually referred to simply as Lyt-2,3$^+$.

Until quite recently, the Ly-1 antigen was thought to be found only on T cells, and it was accordingly designated Lyt-1. However, it is now quite clear that this antigen is found on a subset of B cells as well, and this antigen has reverted to its original designation of Ly-1.

The structure of molecules bearing the Lyt-2 and Lyt-3 antigens is beginning to be elucidated. Molecules precipitated from thymocytes by antisera to either antigen contain three types of disulfide-linked peptides: 29 kd, 33 kd, and 37 kd. The 33-kd peptide appears to be a cleavage product of the 37-kd peptide; both display the

Table 11-8 The Ly Antigen System in Mice

Antigen	Tissue distribution	Chromosomal location	Functional associations
Ly-1	All T cells; some B cell subsets	19	Can be useful in identifying Th cells
Lyt-2	90% of thymocytes; ca. 50% pTC[a]	6	Marker for CTL and suppressor T cells
Lyb-2	>95% pBC; ca. 50% bone marrow cells	4	None apparent
Lyt-3	90% of thymocytes; ca. 50% pTC	6	Marker for CTL and suppressor T cells
Lyb-3	Ca. 50% of pBC; 5% marrow cells	?	None apparent
Ly-4	Mostly B cells; some T cells	2	None apparent
Lyb-4	B cells only	4	None apparent
Ly-5	Mostly T cells; some B, NK cells	1	So called T200 molecule
Lyb-5	Ca. 50% pBC[b]	?	B cell differentiation marker
Ly-6	All mature T and B cells	4	None apparent
Lyb-6	B cells only	4	None apparent
Ly-7	Most T and B cells	12	None apparent
Ly-8	Thymocytes; most T and B cells	4?	None apparent
Ly-9	Thymocytes; T and B cells	1	None apparent
Ly-10	T cells; some B cells	19	None apparent
Lyt-11	Thymocytes	?	None apparent
Ly-12	Most lymphocytes	19	None apparent
Ly-13	Most lymphocytes	?	None apparent
Ly-14	Thymocytes; most lymphocytes	7	None apparent
Ly-15	Thymocytes and lymphocytes	?	Probably same as LFA-1 molecule
Ly-16	Most lymphocytes	?	None apparent
Lyb-17	All pBC; 50–60% bone marrow cells	?	None apparent
Ly-18	Most lymphocytes	?	None apparent
Lyb-19	Most B cells	4	None apparent
Ly-20	Most lymphocytes	1	None apparent
Ly-24	B cells, macrophages	?	None apparent

[a]Peripheral T cells.
[b]Peripheral B cells.

Table 11-9 Distribution of Lyt-1, 2, 3 Antigens[a]

Organ	Newborn			Adult		
	Lyt-1,2,3	Lyt-1	Lyt-2,3	Lyt-1,2,3	Lyt-1	Lyt-2,3
Thymus	95	<5	<5	95	5	5
Lymph node	95	<5	<5	40–60	20–35	5–15
Spleen	95	<5	<5	40–60	20–35	5–15

[a]Numbers shown are percentages of Thy-1[+] cells in that particular organ displaying the indicated antigen.

Lyt-2 antigenic determinant. All three peptides are glycosylated and are embedded in the plasma membrane, although whether any or all are transmembrane is unknown.

In thymocytes, the Lyt-2,3 molecule is present as two heterodimers in which the 29-kd subunit is disulfide bonded to one or the other of the larger subunits. It seems likely that both types of molecule are expressed on each cell. In lymph nodes, only a single type of Lyt-2,3 molecule is expressed on T cells, namely the 29-kd–37-kd dimer.

Ontogenetically, the appearance of Lyt-2,3[−] and Lyt-2,3[+] T cells occurs over the first 10 weeks of postnatal life. The proportion of Ly-1[+],Lyt-2,3[+] cells is sensitive to the presence of a functional thymus, even in adult life. Thymectomy results in a significant decrease in the relative proportion of triply positive cells and a corresponding increase in the relative proportion of Lyt-2,3[−] and Lyt-2,3[+] cells. Currently available evidence suggests that the triply positive cells are developmentally more primitive and probably are a pool from which Lyt-2,3[−] and Lyt-2,3[+] cells mature. Ly-1[+],Lyt-2,3[+] cells may also participate directly in immune responses, perhaps in a regulatory role.

A major breakthrough in analyzing T-cell diversity came with the correlation of Ly surface phenotype with T-cell function. Cantor and Boyse carried out an elegant experiment to answer a simple but important question about T-cell differentiation: Is it the case that commitment to the cytotoxic versus T helper pathways occurs at some step *prior* to encounter with antigens, or is this decision made only *after* encounter with antigens? Their experiment is diagrammed in Figure 11-4. Enriched starting populations of T cells were treated either with Ly-1 antiserum plus complement, to produce a population of predominantly Lyt-2,3[+] cells, or with Lyt-2 or Lyt-3 antiserum plus complement, to produce a population of predominantly Lyt-2,3[−] cells. Each group of T cells was then tested independently for its ability to act as a potential source of helper T cells, or a source of cells capable of mounting a graft-type reaction (cytotoxicity). It was found that Lyt-2,3[−] cells could provide T-cell help, but could not become cytotoxic effector cells. Lyt-2,3[+] cells, on the other hand, could be used to generate cytotoxic effector cells, but could not provide T-cell help. This experiment established conclusively that differentiation of T cells

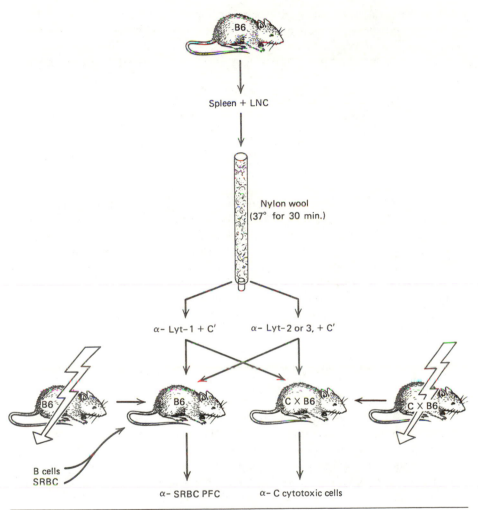

Pretreatment	Results PFC/Spleen	Cyto-toxicity
NMS	2160	60
α-Lyt-1 + C′	35	64
α-Lyt-3 + C′	2360	8

Figure 11-4 The Cantor-Boyse experiment showing that functional T-cell subpopulations committed to help or cytolytic pathways exist prior to encounter with antigen. In any given experiment, an animal received *either* α-Lyt-1 treated cells, *or* α-Lyt-2 or 3 treated cells, not both. B6 mice are H-2^b; C mice are H-2^k

into prehelper or precytotoxic cells occurs early in T-cell differentiation, independently of exposure to antigen. Subsequent experiments showed that in order for Lyt-2,3$^+$ cells to develop *efficiently* into cytotoxic cells, they, like B cells, require help from Lyt-2,3$^-$ helper cells. This interaction is discussed in greater detail in Chapter 14.

The L3T4 Antigen

The presence of the Lyt-2 antigen on murine T cells correlates very well with cytolytic/suppressor T-cell function. Although the Ly-1 antigen was initially used to identify helper T-cell subsets in mice, as pointed out in the previous section, its distribution is not strictly correlated with T helper function. A more useful antigen, L3T4, was described in 1983 by several laboratories. L3T4 seems to correlate very strictly with T helper function in mice and is probably the functional and structural homolog of the T4 antigen in humans (see following section). Very recent evidence by Greenstein et al. demonstrates that L3T4 in mice (and presumably T4 in humans) interacts with nonpolymorphic determinants on class II antigens on antigen presenting cells, although L3T4 is distinct from the primary T cell receptor for MHC antigens (Figure 11-5). The L3T4 molecule appears to be important in stablilizing the interaction between T helper cells and antigen presenting cells, particularly when the interaction through the T-cell receptor is weak.

Human T-Cell Antigens

Recently, monoclonal antibodies have been generated that identify differentiation and perhaps function-associated antigens on human T cells (Table 11-10). The T-1 antigen is present on all thymocytes and peripheral T cells, although it is highest on T cells that serve as amplifiers for both B cells and cytotoxic T cells. An almost identical pattern is found for the T-4 antigen. The T-3 antigen is always found in intimate association with the T-cell receptor, on both helper and cytotoxic T cells. A similar antigen has recently been detected in mice as well, although as of this writing it has not yet received a formal designation. T-6 is almost certainly the homolog of the murine TL structure. The T-5 and T-8 antigens are associated with human cytotoxic T cells and suppressor cells. T-8 may also be present on human NK cells. Antibodies to T-8 precipitate molecules structurally very similar to those precipitated by antibodies to Lyt-2 or Lyt-3 in the mouse.

Macrophage Surface Markers—the Mac-1 Antigen

A useful marker for murine macrophages has been described by Tim Springer and his colleagues. The so-called Mac-1 antigen is displayed as a dimeric membrane protein consisting of a 170-kd α chain and a 95-kd β chain. This molecule, which is most likely the membrane receptor for complement fragment C3b, is related to the

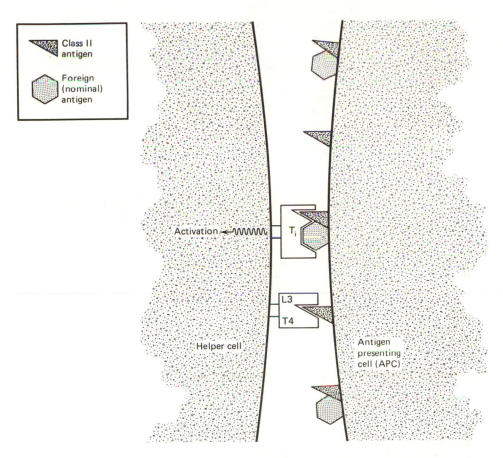

Figure 11-5 The T helper cell-specific L3T4 molecule is probably a secondary receptor for class II antigens. As will be discussed in detail in Chapters 12 and 13, T helper cells have a primary receptor (T_i) that recognizes foreign (nominal) antigen in the context of class II antigen. The interaction of T_i with the class II-nominal antigen complex leads to activation of the T helper cell. L3T4 molecules are able to interact with class II molecules by themselves, most likely through different portions of the molecule than are recognized by T_i. This interaction (L3T4-class II) does not lead to T helper cell activation. It appears to be most important when the amount of nominal antigen is very low, leading to an otherwise unstable T helper–APC association.

LFA-1 molecule described in Chapter 14. LFA-1 and Mac-1 share the same β chains, but have different (although related) α chains. Mac-1 is found in high concentration on virtually all macrophages (ca. 10^5 molecules/cell), and in lower concentrations on granulocytes and possibly NK cells. It is absent from T cells, B cells, and dendritic cells. A homologous molecule is found on human macrophages; it displays the M-1 antigen. The human and murine molecules are closely related.

Table 11-10 Differentiation Antigens on Human T Cells

Antigen	Molecular weight	Distribution		Functional associations
		Thymus	PBTL[a]	
T-1	67 kd	High-density medulla Low-density cortex	100%	None; found in higher concentrations on T_h cells
T-3	67 kd	20–30% thymocytes positive	100%	Intimately associated with human T-cell receptor
T-4	64 kd	80% of thymocytes positive	60%	Marker antigen for T helper cells
T-5				Marker for CTLs and T suppressor cells
T-6	48 kd	Cortex only	Absent	Found in association with β-2m; could be TL analog
T-8	76 kd	80% of thymocytes positive	35%	Marker antigens for CTLs and T suppressor cells
T-9	94 kd	Small proportion of cortical thymocytes	Absent	Ferritin receptor
T-10	45 kd	100% positive	Positive	None
T-11	55 kd	95% positive	100%	Generalized T-cell marker

[a]Peripheral blood T lymphocytes (i.e., those T cells found circulating in the blood).

Summary

In this chapter we examined, in a more or less chronological fashion, the flow of experimental information that led to what is now generally accepted as one of the foundation stones of modern immunology: the concept of two distinct but interacting compartments within the immune system.

The thymus is now known to control the function of a particular line of lymphoid cells into what are commonly referred to as "T cells." Details of the ontogeny and function(s) of T cells are presented in the next chapter but the broad outlines of this subject are already clear. The T-cell compartment is apparently solely responsible for initiating reactions of the graft rejection and delayed hypersensitivity type (see also Chapter 14 and 17). T cells are also crucial in helping to effect antibody responses to many antigens; we will examine possible mechanisms for T-cell collaboration with antibody-forming cells in more detail in Chapter 13.

The bursa in chickens plays a key role in the development of B cells, now known to be the immediate precursors of the antibody-producing and -secreting plasma cells. The mammalian equivalent of the bursa is still unidentified. Various gut-associated lymphoid tissues (tonsils, Peyer's patches, appendix, etc.) have been suggested as candidates, but to date no convincing evidence in support of any of these sites has been forthcoming. Many investigators feel it is entirely likely that the bone marrow itself may be the site of maturation of B cells in mammals. Although no mature T cells can be identified in bone marrow proper, one can find at this site a substantial proportion of morphologically and functionally mature B cells. As far as is known at the present time, B-cell function in response to antigen is limited to maturation to plasma cells and the production and secretion of antibodies. In many cases, B cells alone are capable of responding to antigen and maturing to plasma cells, without the help of T cells (see Chapter 12); this is true for most bacterial antigens, and of certain protein antigens as well.

The role of the thymus and the bursa or its equivalent in development of immune function diminishes soon after puberty in mice and chickens, and probably even earlier in humans. Thus, removal of these organs in adult animals has virtually no impact on immune responsiveness in either compartment, unless such extirpation is accompanied or followed by destruction of existing lymphoid cells by radiation or chemical damage. When unoperated adult animals are rendered immunoincompetent by high levels of whole-body irradiation (500 to 1000 R) or by cytocidal agents, immune function can be restored by reconstitution of the animal with a source of lymphopoietic stem cells, such as bone marrow. However, if the animal has had its thymus removed prior to treatment, no T-cell function will redevelop after stem cell transfer. (The corresponding experiment with the bursa is difficult to do, because sources used for stem cells almost always contain mature B cells, and it is difficult to interpret the cellular history of functional B cells after such transplantation. Nevertheless, there is good evidence for the existence of stem cells, capable of maturing to B cells, in bone marrow.) Advantage is often taken of these facts to produce an animal with B-cell function only, by a sequential combination of adult thymectomy, irradiation, and bone marrow reconstitution.

The classification of human immunodeficiency diseases presented earlier in this chapter can also be interpreted in cellular, although not yet in molecular, terms. The category of diseases characterized by the inability to produce specific antibodies involve various defects in the development of B cells. There may be a complete absence of some crucial developmental intermediate, such as the so-called "pre-B cell" (p. 303), or otherwise apparently normal, mature B cells may fail to carry out appropriate Ig gene rearrangements. Those immune disorders related to deficiencies in graft-type reactions are characterized by a lack of functional T cells. The defect in this case may be related to faulty epithelial components of the thymus, which could not then support the proper maturation of appropriate stem cells to T cells. Any one of the intermediate developmental forms of T cells could be defective. Immunodeficiency diseases of either the T-cell or B-cell variety could also result from a failure, at some earlier point in ontogeny, to develop an appropriate subclass of stem cells for either the thymus or the bursa to act upon. The severe combined immunodeficiency diseases probably involve a defect at an even earlier stage of lymphoid development, perhaps representing a failure to develop an adequate line of lymphopoietic stem cells providing precursors to both the T- and B-cell branches of the immune system. Thus, current efforts to correct this condition center on bone marrow transplants to provide a source of stem cells. Although usually successful, in many cases the transplanted cells, upon maturing in the new host, will mount an immune response against the host (graft-versus-host disease—see Chapter 14), which is occasionally fatal. Recent progress in donor-recipient matching and cell fractionation techniques, however, have improved the prognosis somewhat for management of these complications in humans.

Bibliography

General

Cooper, M. D. et al., Second international workshop on primary immunodeficiency diseases in man. *Clin. Immunol. Immunopath. 2,* 416 (1974).

Good, R. A., and A. E. Gabrielson (eds.), *The Thymus in Immunobiology,* Harper & Row, New York (1964).

Greaves, M., Surface markers for human T and B lymphocytes, current titles in immunology. *Transplantation and Allergy 1,* 93 (1973).

Haynes, B. F., Human T lymphocyte antigens defined by monoclonal antibodies. *Immunol. Rev. 57,* 127 (1981).

Hitzig, W. H., Congenital immunodeficiency diseases: Pathophysiology, clinical appearance and treatment. *Pathobiol. Annu. 6,* 163 (1976).

McKenzie, I. F. C., and T. A. Potter, Murine lymphocyte surface antigens. *Adv. Immunol. 27,* 179 (1979).

Miller, J. F. A. P., A. H. E. Marshall, and R. G. White, The immunological significance of the thymus. *Adv. Immunol. 2,* 111 (1962).

Raff, M. C., Surface antigenic markers for distinguishing T and B lymphocytes in mice. *Transplant Rev. 6,* 52 (1971).

Shortman, K., H. von Boehmer, J. Lipp, and K. Hopper, Subpopulations of T lymphocytes. *Transplant. Rev. 25,* 163 (1975).

Springer, T. A., and J. C. Unkeless, Analysis of macrophage differentiation and function with monoclonal antibodies. *Contemp. Topics Immunobiol. 13,* 1 (1984).

Research

Bruton, O. C., Agammaglobulinemia. *Pediatrics 9,* 722 (1952).

Campbell, D. G. et al. Rat brain Thy-1 glycoprotein. Amino acid sequence, disulfide bonds and an unusual hydrophobic sequence. *Biochem. J. 195,* 15 (1981).

Claman, H., E. Chaperon, and R. Triplett, Thymus-marrow cell combinations. Synergism in antibody production. *Proc. Soc. Exp. Biol. Med. 122,* 1167 (1966).

Friedman, S. M., S. B. Hunter, O. H. Irigoyen, P. C. Kung, G. Goldstein, and L. Chess, Functional analysis of human T cell subsets defined by monoclonal antibodies. II. Collaborative T-T interactions in the generation of TNP-altered-self-reactive cytotoxic T-lymphocytes. *J. Immunol. 126,* 1702 (1981).

Glick, B., T. S. Chang, and R. G. Jaap, The bursa of Fabricius and antibody production. *Poultry Science 35,* 224 (1956).

Gowans, J. L. et al., Initiation of immune responses by small lymphocytes. *Nature 196,* 651 (1962).

Huber, B., H. Cantor, F. W. Shen, and E. A. Boyse, Independent differentiative pathways of Lyl and Ly23 subclasses of T cells. *J. Exp. Med. 144,* 1128 (1976).

Ledbetter, J. A., R. L. Evans, M. Lipinski, C. Cunningham-Rundles, R. A. Good, and L. A. Herzenberg, Evolutionary conservation of surface molecules that distinguish T lymphocyte helper/inducer and cytotoxic/suppressor subpopulations in mouse and man. *J. Exp. Med. 153,* 310 (1981).

Manohar, V. et al., Expression of Lyt-1 by a subset of B lymphocytes. *J. Immunol. 29,* 532 (1982).

Miller, J. F. A. P., Effect of neonatal thymectomy on the immunological responsiveness of the Mouse. *Proc. Roy. Soc. Lond.* B156, 415 (1962).

Miller, J. F. A. P., and G. F. Mitchell, Immunological activity of thymus and thoracic duct lymphocytes. *Proc. Natl. Acad. Sci. USA 59,* 296 (1968).

Mitchell, G. F., and J. F. A. P. Miller, Cell-to-cell interaction in the immune response II: The source of hemolysin-forming cells in irradiated mice given bone marrow and thymus or thoracic duct lymphocytes. *J. Exp. Medicine 128,* 821 (1968).

Mitchison, N. A., The carrier effect in the secondary response to hapten-protein conjugates. I. Measurement of the effect with transferred cells and objections to the local environment hypothesis. *Eur. J. Immunol. 1,* 10 (1971).

Mosier, D. E., A requirement for two cell types for antibody formation in vitro. *Science 158,* 1573 (1967).

Naim, H. et al., The mouse Lyt2,3 complex. Structural analysis of the subunits. *Molecular Immunology 21* 337 (1984).

Rajewsky, K. V., V. Schirrmacker, S. Nase, and N. K. Jerne, The requirement of more than one antigenic determinant for immunogenicity. *J. Exp. Med. 129,* 1131 (1969).

Stashenko, P., L. M. Nadler, R. Hardy, and S. F. Schlossman, Characterization of a human B lymphocyte-specific antigen. *J. Immunol. 125,* 1678 (1980).

Taylor, R., P. Duffus, M. Raff, and S. dePetris, Redistribution and pinocytosis of lymphocyte surface Ig molecules induced by anti-Ig antibody. *Nature New Biology 233* 225 (1971).

CHAPTER 12

The Basic Biology of T Cells and B Cells

The Biology of T Cells

T-Cell Ontogeny in the Embryo

In the mouse, as in vertebrate embryos generally, the first blood cell progenitors are found in the yolk sac, and the principal site of hematopoiesis shifts to the fetal liver as this organ gradually atrophies. Cells from both these sites can be shown to migrate into the primitive thymus. Soon after their formations, the spleen and bone marrow also become active sites of both erythropoiesis and lymphopoiesis. It has been observed that in the mouse embryo, immunocompetent T cells appear in the thymus first, and only later in the peripheral lymphoid organs, suggesting a key role for the thymus in T-cell maturation during embryogenesis. We examine this question in detail in Chapter 15.

The question of whether the thymus itself is truly lymphopoietic was formerly the subject of much controversy. It was observed some years ago that thymic rudiments explanted from 12- to 13-day mouse embryos, a state at which no lymphoid elements could be identified in the thymus, could develop such lymphoid elements if left in culture for 6 to 8 days. Although the initial conclusion drawn was that the lymphoid cells were differentiating from epithelial elements of the thymus, subsequent work in developing chick embryos (and later in early mouse embryos) made it seem more likely that the early thymic rudiments had already been seeded by lymphoid stem cells. Nevertheless, the fact that these putative stem cells seemed to give rise to a restricted spectrum of lymphoid cells suggested the possibility that some developmental commitment to T-cell function may already have been made. When T cells are examined at various stages of development for the ability to function in different thymus-influenced reactions, it has been found that the ability to generate a cytotoxic response normally appears in the thymus 48 hours after birth. This capacity is low or absent in the peripheral lymphoid organs until about one week postpartum. T-cell helper function is also present in the thymus 1 to 2 days after birth, appearing several days later in the spleen.

The question of immunocompetency during ontogeny, particularly for T cells, is intimately tied up with the question of the ability to distinguish self from nonself. Obviously, this ability must be acquired before the immune system begins to function. We know from a variety of experiments that T cells learn to distinguish self from nonself during their maturation in the thymus. It is not yet clear during ontogeny when this distinction is operational. Details of the role of the thymus in development of the ability to distinguish self from nonself is discussed in Chapter 15.

T-Cell Ontogeny in the Adult

Lymphoid cells, like other cells of the blood system, must continually be renewed throughout adult life. The scheme for T-cell ontogeny in adult mammals is shown in Figure 12-1. Bone marrow is known to contain stem cells capable of giving rise to T cells, since adoptive transfer of bone marrow cells into irradiated recipients

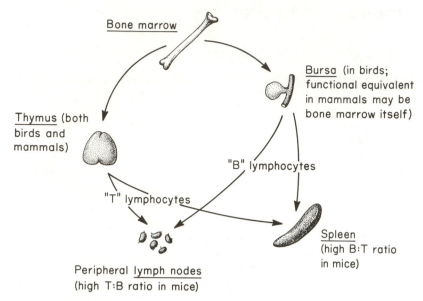

Bone marrow

Bursa (in birds; functional equivalent in mammals may be bone marrow itself)

Thymus (both birds and mammals)

"B" lymphocytes

"T" lymphocytes

Spleen (high B:T ratio in mice)

Peripheral lymph nodes (high T:B ratio in mice)

Figure 12-1 Developmental pathways for bone marrow lymphocyte precursor cells.

results in replenishment of all blood cell compartments, including the full spectrum of T cells. That separate populations of T and B precursors exist in the bone marrow is shown by physical fractionation experiments in which bone marrow cells enriched 2- to 4-fold for B stem cells are 5- to 10-fold depleted in T-cell precursors. Cells from adult bone marrow migrate to or are in some way acted upon by the thymus and caused to mature into thymocytes bearing Lyt, Thy-1, and TL differentiation antigens. (However, the TL antigen is lost before the cells leave the thymus to join the peripheral T-cell population.)

An understanding of what occurs in the thymus during thymocyte maturation is crucial for understanding a number of immune phenomena. As noted earlier, most of the cells proliferating in the thymus never leave it. Only about 1 percent of the thymocyte population leaves the thymus each day, yet turnover time for the entire population is a matter of only a few days, suggesting that about 95 percent of thymocytes die in the thymus. The basis on which some thymocytes are selected for survival, and others are killed off, is one of the major unresolved questions in immunology.

Weissman's classic early experiments (Figure 12-2) established the following facts about the relationship of thymic architecture to the maturational process. Prethymocytes apparently enter the thymic cortex across specialized endothelium of blood vessels that are in contact with the thymic capsule. They then migrate over several days to the medullary region of the thymus, becoming increasingly mature as they progress from the subcapsular cortical region to the medulla. Within hours after entering the thymus, the cells begin to divide and to express the Lyt, Thy-1,

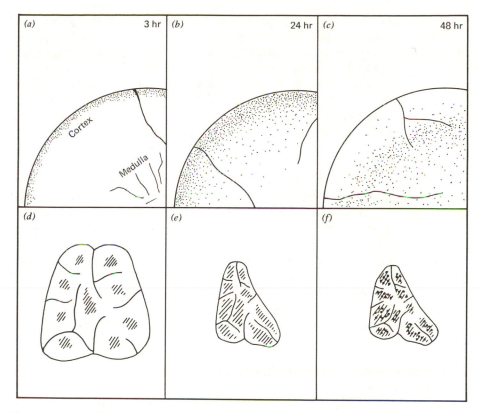

Figure 12-2 Proliferation and maturation of lymphocytes in the thymus. The relationship of lymphocytes in the cortical and medullary compartments of the thymus was worked out in an elegant series of experiments by Irving Weissman. When ^{3}H-TdR was placed on the surface of young mouse thymuses *in vivo*, the labeling patterns in Figures *a* to *c* were obtained. After 3 hours (*a*), the label was incorporated only into the first few layers of cells in the outer cortex, as seen by black dots in a photographic emulsion painted over slices prepared from the thymuses (autoradiography). By 24 hours (*b*), the label was apparent mostly in cells several millimeters into the cortex, but also in a few cells in the medullary region. By 48 to 72 hours (*c*), few cells in the outer cortex were labeled; most of the label was found in the medulla or its immediate vicinity. These results suggested that the cells in the medulla were migratory descendants of the rapidly dividing cells in the cortex.

Further support for this idea was obtained by Weisman from experiments with hydrocortisone (HC). It was known that cells in the medullary regions of the thymus are HC resistant, whereas the thymocytes of the cortex are killed by HC in 12 to 24 hours. Thymuses were treated with HC (systemic injection) at the time of ^{3}H-TdR labeling (t_o) or 3 days afterwards. (*d*) Untreated thymus (hatched areas = medulla); (*e*) thymus exposed to both HC and ^{3}H-TdR at *to*; (*f*) thymus exposed to HC 3 days after exposure of thymus to ^{3}H-TdR. Parts (*e*) and (*f*) were analyzed by autoradiography 24 hours after HC treatment in each case. Part (*e*) shows the cortical atrophy typical of HC treatment, but no labeled cells have reached the medulla. Part (*f*) also shows typical HC-induced cortical atrophy but has labeled medullary cells as well. These experiments established that the HC-resistant thymocytes of the medulla derived from the HC-sensitive cells of the cortex.

and TL antigens (in that order). As the cells approach the medullary regions, they express (as a population) reduced amounts of Thy-1, increased amounts of class I MHC antigens, rearrange at least the β gene of the T-cell receptor, lose the TL antigen, and some of them mature from Lyt-1,2,3$^+$ cells to cells expressing Lyt-2,3 antigens only, or Lyt-2,3 antigens plus reduced amounts of Lyt-1 antigens (Table 12-1). Loss of the TL antigen by the maturing thymocyte population may be a reflection of the fact that individual cells that retain the TL antigen are scheduled to die in the thymus, thus enriching the surviving population for TL$^-$ cells. How retention or loss of TL may be related to the mechanism of thymocyte death is unknown.

One possible mechanism for thymocyte elimination may resolve around sensitivity to hydrocortisone. At some point shortly after entering the thymus, the cells become sensitive to physiological levels of corticosteroids. A subpopulation of these are somehow selected for survival, based possibly on their ability to "properly" recognize self class II MHC antigens on the thymic epithelium (see Chapter 15). These cells, which lack the TL antigen, would appear to have reacquired steroid resistance. Those cells not selected die, probably under the influence of corticosteroids: in animals from which the adrenal glands have been removed, no thymocytes are killed, and the thymus hypertrophies. On the other hand, chronically stressed animals (or people) may suffer from a prematurely atrophied thymus, because of elevated levels of systemic steroids. However, it must be emphasized that both the means of thymocyte selection for survival, and the mechanism of elimination of unselected thymocytes, are still very much open questions.

The question arose as to the relationship between the mature medullary thymocytes and peripheral T cells. In most ways they are indistinguishable—both are immunocompetent, hydrocortisone resistant, TL$^-$, etc. It was tempting to assume that thymocytes proceed through the necessary maturational steps in the various thymic compartments, a few of them ending up in the medulla from where they migrate to the periphery and take up residence as mature T cells.

This simple view was soon challenged by Weissman himself. By following the longer range fate of the ^{3}H-TdR-labeled cortical thymus cells (Figure 12-2), Weissman showed that at least some of them eventually did show up in the T-dependent areas of the spleen and lymph nodes. These cells were Thy-1$^+$, Ig$^-$, and responded to antigen in situ. He then carried out experiments in which the entire thymus was infused with ^{3}H-UdR. As a result of this type of treatment, *all* thymic compartments are equally labeled within a very short time, since all cells are making RNA simultaneously. Labeled cells from ^{3}H-UdR-treated thymuses can be followed out to peripheral tissues just as with ^{3}H-TdR labeling. When the thymus was first exposed to hydrocortisone for 24 hours (leaving only medullary thymocytes) and then infused with ^{3}H-UdR, none of this label was subsequently detected in the T-dependent areas of lymph node or spleen. Most of the cells in the residual medulla were fully labeled, however. These results suggested that mature, medullary thymocytes do not provide a major source of immunocompetent T cells for the peripheral lymphoid organs.

Table 12-1 Characteristics of Thymocytes and T Cells at Various Stages of Differentiation

Thymic region	Percentage of total thymocytes	Size	DNA synthesis	Immuno-competent	Hydrocortisone sensitivity	Surface antigens			
						Thy-1	TL	H2	Ly
Subscapular cortex	5–10	Large	++++	No	High	++++	+	++	Lyt-1,2,3+ only
Midcortex	85–90	Small	+++	No	High	++++	+	++	Lyt-1,2,3+ only
Medulla	5	Medium	±	Yes	Low	++	−	++++	Lyt-1,2,3+; Lyt-1+; Lyt-2,3+
(Lymph nodes and spleen)	—	Small	−	Yes	Low	++	−	++++	Lyt-1,2,3+; Lyt-1+; Lyt-2,3+

Subsequent experiments by Weisman provided evidence that hydrocortisone treatment was not affecting the migration process per se.

The existence of cells in the peripheral lymph tissues that appear to have been at least partially matured in the thymus has been detected by various investigators, but has been studied most closely by Osias Stutman and his co-workers. When a mouse is thymectomized at birth, no *immunocompetent* T cells show up in the periphery, although some Thy-1$^+$ cells do appear in T-dependent areas of the lymph nodes or spleen. In the adult, however, the areas of these organs identifiable as T dependent have much fewer than normal Thy-1$^+$ cells, and the animal is totally deficient in all T-cell-associated functions (graft rejection, help, suppression, etc.) If the thymus is implanted into a mouse that was neonatally thymectomized, mature *competent* T cells can be found in the spleen and lymph nodes a few days later. The same results are obtained if the thymus is enclosed in a cell-tight diffusion chamber, or if the mice are injected with the hormone thymopoietin extracted from the thymus, within 60 days of the thymectomy. It can be shown that in either case the T cells that develop are of host, not thymus graft donor, origin. This suggests that immature T cells had been seeded from the thymus into the periphery prior to birth, but their further maturation into competent T cells requires additional development under the influence of the thymus.

It could be argued that perhaps these cells (Thy-1$^+$, immunoincompetent) migrated directly from the bone marrow to the lymph nodes or spleen and never actually passed through the thymus. This seems unlikely, based on Stutman's observation that they disappear 40 to 60 days after neonatal thymectomy. If a chamber-enclosed thymus is implanted or thymopoietin is administered after this time, no T cells subsequently appear. Because migration of bone marrow cells directly to the lymph nodes or spleen should not be affected by removal of the thymus, it was concluded that they first had to pass through the thymus before taking up residence as immature or partially differentiated T cells.

In contrast to these results, other investigators, most recently Scollay and Shortman, find that all cells leaving the thymus are fully mature and competent within a few hours at most. Thus the questions of how cells are selected to live or die within the thymus, and the exact state of cells leaving the thymus, are still being actively investigated.

The differentiation in the adult thymus of bone marrow T-cell precursors has become of increasing interest because of the use of bone marrow chimeras to study development of the ability of T cells to recognize antigen (Chapter 15). Such studies are complicated by the fact that when bone marrow is removed from bones for study, blood vessels are broken, releasing mature blood cells into the marrow. Under normal conditions, there are no cells in bone marrow per se identifiable as fully mature T cells by unique surface antigenic determinants. It has been shown that the precursors of T cells in the bone marrow can be distinguished from other hematopoietic stem cells on the basis of their buoyant density. However, it is not clear whether the cells dealt with in these studies were marrow derived or blood contaminants, or both. As we will see later, great care must be taken, when using bone marrow as a source of T-stem cells, to remove postthymic T-cells. This can usually be done by treatment with a strong anti-Thy-1 antiserum plus complement.

The Nude Mouse—A Model for the Role of the Thymus in T-Cell Differentiation

Nude mice have a genetic defect, controlled by two or more closely linked loci, that in the homozygous state results in abnormal development of the thymus, and, apparently independently, failure to develop fur (Figure 12-3). The chromosomal region containing these loci can be genetically "grafted" onto different inbred strains, to create nude congenics, which also fail to develop fur and fail to develop a functional thymus. The B-cell and macrophage compartments in nude mice are normal. Substantial resistance to viral infections and tumors is provided by a particularly vigorous NK cell compartment (see Chapter 14), partially alleviating the T-cell deficiency. However, nude mice are unable to reject grafts or to provide T-cell help to B lymphocytes.

The secondary lymphoid organs of nude mice are characterized by the absence of cells in the so-called thymus-dependent areas (see Chapter 2). There is also a severe reduction of circulating small lymphocytes, and those remaining are nearly all B cells. Strongly Thy-1$^+$ cells are essentially absent from nude mice. However, there does exist a significant proportion of cells (about 20 percent) with very weakly Thy-1$^+$ surfaces; these can be converted to strongly Thy-1$^+$ cells by culturing them on monolayers of thymic epithelial cells, or by exposing them to supernates of cultures of activated T cells. Nude mice are also abnormal in that they continue to express the TL antigen on peripheral T cells.

Nude mice clearly have normal *pre*thymic T-cell precursors. Nude bone marrow cells are perfectly capable of restoring an irradiated syngeneic mouse (if the thy-

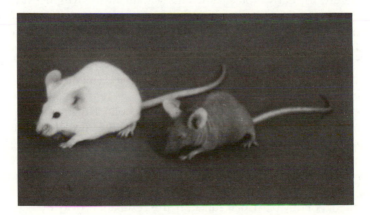

Figure 12-3 Nude mouse and normal littermate. (Courtesy Jackson Laboratories, Bar Harbor, Maine.)

mus is undamaged), and nude mice can be restored to normal immunological function by implanting a viable, histocompatible thymus. The hairless condition is not affected by this latter treatment. It has been demonstrated that restoration in the case of thymus implants involves maturation of host T-cell precursors and not simply replacement of T-cell function by donor thymocytes. On the other hand, it has been difficult to demonstrate restoration of immune function in nude mice with thymus hormone alone, suggesting that donor thymocytes or stromal cells may play some direct role in the maturation of incoming prethymocytes.

Experiments have been carried out both *in vivo* and *in vitro* to examine the cellular defect in nude mouse T cells. Although nude mice cannot respond directly to antigenic challenges by developing either helper or cytotoxic T cells, they can do so if they are provided with a source of the T-cell activating substance IL-2 (see Chapter 13). Injection of IL-2 by itself (or addition of IL-2 alone to cultured nude T cells) does not restore functional competency; the IL-2 must be given together with antigen. Thus it seems that IL-2 is not acting to push cells past a developmental block in nude mice but rather is acting together with antigen as a costimulating signal for T-cell activation. This is consistent with the role proposed for IL-2 generally. The most straightforward explanation of these results is that nude mice fail to develop cells that, on antigenic presentation, produce IL-2. This is the functional normally associated with Lyt-2$^-$ amplifier T cells.

Polyclonal Activation of T Cells by Mitogens

A number of substances, principally plant lectins of various sorts, have been shown to activate T cells. These lectins are specific for particular arrays of carbohydrate moieties, with which they can react either freely in solution or at a cell surface. Originally, it was thought that such substances served merely as mitogens, triggering the cells to divide and synthesize DNA. From this point of view, they were used primarily to study the early molecular events accompanying lymphocyte activation. However, it was subsequently shown that in fact such substances, principally phytohemagglutinin (PHA) and concanavalin A (Con A), could also trigger the expression of cell-specific function. Con A, for example, can be used to generate T-cell help, T suppressor celsls, and cytotoxic effector cells. Furthermore, Con A (and PHA) can activate either unprimed or previously primed (memory) cells for helper or cytotoxic effector function.

As far as can be determined, the sequence of events triggered in individual T cells, leading to expression (or reexpression) of the differentiated function, is indistinguishable whether the cell is activated by antigen or mitogen. The major difference is seen at the population level. When a T-cell population is treated with an appropriate lectin the resultant activation is both polyfunctional and polyclonal. At most concentrations of lectin, helper cells, suppressor cells, and cytotoxic cells are all activated. For any particular function, the resultant activity in the population is expressed toward a wide spectrum of antigenic determinants. For example, if an H-2^b spleen cell population is activated by Con A over a 72-hour period, one will find in the resultant cultures cytotoxic T lymphocytes specific for H-2^d, H-2^k, H-2^a, H-2^s, etc. target cells. These individual CTL behave exactly as would individual CTLs generated by the corresponding antigen, and the population behaves exactly as would a mixture of individual antigen-stimulated CTLs.

The T-Cell Receptor for Antigen

Although it has been clear for a number of years that the B-cell surface receptor for antigen is a form of that immunoglobulin molecule that the cell is programmed to synthesize and secrete, the molecular nature of the T-cell receptor has only recently been determined. The most obvious and attractive candidate for the T-cell receptor would also be immunoglobulin. All of the functional subclasses of T cells respond to antigen in an immunologically specific way, and it would seem logical and efficient to use the same molecule for this purpose on both T and B cells. However, it was clear very early on that the T-cell receptor is not classical Ig. T cells have very little immunoglobulin isotype associated with the plasma membrane, and there is good evidence to suggest that what little there is is passively acquired rather than synthesized by the T cell displaying it. Antisera against the known Ig isotypes have no effect on any of the T-cell functions. And a number of investigations have suggested that what the T-cell receptor "sees" includes a larger portion of the antigen molecule than what is recognized by immunoglobulin, plus a portion of an MHC molecule.

Definition of the Murine T-Cell Receptor at the Protein Level

Two experimental approaches were important in elucidating the structure of the T-cell receptor. In the first approach, cloned T-cell lines, or T-cell hybridomas, were used to immunize suitable recipients in an attempt to produce antiidiotypic T-cell receptor antibodies. The rationale behind this approach is that because cloned T-cell lines and hybridomas are monoclonally derived, then the antigen receptor that they display should also be monoclonal, similar to myeloma proteins or experimentally generated monoclonal antibodies. When such monoclonal immunoglobulins are used for immunization, antibodies specific for the antigen binding regions are readily produced. The same should be true for monoclonal surface receptors.

The results shown in Table 12-2, from the laboratory of Marrack and Kappler at Denver, are typical of those obtained using this approach. D011.10 is a T-cell hybridoma with helper function. It was produced by fusing BALB/c (H-2^d) helper T cells, specific for chicken ovalbumin (OVA), with H-2^k tumor cells. "Help" in these experiments is defined as the production of IL-2 by the hybridoma in response to an appropriate antigenic challenge. D011.10 will produce IL-2 when presented with OVA on a presenting cell bearing IA^d class II molecules. Using D011.10 cells to immunize (Balb.B × AKR)F$_1$ mice, these researchers were able to derive a mono-

Table 12-2 Specificity of the Marrack-Kappler
T-Cell Receptor mAb KJ1-26

Hybridoma tested	Specificity	Units of IL-2 produced[1]	
		−KJ1-26	+KJ1-26
D011.10	OVA/IA^d	2560	<10
3DT-18.11	TGAL/IA^d	3700	2560
AODH-3.4	OVA/IA^k	160	160
4DO-11.7	OVA/IA^d	2560	5120
3DO-52.8	OVA/IA^d	1000	1800
3DO-52.6	OVA/IA^d	800	1000

[1]Values differing by less than a factor of 4 may not be significantly different.

clonal antibody (KJ1-26) that blocked the ability of D011.10 to respond to OVA presented on an H-2^d B-cell lymphoma. (Although antigen is normally presented to T cells on macrophages, under some experimental conditions B-cell lines can be used.) However, KJ1-26 would not block the responsiveness of hybridomas recognizing other antigens in the context of IA^d, or OVA in the context of other class II molecules. KJ1-26 would not even block the response of three other T-cell hybridomas reactive to OVA in the context of IA^d. Thus this monoclonal antibody appeared to be reacting with highly idiotypic determinants within the D011.10 receptor.

The Marrack-Kappler group also used KJ1-26 to immunoprecipitate the D011.10 receptor molecule. They identified a dimeric 80 to 90 kd molecule composed of approximately 40 to 44 kd subunits held together by a disulfide bond. This molecule appeared to be present in about 15,000 copies per hybridoma cell. Other researchers, using a peptide mapping approach similar to that used in the early studies on Ig L chains, showed that the component chains (called α and β) had variable and constant regions.

Molecular Genetic Studies

The second approach that has been used to characterize the receptor on T cells is to isolate and study the genes that code for it. Various strategies have been used in identifying the receptor genes. One rather imaginative approach that paid off was that used by Mark Davis and colleagues. They reasoned that since T cells and B cells must interact with essentially the same antigenic universe (at least in terms of size), then the T-cell receptor would very likely share some of the features of immunoglobulins with respect to mechanisms for generating diversity. They therefore examined several cloned murine helper T-cell lines for genes that undergo rearrangement between germ-line and mature T-cell DNA. They began by making cDNA copies of membrane-bound polysomal mRNA from cloned cells. Polysomal mRNA was used to increase the likelihood of isolating an mRNA for an integral membrane protein. These cDNA copies were then subjected to "subtraction hybridization" with B-cell mRNA (Figure 12-4) to enrich for T-cell specific sequences. The nonhybridized cDNA was used to screen a second T helper cell cDNA library. Of 10 cDNA clones that were identified as T helper cell specific, one hybridized to a region of the genome that is rearranged in all mature functional T cells (Figure 12-5), but not in B cells or nonlymphoid cells. By comparison with preliminary sequence information obtained with isolated receptor proteins, this clone turned out to react with a group of gene segments coding for the β subunit of the T-cell receptor.

The β-chain gene has now been characterized by several different labs, and is the most intensely studied of the three receptor chains identified so far. It codes for a 32-kd peptide, and its general organization in the genome is shown in Figure 12-6. It is found on chromosome 6 in the mouse, which thus links it karyologically to the Ig kappa gene family. Although a possible evolutionary relationship to kappa cannot be rigorously ruled out, at present there is nothing to suggest that its presence on the same chromosome with kappa is anything more than coincidence. The human β gene, for example, is unlinked to any of the human Ig gene families. Molecular genetics thus confirms what immunologists had concluded from other experimental evidence: the T-cell receptor is not classical Ig.

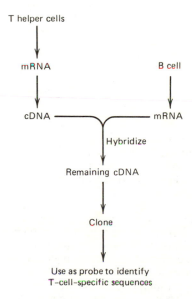

Figure 12-4 Enrichment of T-cell-specific cDNA by subtraction–hybridization with B-cell mRNA.

One immediately striking feature of the organization of the T-cell receptor β gene is its similarity to Ig genes. A small but unknown number (20 to 30) of V-region segments lies upstream of two complete sets of D, J, and C segments. A selected V segment can apparently combine with elements of either set. For the β chain, only a single D segment is present in each set. Each J cluster is composed of six J_β segments, located about 0.5 kb upstream of the single C segment associated with each set.

The two murine C_β gene segments differ by only 4 to 5 amino acids, and the inferred human and mouse C_β amino acid sequences show greater than 80 percent homology. On the other hand, the two clusters of J_β segments in mice show almost no sequence homology. Interestingly, the two C_β segments show about 30 percent homology with some Ig domains, and have a potential internal disulfide bond separated by 60 or so amino acids.

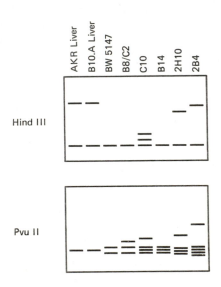

Figure 12-5 Southern blot analysis showing rearrangement of T-cell-specific DNA. One of the cDNAs derived from the experiment shown in Figure 12-4 was made radioactive and used to probe DNA from several different mouse cell sources. The DNA was first digested either with HindIII or PvuII, electrophoresed, and then reacted with the cDNA. The first two lanes show the hybridization pattern of the labeled probe with digested liver DNA, which may be taken as characteristic of the germline (unrearranged) pattern. Hybridization patterns with DNA from three different B cell lymphomas showed the same pattern as liver DNA (data not shown). This would be expected if the cDNA probe is reacting only with T-cell receptor genes, which should not be rearranged in B cells. On the other hand, the probe showed a variety of different hybridization patterns with digested DNA from each of 6 different mature T-cell lines (lanes 3 to 8). Different patterns for each of the six lines would be expected if each is expressing a different T-cell receptor (related to differing antigen specificities). The probe turned out to represent a portion of the β-chain gene. [From data presented in S. Hedrick et al., Sequence relationships between putative T cell receptor polypeptides and immunoglobulins. *Nature, 308,* 153 (1984).]

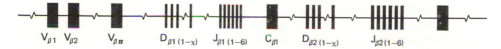

Figure 12-6 Prototypical gene for the β chain of the T-cell receptor.

The V_β genes sequenced so far seem to display slightly more structural diversity than do Ig V regions, but this may be biased by the small number of V_β sequences studied. In general, homology among Ig V_H genes ranges from 35 to 75 percent whereas T-cell receptor V_β gene homology ranges from 18 to 51 percent. The hypervariability plots for V_β sequences are similar to those for Ig V regions (Figure 4-12). In terms of three-dimensional structure, V_β also seems to fold like an Ig domain.

Moreover, the combinatorial modes with D and J segments may differ in β genes from that seen in immunoglobulin H chain genes. The flanking sequences around D and J segments should allow for direct V–J joining, and for joining of a V segment with more than one D segment. How often this actually happens will have to await analysis of more V_β gene sequences.

To date, about 20 rearranged V_β segments have been sequenced. Of these, only 9 different sequences have been found; one sequence was represented 5 times, and several others had two to three repeats. Assuming that the sequences studied were random and statistically representative, it seems likely that there may be no more than 20 to 30 or so different germ-line V_β sequences. We return to this point again in the section on the biology of the T-cell receptor.

Another unusual feature of the β-gene coding segments is the presence of a promotor region upstream of the D segments. As in B-cell heavy chains, the first rearrangement involves joining of a D and J segment, normally followed by translocation and joining of a V segment to the D–J couplet. However, at least in immature T cells in the thymus, the D–J–C unit is, in fact, transcribed and can be found in the cytoplasm. The function of such transcripts is completely unknown at present.

The second T-cell receptor gene to be described was at first thought to be the gene for the α chain, but has since been renamed the γ gene. It appears to be transcribed only in CTL. Although quite similar in structure to the true α gene (see below), the γ gene is not glycosylated and is transcribed at a very low level with respect to the α and β genes. Preliminary evidence suggests that there may be even fewer V-gene segments than for the β gene, and perhaps only a single J segment.

The gene segments coding for the α chain of the T-cell receptor have only recently been isolated and studied. These segments code for a 27-kd peptide with three potential *N*-glycosylation sites that is found in both CTL and T_h cells in approximately equal amounts. Although the overall organization of the α-gene segments is similar to the β-gene group, there are some interesting differences. The number of V_α segments is somewhat larger, perhaps 50 to 100. Variability plots for the known V_α segments appear similar to V_β and the V_{Igs}. There is only one set of J_α and C_α segments. So far a D_α segment has not been identified. However, there are at least 18 J_α segments, and perhaps as many as 50. These are located quite far upstream from the C_α segment (20 to 40 kb versus 1 to 6 kbp in β and Ig gene families) and are loosely dispersed across a wide region (50 to 60 kb) of DNA. One consequence of this arrangement is that a rather large primary nuclear transcript is required to contain a complete coding sequence.

A comparison of V_α, V_β, and the three immunoglobulin V-region amino acid sequences shows several regions of homology. V_α and V_β share with V_H, V_κ, and V_α some of the same amino acid sequences the latter three share with each other. These amino acids in the immunoglobulins are known to be critical for V-domain folding, and for V_H–V_L interactions. The fact that V_α and V_β show homologies to V_H and V_L in these same regions suggests that the V segments of the T cell receptor and of immunoglobulins are evolutionarily related and suggests that they fold and interact in a similar manner.

A proposed structure for the T-cell receptor, as inferred from the α and β gene sequences, is shown in Figure 12-7.

The T-3 Complex

On human T cells, an additional complex of three noncovalently linked peptides is associated with the T-cell receptor. The function of this complex, referred to as T-3 because at least one of the three peptides bears the T-3 antigen (p. 282), is unknown, but it must be present for the T-cell receptor to function properly. The T-3 peptides almost certainly do not interact directly with antigen. They could be involved in maintaining the conformation of the α–β-receptor complex, or, as seems more likely, they may be involved in transmitting the signal generated by the α–β-antigen complex to the interior of the cell. The three peptides range in size from 20 to 28 kd, and will likely be labeled the γ, δ, and ϵ chains of the T-cell receptor. Just recently, a T-3 complex equivalent has been found to be associated with the mouse T-cell receptor.

Biology of the T-Cell Receptor

Ontogeny

Rearrangement and expression of T-cell receptor genes in the mouse thymus begins on day 17 of development (gestation—21 days). The first rearrangement to be seen is a D_β segment joining to a J_β segment. The V_β to D_β–J_β joining event follows about 24 hours later. The α gene may not rearrange before birth, but during T-cell ontogeny in the adult, rearrangement does occur in the thymus.

The development of various T-cell differentiation markers in the human thymus was indicated in Table 12-1. Pre-T cells entering the thymus display only T-11 antigens. Immediately upon taking up residence in the cortex of the thymus, they

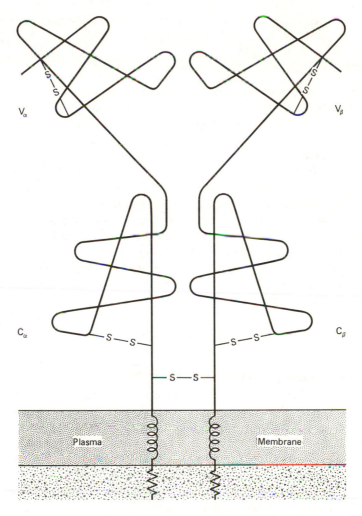

Figure 12-7 Hypothetical model of the murine T-cell receptor for antigen, predicted from gene sequence studies. The actual positions of the inferred disulfide bonds are V_α, 21 to 94; V_β, 23 to 91; C_α, 151 to 207; C_β, 140 to 201.

begin to display the T-cell markers T-6, T-4, and T-8. As the thymocytes migrate down into the medullary areas of the thymic lobes, they undergo several changes. They rearrange their β- (and presumably α-) chain gene segments and begin to display β chains on their surface, together with the T-3 antigen. T-3 is a determinant found on a cluster of three proteins that are intimately associated with the T-cell receptor. At the same time, the thymocytes lose either the T-4 or T-8 marker, probably signaling their commitment to either the T_h or CTL pathways. So far it is unclear just when in thymic development the α chain is expressed on the thymocyte surface, although it is probably later than β. Events similar to these appear to take place during murine T-cell differentiation as well.

Diversity

The question of diversity of the T-cell receptor repertoire is currently under investigation. Because T cells interact with the same range of antigens as do B cells, plus MHC structures, the T cell receptor might be expected to display a level of diversity at least equivalent to immunoglobulin. Initial data coming from studies of the β gene (the first to be studied in detail) generated considerable concern. There is a very small number of germ-line V_β genes in the mouse, probably not more than 25 to 30. Moreover, the same V_β gene segment has been found in T cells with widely divergent antigenic specificities. In one case, the same V_β gene was found to be rearranged in a T_h cell and in a CTL, in the one case presumably facilitating recognition of a class II molecule plus nominal antigen, and in the second case facilitating recognition of a class I antigen plus virus.

The concern generated by these initial findings has been alleviated by subsequent observations. First of all, combinatorial diversity of V, D, and J segments is considerably greater in both α and β than in the immunoglobulin V families. The α and β sets use the same type of 7mers and 9mers, plus 12 or 23 base spacers, as do the immunoglobulins (p. 108) for joining V, D, and J segments. However V_α and V_β can join either to D or directly to J segments, and more than a single D segment may be interspersed between V and J. And as with the Ig V genes, there is imprecision of segment joining (p. 111).

The problem of diversity has been helped considerably by the finding of a reasonable number of V_α segments (at least 21 so far, with statistical arguments making a final number of about 100 quite reasonable). Although no D_α segments have been identified, the large number of J_α segments (18 identified so far, but probably more like 50 total), together with junctional diversity allows a large number of different complete V_α sequences to be generated. The estimates of T-cell receptor V-region diversity emanating from the most recent data yield numbers quite close to those estimated for immunoglobulins.

T-Cell Activation

Some antibodies to the T-cell receptor have been shown to activate the cell rather than to block its function. For example, some antibodies (including mAbs) made against a cloned T helper cell receptor were shown to trigger the T cells to proliferate, and to secrete lymphokines able to promote B-cell proliferation and differentiation in the absence of accessory cells. Presumably these antibodies were recognizing antigenic determinants lying within the actual antigen-combining site of the receptor, and were mimicking antigen. Such determinants would be analogous to idiotypic determinants associated with the antigen combining site of antibody molecules. One implication of this finding is that, at least with cloned T_h cells (which are probably analogous with memory cells *in vivo*), extensive cross linking of T-cell receptors may not be a requirement for activation. Monoclonal antibodies would be unlikely to be able to crosslink more than two receptors, unless the same idiotypic determinant were present more than once per receptor binding site. Moreover, at least with memory-type T cells, antigen presenting cells may play no role beyond simple gathering and physical presentation.

The Biology of B Cells

Fetal Ontogeny of B Lymphocytes

The early stages of B lymphocyte development are identical with T-cell ontogeny. B cells derive from pluripotent hematogenous stem cells that appear sequentially in the yolk sac, liver, bone marrow, and spleen of the fetus. It is not known at which stage of lymphoid stem cell maturation that T and B cells become distinct. In bird embryos, which have a bursa, B-stem cells appear in the bursa before they can be detected in the bone marrow. B lymphocytes are functionally less heterogeneous than are T cells, their apparently principal, if not sole, *raison d'être* being the production and secretion of immunoglobulin. Most studies of B-cell ontogeny have thus focused on the development of the ability to produce Ig.

The existence of cells in the early mouse embryo with B lymphocyte characteristics has been reported by many investigators (Table 12-3). The basic scheme for the fetal ontogeny of B cells in mice is shown in Figure 12-8. Blood stem cells form from the embryonic mesoderm, probably 5 to 6 days after fertilization. These cells are found progressively in the yolk sac, liver, bone marrow, and spleen. Throughout life, the bone marrow remains the major repository of blood stem cells.

On about day 12 or 13 of fetal development (term: 20 to 21 days), the first definitive step in the differentiation of B cells occurs. This involves the rearrangement of a D_H segment to J_H-C_μ, followed almost immediately by rearrangement of a V_H–J_H unit to form a complete μ chain coding sequence. The result is a cell (called a pre-B cell) that has detectable levels of the secreted form of μ chain in the cytoplasm, but no detectable surface IgM. This form is present in the embryo for several days. The cell in which this initial event takes place may have undergone some previous event signaling its commitment to the B-cell pathway, but if so at present we have no means of detecting it.

By day 16 to 17 of development, a second event takes place that converts the pre-B cell to what we might call an immature B cell. Concomitant with rearrangement of one of the light-chain genes, a completed IgM molecule appears on the B-cell surface. We do not know if expression of the L-chain gene itself controls insertion of IgM into the membrane, or if these two events are independent and simply concomitant. It would appear that in addition to L-chain gene expression, there is also a switch from transcription of the secreted form of μ-chain gene, to the membrane form (p. 113).

Table 12-3 Appearance of Cell-associated Ig during Embryonic Development in the Mouse

Organ	Fetal								Birth	Neonatal				
	11	12	13	14	15	16	17	18		1	2	3	4	5
Liver (cytoplasm)	+	+	+	+	+	+	+	+	+	+	+	+	±	±
Liver (surface)	–	–	?	?	?	?	+	+	+	+	+	+	±	±
Spleen (cytoplasm)	–	–	+	+	+	+	+	+	+	+	+	+	+	+
Spleen (surface)	–	–	–	–	–	–	+	+	+	+	+	+	+	+
Lymph node (surface)	–	–	–	–	–	–	–	–	–	–	±	+	+	+

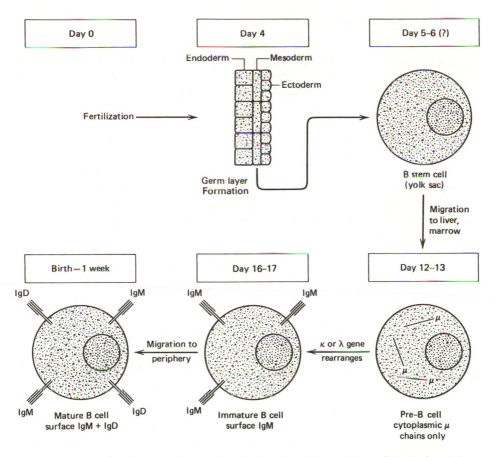

Figure 12-8 B-cell ontogeny. (See text for details). The differentiation of B cells in adult bone marrow follows essentially the same pathway, but the overall developmental time may be shorter.

As we will discuss later, B cells at this stage are competent to bind antigen, but they probably are not competent to respond to antigen by producing antibody. This capacity may not appear until another event that occurs at or shortly before birth, after migration of the cells to peripheral lymphoid tissue—the production and surface expression of membrane IgD. As with the decision to produce surface versus membrane forms of immunoglobulin molecules, the decision to produce membrane IgD in addition to membrane IgM is executed at the level of RNA splicing rather than DNA transcription (p. 115). The expression of other isotypes of immunoglobulin also occurs shortly after birth, and may be the result of antigen-induced isotype switching (p. 111).

B-Cell Ontogeny in the Adult

There are two classes of lymphocytes bearing surface Ig in adult mice, based on circulation pattern and turnover. One class is found mostly in solid lymphoid tissue and is continuously and rapidly renewed throughout adult life. These are mature, immunocompetent B cells that have not yet encountered antigen (virgin B cells). The average turnover time of virgin B cells, as determined by ^{3}H-thymidine/auto-radiography studies, is on the order of two to three days. The second class is relatively long lived and is found mostly in the circulation. These are memory cells generated from virgin B cells previously triggered by antigen.

The sequence of differentiative events for B cells in adult organisms is essentially a compressed version of what happens during fetal ontogeny (Figure 12-8). B-stem cells in bone marrow undergo sequential μ- and L-chain rearrangements, probably without a four- to five-day lag period between the two events. On the other hand, several percent of nucleated marrow cells may be pre-B cells, so some delay between H and L chains may in fact occur. The expression of surface IgD, which takes place only after the B cells migrate from the marrow to peripheral lymphoid tissue, appears to be necessary in order to produce a fully mature, antigen-responsive B cell. Further differentiation of the B cell to a plasma cell requires interaction with antigen, and T-cell help. This pathway is discussed in detail in Chapter 13.

The bone marrow of most adult mammals contains the full spectrum of developmental stages of B lymphocytes. As noted earlier, pre-B cells can be found in bone marrow that make (and possibly) secrete μ chains, but display μ only in the cytoplasm and not on the surface. Available evidence suggests these cytoplasmic μ chains are predominantly of the secretory rather than the membrane type. At about the time of rearrangement of L-chain gene segments, pre-B cells begin to synthesize membrane μ, to assemble full molecules of at least membrane IgM, and to display IgM on their surfaces. Similar stages of maturation can also be identified in the spleen. The exact locus of final B-cell maturation is not really known. In lethally irradiated mice in which the bone marrow has also been selectively destroyed with ^{91}Sr, transplanted syngeneic bone marrow cells are still capable of maturing to fully competent B cells, probably in the spleen. Intermediate and advanced stages of B-cell differentiation may also take place in the spleen, and perhaps in the lymph nodes.

The Role of the Bursa in Avian B-Cell Development

In birds, a great deal of controversy has centered around the exact role of the bursa in B-cell ontogeny in both the embryo and the adult. It had been assumed that the embryonic bursa promotes the differentiation of B-lymphocyte precursors from bone marrow, much as the thymus serves as a site of maturation for bone marrow T-cell precursors. It had also been assumed that the bursa serves as a site for maturation of appropriate bone marrow-derived B-cell precursors in the adult.

However, this assumption has been challenged. In studies using karyotypically distinguishable syngeneic bone marrow cells injected into normal adult chickens, donor cells were subsequently found in the host bone marrow and thymus, but not in the bursa. Apparently there is no route for stem cells from the marrow to the bursa. In these same studies, mature donor T cells were also found in the circulation, suggesting that stem cells had been acted on by the thymus, but no circulating cells of donor origin with surface Ig could be identified. Thus it may be that at least after hatching (and perhaps in embryonic life as well) the bursa is in fact a self-contained system of B-lymphocyte stem cells and maturational apparatus.

The nature of the defect in bursectomized birds has recently been reexamined in some detail. Embryonic chicks were bursectomized *in ovo* at 60 hours of development, and spleen cells from the resulting chickens after hatching were analyzed for B-cell function (Figure 12-9). Shortly after hatching, the spleens of the bursectomized chickens were somewhat smaller than sham-operated controls, and the spleen cells responded poorly to polyclonal B-cell activators (PBAs) *in vitro* as measured by total Ig secretion. (PBAs trigger all mature B cells and drive them to a state of immunoglobulin secretion.) By 10 weeks posthatching, spleen cells from bursectomized and control chickens gave equal responses to PBAs *in vitro*. Moreover, the bursectomized birds had normal spleen architecture, including B cells displaying various surface Ig classes, and had normal levels of serum immunoglobulins. Nevertheless, as Bruce Glick observed many years ago, the bursectomized birds are completely unable to produce antibodies to specific antigenic

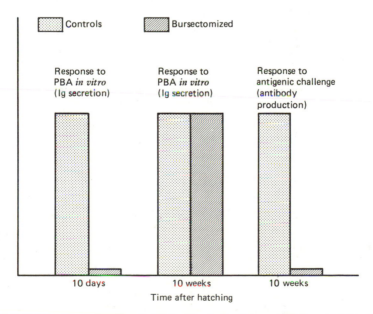

Figure 12-9 Spleen B-cell function in birds after bursectomy at 60 hours of development.

challenges. This series of experiments was very important in leading to the conclusion that the role of the bursa may be more crucial in facilitating B cell responses to antigen than in B-cell ontogeny.

B-Cell Surface Markers

As was pointed out earlier, B cells seem to be functionally rather homogeneous, at least compared to T cells. However, B-cell subpopulations have been defined by a number of other criteria; size, turnover, and circulating patterns have already been mentioned. An additional way of grouping B cells into subpopulations is on the basis of surface markers that are more or less restricted to B lymphocytes. The most often used markers are surface Ig, the Fc receptor (FcR), the complement receptor (CR), class II antigens, and Lyb-5 antigen. These various markers make an ordered developmental appearance in mice (Table 12-4). Recently it has been shown that the surface antigen Ly-1, previously thought to be present only on T cells, is also found on a subset of B cells. This particular subset displays low levels of δ and high concentrations of surface μ. Interestingly, this particular subset is very prominent in NZB mice that develop spontaneous autoimmune disease (Chapter 18).

The various classes of Ig isotype markers appearing on the surfaces of developing B lymphocytes are particularly useful in studying functional maturation of these cells. In both fetal and adult B-cell differentiation, IgM appears on the cell surface

Table 12-4 B-Lymphocyte Subpopulations Defined by Surface Antigenic and Functional Markers

Organs where first detected	Organs where found in adult	sIgm	Fc	Ia	sIgD	CR	Mls	Lyb-5
17-Day fetal liver	Newborn-3 week bone marrow and spleen	+	+	−	−	−	−	−
Newborn spleen	Bone marrow	+++	+	+	−	−	−	−
7- to 14-Day spleen	Spleen	+++	+	+	+	−	−	−
7- to 14-Day spleen	Spleen	++	+	+	++	+	−	−
7- to 21-Day spleen	Spleen	+	+	+	+++	+	+	+

Adapted from I. Scher et al., Murine B-lymphocyte heterogeneity. *J. Immunol. 119,* 1938 (1977).

before any other Ig class. It is not certain at present whether B cells with *only* IgM on the surface (μ^-) can respond to antigen- and produce antibody-forming cells. Cells with both IgM and IgD on the surface ($\mu^+\delta^+$) are clearly capable of responding in a primary humoral reaction and secrete IgM. There is some evidence to suggest that $\mu^+\delta^+$ cells can respond to certain T-independent antigens and that the acquisition of IgD is required for the cells to respond to T-cell help. Bone marrow cells with only IgM on the surface are thought to be particularly susceptible to tolerance induction. In cells that are $\mu^+\delta^+$, it has been shown that both immunoglobulins bear the same idiotype and have the same antigenic specificity. This is, of course, what we would expect based on our knowledge of transcription and subsequent processing of the μ and δ genes (Chapter 5). The fact that the δ isotype seems always to be lost from cells after further, antigen-dependent maturation suggests the possibility that the IgD molecule may play some role as antigen receptor for virgin B cells; however, this has not yet been proved.

The B-Cell Receptor for Antigen is Immunoglobulin

One of the cardinal predictions of the clonal selection theory is that a cell competent to respond to antigen by producing antibody should display on its surface a copy of the antibody it is programmed to make. Experimental evidence in support of this concept was sought almost immediately after the clonal selection theory was enunciated, but nearly 10 years passed before meaningful data began to be assembled. Then, in a matter of 2 years or so, the question was resolved to everyone's satisfaction.

In the late 1960s several investigators showed that a radioactive antigen such as bovine serum albumin or bacterial flagellin would react with (bind to) about 1/5000 or 1/10,000 mouse spleen cells. This seemed to be in accord with the notion that relatively few lymphocytes should recognize and respond to any given antigen. But were the cells binding a particular antigen the same as the cells that produced antibody to that antigen?

This question was addressed in an experiment carried out by Ada and Byrt in 1969 (Figure 12-10). They incubated mouse spleen cells with unlabeled or with [125]-I-labeled polymerized flagellin from Salmonella. After a brief incubation the cells were washed to remove antigen not specifically bound to cell-surface receptors. The [125]-I-labeled flagellin was quite "hot"; the washed cells were allowed to incubate with the antigen for 16 to 20 hours, to maximize the possibility of radiation damage to cells that had bound antigen. The cells were then transferred into irradiated syngeneic animals and challenged with an immunogenic dose of either the same polymerized flagellin used in the preincubations, or with an immunologically distinct flagellin. The results are shown in Table 12-5. These data demonstrated clearly that cells that bind antigen are the ones that would ordinarily go on to produce antibodies.

That the receptor for antigen on the putative antibody-producing cell is immunoglobulin had been suggested indirectly by experiments showing that antigen binding could be blocked by antiimmunoglobulin antibody. Interestingly, nearly 10 years after publication of the clonal selection theory, no one had yet demonstrated immunoglobulin molecules on lymphoid cell surfaces. Part of the reason for this was that until the late 1960s no one was sure that lymphocytes were, in fact, the precursors of antibody-producing cells. Another problem was that most investigators used fluorescent antibodies, the only means for visualizing molecular structures, on fixed tissues or cells. In such cases, cells making or capable of making immunoglobulin would provide a much stronger signal from their cytoplasm than

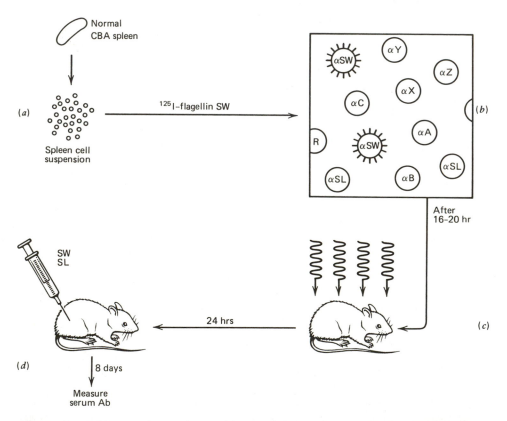

Figure 12-10 The Ada-Byrt "antigen suicide" experiment. Spleen cells are prepared from a CBA mouse (a) and incubated with ^{125}I-flagellin SW-1338. Some of the spleen cells (presumably those committed to producing anti-SW-1338 antibody) bind the hot flagellin (b). Cells committed to making other antibodies (e.g., against flagellin SL-871, or antigens A, B, C, etc.) do not bind hot SW-1338. Over the next 16 to 20 hours at 37°, the cells binding ^{125}I-flagellin will die. At the end of the incubation, the remaining cells are injected into an irradiated CBA mouse (c), and 24 hours later this mouse is injected with either SW-1338 or an immunologically non-cross-reactive flagellin, SL-871 (d). Eight days later the mice are tested for anti-flagellin antibody (see results in Table 12-5).

Table 12-5 Results of Ada and Byrt's Experiment

Experiment	Antigenic pretreatment of spleen cells before transfer	Mean antibody titer ($\log_2$) in recipient animal after challenge with	
		SW1338	SL871
1	SW1338, labeled	< 0.5	5.4
	SW1338, unlabeled	2.9	4.3
2	SL871, labeled	0.82	< 0.5
	SL871, unlabeled	1.6	4.8
3	SL871, labeled	2.0	1.1
	SL871, unlabeled	3.3	4.2

from their membranes; the latter, in fact, would not be at all discernible. Only in 1970 did Raff, Sternberg, and Taylor attempt to stain and observe living cells with fluoresceinated anti-Ig antibodies. They described a spleen cell subpopulation that was Ig$^+$.

All available evidence suggests that the antigen receptor on B cells is in fact a form of the immunoglobulin that the B cell is programmed to produce and secrete. B cells have large quantities of Ig on their surfaces, and it is now clear that membrane and secreted Ig in the same cell are identical. Binding antigen to the B-cell surface is inhibited by antibodies to Ig. If surface Ig is capped (Chapter 6) on B cells, they fail to bind antigen; when Ig is regenerated on the B-cell surface, the antigen-binding capacity of the cell is restored.

Allelic Exclusion

At maturity, each B cell is programmed to secrete only one species of immunoglobulin molecule. Although more than one heavy-chain isotype may be present on the B-cell surface, the available evidence suggests that all surface Ig molecules display the same V region. As noted in Chapter 4, in all immunoglobulin molecules both light chains are identical, as are both heavy chains. This would, of course, be expected in a homozygous animal where both sets of chromosomes carry identical Ig genes. Surprisingly, this is also true in heterozygotes where a different set of genes for V and C regions is inherited from each parent. Theoretically, light and heavy chains could be produced from genes on either parental chromosome; because light- and heavy-chain gene families are on different chromosomes within the haploid set, one might expect to see Ig molecules in heterozygotes with light and/or heavy chains contributed by both parents. This is never observed. This phenomenon was first described as a result of studies on the expression of light-

and heavy-chain alleles in rabbit immunoglobulin molecules. In heterozygotes where each parent contributes a different allele for a particular H- or L-chain marker, it was found that all of the Ig molecules present on cell surfaces and in the serum carried one or the other allele, but never both. Both parental markers were, however, represented in the total population of molecules and cells. For this reason, the phenomenon was referred to as "allelic exclusion." This type of exclusion is apparently restricted to the immunoglobulins and to the T-cell receptor. In all other cases, parental somatic genes are codominantly expressed in all cells.

One obvious advantage of allelic exclusion is that it restricts the B cell to a single antigenic specificity. If V regions from each parent of a heterozygote were expressed, then each B cell could express at least two, and perhaps four, different antigenic specificities. This would pose serious problems in terms of regulation of the immune response, including adequate control of antiself reactivity without impairing expression of a full repertoire of responses against foreign antigens. Although allelic exclusion makes good biological sense, at present there is no satisfactory genetic or molecular explanation for how allelic exclusion works.

Autonomous B-Cell Responses

In order to be triggered by and produce antibodies to most immunogens, both soluble and cellular, B lymphocytes require help provided by T lymphocytes. However, a few immunogens, called thymus-independent antigens, are capable of triggering B cells directly. A partial list of T-independent antigens is presented in Table 12-6. Many of these antigens are associated with bacterial cell wall products, suggesting the possibility that this mode of immune reactivity may have evolved to facilitate rapid responses to bacterial invasion. The one common feature for such antigens at the molecular level is that they are composed of repetitive subunits. This has led to speculation that they trigger B cells by cross-linking large numbers

Table 12-6 Representative Thymus-independent Antigens

Antigen	Source
LPS	Lipopolysaccharide from *E. coli*
FLA	Polymerized flagellin from *S. adelaide*
SIII	Pneumococcal polysaccharide
PVP	Polyvinyl pyrrolidone (synthetic polymer)
Dextrans; levans	Natural polysaccharides
Ficoll	
Polyglutamic acid	Synthetic polypeptide of *d*-glutamic acid
Hyaluronic acid	

of surface Ig receptors. Although no definitive proof of this has been developed, it is consistent with at least two other observations. (1) The response to most defined haptens (which must be coupled to carriers in order to be "seen" by the immune system) is ordinarily T dependent. However, if the haptens are closely spaced together on polymeric "backbones" such as agarose or ficol, they can activate B cells directly. It has not been determined whether the B cells responding to a hapten in polymerized form are the same as those that would respond to the same hapten in a T-cell-reactive carrier. (2) In most species, B cells can be activated polyclonally by antibodies to Ig. If surface Ig is assumed to be the B-cell receptor for antigen, then antibodies to Ig determinants could mimic T-independent antigen by cross-linking B-cell receptors. We return to this point in the next chapter.

T-independent antigens only trigger IgM responses in B cells and do not usually promote production of memory cells. There is now evidence to suggest that B cells responding to T-independent antigens may be a separate and distinct subpopulation of B cells, which may be inherently restricted to IgM production. Alternatively, they may fail to switch to IgG production because they fail to receive T-cell help. The evidence for separate B-cell subpopulations responding to T-dependent and T-independent antigens comes mainly from two types of experiments. Gorczynski and Feldmann separated B lymphocytes into size classes by sedimentation and showed that the cells responding to a T-dependent antigen (TNP–KLH) were predominantly smaller B cells, whereas the B cells responding to a T-independent antigen (DNP–POL) tended to be larger. Some investigators have speculated that the large and small subclasses of B cells may represent relatively immature and mature cells, respectively. A second approach to defining separate B-cell subpopulations for thymus-dependent and -independent responses has come from studies with the CBA/N strain of mice. These mice have an X-linked, recessive defect in development of their B cells. None of the CBA/N B cells display the LyB-5 marker, which appears fairly late in B-cell ontogeny (Table 12-4). These mice are able to respond to all T-dependent antigens but respond to only a portion of those antigens eliciting T-independent responses in other strains. Using antisera produced in CBA/N mice against spleen cells from normal mice, both Lyb-5$^+$ and Lyb-5$^-$ subpopulations of B cells were found to be present in all mouse strains. Thus T-dependent and at least some T-independent responses are mediated by different B-cell subpopulations.

Many T-independent antigens are also more or less indiscriminately mitogenic for B cells at higher concentrations. When used in this fashion they are usually called polyclonal B-cell activators (PBAs), reflecting the fact that activation is independent of the antigenic specificity of the B cells. PBAs can activate B cells that would ordinarily require T-cell help, but in most cases they also trigger IgM production and do not stimulate memory cell production. Different PBA appear to activate different subpopulations of B cells. However, these subpopulations are not distinguished by antigen specificities and the CBA/N data suggest they do not represent distinct functional subpopulations; they appear to represent different stages in B-cell maturation.

The relationship of T-independent antigens as antigens, to their PBA activity, is illustrated by the elegant experiment shown in Figure 12-11, carried out by Coutinho, Gronowicz, Möller, and their colleagues. A nonmitogenic, T-dependent hapten (NNP) was coupled to a highly potent and specific T-independent antigen and B-cell mitogen (LPS). The resulting conjugate was cultured with spleen cells at differing concentrations for two days, and the subsequent development of PFCs specific for the hapten was assayed. PFCs specific for sheep red blood cells were also assayed, as a measure of nonspecific (polyclonal) B-cell activation. Optimal culture concentrations for the induction of specific, high-affinity anti-NNP antibody responses were in the range of 2.5 to 12.8 $\times$ 10^{-3} μg/ml. At these concentrations, no polyclonal activation could be detected; the polyclonal response was induced beginning at about 0.1 μg/ml with a plateau at about 10 μg/ml. This is precisely the range previously observed for optimal polyclonal stimulation by LPS alone, showing that the PBA activities of LPS are not altered by conjugating it with hapten. At these higher concentrations of conjugate, the high-affinity antibody response to NNP is actually inhibited, although the low- and intermediate-affinity responses increase. The authors interpreted their results in the following way. At low concentrations of conjugate, the NNP binds preferentially and tightly to those B cells

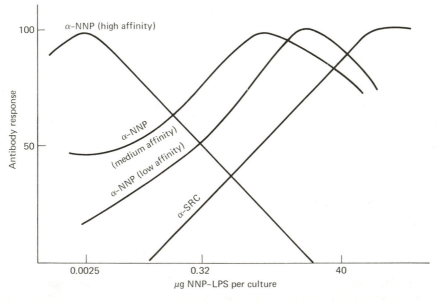

Figure 12-11 Dependence of antibody affinity and specificity on immunizing dose of hapten–mitogen complex. [From A. Coutinho et al., Mechanism of thymus[independent immunocyte triggering. *J. Exp. Med.* *139*, 74 (1974). Copyright by the Rockefeller University Press and the author (A. Coutinho), 1974.]

with high-affinity receptors for NNP. This association in effect concentrates LPS at these B-cell surfaces, and allows delivery of a mitogenic signal that activates the cell. This signal presumably replaces the T-cell help that would ordinarily be required to activate NNP-specific (T-dependent) B cells. As the concentration of conjugate is increased further, it binds to NNP-specific cells of intermediate and low affinity, leading to their activation as well. As the concentration of conjugate is increased still further, a level of LPS concentration in solution is reached that facilitates general, polyclonal B-cell activation. However, as the concentration of LPS in solution is increased through this higher range, the total concentration of LPS at the surface of NNP-specific cells is now supraoptimal, and the cells become immunologically paralyzed. This paralyzing effect of high B-cell mitogen concentrations is well established.

B-cell mitogens generally can serve both as specific antigens at low concentrations and as PBA at higher concentrations. The nature of the surface receptor for mitogenic activity is unknown. The fact that as PBA they can stimulate production of antibody to T-dependent antigens led Coutinho et al. to postulate that the help contributed by T cells may consist of nothing more than a mitogenic signal. In fact, Coutinho et al. suggest that the only role of the surface Ig receptor on B cells is to focus the T-helper mitogenic factor (or the mitogenic portions of the T-independent antigen) onto the surface of the B cell. In either case, it is actually a single, nonspecific mitogenic signal that triggers the B cell. The only purpose of the surface Ig receptor, in their view, is to allow selection of the appropriate B-cell clones; the receptor itself would play no role in cellular activation. Although various difficulties inherent in this model have been pointed out (particularly the direct activation of B cells by anti-Ig antibody) it remains one of the more coherent and attractive models for B-cell activation.

Another view of B-cell activation is the cross-linking hypothesis. According to this view, the key feature in B-cell activation is the cross-linking of B-cell receptors (sIg) by antigen. Thymus-independent antigens, as we have already noted, are usually characterized by a polymeric, repeating unit structure, which could serve to cross-link B-cell receptors. Cross-linking of sIg would also occur when B cells are treated with anti-Ig antibodies. According to this model, what the T cell and macrophage may contribute are assembly and presentation of antigen in some closely spaced, repeating pattern on a presenting cell surface, capable of cross-linking B-cell receptors. (Thymus-independent B-cell responses are also usually macrophage independent.) What PBA would do is to cross-link surface receptors for mitogen, which would also lead to B-cell activation. Just how cross-linking would lead to B-cell activation is unclear, but it has been postulated that redistribution of surface receptors (either for antigen or for mitogen) through patching and capping may provide an activating signal.

At present it is not possible to distinguish between these two models for B-cell activation. There is good evidence in support of both. The question of activation signals for B cells needing T-cell help is addressed more fully in Chapter 13.

Bibliography

General

Boyse, E., and J. Abbott, Surface reorganization as an initial inductive event in the differentiation of prothymocytes to thymocytes. *Fed. Proc. 34,* 24 (1975).

Cantor, H., and I. Weissman, Development and function of subpopulations of thymocytes and T lymphocytes. *Progress in Allergy 20,* 1 (1976).

Crone, M., C. Koch, and M. Simonsen, The elusive T Cell receptor. *Transplant. Rev. 10,* 36 (1972).

Haskins, K., J. Kappler, and P. Marrack, The MHC-restricted antigen receptor on T cells. *Annual Review of Immunology 2,* 51 (1984).

Kindred, B., Nude mice in immunology. *Progress in Allergy 26,* 137–238 (1979).

Klinman, N., D. Wylie, and J. Teale, B Cell development. *Immunol. Today 2,* 12 (1981).

Meuer, S. et al., The human T cell receptor. *Annual Review of Immunology 2,* 13 (1984).

Mosier, D. E., and B. Subbarao, Thymus-independent antigens: Complexity of B lymphocyte activation revealed. *Immunol. Today 3,* 217 (1982).

Scher, I., B lymphocyte development and heterogeneity. Analysis with the immune defective CBA/N mouse strain. In E. Gershwin and B. Merchant, eds., *Immune Defects in Laboratory Animals,* Plenum Press, New York, 1981, p. 163.

Whitlock, C., K. Denis, D. Robertson, and O. Witte, In vitro analysis of murine B cell development. *Annual Review Immunol. 3,* 213 (1985).

Research

Ada, G. L., and P. Byrt, Specific inactivation of antigen-reactive cells with ^{125}I-labeled antigen. *Nature 222,* 1291 (1969).

Arden, B. et al., Diversity and structure of genes of the alpha family of the mouse T cell antigen receptor. *Nature 316,* 783 (1985).

Barth, Richard K. et al., The marine T cell receptor uses a limited repertoire of expressed V_β gene segments. *Nature 316,* 517 (1985).

Dennert, G., and R. Hyman, Functional Thy-1 + cells in cultures of spleen cells from nu/nu mice. *Eur. J. Immunol. 10,* 583 (1980).

Eerola, E. et al., Immune capacity of the chicken bursectomized at 60 hours of incubation: Mitogen-induced cell proliferation and immunoglobulin secretion. *J. Immunol. 131,* 120 (1983).

Hardy, R. R. et al., Murine B cell differentiation lineages. *J. Exp. Med. 159,* 1169 (1984).

Haskins, K. et al., The MHC-restricted antigen receptor on T cells. I. Isolation with a monoclonal antibody. *J. Exp. Med. 157,* 1149 (1983).

Hedrick, S. et al., Rearrangement and transcription of a T cell receptor β chain gene in different T cell subsets. *PNAS, 82,* 531 (1985).

Ikehara, S. et al., Functional T Cells in athymic nude mice. *Proc. Natl. Acad. Sci. USA 81,* 886 (1984).

Kaye, J., et al., Both a monoclonal antibody and antisera specific for determinants unique to cloned T helper cells can substitute for antigen and APC in the activation of T cells. *J. Exp. Med. 158,* 836 (1983).

Levitt, D., and M. Cooper, Mouse pre-B cells synthesize and secrete μ heavy chain but not light chains. *Cell 19,* 617 (1980).

Lindsten, T., and B. Andersson, Ontogeny of B cells in CBA/N mice. Evidence for a stage of responsiveness to thymus-independent antigens during development. *J. Exp. Med. 150,* 1285–1292 (1979).

Marrack, P., R. Shimonkevitz, C. Hannum, K. Haskins, and J. Kappler, The major histocompatibility complex-restricted antigen receptor on T cells. IV. An antiidiotypic antibody predicts both antigen and I-specificity. *J. Exp. Med. 158,* 1635 (1983).

Raff, M. C., M. Sternberg, and R. B. Taylor, Immunoglobulin determinants on the surface of mouse lymphoid cells. *Nature 225,* 553 (1970).

Scollay, R., E. Butcher, and I. Weissman, Thymus cell migration. Quantitative aspects of cellular traffic from the thymus to the periphery in mice. *Eur. J. Immunol. 10,* 210 (1980).

Scollay, R., W.-F. Chen, and K. Shortman, The functional capabilities of cells leaving the thymus. *J. Immunol. 132,* 25 (1984).

Stutman, O., Two main features of T-cell development: Thymus traffic and postthymic maturation. *Contemp. Topics Immunobiol. 7,* 1–46 (1977).

Weissman, I. L., Thymus cell migration. *J. Exp. Med. 126,* 291 (1967).

CHAPTER 13

The Humoral Immune Response

In Chapter 11 we examined the evidence indicating that the response of B cells to most antigens requires T-cell help. In order to discuss the nature and possible loci of action of this helper function, we first need to have some impression of what happens to a B cell after it is triggered by an antigen and T-cell help. Once this is clear, we will explore in more detail the nature of the interaction of T cells with B cells and with other cells of the immune system in the induction, development, and regulation of antibody production.

318

Maturation of the B-Cell Response

Kinetics of Antibody Production

Typical profiles for primary and secondary antibody responses are shown in Figure 13-1. In the primary response, several days often elapse after administration of antigen before specific antibodies appear in the serum, or before specific PFC can be detected in lymphoid tissue. This represents the period necessary to bring the virgin, immunocompetent, $\mu^+\delta^+$ B cell from the resting state to the fully active, antibody synthesizing and secreting state (plasma cell). The cells must switch from production of mRNA for membrane-bound Ig to secreted Ig (Chapter 5); ribosomes must be assembled; the cell's energy-producing apparatus must be geared up; and DNA synthesis and mitosis must be initiated. Proliferation is a critical aspect of the maturation phase of the primary response. If either DNA synthesis or mitosis is inhibited, the quantity of both PFCs and antibody subsequently produced is drastically reduced. This is related to the important process of clonal expansion—those B cells that receive an appropriate antigenic signal begin to divide and produce genetically identical daughter cells, thus expanding the total number of cells responding.

Within 24 hours of contact with an appropriate form of antigen, the cells become blastoid, begin to synthesize DNA, and then enter mitosis. The average cell cycle time for activated B lymphocytes is about 12 to 15 hours, but it is unknown how many rounds of cell division ensue for a given activated cell. Since a substantial portion of the rise in antibody production after B-cell activation must be due to this clonal expansion, it is not surprising that inhibition of proliferation affects the total amount of antibody produced. However, such inhibition also prevents the differentiation of the initially triggered B cell into a fully functional plasma cell; in some step not fully understood, one or more rounds of cell division are required for this maturational event to occur. Successive generations of B-cell progeny acquire increasing ability to synthesize and secrete antibody until the fully mature and functional plasma cell stage is reached.

Levels of specific antibodies in the blood, and of PFCs in lymph tissue, usually reach a peak in the primary reaction in about five to seven days. Depending on the degree to which antigen is retained in the lymph organs, the response may fall off sharply thereafter, or it may persist for several weeks or months. The fall in serum antibody occurs as the antigen is cleared from the system, either by direct degradation and excretion, or as the result of neutralization by antibody and clearance through the reticuloendothelial system.

Two types of cells may be produced as the result of primary B-cell stimulation: the antibody-forming cell (AFC or plasma cell), which is a terminal cell type (i.e., it does not survive beyond the antibody production and secretion stage), and the memory B cell, which enters the circulating lymphocyte pool and is relatively long lived. The memory B cell, which is generated only in a T-dependent primary response, serves as the reacting cell in secondary antibody responses. It is similar

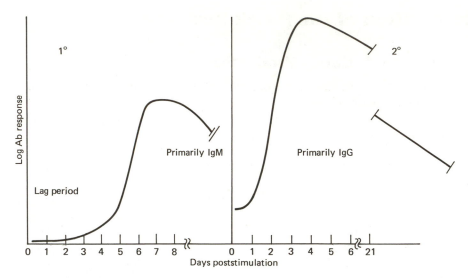

Figure 13-1 Kinetics of development of primary and secondary antibody responses.

in size and general features to the virgin B cell. However, it has lost the δ and μ surface isotypes, and acquired either surface γ or α. The antibody response is more rapid and of greater magnitude when memory cells are restimulated with antigen. This reflects the shorter time required to bring memory cells to their maximum synthetic/secretory capacity, compared to virgin B cells, and the fact that the frequency of cells responding to antigen in the secondary reaction has been greatly increased as a result of selective clonal expansion in the primary reaction.

Isotype Switching during Maturation of the Antibody Response

In the early stages of a primary humoral response, only antibodies of the IgM class are detectable either in serum or in an *in vitro* PFC generating system. However, as the primary response (to T-dependent antigens-) progresses, IgG or IgA antibodies can be detected as well, and toward the end of the response are usually the predominant antibody class. In the secondary response, relatively little IgM is produced; IgG or IgA antibodies predominate from the beginning. The IgM produced in secondary responses most likely represents *de novo* stimulation of virgin B cells reactive to the antigen used, since IgM-producing memory cells are probably not generated in primary responses. The genetic basis for isotype switching was discussed in detail in Chapter 5.

Two types of experiments have shed light on the cellular basis of μ → γ switching during the course of maturation of the B-cell response. The first, carried out by Nossal and his colleagues in Australia in the 1960s, involves culturing single activated B cells in individual microdroplets and analyzing the classes of antibody secreted into the droplet. Although the vast majority of droplets contained only IgM or IgG, 1 to 2 percent contained both IgM and IgG. This proves that at least some normal activated B cells are able to produce two Ig classes simultaneously, probably through concomitant translation of previously transcribed μ mRNA, and newly transcribed α mRNA.

A subsequent study by Andersson, Coutinho, and Melchers provided additional evidence for a $\mu \rightarrow \gamma$ switch within a single clone. They used the polyclonal B-cell activator LPS to trigger differentiation of B lymphocytes and then carried out cultures of individual B cells. They observed that about 30 to 40 percent of all B cells were activated to IgM production by LPS, but that only about 3 to 4 percent of these matured to IgG production. They were able to conclude from their studies that every IgG-secreting clone had derived from an IgM-secreting precursor.

These two studies, together with various indirect observations, have led to the generally accepted conclusion that the switch from μ to γ to α is a normal event in the life of most B-cell clones. So far, isotype switching during a specific antigen response has only been observed in T-cell-facilitated reactions, leading to speculation that helper T cells play some critical role in triggering the switch. Those clones that do not make the switch from μ or γ or α apparently do not generate memory cells, so it is tempting to speculate that isotype switching and generation of memory, both of which are also T cell dependent, are functionally connected events.

Affinity Maturation

In addition to a change in antibody class during maturation of the humoral immune response, there is also a change (increase) in the average affinity of the antibodies produced as the response progresses. However, whereas all evidence points to the maturation-related change in isotype occurring within individual cells, the change in antibody affinity occurs only at the population level and represents a change in the overall clonal makeup of the cells actually producing and secreting the antibody.

Eisen was among the first to show that the population of antibodies produced in response to even a simple antigen is heterogeneous with respect to affinity. He added increasing amounts of antigen to a sample of antiserum and collected the precipitate at each step. He dissociated the antigen–antibody complex in each sample, recovered the antibody, and measured its affinity by equilibrium dialysis (Chapter 6). He found that antibodies precipitated at low antigen concentration had high affinity for antigen, whereas antibody precipitated at the highest antigen concentration was of low affinity. The affinities measured in a single sample of antiserum in some cases differed by a factor of 10^4.

If one examines in detail the average affinity of antibodies produced in response to a given antigen, it can be seen that changes in affinity are both time and dose dependent. Highest affinity antibody is produced when animals are immunized with low doses of antigen. In all cases, the average affinity of antibody produced increases as a function of time after immunization. Interestingly, only IgG shows affinity maturation; little change of affinity with time is seen during primary, mainly IgM, reactions.

These observations formed the basis for the antigen selection hypothesis proposed by Siskind and Benacerraf in 1969. They suggested that at low concentrations of antigen, only B cells bearing high-affinity receptors will be stimulated; these cells will expand clonally and produce high-affinity antibodies. As the response matures, antigen will be cleared from the system, lowering its effective concentration. As a result, only clones of very high affinity will continue to be stimulated and expanded toward the end of the response. On the other hand, with a high initial dose of antigen (or continuous administration of even moderate doses of antigen), medium- to low-affinity clones will continue to be stimulated further into the response, lowering the average affinity of circulating antibody at any given point in time.

The affinity maturation effect can also be studied at the plaque-forming cell level (Figure 13-2). In the PFC assay, individual plasma cells secrete antibody into their immediate vicinity, which is occupied by antigen-coated red blood cells and free complement. The antibodies attach to the RBC, bind complement, and lyse the red cells, forming clear areas or plaques. If free antigen is also added to this system, it will compete with RBC-bound antigen for antibody secreted by the PFCs. According to the antigen selection theory, one would predict that plaques formed by secretion of high-affinity antibody would be inhibited by low concentrations of free antigen, whereas low-affinity plaques would require high concentrations of free antigen to be inhibited.

This is what is seen in Figure 13-2. The hapten DNP, coupled to an appropriate carrier, was used to immunize mice. At various times after immunization, spleens were removed and the cells tested in a plaque assay using DNP-coated SRBC as target cells. The affinity of secreted anti-DNP antibody was estimated from the concentration of free DNP (actually, DNP coupled to lysine) required to inhibit lysis of DNP-coated red cells. Both IgG- and IgM-producing PFCs were analyzed. It was found that in the primary response, very little change in average affinity of PFCs was noted, the only change being in the small number of IgG-producing PFC, from animals immunized with low levels of antigen. In the secondary response, where IgM PFCs were too infrequent to be meaningfully analyzed, a dramatic, time-dependent increase in the average affinity of IgG-secreting PFCs was observed. These studies thus parallel exactly the observations made concerning whole serum antibody.

The fact that affinity maturation does not affect the IgM response is puzzling. It may mean that the V regions associated with IgM antibody represent a restricted, fixed number of V-region genes, perhaps those associated with the germ-line repertoire. IgG antibodies, on the other hand, may be predominantly associated with a pool of V-region genes that can be mutated somatically during the course of clonal expansion. Alternatively, V-region somatic mutation processes may only be turned on in cells that have undergone isotype switching from μ to γ or α.

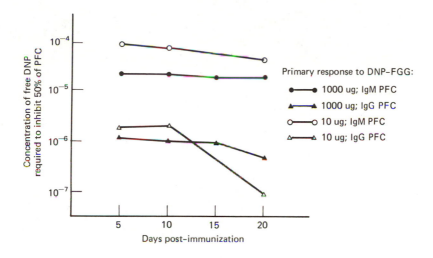

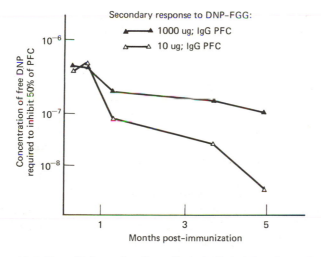

Figure 13-2 The affinity maturation effect studied at the plaque-forming cell level. [Adapted from R. Huchet and M. Feldmann, Studies on antibody affinity in mice. *Eur. J. Immunol.* **3**, 49 (1973).]

Cooperation of T Cells and B Cells in the Humoral Response

Having thoroughly documented in Chapter 11 the existence of separate T and B lymphocyte populations, and the requirement for their collaboration in most humoral immune responses, we are now ready to examine the nature of this collaboration and its consequences.

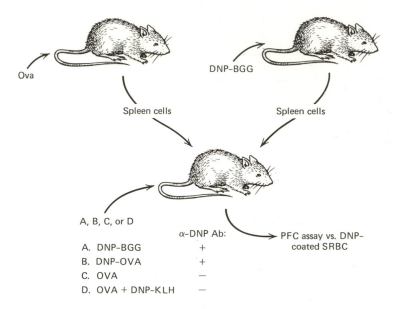

Ova

DNP–BGG

Spleen cells

Spleen cells

A, B, C, or D

α–DNP Ab:

A. DNP–BGG   +   PFC assay vs. DNP–
B. DNP–OVA   +   coated SRBC
C. OVA   –
D. OVA + DNP–KLH   –

Figure 13-3 The Mitchison-Rajewsky experiment showing that hapten and carrier (used to challenge a passively primed animal) must be physically coupled.

Antigen-specific T—B Collaboration

About 1969, after it had become clear that T and B cells did, in fact, collaborate in Ab production, it became important to define a mechanism by which they could do so. Mitchison and Rajewsky (Figure 13-3) carried out a key early experiment. This experiment showed that recognition of the hapten–carrier complex is a "linked recognition" phenomenon. That is, the induction of an antibody response from a mixture of carrier-primed T and hapten-primed B cells is much more efficient when the carrier and hapten are physically linked. Injection of a mixture of un-linked carrier and hapten gives virtually no response. (However, under special conditions *in vitro,* a response may be induced by unlinked carrier and hapten; see section later on T-cell replacing factor.)

This was a crucial observation because it established an important restriction on any explanation of T-cell–B-cell collaboration. Mitchison and Rajewsky proposed that the carrier–hapten complex actually forms a bridge linking T cells and B cells. They suggested that B cells could only be triggered by antigens if they were physically coupled to T cells. At the time, this model satisfied all of the known data and for at least a year or two was generally accepted. On the other hand, it was pointed out by a number of people that the model suffered from at least one theoretical drawback. Because the fraction of T cells or B cells recognizing a carrier–hapten complex should be very small (possibly 10^{-5} in each case), then the probability of having a T cell and B cell recognizing the carrier–hapten complex actually in physical proximity to one another at any given time is also quite small. This requirement for a T cell and B cell to be in physical proximity to one another could provide an extremely rate-limiting step in the overall response.

Another possible explanation of the results in Figure 13-3 is that the complex does in fact link the T and B cell but that the T cell then makes a separate non-specific signal that it transmits to activate the B cell. In other words, binding a B cell to a T-cell-bound antigen would be insufficient to trigger the B cell; it also needs to receive a "second signal" from the T cell, which is likely to be relatively non-specific. It would have to be a part of such a model that the nonspecific signal was only effective over a very short distance; otherwise, it would activate many other types of B cells in its immediate vicinity.

Another possibility consistent with the observation that the carrier and hapten must be covalently linked is that a T cell may recognize, bind, and somehow process the carrier–hapten complex and then release it. The complex plus information contributed by the T cell could then diffuse into the surrounding area and "find" an appropriate B cell. This would get around the requirement for T cells and B cells to be in precisely the same place at the same time, in order to be physically linked by the complex. It effectively increases the "sphere of influence" of a helper T cell and assures that only B cells specific for the processed antigen are activated.

The question then became how to test these various models for T–B collaboration. Two of these models predict that T cells and B cells must be physically bridged by a hapten–carrier complex as a prerequisite for B-cell activation. The third model predicts that T cells and B cells can collaborate at a distance. Mark Feldmann and Tony Basten in 1971 began to design experiments to distinguish between these two possibilities. The unique feature introduced by their system was the possibility of physical separation of T- and B-cell populations across a cell-impermeable (1-μm pore size) membrane (Figure 13-4).

In their initial experiments, Feldmann and Basten cultured carrier-primed T

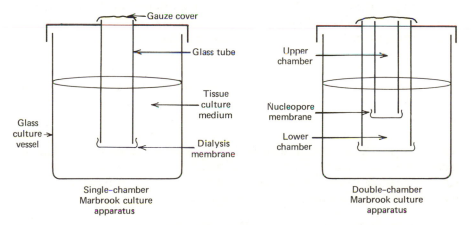

Figure 13-4 Marbrook culture chambers used for generating a humoral immune response *in vitro.*

Table 13-1 Collaboration of T and B Cells Across a
Cell-impermeable Membrane

Upper chamber	Lower chamber	Antigen	PFC/10^6 spleen cells versus	
			DNP–SRBC	**DRBC**
None	$T_{KLH} + B_{DNP-KLH}$	DNP–KLH	960	14
None	$B_{DNP-KLH}$	DNP–KLH	72	26
T_{KLH}	$B_{DNP-KLH}$	DNP–KLH	1011	38
T_{KLH}	$B_{DNP-KLH}$	None	94	16

Compiled from data presented in M. Feldmann and A. Basten, Cell interactions in the immune response *in vitro. J. Exp. Med. 136,* 49 (1972).

cells and hapten-primed B cells either together in one of the chambers, or separately on opposite sides of the membrane. The antigen to be tested was present in both chambers. Typical data for this type of experiment are shown in Table 13-1. The antihapten antibody response obtained with T and B cells separated by a cell-impermeable membrane was, in most cases, as good as the response obtained with the T and B cells mixed together. The data in Table 13-1 show that the signal sent across the membrane by carrier-primed T cells is specific; B cells with potential reactivity toward an unrelated antigen (donkey red cells in this case) were not activated. In other experiments not shown here, it was also found that the response was the same whether or not T cells were removed from the primed B-cell population, demonstrating that the primed T-helper cells were acting directly on B cells, and not activating T cells. Finally, it was found that if the 1-μm pore membrane was replaced with a dialysis membrane, collaboration between T and B cells did not occur. Because dialysis membranes will only pass molecules with a molecular weight less than about 10,000 it was concluded that the soluble T-cell factor must be greater than that in size. In subsequent experiments, the factor was found to have both hapten and carrier determinants associated with it.

Although these experiments show that helper T cells and B cells *can* interact at a distance, they do not rule out the possibility that these cells may interact directly *in vivo*. Given the rather low frequencies of both T and B cells specific for a particular antigen, the probability of an appropriate T and B cell being in the same place at the same time may seem *a priori* prohibitively low. On the other hand, a factor secreted by a T cell into the total circulatory volume of even a small animal represents an enormous dilution. Most immune reactions, however, take place in highly compartmentalized lymph tissue, and it may be that such factors need only be effective within a relatively small radius from the T cell producing them.

Antigen-nonspecific T–B Collaboration

The experiments of Feldmann and Basten demonstrated that, at least under certain experimental conditions, T cells can help B cells mature to the antibody-secreting stage without being in physical contact with them. In their system, the T-cell help provided appeared to be an antigen-specific soluble factor. Since those pioneering experiments, a few labs have gone on to try to characterize antigen-specific factors and to deduce their mode of action. We discuss these later in this chapter. But perhaps somewhat more attention has been devoted to a secondary category of factors that also help B cells at a distance but that do so in an antigen-*non*specific manner. Two of the earliest examples of this were T-cell replacing factor (TRF), and allogeneic effect factor (AEF).

T-Cell Replacing Factor

T-cell replacing factor (TRF) was defined most clearly in experiments carried out by Schimpl and Wecker in 1977. Like Feldmann and Basten, Schimpl and Wecker were looking at the response of *in vivo*-primed spleen cells to the immunizing hapten–carrier complex *in vitro*. They were examining the ability of free hapten and free carrier to *block* the response of primed cells to the linked hapten–carrier complex. Although free hapten very efficiently inhibited the response to hapten–carrier, presumably by blocking antigen-specific receptors on the surface of potentially responsive B cells, free carrier had no corresponding inhibitory effect on T cells, even at very high concentrations (Figure 13-5). It seemed quite

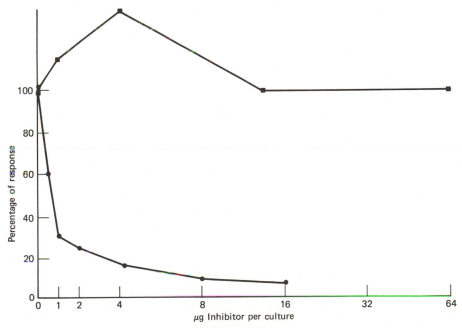

Figure 13-5 Inhibition of the antibody response to DNP–KLH by free hapten and free carrier. Spleen cells from mice primed and boosted once with DNP–KLH were cultured in the presence of 0.01 μg DNP–KLH and increasing amounts of either DNP-gly-gly (●——●) or KLH (■——■). Anti-DNP IgG PFC were tested on day 5 of culture. Results are expressed as percentage of the response in the absence of either inhibitor.

reasonable to expect that free carrier would tie up carrier-primed helper T cells, preventing their "seeing" and effectively processing the hapten–carrier complex for presentation to B cells. Yet this seemed not to happen.

One possible explanation of these results is that, under appropriate experimental conditions, primed T and B cells may not need to see hapten and carrier determinants on the same molecule in order to mount an antihapten response. This point was tested in the following way. Spleen cells from DNP–KLH-primed mice were cultured *in vitro* in the presence of DNP on a heterologous carrier (either BGG or OVA), plus free homologous carrier (KLH). The results of three such experiments are shown in Table 13-2. A response to DNP can clearly be induced when DNP is presented on a heterologous carrier, *provided that* the homologous carrier is also present in the system. It has subsequently been shown that both primed and unprimed T-helper cells—on stimulation by antigen—produce soluble factors, called T-cell-replacing factors (TRF), that are not antigen specific yet that are required by B cells in order to mature to antibody-producing cells (plasma cells). TRF is almost certainly a complex of factors needed by B cells to mature to plasma cells. We discuss some of these factors more fully on page 333.

Allogeneic Effect Factor

Another example of nonspecific activation of B cells by T cells was reported by Katz and Benacerraf and their co-workers in 1971. They made the interesting observation that antigen-primed animals undergoing a graft-versus-host (GVH) reaction spontaneously produce a secondary response to the priming antigen *in the absence of secondary stimulation by the antigen.* GVH rections, described in detail in Chapter 14, involve the attack of lymphocytes from one animal (the graft) on the cells and tissues of a second animal into which they are transfused (the host). T cells in the donor graft recognize the host tissues as foreign and attack the host in what is, in effect, a transplant rejection reaction. If donor T cells are recovered from the host after several days, they can be shown to be fully activated and highly cytotoxic to host-strain cells.

Data from a typical experiment showing the GVH effect is presented in Table 13-3. These *in vivo* experiments were all concerned with the secondary antibody response to a defined hapten. There are three particularly striking features of these results. First, the transfer of allogeneic cells into the host greatly enhances the secondary antibody response to a priming hapten coupled to the priming carrier. Second, allogeneic cells facilitate a secondary response to the same hapten coupled to a heterologous carrier. (It will be remembered from Chapter 11 that ordinarily there is virtually no secondary response to hapten coupled to a heterologous carrier. This presumably reflects the lack of helper T cells specific for the new carrier.) Finally, as mentioned earlier, it was found that simply the transfer of allogeneic cells alone into a hapten-primed animal would result in antibody production in the *absence* of a secondary challenge with a hapten–carrier complex.

These phenomena, collectively and commonly referred to as the *allogeneic effect,* were shown to be due to a specific attack of graft cells on host tissues. A

Table 13-2 Stimulation of the Anamnestic Antihapten IgG Response by Simultaneous Addition of a Heterologous Carrier-Hapten Conjugate and Homologous Carrier

	Exp. I	Exp. II	Exp. III
No addition	189	106	292
0.1 μg DNP–KLH	11,533	6,684	27,798
0.1 μg DNP–BGG	528	250	674
1 μg KLH	747	433	901
0.1 μg DNP–BGG + 1 μg KLH	6,855	5,764	11,400
0.1 μg DNP–OVA	ND	ND	869
0.1 μg DNP–OVA + 1 μg KLH	ND	ND	6,889

Reprinted from Th. Hünig, A. Schimpl, and E. Wecker, Mechanism of T-cell help in the immune response to soluble protein antigens. I. Evidence for in situ generation and action of T-cell-replacing factor during the anamnestic response to dinitrophenyl keyhole limpet hemocyanin in vitro. *J. Exp. Med. 145*, 1216–1227 (1977) by copyright permission of the Rockefeller University Press.

Spleen cells from DNP–KLH-primed and boosted mice were cultivated in the presence of a heterologous DNP-protein conjugate with or without simultaneous addition of the homologous carrier KLH. Results are given as anti-DNP IgG-PFC/10^6 recovered cells tested on day 5 of culture.

ND, not done.

Table 13-3 The Allogeneic Effect

Experiment	Animal primed with	Animal challenged with	Cells transferred into primed animal	Anti-DNP response (μg/ml serum)
1	DNP–OVA	—	—	15
	DNP–OVA	—	Allogeneic lymphocytes	180
	DNP–OVA	DNP–OVA	Allogeneic lymphocytes	605
2	DNP–OVA	—	—	20
	DNP–OVA	—	Allogeneic lymphocytes	200
	DNP–OVA	DNP–BGG	Allogeneic lymphocytes	530

Based on data discussed in D. Katz and B. Benacerraf, The regulatory influence of activated T cells on B cell responses to antigen. *Adv. Immunol. 15*, 1 (1972).

molecular basis for this cellular effect was subsequently postulated by Katz and his colleagues. They found (as did many others) that if two populations of allogeneic cells are cultured together *in vitro,* such that one population (the "graft") was specifically recognizing the other population (the "host") as foreign, then the "graft" T cells produce and secrete a variety of soluble factors into the medium that can exert a nonspecific activating effect on primed B cells, thus leading to secondary antibody responses *in vitro.* One of these factors, called allogeneic effect factor or AEF, is a protein of molecular weight 30,000 to 40,000 that can facilitate either primary or secondary reactions, under appropriate conditions, to a wide range of antigens. Many other factors, or lymphokines, are produced at the same time.

How does all of this fit together, and what does it tell us about T–B collaboration in the real world?

The Mitchison-Rajewsky experiment tells us that *in vivo,* T cells and B cells respond best if each interacting T and B cell pair are physically proximal, either joined directly by an antigen bridge or perhaps clustered about on the same antigen-presenting macrophage. Most immunologists would probably agree that this is, in fact, what does happen *in vivo.* But that doesn't tell us anything at all about *how* the physically linked T cells and B cells interact. Both the TRF and AEF experiments suggest that antigen-activated T cells elaborate soluble factors that can promote B-cell differentiation. B cells do not *necessarily* have to be in contact with T cells to utilize these factors.

This is precisely the view most commonly held at present. T cells bind to antigen via one determinant on a molecule, and B cells bind to the same antigen molecule via a different determinant. The T cell then secretes a variety of factors needed by the B cell to complete its differentiation.

But before examining in detail the nature of these factors and exactly how B cells use them, we must first describe one of the most important features of T-cell–B-cell-macrophage interactions: the phenomenon of MHC restriction.

MHC Restriction of Cell Interactions in the Humoral Immune Response

Shortly after the notion of collaboration between T and B lymphocytes in the production of antibody had been established, cellular immunologists began to explore various parameters affecting this interaction. A number of laboratories noted that thymus-derived cells from one strain of animal did not seem to function well when transferred into other strains. One of the first studies to address this question in a systematic way was that of Kindred and Shreffler in 1972. Using nude mice as an immunologically neutral host, they showed that only T and B cells that were identical at H-2 could cooperate in a humoral immune response. This was proved very nicely by using congenic strains differing only in H-2. Use of the nude mouse host eliminated problems of host rejection of one or the other populations of collaborating cells, a problem that had made interpretation of previous experiments of this type difficult.

Another early system in which restrictions on T–B collaboration were studied was that of Katz and Benacerraf. They too found that only MHC-identical T and B cells would cooperate to mount an antibody response. A typical experiment illustrating this effect is shown in Figure 13-6, and the results are summarized in Table 13-4. Normal or carrier-primed (helper) spleen cells from one of the parents of an F_1 hybrid mouse were injected into an untreated F_1 recipient. Following this transfer, the recipients were irradiated with 600 R. Previous experience had shown that unstimulated T cells are severely depleted by this treatment, whereas already primed T cells, and host B cells and macrophages, are only marginally affected. The irradiation thus prevents two potential problems: development of a primary response by unprimed cells transferred with the carrier-primed T cells, when the system is subsequently challenged with antigen, and prevention of a graft-versus-host (GVH) reaction by unprimed T cells from parent 1 recognizing parent 2 antigens present on the F_1, or on the passively transferred B cells. Such a GVH reaction (see Chapter 14) in itself would not pose a threat to the recipient but could result in the production of AEF by the donor T cells that could potentially activate B cells in a nonspecific manner. After the irradiation, the F_1 mice received an inocu-

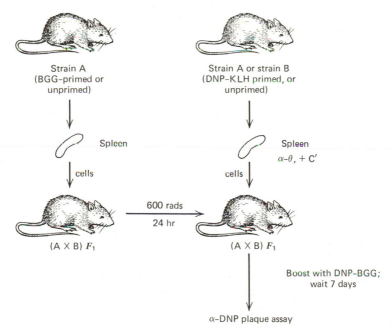

Figure 13-6 Protocol for experiment to test whether histoincompatible T and B cells can cooperate in an antibody response. The mouse on the lower right is the same as the one on the lower left after irradiation.

Table 13-4 Results of an Experiment of the
Type Shown in Figure 13-6

Group	Source of T_h-BGG	Source of B_{DNP}	α-DNP response (μg Ab/ml serum)
A	(Normal B10.A)	B10.A	100
B	B10.A	B10.A	600
C	(Normal A)	B10.A	175
D	A	B10.A	1500
E	(Normal B10)	B10.A	220
F	B10	B10.A	170
G	(Normal A.By)	B10.A	210
H	A.By	B10.A	185

Based on data presented in D. Katz et al., Cell interactions between histoincom-
patible T and B lymphocytes. *J. Exp. Med. 137* (1973), p. 1405. Recipient was an
(A × B10) F_1 hybrid mouse. H-2 haplotypes: B10.A, H-2^a; A, H-2^a; B10, H-2^b;
A.By, H-2^b.

lum of hapten-primed B cells from either the same or the opposite parent. The F_1
mice were then injected with the relevant hapten–carrier complex and tested for
antihapten antibody one week later.

Groups A and B in Table 13-4 demonstrate the effect of carrier priming on the
antihapten response when both hapten- and carrier-primed cells are syngeneic.
Groups C and D suggest that syngeneity at H-2 is sufficient, because a difference in
non-H-2 background between the cooperating cells does not interfere with their
ability to interact in the production of antibody. On the other hand, as is evident
from groups E to H in this experiment, dissimilarity at H-2 alone results in a total
inability of the T and B populations to interact.

A detailed analysis of this H-2 restriction effect, using intra-H-2 recombinant
strains, showed that the portions of the H-2 regions in which identify between
carrier and hapten-primed cells was crucial for their subsequent interaction, was in
the IA subregions. Other immune response systems (utilizing different strains and
antigens) showed a requirement for identity at either IA or IE. Other (non-I)
regions of H-2, in the absence of IA or IE identity, failed to support cell interaction.
It seemed logical to assume that genetic regulation of the interaction of two cells
must occur via cell surface structures. Therefore, the existence of I-region-coded
genes, called at the time CI (cellular interaction) genes, to code for such structures,
was inferred. We now know that these are, in fact, class II genes that code for the
α-β dimers, described in Chapter 9, that are present on B cells and macrophages.

The foregoing experiments demonstrated a requirement for class II identity
between T cells and B cells in mounting an antibody response. But these experiments did not take into account an important element of immune responsiveness—

the macrophage. In fact, as we will see in the following section, one of the principal sites of MHC restriction is between T cells and macrophages.

The Interaction of T Cells, B Cells, and Macrophages in the Production of Antibodies

The overall scheme for T–B–M interactions is shown in Figure 13-7. The first point of contact of antigen with the immune system is through macrophages, or perhaps dendritic cells (antigen-presenting cells, or APC). APC pick up antigen and display it on their surface membranes. If the antigen is large (cells; bacteria; macromolecular complexes) the APCs may first break it down into smaller fragments. This is called *antigen processing,* and probably involves the phagocytic/degradative apparatus of these scavenger cells (Chapter 17). The macrophages display the native or processed antigen on their surface membranes in the context of their class II antigens. We do not know what "in the context of" means; it simply defines the requirement

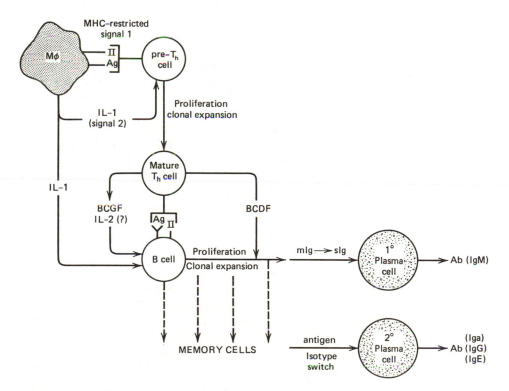

Figure 13-7 Cellular interactions in the production of antibody.

of T cells to react to both foreign ("nominal") antigen, and class II antigen simultaneously in order to be activated.

Macrophages produce an important soluble factor called interleukin 1, or IL-1. This lymphokine[1] is probably a collection of functionally related peptides. Recent gene sequencing studies in humans suggest that there are at least two IL-I molecules that are posttranslationally modified to produce active peptides of about 18,000. IL-1 appears to play an obligatory role in the activation of previously unstimulated T helper cells. Thus macrophages can provide two crucial signals for T_h cell induction: a processed antigenic signal, presented in the context of a self class II molecule, and a soluble growth and/or differentiation promoting factor (IL-1). Current evidence suggests that previously activated, memory T_h cells may not need Il-1, or certainly not as much of it, in order to be reactivated by processed antigen. For example, memory T cells can be reactivated by antigen (in an appropriate form) presented on the surface of B cells, which have class II molecules but appear not to secrete IL-1. There is also some evidence that differentiating B cells themselves utilize IL-1 provided by macrophages.

Macrophages present the nominal antigen to pre-T_h cells. Pre-T_h cells recognize the complex of nominal antigen, using the T-cell surface receptor described in the last chapter. The class II antigen on the macrophage is normally of the same H-2 haplotype as the T cell. This is the first point where we see MHC restriction. The complex of nominal antigen and self class II antigen acts as "signal 1," partially activating the T helper cell. "Signal 2," needed to complete the activation of the T_h cell, is IL-1. It may be that one result of signal 1 is the subsequent display, on the pre-T_h, of a receptor for IL-1. One would not want pre-T_h that had *not* been activated by antigen to respond to IL-1 released in the course of neighboring reactions to other antigens.

Once pre-T_h have been acted on by both signal 1 and signal 2, they synthesize DNA, divide, and clonally expand into antigen-specific, fully mature T helper cells. They are now ready to interact with B cells.

B cells of course have antigen-specific receptors on their surfaces in the form of the immunoglobulin they are prepared to synthesize and secrete. Thus they are able, in a very specific way, to pick up antigen from the environment and display it on their surface. B cells also display surface class II antigens, and again nominal antigen is presented to the outside world "in the context of" class II antigens.

B cells with nominal antigen displayed on their surface are prepared to receive T-cell help. In fact, we know that the binding of antigen to the B cell is itself a partially activating signal, a "signal 1," that prepares the B cell to be responsive to factors that will soon be provided by the T helper cell. This help can be provided by T_h cells that were previously activated and clonally expanded in response to some

[1]Because IL-1 is produced by macrophages and monocytes, some investigators refer to it as a "monokine." However, cells such as keritinocytes and synovial cells also produce IL-1, and IL-1 has been implicated in other functions such as induction of fever, trace metal clearance in the liver and plasma, and various aspects of the inflammatory sequence. Thus, both lymphokine and monokine may be rather parochial terms for IL-1.

portion of the same nominal antigen (obviously not the same as the B cell recognizes and binds to) in the context of the class II antigen displayed by the B cell. This is thus the second locus of MHC restriction: The B cell class II antigen must be the same as the macrophage class II antigen, and both must be perceived as "self" by the T helper cell.

After the T_h cell binds to the B cell it is able to deliver T-cell help. This takes the form of at least two lymphokines and quite probably more. The first lymphokine ("signal 2," if you will) is B-cell growth factor (BCGF). BCGF causes B cells that have been activated by antigen to start proliferating and clonally expanding. It is possible that another T-cell lymphokine, interleukin 2 (IL-2), also promotes B cell proliferation. In order to differentiate further into antibody-producing plasma cells, the B cells must receive a qualitatively different T helper cell factor, BCDF (B-cell differentiation factor). This factor triggers a switch diverting the cell from processing membrane forms of immunoglobulin transcripts to producing the secreted form of IgM.

These and perhaps other soluble factors can be utilized by appropriately activated B cells in the absence of T cells per se. B cells are most easily activated by antigens that can cross-link the B cell receptor Ig; this can be mimicked in some instances by anti-Ig antibody.

Tolerance

Immunological tolerance can be defined as the inability of an animal to mount an immune response against a specific antigen. It should be distinguished from immunosuppression, in which entire segments of the immune system may be rendered dysfunctional, leading to a more generalized, non-antigen-specific unresponsiveness. Antigen-specific tolerance may be induced in both T cells and B cells. In a sense, tolerance is a form of immunological memory in that it represents an altered state of immune responsiveness resulting from previous exposure to a particular antigen.

A prime example of tolerance is tolerance of self. It is absolutely essential that the immune system not react against self-components; it is also essential that the immune system not become tolerant of foreign antigen. In the case of self-tolerance, we guess that as T cells (particularly CTLs) with potential antiself reactivity mature in the thymus, those with antiself reactivity are activated and eliminated, perhaps by hydrocortisone. Or perhaps they are allowed to mature but are somehow suppressed. This is only speculation. Whatever the mechanism for antiself T-cell elimination (or suppression; see below), it is not the case that self-reactivity is eliminated once and for all during fetal development. Whatever mechanism is employed, it must be activated and utilized over and over again throughout life as new T cells mature to replace old T cells. We also don't know how antiself reactivity is regulated in B cells. There is good evidence that B cells with antiself reactivity exist but fail to turn on because of the absence or suppression of appropriate T-cell help.

The phenomenon of tolerance has been studied experimentally for many years. One of the first observations was made by Ray Owen in 1945. He was studying genetically distinct dizygotic cattle twins that share a single, vascularly fused placenta. As adults, these cattle share a common pool of two distinct blood lymphocyte haplotypes and use both equally well. If one tried to mix the two blood types in adults, the result would be rapid mutual rejection. The fact that two distinct cell types were functioning in the same animal suggested to Owen that the cattle had somehow become immunologically tolerant of one another because of their shared placenta. This led to the speculation that antigen exposure during fetal life led to tolerance. This was verified for transplanted cells and tissues a few years later when Medawar tried to exchange skin grafts between such cattle and found that they were accepted.

This notion was first tested in a truly experimental fashion by Billingham, Brent, and Medawar in 1953 (Figure 13-8). They exposed CBA mice at birth to a mixture of cell types from an A-strain mouse. When the CBA mice were eight weeks old, they tried to transplant it with skin from an A-strain mouse. The grafts were successful. However, the CBA mice were able to reject a third-party graft in the normal fashion. There was some speculation that the A-strain graft, when placed on the treated CBA mouse, might lose (or have covered up) its antigens. This was disproved by transferring into the CBA mouse that had been grafted with the A strain skin, some lymph node cells from a CBA mouse that had previously rejected a skin graft from an A strain mouse. In this case, rapid rejection of the A-strain skin graft occurred.

Several points should be made about this experiment. First of all, the donor and recipient differed only at the H-2D region. There were no class II differences between them. This was probably important in avoiding graft-versus-host disease

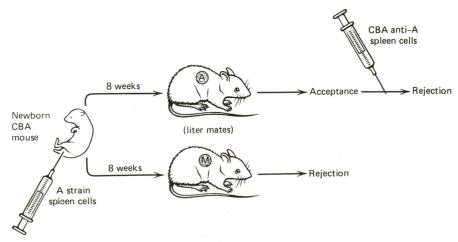

Figure 13-8 The Billingham-Brent-Medaway experiment demonstrating neonatal tolerance to allogeneic cells.

(see Chapter 14). It may also be important in the induction of tolerance. Moreover, one can demonstrate in such situations the persistence of donor strain cells in the adult mouse. *This persistence of the tolerizing antigen turns out to be very important in maintaining the tolerant state.*

These experiments show that with tissue grafts, there is a period around the time of birth (the exact time is different in different species) when it is relatively easy to induce tolerance in an animal. A short time later it is very difficult (in fact impossible) to induce tolerance in this fashion to tissue transplants. It seems that the maintenance of the tolerant state requires the persistence of antigen in the tolerized animal (i.e., it must be a chimera). This is probably necessary because of the constant turnover of T cells in the body. There is no way to pass on tolerance from old T cells to new ones: each generation must learn tolerance (or immunity) on its own.

Tolerance has also been studied using nontissue antigens. Among the earlier studies of this type were those of Felton. He used purified pneumococcal polysaccharide, the normal immunizing dose for which is 0.5 μg/mouse. Doses of 5 μg or higher induce a state of unresponsiveness to subsequent immunizing doses of this antigen. This phenomenon was called "immune paralysis." Such paralysis seemed to last for the lifetime of the animal. Felton later showed that tolerance lasted as long as residual antigen remained in the tissues; this turned out to be a key observation.

Other investigators studied protein antigens as inducers of immune paralysis. They found that in order to induce paralysis with protein antigens, about 100 mg was required. Moreover, the paralysis thus induced was usually quite short lived, a fact consistent with the observation that protein antigens rarely persist in the immunized animal. The state of unresponsiveness can, however, be maintained by repeated exposure to antigen during the paralytic state.

It was also observed with protein antigens that the *physical state* of the antigen is important in tolerance induction. Soluble antigens, as opposed to aggregated or denatured antigens, are much more effective in inducing tolerance. Aggregated forms of antigen are most likely processed more efficiently by macrophages, and presented as an inducing signal to T cells. It may also be the case that antigen interacting directly with B cells may paralyze them. However, even with soluble antigens as tolerogen, it is necessary to reexpose the animal periodically to the tolerogen or else the paralysis wanes.

The effect of *antigen dose* on tolerance versus immunity is a rather complex phenomenon. Soluble antigens are not always tolerogenic. In fact, whether they induce tolerance or immunity depends upon the dose at which they are administered. One of the earliest reports of this phenomenon was that of Mitchison. He gave mice a course of injections of soluble BSA over a 10-week period, waited 2 weeks, and then challenged them with an immunogenic dose of BSA. His results are shown in Figure 13-9. He found that solubilized, free BSA administered at extremely low doses (10^{-12}g) did not impair the immune response to a subse-

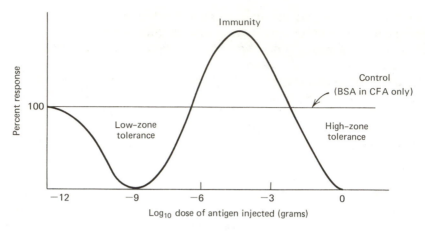

Figure 13-9 Effect of antigen dose on the induction of immune responsiveness.

quent challenge with BSA in adjuvant. As the dose of antigen was increased, the response to subsequent challenge decreased, even when the tolerizing dose was still only in the nanogram (10^{-9}g) range. As the dose was increased further the free BSA again became immunogenic and in fact induced a memory effect for the BSA in CFA. Finally, as the dose was increased still further, the free BSA became again tolerogenic. Thus, two zones of tolerance could be discerned: a low-zone tolerance, peaking at a dosage of 10^{-9}g/animal, and a high-zone tolerance range above about 10 mg/animal.

Mitchison went on to show that tolerance can be induced in both T and B cells. In further examination of the phenomenon illustrated in Figure 13-8 it was found that low-zone tolerance produced a defect in T cells only and that the B cells were perfectly active; high-zone tolerance was induced in both T cells and B cells. One piece of evidence suggesting that low-zone tolerance to BSA is restricted to the T-cell population comes from an experiment carried out by Weigle. Weigle showed that tolerance to BSA in the low zone could be broken by exposure of the animal to a cross-reacting albumin, porcine serum albumin (PSA). If BSA can be represented as a molecule with six determinants (Figure 13-10), then PSA could be represented as a molecule with determinants 1 to 4 of BSA plus, say, two additional determinants (8 and 9) not found on BSA. When PSA was given to animals made tolerant by a low-zone treatment with BSA, it was found that antibodies were produced to those determinants on BSA shared with PSA (i.e., determinants 1 to 4). Thus, the B cells capable of producing antibody to determinants 1 through 4 were clearly not tolerized by the exposure to tolerogenic doses of BSA. Presumably the PSA molecule is recognized by T cells through the new (nontolerized) determinants (8 and 9). The T cells are able to interact with the PSA molecule and present it to B cells capable of responding to the determinants 1 to 4. One possible explanation of the restriction of low-zone tolerance to T cells is that T cells may have higher affinity receptors for antigen, at least with respect to tolerance induction, than do B cells. Judging from the data this would be by a factor of about 10^3.

The distinct properties of T and B cells, with respect to tolerance induction, were further emphasized in a study of Chiller et al. in 1971. They were among the first to investigate unresponsiveness in the newly defined T- and B-cell subsets and

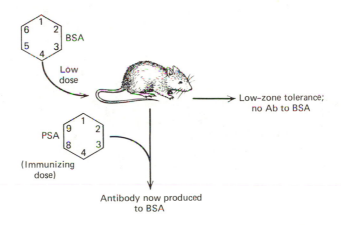

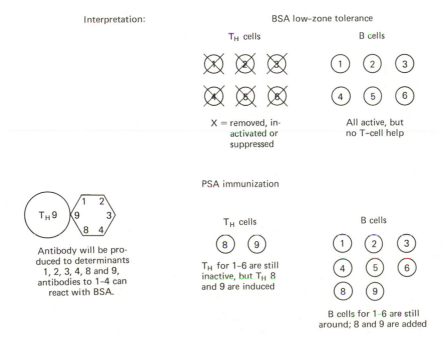

Figure 13-10 Abrogation of tolerance by exposure to a cross-reactive antigen.

had shown in 1970 that tolerance in either cell type was sufficient to block antibody production. In the study in Figure 13-11, they injected mice with disaggregated human IgG, which induces tolerance rather than immunity. The mice were killed at various times thereafter, and thymus or bone marrow cells were isolated. These were each injected together with normal partner cells (T or B) into an irradiated syngeneic mouse, and the immune response to aggregated IgG in the reconstituted mouse was tested as a function of time. As can be seen in Figure 13-11, thymus cells are rendered tolerant almost immediately on exposure to the tolerogen and remain so for a long time. B cells require a week or more to become tolerized, but by seven weeks have recovered and are able to cooperate with normal T cells in the response to immunogen. Moreover, the T cells could be rendered tolerant with 10 times *less* tolerogen than required to tolerize B cells (data not shown).

A possible basis for tolerance induction in B cells is suggested by experiments carried out by Vitetta and co-workers in the late 1970s. Neonatal B cells are μ^+ and δ^-. Shortly after birth, they become μ^+ and δ^+. Neonatal B cells are easily tolerized to many thymus dependent antigens whereas adult B cells are very difficult to tolerize. This was demonstrated in an *in vitro* system devised by Vitetta and

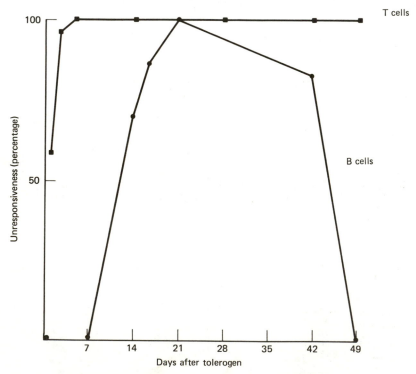

Figure 13-11 Kinetics of induction and spontaneous loss of unresponsiveness in thymus and bone marrow cells. [From J. Chiller et al., *Science, 171,* 813 (1971).]

her co-workers. They then asked whether the presence or absence of δ on a B-cell surface may be related to the susceptibility of the B cell to tolerance induction. In a first series of experiments, they removed surface δ by selective papain treatment (δ chains have a highly papain-sensitive region near the membrane). Adult B cells treated this way became much more susceptible to tolerance induction (like newborn B cells) in their *in vitro* system. The same thing was observed when IgD was selectively capped off of adult B cells; they again became more like newborn B cells in terms of their susceptibility to tolerance induction.

We can imagine that B cells maturing in the presence of antigen (at the μ-only stage) will be readily tolerized, particularly in the presence of persisting antigen. It would thus be possible to tolerize B cells only as they mature from stem cells. This may be the explanation for the requirement of a week or so before tolerance in B cells is apparent. During the first week, the more difficult to tolerize adult B cells will continue to participate in responses to antigen. As those mature B cells turn over, incoming B cells at the μ only stage will be immediately tolerized by antigen and never be able to participate in antibody responses to that antigen. An interesting and possibly related feature of B cells is that the μ on $\mu^+\delta^-$ B cells, when capped off, does not reappear. When the μ on $\mu^+\delta^+$ B cells is capped off, it returns after a few hours in culture. If antigen caused partial or complete capping of B cells at the $\mu^+\delta^-$ stage, those particular B cells would be effectively tolerant for life.

Suppressor T Cells

Until about 1970 it was more or less assumed that tolerance implied clonal deletion; that is, in both T- and B-cell tolerance it was assumed that cells responding to a particular antigen were actually deleted as a result of tolerance induction to that antigen. In 1970, a critical experiment carried out by Gershon first introduced the notion that tolerance may not be clonal deletion but may represent clonal suppression through the agency of a subpopulation of T cells called suppressor T cells. Gershon's experiment is illustrated in Figure 13-12. This experiment shows that T cells must be present during the tolerizing regimen if tolerance is to be induced. If T cells are absent during this time, no tolerance is induced; subsequent challenge with the immunogen leads to a perfectly normal response. However, if T cells are present during the tolerizing regimen, tolerance is induced and a subsequent challenge with an immunizing dose of the antigen in question gives no antibody response. Furthermore, if T cells are recovered from the animal at the end of the tolerizing regimen, it can be shown that they are able to suppress the response of either virgin or primed T helper cells. A vast body of experimental evidence has accumulated that demonstrates that antigen specific suppression plays a very important role in immune regulation. It is thought to be a major factor behind tolerance to self. It can be demonstrated that there are both T helper cells and B

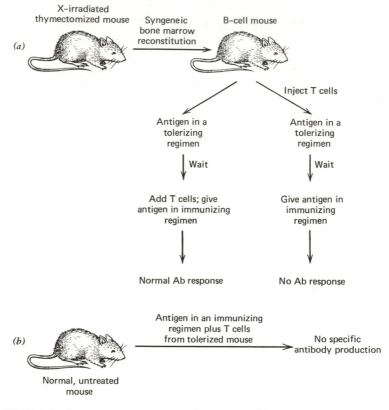

Figure 13-12 Experiments demonstrating existence of suppressor T cells. Experiment *a* shows that a thymectomized, irradiated, BM-reconstituted mouse (B-cell mouse; no T-cell function) cannot be made tolerant in a standard tolerance-inducing regimen unless provided with a source of competent T cells during the regimen. Experiment *b* demonstrates that the suppression generated in a tolerizing regimen resides in and can be specifically transferred with peripheral T cells.

cells within the body capable of reacting with self-components. The development of autoimmune disease is very often accompanied by a defect in suppressor T cells (Chapter 18).

As seen in Chapter 11, T helper cells are characterized by the absence of the Lyt-2 antigen on the surface. The T-suppressor cells described above are Lyt-2$^+$ just like cytotoxic T cells. However, there is good evidence to show that T suppressor cells and cytotoxic T cells are distinct T-cell subsets. The significance of the presence of Lyt-2 antigen on both cell types is not fully understood.

Low-zone tolerance is probably due to suppressor T cells. It may be that at low-antigen doses, T suppressor cells are selectively induced, rather than T helper cells. The nature of the T-cell defect in high-zone tolerance is not understood at present.

As mentioned earlier, high-zone tolerance also involves B cells. It is known that with a high-zone tolerizing regimen, the T cells are rendered tolerant for a long period of time, whereas tolerance in the B cells is for a much shorter period of time. This may reflect a more rapid turnover rate in virgin B cells.

The involvement of suppressor T cells has been demonstrated in a variety of experimental systems *in vivo* and *in vitro*. Certain strains of mice fail to respond to certain antigens. This could happen for a variety of reasons, one of which may be that the combination of a given antigen with a particular APC class II gene product induces the formation of suppressor rather than helper T cells.

One of the first such systems to be described involves the humoral response in mice to the linear terpolymer GAT ($Glu_{60}Ala_{30}Tyr_{10}$). The response to GAT is all or none at the level of primary immunization. Responder haplotypes ($H-2^{a,b,d,k}$) produce a prompt, vigorous antibody response to soluble GAT. Nonresponder haplotypes ($H-2^{p,q,s}$) never produce antibodies in response to soluble GAT, even on repeated stimulation. However, nonresponder strains will produce GAT antibodies if immunized with GAT bound to methylated bovine serum albumin (MBSA) as a carrier. This finding indicates immediately that the defect in the system is not in B cells specific for GAT, since antibodies to GAT can be produced if GAT is presented in an appropriate manner. The problem most likely lies either with T cells or with antigen-presenting cells (APC) involved in processing of the GAT signal.

Two possibilities could account for the failure to generate a GAT-specific antibody response in this system. It could be that helper T-cell precursors capable of recognizing GAT do not exist in nonresponder mouse strains; alternatively, GAT could induce T-cell help in responder strains, but T-cell suppression in nonresponder strains. The data shown in Table 13-5 support the latter interpretation. As noted previously, when nonresponder mice are immunized with GAT–MBSA, they produce a vigorous anti-GAT antibody response. However, when they are first exposed to soluble GAT, and then to GAT–MBSA, they fail to develop an anti-GAT response. Moreover (data not shown), when spleen cells from a GAT-treated nonresponder are passively transferred to mice of a responder strain, the latter are incapable of responding to either GAT or GAT–MBSA. If the GAT-suppressed spleen cells are treated with anti-Thy-1 plus complement before transfer, this effect is not seen. All of these results are most compatible with the selective activation by GAT of suppressor T cells in nonresponder strains.

In addition to suppression of the GAT response by GAT-primed nonresponder T cells, suppression can also be achieved utilizing a sonicated extract of such cells. This probably represents the activity of a suppressor factor residing in suppressor T-cell membranes (see next section).

Thus in the GAT system, regulation of responsiveness is determined by a balance between help and suppression. Careful analysis of the sequence of events in nonresponder mice using GAT–MBSA showed that GAT-specific T helper cells do exist and can be activated. However, soluble GAT presented to nonresponder strains of mice

Table 13-5 Effect of GAT on Responses to GAT–MBSA by Responder (C57BL/6; H-2^b) and Nonresponder (DBA/1; H-2^q) Mice *in Vivo*

	Immunizing regimen	
Strain	GAT–MBSA	GAT Day 0 GAT–MBSA Day 3
C57BL/6	10,000	10,400
DBA/1	8,000	600

Mice were injected either with GAT–MBSA only, or with GAT followed three days later by an injection of GAT–MSBA. Spleens were removed on day 7. Values shown are GAT-specific PFC/spleen.

seem to activate suppressor cells preferentially. Because GAT-specific pre-T$_h$ exist in nonresponder strains, it is not clear why suppressor cells are preferentially activated.

A particularly intriguing observation was made in this system by Pierres et al. When spleen cells from GAT-responder mice were depleted of macrophages, administration of even small amounts of GAT induced not responsiveness but suppression. Thus presentation of GAT directly to lymphocytes, bypassing macrophages, can induce T suppressor cells. The same effect can be achieved by flooding the system of responder mice with high concentrations of GAT, perhaps by saturating the macrophage system and leaving free GAT to interact with T cells. These observations suggest that the defect in nonresponder mice may be the absence of macrophages able to present GAT to T cells.

The notion of selective activation of helper or suppressor pathways has been extended to more complex biological molecules by several investigators, including Sercarz and his colleagues at UCLA. Whereas synthetic polypeptide antigens have the advantage of a very limited number of (often only one) different immunogenic determinants, the precise structure of the overall molecule and thus the three-dimensional organization of the determinants, can never be known for certain and may not be entirely reproducible from batch to batch. Biological macromolecules, although antigenically more complex, have the advantage of being absolutely reproducible structurally. Moreover, by using homologous forms of the same molecule from different species, one can obtain a collection of molecules with varying but reproducible degrees of structural variation.

One of the systems explored by Sercarz and co-workers is the lysozyme molecule, obtained from the egg whites of various bird species. This monomeric, globular protein (14,400 MW) has been characterized extensively in terms of primary, secondary, and tertiary peptide structure in most of the species studied. The immune response to gallinaceous lysozyme in mice was shown to be under I-region control. For example, I^a and I^d haplotypes are responders to hen egg white lysozyme (HEL), whereas mice of the I^b haplotype are nonresponders. In responder strains, the majority of antibody produced (70 to 95 percent) is directed toward the region of the molecule defined by the amino and carboxy termini, which lie close together in the native molecule (Figure 13-13). Antibodies specific for this determinant (N–C) can be induced in H-2^b mice primed with HEL coupled to SRBC but not by HEL alone. By analogy with the GAT system, the possibility of suppression induced in H-2^b mice by native HEL was investigated. T cells from HEL-primed H-2^b mice were shown specifically to suppress the production of antibody to the N–C determinant of HEL. A subset of T cells displaying IJ region-associated antigens was subsequently found to be responsible for the suppression.

Interestingly, ring-necked pheasant lysozyme (REL) does not induce suppression in H-2^b mice, but rather induces normal quantities of N–C determinant antibody that crossreacts almost completely on HEL. REL and HEL differ at only 9/129 residues. This suggested that specific regions of the molecule may be involved in the induction of suppression versus tolerance. This notion was confirmed by studies in which the response of H-2^b mice to individual fragments of HEL was analyzed. The N–C fragment generated by mild acid treatment of the intact molecule (Figure 13-13) was found to induce suppressor T cells in H-2^b mice with the same efficiency as intact HEL. The LII fragment, on the other hand (amino acids 13 to 105), activated T cells equally well in nonresponder (H-2^b) and responder (H-2^a) mice. The LII fragment is essentially the HEL molecule without the N–C portion. These experiments suggested that some part of the N–C structure was responsible for inducing suppression in H-2^b mice.

The exact location of the determinant in the N-C fragment responsible for suppressor induction was first inferred by a close study of the amino acid sequences in this region of the molecule among different lysozymes. It was found that all of the lysozymes immunogenic in H-2^b had tyrosine at position 3, whereas all suppressor-inducing lysozymes had phenylalanine at this position. Subsequent studies showed that removal of the first three H-terminal amino acids from "suppressor" lysozymes abolished their ability to induce suppression in H-2^b mice, although interestingly this treatment did not convert them to fully immunogenic molecules. Thus the extreme N-terminal end of the molecule, and perhaps only a single amino acid position, determines in H-2^b mice whether the suppressor pathway is activated.

At present we do not know how such a restricted portion of a molecule could control induction of suppression. It may be that in H-2^b mice, the T_s-receptor repertoire is slightly different from the T_h-receptor repertoire. Particular T_s subclones may directly recognize the N-terminal portion of those molecules with phenylalanine at position 3, whereas N-2^b T_h clones recognize HEL molecules with tyrosine at this position. Alternatively, this position may be crucial in macrophage association. The role of antigen-presenting cells has not been studied yet in this

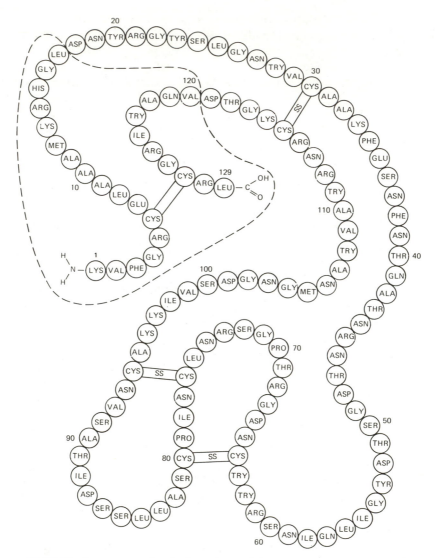

Figure 13-13 The lysozyme molecule from domestic hens. The N–C fragment, against which antibody is produced in responder strains, and which contains the suppression-inducing determinant in nonresponder strains, is enclosed within the broken line. Drawing courtesy Dr. Eli Sercarz, UCLA.

system, but it is possible that H-2^b APC may not pick up, process, or present HEL, allowing it to interact directly with T cells, a condition which in the GAT system leads to suppression induction. Because the response to HEL is definitely under control of a gene in the IA subregion, it is possible that the $A_\alpha^b A_\beta^b$ dimer may be involved. The relationships between IA-region genes and the restricted region of the HEL molecule involved in selection of help versus suppression are currently the subject of intense investigation.

Antigen-specific Helper T-Cell Factors

The existence of soluble factors involved in T–B-lymphocyte cooperation was clearly indicated by the experiments of Feldmann and Basten, described earlier in this chapter. Their factor could pass through a cell-impermeable membrane but not through a dialysis membrane. It was produced by T cells and was antigen specific in that only B cells capable of producing antibody to the antigen processed by the T cells were activated.

The discovery of a factor produced by T cells, which has the ability to activate B cells in an antigen-specific manner, suggested a way in which Ir gene control of antibody responses might possibly be expressed. If Ir genes code for factors on T helper (T_h) cells, which are obligatory in the processing of antigen for B-cell activation, then the presence, absence, amount, or properties of T_h factors would have an obvious regulatory effect on specific antibody production. The first strong evidence that such factors might indeed be under I-region control came from the work of Munro and Taussig in 1973–1974. Using *in vivo*-generated, (T,G)-AL-specific helper cells restimulated with (T,G)-AL *in vitro,* they were able to produce T_h factors that (1) contained specific antigen as a part of the factor, (2) did *not* contain immunoglobulin, in contrast to the factor described by Feldmann and Basten, (3) reacted with anti-Ia antisera, particularly antisera directed against IA-coded Ia antigens, and (4) replaced the need for T helper cells in the response to (T,G)-AL *in vivo.*

The involvement of antigen-specific factors has now been demonstrated in a number of experimental systems (Table 13-6). The (T,G)-AL factor remains one of the most intensely studied of these factors. It is produced by Lyt-2$^-$ T cells, but not by Lyt-2$^+$ T cells. Although the (T,G)-AL factor binds antigen fairly avidly, it is not quite as restricted in its specificity as the intact T helper cell. T helper cells specific for (T,G)-AL will not facilitate the response to closely related antigens such as (H,G)-AL. The (T,G)-AL factor, however, will promote a response to (H,G)-AL and (Phe,G)-AL almost as efficiently as to (T,G)-AL. Moreover, whereas T helper cells are usually MHC restricted when responding to antigens under Ir gene control, most helper factors are not MHC restricted.

The possibility that antigen-binding T-cell factors might be related to the T-cell receptor excited great interest in their structure. Until recently, $T_h F$ have been available in quantities too small to permit biochemical studies more refined than determining approximate molecular weights. In recent years, however, T helper cell hybridomas have been produced that secrete $T_h F$ in response to antigenic challenge. We may expect more detailed information on the structure of $T_h F$, and its relation (if any) to the T-cell receptor, in the near future.

Another aspect of T helper factors that has created interest in their molecular

Table 13-6 Antigen-specific Factors

	Producer cell	Target cell	Function	Works in 1°	Works in 2°	MHC restricted/	Ia	Ig idiotype	MW
Feldmann-Basten	T cell	B cell	Help	+	+	?	?	?	>10,000
Taussig-Mozes	Ly1 T cell	B cell (Mφ)	Help	+	+	No	IA	+	~50,000
Erb-Feldmann	Mφ	T cell		+	?	Yes	?	?	~50,000
Tada	Ly2,3 T cell	Ly1,2,3 T cell	Supp	+	+	Yes	I-J	?	~50,000
Feldmann	Ly2,3 T cell	Ly1+,2− T cell	Supp	+	+	No	I-J	?	?
Kapp	T cell	Ly1 T cell	Supp	+	?	No	I-J	+	45,000

structure is the presence of antigens coded for by the IA subregion. The Ia antigens found on T_hF and on activated T helper cells, are not, however, class II antigens. Antiserum made between IA-disparate strains can be bound to a solid substrate and used to remove T_hF from culture supernates. If the antiserum is absorbed extensively with B cells before use, it loses the ability to bind class II antigens, but its ability to bind T_hF is undiminished. Conversely, if the antiserum is absorbed with activated T cells, it can no longer absorb the factor but still reacts with class II MHC antigens. Thus we can infer the existence of another IA locus in the Ia subregion, distinct from A_α, A_β, and E_β. The nature of the I-region gene product may also become apparent from studies of the hybridoma T_h mentioned previously.

Factors must of course be able to act specifically on target cells. In the case of B cells, this "acceptor" molecule could certainly be sIg, since T_hF only works when it has antigen bound to it. However, T_hF is also picked up by macrophages, which do not have sIg. Moreover, B-cell acceptance of T_hF can be blocked with antiserum specific for class II MHC molecules. This led Munro and Taussig to propose that two MHC-linked genes may actually be involved in this type of Ir gene control: one gene coding for the nonclass II Ia element on the T_hF, and a second gene coding for the T_hF-acceptor molecule, presumed to be a class II MHC molecule. Because T_hF never works unless bound with antigen, it seems unnecessary to postulate a B-cell acceptor molecule other than sIg. On the other hand, as we have seen in previous chapters, antigen may well need to be associated with class II MHC products on the surface of antigen-presenting cells. Although in previous cases we have been concerned mostly with presentation of antigen to T cells, it is certainly possible that transmission of T_hF from T cell to B cell may also require association of T_hF with class II molecules on the macrophage surface. If macrophages are involved in presenting T_hF to B cells, then the ability of anti-Ia sera to block T-cell utilization of T_hF could be explained at the level of the macrophage rather than the B cell itself. Absence of an "appropriate" Ia molecule on the macrophage surface could result in an apparent Ir gene defect.

Antigen-specific Suppressor T-Cell Factors

Several laboratories have carried out extensive characterization of factors associated with suppressor T cells. The first T_s factor to be well characterized was described by Tada and his associates. Unlike the helper factors just described, the T_s factor of Tada et al., is not readily shed from the surface of spleen or lymph node T_s cells after binding of antigen. Mice are given carrier molecules in a regimen known to favor the induction of T_s cells rather than T_h cells. Lymphocyte suspensions are prepared from the spleens or thymuses of such mice, and then sonicated to liberate suppressor factor into a soluble extract form. Soluble extracts are defined as the supernate obtained after centrifuging the sonicate for one hour at

40,000 × gravity. It is presumed that the factor actually resides as an integral protein in the T_s cell plasma membrane. The cell producing the suppressor factor is of the Lyt-2$^+$ phenotype.

Typical experimental results using this factor to suppress secondary humoral responses *in vitro* are shown in Table 13-7. In experiment 1, we see that DNP–KLH-primed spleen cells are suppressed in their response to DNP–KLH by T_s factor extracted from thymuses of KLH-suppressed mice but not by extracts of thymus cells from normal mice or mice suppressed in their response to the unrelated antigen ovalbumin (OA). The data in experiment 2 are particularly illuminating. Here the test spleen cells are primed to DNP–OA. A good PFC response is obtained in response to DNP–OA, and a small but significant response is obtained in re-sponse to DNP–KLH, perhaps because of minor cross-reactivity of determinants on the two carriers. The simple presence in the culture medium of DNP–KLH does not seem to inhibit the response of the spleen cells to DNP–OA. When T_s factor obtained from OA-suppressed thymuses is added together with the two antigens, the anti-DNP response is strongly suppressed, but no suppression occurs when the T_s factor from KLH-suppressed thymuses is used. (Remember that only helper T cells primed to DNP–OA are present.) Besides demonstrating the specificity of the factor, these data also show that the locus of action is probably not the DNP-sensitized B cell. The DNP primed B cells can bind DNP–KLH and DNP–OA equally well (data not shown). If the suppressor factor were acting on B cells, then either factor would produce suppression when a mixture of the two antigens is present. Thus the most logical conclusion is that the T_s factor acts on some species of carrier-specific T cell. Subsequent work from Tada's group suggested that the specific T cell on which the factor works is Lyt-1,2,3$^+$. This cell is also IJ$^+$; pretreat-ment of this cell with anti-IJ serum blocks its ability to be acted on by factor. There has been a suggestion that a specific subset of Lyt-1,2,3$^+$ T cells, bearing the Qal locus marker, may give rise to Lyt-2$^+$ suppressor cells. It is possible (but only speculation at this point) that Tada's factor may act to drive the differentiation of

Table 13-7 Effect of T_s Factor on *in Vitro* Secondary Humoral Responses

Experiment	Spleen cells (unfractionated) primed to	T_s factor specific for	Antigen added	α-DNP PFC
1	DNP–KLH	None	DNP–KLH	++++
	DNP–KLH	KLH	DNP–KLH	+
	DNP–KLH	OA	DNP–KLH	++++
2	DNP–OA	None	DNP–OA	++++
	DNP–OA	None	DNP–KLH	+
	DNP–OA	None	DNP–OA + DNP–KLH	++++
	DNP–OA	OA	DNP–OA + DNP–KLH	±
	DNP–OA	KLH	DNP–OA + DNP–KLH	++++

suppressor precursors, thus providing a sort of "amplification loop" for suppressor regulation of antibody production.

In further experiments, it was shown that the T_s factor (1) binds specifically to the original suppressing antigen, (2) bears no detectable antigenic determinants related to the constant regions of mouse Ig, and (3) could be removed from solution by anti-Ia antibodies, specifically anti-IJ subregion antibodies. This factor is thus very similar in its overall properties to the T_h factor described by a number of laboratories. However, a major difference noted by Tada is that the T_s factor is genetically restricted, that is, it can only suppress IJ subregion-syngeneic T cells. No such genetic restriction applies to the interaction of T_h factors and B cells.

A suppressor factor similar to Tada's has been found for the GAT system described earlier. Nonresponder strains ($H\text{-}2^{p,q,s}$) fail to produce antibodies after immunization with GAT, and this failure can be traced to the induction of antigen-specific suppressor T cells. Isolation and culture, in the presence of GAT, of these suppressor T cells does not lead to the production of a GAT-specific T-cell factor. However, sonication of the T_s cells does result in the liberation of such a factor. This factor is a protein, 40,000 to 50,000 daltons bearing IJ determinants. It binds GAT specifically, but lacks isotypic and allotypic determinants. Like Tada's factor, GAT T_sF acts on an Lyt-1,2,3 cell to induce suppressor T cells. Unlike Tada's T_sF, however, GAT T_sF acts across IJ barriers, that is, it is not genetically restricted.

As discussed earlier, T suppressor cells can also be induced by GAT in responder strain spleen cells if the latter are depleted of macrophages. These T cells also produce a GAT specific T_sF. Interestingly, however, this factor appears to act directly on T_h cells, rather than by inducing suppressor differentiation from Lyt-1,2,3 cells.

Cloned T-cell lines and hybridomas have now been generated by both the Tada and Kapp/Pierce labs. These have provided large amounts of factor suitable for biochemical work. Interestingly, most of these suppressor cell lines secrete their factors into the cell medium without sonication, some doing so constitutively, in the absence of antigen. Work to characterize in more detail the molecular nature of these factors is now in progress.

A T_s factor different from those reported by Tada and Kapp et al. was described by Marc Feldmann. This factor is different in that it is released in soluble form by Lyt-2$^+$ T_s cells after incubation with antigen, much like the T_h factors described earlier. A second major difference from at least Tada's factor is that the Feldmann factor appears to act directly on the T cell (Lyt-2$^-$) that produces T_h factor. How the two types of factors interact, if at all, is not clear, but it has been proposed that Feldmann factor may act on T_h cells directly to suppress primary immune reactions, whereas the Tada-Kapp type factor may act on Lyt-1,2,3 lymphocytes in a sort of amplification loop to drive the differentiation of more suppressor cells.

Feldmann's factor is ca. 50,000 daltons in size and is controlled by genes mapping to IJ. However, its mode of action and general physical properties suggest it is distinct from the Tada factor. There may thus be a number of genes in IJ coding for or controlling suppressor factor. Because the Tada-Kapp factor must be physically extracted from T_s-cell membranes, it is possible that it may work in direct cell–cell contact. If the Feldmann factor indeed directly mediates suppression, it would make sense for it to be truly soluble; this would be most consistent with the observation that a relatively few suppressor cells are capable of suppressing an entire antibody response.

Soluble Factors Involved in Macrophage–T-Cell Interaction

In 1975, Erb and Feldmann described a system for the primary generation of T helper cells (T_h) to soluble antigens *in vitro,* which displayed an absolute requirement for macrophages (M). Antigen presented to T cells depleted of M failed to induce T_h. However, M incubated with antigen alone for several days released a cell-free factor into the supernate that was by itself able to induce antigen-specific T helper cells in M-depleted T cells. Thus, direct M–T cell contact was unnecessary. However, the factor would only work if the M and T cells were identical at the IA subregion of the H-2 complex. The factor itself, which has a molecular weight of about 50,000, contained both class II antigens and determinants of the specific antigen used for induction. It did not display Ig antigenic determinants or K or D determinants. The I region-coded portion of the factor is a protein or glycoprotein.

Bibliography

General

Dorf, M. E. (ed.), *The Role of the Major Histocompatibility Complex in Immunobiology,* Garland STPM Press, New York (1981).

Gillis, S., and F. P. Inman (eds.), The interleukins. *Contemp. Topics in Molec. Immunol. 10* (1985).

Kishimoto, T., Factors affecting B cell growth and differentiation. *Annual Review Immunol. 3,* 133 (1985).

Malkovsky, M., and P. Medawar, Is immunological tolerance a consequence of IL-2 deficiency during the recognition of antigen. *Immunol. Today 5,* 340 (1984).

Miller, J. F. A. P., Immunological Memory, *Contemp. Topics Immunobiol. 2,* 151 (1973).

Research

Armerding, D., D. H. Sachs, and D. H. Katz, Activation of T and B lymphocytes in vitro. III. Presence of Ia determinants on allogeneic effect factor. *J. Exp. Med. 140,* 1717 (1974).

Asano, Y., A Singer, and R. Hodes, Role of the major histocompatibility complex in T cell activation of B cell subpopulations, MHC-restricted and -unrestricted B cell responses are mediated by distinct B cell subpopulations. *J. Exp. Med. 154,* 1100 (1981).

Ashwell, J., A. de Franco, W. Paul, and R. Schwartz, Antigen Presentation by Resting B Cells. *J. Exp. Med. 159,* 881 (1984).

Billingham, R. E., L. Brent, and P. Medawar, Quantitative studies on tissue transplantation immunity. III. Actively acquired tolerance. *R. Soc. (London) Phil. Trans. Series B, 239*, 357 (1956).

Chiller, J., G. Habicht, and W. Weigle, Kinetics differences in unresponsiveness of thymus and bone marrow cells. *Science 171*, 813 (1971).

Dekruyff, R. H., Clayberger, C., and Cantor, H., Hapten reactive inducer T cells. II. Evidence that a secreted form of the T cell receptor induces antibody production. *J. Exp. Med. 158*, 1881 (1983).

Dresser, D. W., Specific inhibition of antibody production. I. Protein overloading paralysis. *Immunology 5*, 161 (1962).

Erb, P., B. Meier, T. Matsunaga, and M. Feldmann, Nature of T-cell macrophage interaction in helper-cell induction in vitro. II. Two stages of T-helper-cell differentiation analyzed in irradiation and allophenic chimeras. *J. Exp. Med. 149*, 686 (1979).

Feldmann, M., Cell interactions in the immune response in vitro. V. Specific collaboration via complexes of antigen and thymus-derived cell immunoglobulin. *J. Exp. Med. 136*, 737 (1972).

Feldmann, M., and A. Basten, Cell interactions in the immune response. Specific collaboration across a cell-impermeable membrane. *J. Exp. Med. 136*, 49 (1972).

Felton, Lloyd, D., The significance of antigen in animal tissues. *J. Immunology 61*, 107 (1949).

Germain, R. N., J. Theze, J. A. Kapp, and B. Benacerraf, Antigen-specific T-cell-mediated suppression. I. Induction of L-glutamic acid^{60}-L-alanine^{30}-L-tyrosine^{10} specific suppressor T cells in vitro requires both antigen-specific T-cell-suppressor factor and antigen. *J. Exp. Med. 147*, 123 (1978).

Gershon, R. K., T cell control of antibody production. *Contemp. Topics Immunobiol. 3*, 1 (1974).

Gershon, R. K., and K. Kondo, Infectious immunological tolerance. *Immunology, 21*, 903 (1971).

Hünig, Th., A. Schimpl, and E. Wecker, Mechanism of T-cell help in the immune response to soluble antigens. I. Evidence for in situ generation and action of T-cell-replacing factor during the anamnestic response to dinitrophenyl keyhole limpet hemocyanin in vitro. *J. Exp. Med. 145*, 1216–1227 (1977).

Kappler, J. W. et al., Antigen-inducible, H-2 restricted, IL-2 producing T cell hybridomas. Lack of independent antigen and H-2 recognition. *J. Exp. Med. 153*, 1198 (1981).

Katz, D. H., M. E. Dorf, and B. Benacerraf, Cell interactions between histoincompatible T and B lymphocytes. VI. Cooperative responses between lymphocytes derived from mouse donor strains differing at genes in the S and D regions of the H-2 complex. *J. Exp. Med. 140*, 290 (1974).

Kindred, B., and D. Shreffler, H-2 dependence of cooperation between T and B cells in vivo. *J. Immunol. 109*, 940 (1972).

Kitamura, K., H. Nakauchi, S. Koyasu, I. Yahara, K. Okumura, and T. Tada, Characterization of an antigen-specific suppressive factor derived from a cloned suppressor effector T cell line. *J. Immunol. 133*, 1371 (1984).

Kontiainen, S., and M. Feldmann, Suppressor-cell induction in vitro. IV. Target of antigen-specific suppressor factor and its genetic relationships. *J. Exp. Med. 147*, 110 (1978).

Marrack, P. et al., Nonspecific factors in B cell responses. *Immunol. Rev. 63*, 33 (1982).

Mitchison, N. A., Induction of immunological paralysis in two zones of dosage. *Proc. Royal Society (B) 161*, 275 (1964).

Munro, A. J. et al., Antigen-specific T cell factor in cell cooperation: Physical properties and mapping in the left-hand (K) half of H-2, *J. Exp. Med. 140,* 1579 (1979).

Owen, R. D., Immunogenetic consequences of vascular anastomoses between bovine twins. *Science 102,* 400 (1945).

Sercarz, E., and A. Coons, Specific inhibition of antibody formation during immunological paralysis and unresponsiveness. *Nature 184,* 1080 (1959).

Singer, A., K. Hathcock, and R. Hodes, Cellular and genetic control of antibody responses. VIII. MHC restricted recognition of accessory cells, but not B cells, by parent-specific subpopulations of normal F_1 T helper cells. *J. Immunol. 124,* 1079 (1980).

Singer, A., K. Hathcock, and R. Hodes, Self recognition in allogeneic radiation bone marrow chimeras. *J. Exp. Med. 153,* 1286 (1981).

Singer, A. et al., Role of the major histocompatibility complex in T cell activation of B cell subpopulations. Lyb-5 and Lyb-5 subpopulations differ in their requirement for MHC-restricted T cell recognitions. *J. Exp. Med. 154,* 501 (1981).

Taniguchi, M., T. Tada, and T. Tokuhisa, Properties of antigen-specific suppressive T cell factor in the regulation of antibody responses in the mouse. III. Dual gene Control of T cell-mediated suppression of the antibody response. *J. Exp. Med. 144,* 20 (1976).

Taussig, M. J., T cell factor which can replace T cells in vivo. *Nature 248,* 234 (1974).

Taussig, M. J. et al., Antigen-specific T cell factor in cell cooperation. Mapping within the I region of H-2 and the ability to cooperate across allogeneic barriers. *J. Exp. Med. 142,* 694 (1975).

Weigle, W. O., Immunological unresponsiveness. *Adv. Immunol. 16,* 61 (1973).

Wigzell, H., and B. Andersson, Cell separation on antigen coated columns. Elimination of antibody forming cells and memory cells. *J. Exp. Med. 129,* 23 (1969).

Zinkernagel, R. M., and P. C. Doherty, H-2 compatibility requirement for T-cell-mediated lysis of target cells infected with lymphocytic choriomeningitis virus. *J. Exp. Med. 141,* 1427 (1975).

CHAPTER **14**

Cell-mediated Cytotoxicity

The initial discovery and characterization of lymphoid cells that can recognize and destroy allogeneic cells and altered self cells resulted from attempts to understand the mechanism of transplant rejection (Chapter 19). One of the difficulties in establishing an immunological basis for transplant rejection was the apparent absence of a role for antibody and complement, which until the second half of this century was the only recognized immunological effector mechanism. In fact it was not until 1953 that lymphocytes were identified as responsible for graft rejection, and only in 1961 were lymphocytes with cytotoxic properties isolated for *in vitro* study.

The principal mediator of cytotoxicity in graft reactions is the cytotoxic T lymphocyte (CTL); this cell has been the object of intense study for the past two decades. However, cytotoxicity is not unique to CTLs. Another lymphocyte-derived cell, called a "natural killer" (NK), cell has the property of cytotoxicity, as do macrophages, eosinophils and possibly even T helper cells, under special circumstances. In this chapter we examine the phenomenon of cells that kill other cells and try to understand why, how, and under what circumstances they do it.

Cytotoxic T Lymphocytes (CTL)-mediated Cytotoxicity

In 1960–1961, several laboratories provided evidence that allograft-immune lymphocytes are cytotoxic for target cells of the immunizing genotype. Lymphocytes obtained from the lymph node draining an allogeneic skin transplant can attack and destroy target cells bearing the class I histocompatibility antigens of the transplant donor. Cytotoxic lymphocytes can also be demonstrated in the spleens of animals undergoing a GVH reaction (see section below on GVH) or in lymph nodes draining the site of a subcutaneous injection of free allogeneic cells.

Analysis of cell surface antigens has demonstrated conclusively that allograft-generated cytotoxic lymphocytes are T cells, of the Lyt-2$^+$ subset in mice, and the T8$^+$ subset in humans. Available evidence in other species also suggests that graft-generated cytotoxic cells are thymus-influenced lymphocytes. *In vitro* studies in the mouse (see section below on mixed leukocyte culture) have shown that the entire process of generation and expression of CTL-mediated cytotoxicity can be carried out with T cells as responding cells.

A cytotoxic function for CTLs *in vivo* is suggested by the results of the so-called Winn assay. Lymphocytes taken from an allograft-sensitized animal are mixed together with tumor target cells bearing the allograft histocompatibility antigens. The cell mixture is then injected into some physically restricted site (usually subcutaneous) in an animal syngeneic with the tumor. Controls include unsensitized lymphocytes mixed with the same tumor, or the same sensitized lymphocytes mixed with an unrelated tumor. Whereas tumors develop from both control mixtures that are indistinguishable in size and growth rate from those developing from tumor cells injected alone, the experimental test groups develop either no tumors or tumors whose growth curve is drastically retarded in time. These results have been interpreted as evidence for cytotoxicity of the sensitized lymphocytes against the allogeneic tumor target cells, although they might just as easily be interpreted in terms of a cytostatic effect exerted by the lymphocytes.

The cytotoxic nature of allograft-sensitized effector lymphocytes can be readily demonstrated in *in vitro* cytotoxicity assays. The most commonly used technique for measuring cytotoxicity *in vitro* is the ^{51}Cr release assay (Figure 14-1). Cytotoxic lymphocytes are collected from the appropriate lymphoid organ at the peak of the cytotoxic response (between 5 and 11 days in the case of allogeneic graft reactions, depending on the site and method of immunization and the particular lymphoid organ involved). Target cells are prepared from the original graft donor for assay of specific cytotoxicity, and from unrelated individuals as a control. Although almost any cell type bearing class I donor MHC antigens will serve as a target for cytolytic damage, the two most commonly used types are tumors that either grow in the ascites form *in vivo* or in single-cell suspension *in vitro*, and normal lymphoid cells

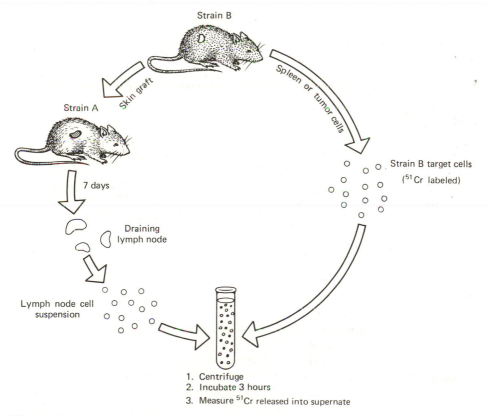

Figure 14-1 The ^{51}Cr release assay.

that have been converted to blast cells by treatment with appropriate mitogens. Both cells types have in common the fact that they are in the blast state and rapidly dividing. Cells that grow attached to a substrate (monolayers) and cells not synthesizing DNA are in general less susceptible to cell-mediated cytotoxic damage.

The target cells are incubated briefly with $Na_2{}^{51}CrO_4$, which enters the cell by passive diffusion. Once inside the cell, the radiochromium is sequestered by binding to cytoplasmic proteins, which retards its spontaneous leakage from the cell. Furthermore, in most cases the chromium is reduced from Cr^{+6} to CR^{+3}. Cr^{+3} enters cells orders of magnitude more slowly than Cr^{+6}; thus ^{51}Cr released from damaged target cells is not significantly reincorporated into undamaged target cells or into effector cells, which would complicate interpretation of assay results. After washing away unincorporated ^{51}Cr from the freshly labeled target cells, they are incubated at 37°C with putative effector cells. The CTLs and target cells are usually centrifuged together to enhance interaction, and incubated at 37° for one to four hours. The amount of ^{51}Cr released during the assay incubation period can be readily related to the number of target cells killed.

Mechanisms Involved in CTL-mediated Lysis

The mechanism by which CTLs kill their target cells has been perhaps one of the most intensely studied questions in cellular immunology and yet is one of the least understood of immunological phenomena. We understand it only in broad outline. Cytolysis requires direct effector cell–target cell contact. Utilizing the T-cell receptor described in Chapter 12, the sensitized CTL is able to discriminate sharply among various allogeneic targets. This has been examined most closely in the mouse. Here it can be shown that in allograft sensitization across an H-2 difference, the CTLs recognize the H-2K and D proteins in both the sensitization and effector phases of the reaction. As illustrated by the experiment in Figure 14-2, separate effector populations are raised against the K and the D antigens. In fact we now know from CTL cloning experiments that just as in the case of T helper cells and class II antigens, a wide range of individual CTL clones is activated toward K, D, or L molecules. The various clones recognize determinants on different portions of the target class I molecule.

The process of cytolysis against alloantigens is currently viewed as being composed of three steps (Figure 14-3). In the first step, the effector cell binds to the target cell through interaction of the T-cell membrane-bound receptor with class I major histocompatibility determinants (K and D in the mouse; HLA-A, B, and C in the human) on the target cell. This is the step that allowed specific adsorption and removal of effector cells in Figure 14-2. The second step in cytolysis is the so-called lytic programming step, which sets in motion the lytic sequence directed against the target cell. The final step in the reaction is the dissolution of the target cell.

The binding of effector cells to target cells (conjugation), unlike the binding of alloantibody to target cells, is inhibited at low temperatures. It is also inhibited by treating the effector cells with a variety of agents that interfere with energy metabo-

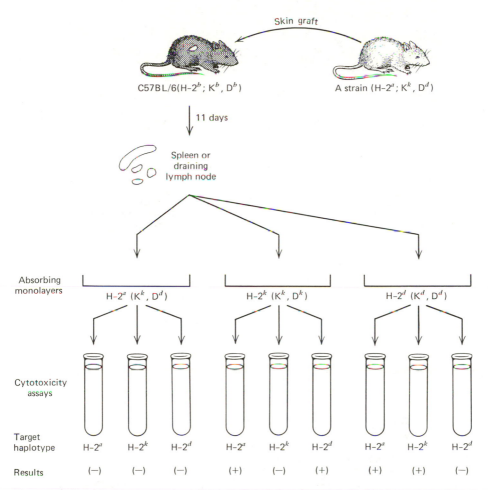

Figure 14-2 Evidence that H-2K and D target antigens are recognized by separate effector cell populations. The H-2^b mouse, when grafted with cells from the H-2^d mouse, produces cytotoxic T cells that can kill target cells bearing either or both K^k or D^d. These effector cells can be absorbed on cell monolayers of various surface phenotypes. If the effector cells recognize surface antigens on the absorbing cells, they will bind to them very tightly. The cells that do not adhere to the monolayer will then be depleted of cells recognizing monolayer antigens. When effector cells were absorbed on an H-2^a monolayer, the nonadhering cells were unable to lyse any of the target cells in the cytotoxicity assay, as would be expected. However, when the effector cells were absorbed on either H-2^k or h-2^a monolayers, the nonadherent cells were able to lyse target cells syngeneic to the opposite monolayer, or H-2^a target cells. This result can only be explained on the basis of two general populations of effector cells, one recognizing K^k, and one recognizing D^d.

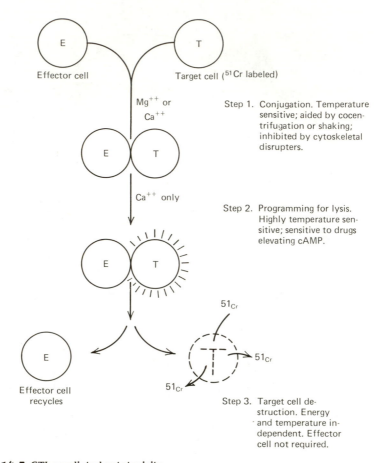

Figure 14-3 CTL-mediated cytotoxicity.

lism or cytoskeletal elements. Thus binding seems to be a process requiring an active, motile cell. Specific interactions of effector and target cells are supported by divalent cations (either Mg^{2+} or, to a lesser extent, Ca^{2+}), and effector–target interactions can be disrupted or prevented by cation-chelating agents. The binding of effectors to targets can be visualized microscopically. If the target cells are in suspension (as opposed to monolayer), individual effector–target complexes, or "conjugates," can be directly quantitated.

The existence of a discrete lytic programming step was first inferred from the fact that disruption of conjugates immediately after formation, and up to 5 to 10 minutes later prevents subsequent lysis of the target cell. Disruption of the conjugates after this time has no inhibitory effect on target cytolysis. Moreover, whereas conjugation occurs best in the presence of Mg^{2+}, the lytic programming step can only be supported by Ca^{2+}. Programming is even more sensitive to temperature than conjugation, suggesting that it may be more energy dependent. This step is also very sensitive to drugs that elevate intracellular cAMP. Such drugs have no effect on conjugation.

The final stage of cytolysis is independent of effector cells, and within most standard conditions used to assay cytotoxicity, independent of temperature and energy. Most available evidence suggests that the lethal event involves permeability changes induced in the target cell membrane as a result of the lytic programming event. Water can diffuse rapidly into the cell after formation of even small lesions, leading to an osmotic imbalance. Early in this stage, only small molecules escape from the target cell into the surrounding medium. As the process continues, larger and larger molecules and molecular complexes leave the cell, suggesting a progressive deterioration of the target cell membrane.

After completion of target cell programming, the CTL can detach and bind to a new target cell, starting the cycle over again. CTLs can recycle many times, as shown by the fact that CTLs mixed with target cells at ratios as low as 1:10 can kill 100 percent of the target cells.

Polarity of Lysis

An important experiment that provides additional information about the relationship of conjugation and lysis was carried out by Golstein in 1974 (Figure 14-4). When A anti-B cytotoxic T lymphocytes (CTL) are incubated with B anti-C CTL as target cells, only the B anti-C CTL is killed. This simple but elegant experiment tells us several important things about CTL-mediated killing. First of all, it tells us that CTL are themselves susceptible to CTL killing. Therefore, mechanisms postulating release of cytotoxic molecules by CTL during killing (see following section) must explain how CTL themselves would escape lysis. Second, this experiment tells us that conjugation per se is not sufficient for lysis. Clearly, the B anti-C CTL was conjugated to the A anti-B CTL in a lytically relevant way, because it was itself lysed. Yet the perfectly cytotoxic B anti-C CTL did not affect the A anti-B CTL. Thus there is

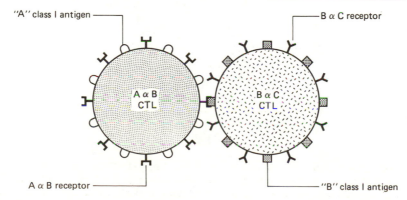

"A" class I antigen ⎯   ⎯ B α C receptor

A α B
CTL

B α C
CTL

A α B receptor ⎯   ⎯ "B" class I antigen

Figure 14-4 The polarity-of-lysis experiment. Only the BαC CTL is killed. Any model to explain killing by CTLs must ultimately explain how the AαB CTL escapes lysis.

a polarity in the lytic event; lysis can only occur in the direction CTL receptor →
class I MHC molecule. This observation has been taken by some to mean that the
lytic apparatus of the CTL is only activated when its MHC receptor is occupied.
Another possibility currently being explored is that the target cell class I MHC
antigen is itself involved in delivery of the lethal hit.

The "Innocent Bystander" Experiment

One of the earliest models for how CTLs kill their target cells envisioned release
of soluble cytotoxic factors, called cytotoxins or lymphotoxins, by the CTL. However, a crucial experiment called the "innocent bystander" experiment (Figure 14-5)
placed sharp restrictions on such a mechanism. CTLs were mixed together with
their specific targets, which they are able to kill with great efficiency. The specific
target cells were not labeled with ^{51}Cr. Third-party target cells, unrelated to the
targets for which the CTLs were specific, were labeled with ^{51}Cr and introduced
into the same assay mixture. When all three cells were cocentrifuged and incubated
at 37° for the usual assay period, the rate of ^{51}Cr release from the third-party cells
was found to be the same (essentially background level) whether the CTL-specific
targets were included in the assay or not.

This experiment eliminates a generalized release of cytotoxic molecules by the

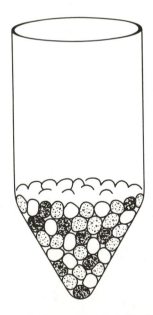

Figure 14-5 The "innocent bystander" experiment. AαB CTL (○) are mixed together with
unlabeled B (◉) and ^{51}Cr-labeled C (●) target cells. Although the B target cells are killed,
no ^{51}Cr is released into the overlying culture medium, indicating that the C targets (the
"innocent bystanders") are not damaged during the reaction leading to lysis of B target
cells.

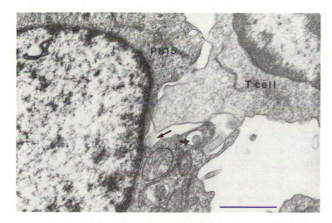

Figure 14-6 Electron micrograph of a CTL-target cell conjugate. The target cell is a P815 mastocytoma of DBA/2 origin. One large CTL projection extends to the nuclear envelope of the target cell; note the close contact between the tip of the projection and the indented target cell plasma membrane overlying the nucleus (straight arrow). A second projection is seen in cross section (curved arrow). Bar = 1 μm. [From C. J. Sanderson and A. M. Glauert, *Immunology 36*, 119 (1979).]

CTL on conjugation with its specific target cell. It can still be argued that cytotoxic molecules are released only into the intercellular spaces at the CTL–target cell conjugation interface. This would explain the innocent bystander effect. However, we are still left with the problem of polarity of lysis. We know that CTLs are susceptible, as target cells, to whatever mechanism CTLs use to kill. Yet, CTLs are themselves not harmed in the lytic reaction, as demonstrated by their ability to recycle through many rounds of target cell killing. If the lytic mechanism involved soluble molecules released into the tightly confined spaces between the CTL and target cell membranes, it is difficult to imagine how the CTLs themselves would escape unharmed.

Current speculations about the lytic mechanism in CMC fall into three general categories.

Mechanical Models.   Both the CTL and target cell partners in a tightly formed conjugate are viable, motile cells with actively flowing membranes. The membranes of the two cells are extensively interdigitated (Figure 14-6). It may simply be that attempts to escape from conjugation result in physical disruption of target cell membranes, whereas CTL membranes may be specially constructed to resist such damage. Highly active target cells (tumor cells, macrophages, etc.) are much more sensitive to CMC than cells that grow in monolayers.

It has also been suggested that cellular processes from the CTL, which have been observed to penetrate deeply into the target cell (Figure 14-6), disrupt organelle systems of the target, leading to eventual target cell death. Another version of a mechanical model suggests that CTL receptors distort target cell class I MHC antigens in the regions of membrane interaction, causing leakage of ions and water at the interface between MHC proteins and surrounding membrane lipids.

Secretion Models. It has also been suggested, on the basis of electron microscopic examination, that granules similar to lysosomal granules exist in lytic cells and tend to localize at the effector cell–target cell conjugation boundary. The granules could contain hydrolytic enzymes or other potentially lytic substances that are exocytosed into the open spaces at the conjugate interface. In support of this idea is the observation that after conjugation there is a reorientation of cytoplasmic organelles possibly involved in secretion in the CTL, but not in the target cell. Such models must, of course, postulate that the effector cells themselves are resistant to attack by the lytic agents. Such a mechanism is almost certainly operative in macrophage-mediated lysis, and in NK cell-mediated lysis (see below).

Membrane Insertion Models. Although it has not been possible to demonstrate a role for complement per se in CMC, insertion of amphiphilic molecules or channel-forming structures of some sort into target cell membranes remains an attractive possibility. Podack and Dennert have recently identified lesions in target cells after CTL attack that look intriguingly like the membrane attack complex lesions caused by complement. As with secretion models, some sort of mechanism must be postulated to explain unidirectionality of killing.

CTL Surface Molecules Involved in CMC

Recent studies in several laboratories using monoclonal antibodies against CTL surface components have identified molecules potentially involved in various of the defined cytolytic steps. One of the first cell surface structures so implicated was the Lyt-2 molecule. Antibodies to Lyt-2 were shown in 1979 to block CTL killing of target cells *in vitro*. Target cells not themselves bearing Lyt-2 were chosen, making it clear that the antibodies were blocking at the level of the CTL. Blocking was shown to occur at the recognition rather than lytic programming stage of cytolysis. This raised hopes that the Lyt-2 antigen might be associated with the CTL receptor. However, the action of Lyt-2 antibodies on CTL function is quite variable. Some CTL are affected at only very high concentrations of Lyt-2 antibody, whereas others are highly sensitive to anti-Lyt-2. Sensitivity to blocking correlates with cytolytic activity of the CTL only in the sense that the most active CTL are least sensitive to Lyt-2 antibody. Moreover, several cloned CTL lines have now been developed that lack detectable Lyt-2, and whose lytic function is not blocked by Lyt-2 antibody at any concentration. Thus Lyt-2 is not involved in an obligatory fashion in CTL lysis. Current speculation about the function of Lyt-2 centers on its possible role in stabilizing CTL-target cell interactions, particularly when the CTL receptor may have a low affinity for target cell antigens.

A second CTL cell surface possibly involved in lysis was described in a similar fashion by Tim Springer and Eric Martz. A rat antimouse CTL antibody was developed that reacts with a CTL structure termed lymphocyte function-associated antigen (LFA-1). The LFA-1 antigen is associated with a molecule composed of 94,000-

and 180,000-dalton subunits. The LFA-1 molecule is not restricted to CTL, but is found on a variety of other lymphoid cells as well. In addition to blocking lysis by CTL, LFA-1 antibodies also block proliferation of T cells in response to antigen. Like Lyt-2 antibodies, LFA-1 antibodies block conjugation rather than the lethal hit, and LFA-1 is also thus thought to promote cell-cell adhesion.

Antibodies to a wide range of other CTL surface molecules such as Thy-1, Qa, H-2K or D, β-2m, etc. have no affect on lysis. Although blocking of both the Lyt-2 and LFA-1 antigens has a strong inhibitory effect on CTL lytic function in most cases, neither one seems likely to represent recognition or lytic molecules. Nevertheless, elucidation of their functions in the lytic sequence will likely shed additional light on the mechanism of CMC, and the search for additional surface molecules involved in CTL lysis continues.

Cloned CTL Lines

One of the major difficulties in studying the mechanism of lysis by CTL has been that the frequency of CTL in most immune populations is not more than 5 to 10 percent at best. Studies of CTL at the biochemical level in such populations are not practical, because 90 to 95 percent of the cells one would be studying would be irrelevant. The same difficulty inhibited for many years study of the molecular nature of the T-cell receptor. This problem is similar to the one faced by researchers who wanted to use homogeneous populations of specific antibodies in their experiments but had only heterogeneous antibody populations from immune serum. The solution to that problem, as we saw in Chapter 4, was the development of hybridoma cell lines that secrete monoclonal antibody. The cellular immunologists have adopted a similar approach, and have developed a number of CTL hybridomas and cloned CTL lines. In these lines, all of the CTL are derived from a single CTL precursor. They are thus identical in terms of both receptor and lytic apparatus.

There are two strategies for developing continuously growing CTL lines: direct cloning of activated CTL and formation of hybridomas. In the latter case, the strategy is the same as that used by the developers of monoclonal antibody-producing cell lines. Populations enriched for CTL are first fused with a T-cell tumor line. Hybrid progeny are selected on HAT medium as described in Chapter 4 for antibody-producing hybrids. The surviving, proliferating hybridomas are then screened for cytotoxic function and subcloned repeatedly by limiting dilution to ensure monoclonality. Although seemingly a straightforward procedure, in fact, after five years only a few laboratories have reported success. The CTL hybridomas that have been generated in most cases have slightly anomalous properties, and, in general, attempts to generate continuously growing CTL lines by this method are falling off.

The technique for direct cloning of CTL into continuously growing lines is illustrated in Figure 14-7. Spleens from alloimmunized mice are restimulated with specific antigen *in vitro*. The frequency of active CTL in such secondary cultures is

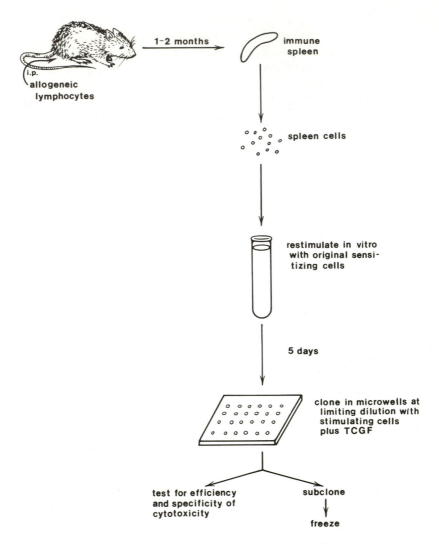

Figure 14-7 Cloning of cytotoxic T lymphocytes. See text for details.

considerably higher than in primary cultures (starting with an unimmunized spleen). At the peak of the secondary reaction (four to six days), the cultures are plated out in microwells with an excess of irradiated stimulating cells, and T-cell growth factor (TCGF). TCGF, the crucial component of which is probably IL-2, can be generated in a number of ways. It is found in the supernate of allogeneic MLC reactions (see following sections), or in the supernate of mitogen-stimulated T-lymphocyte cultures. It can also be secreted by a number of cell lines on appropriate stimulation. The latter often provide a more reproducible source of TCGF than random, *de novo* generated T-cell reactions.

Positive wells from the first culture are subcultured with antigen and TCGF at a sufficiently low density ($<$ 0.3 cells/microwell) to ensure that any positive wells in the second culture derive from single-cell precursors. Additional subclonings may be carried out to provide further assurance of monoclonality.

Generation of Cytotoxic T Cells *in Vitro:* The Mixed Leukocyte Culture (MLC) Reaction

A detailed study of CTL-mediated cytotoxicity *in vivo* is complicated by a number of factors. An intact, living organism is a delicate balance of a large number of interacting systems, and any attempt to alter one system (graft rejection, for example) can have effects on other systems that may affect the system under study in ways not fully understood. Furthermore, a healthy animal may have a number of immune reactions proceedings in parallel with an ongoing graft reaction and often within the same lymph tissues. Thus it is difficult *in vivo* to isolate or even identify just those cells involved in the rejection reaction. It is also difficult to make any sort of quantitative measurements *in vivo* without seriously disrupting the system. Thus most of our detailed knowledge of cellular mechanisms in allograft reactions has come from experiments carried out *in vitro* in the mixed leukocyte culture (MLC) reaction.

MLC reactions occur when two genetically distinct populations of lymphocytes are cultured together under appropriate *in vitro* conditions. If the populations are mutually allogeneic at one or more class II loci, they will each undergo a proliferative reaction. Ordinarily, the reaction is made "one way" so that one population responds, whereas the other serves the apparently passive role of stimulator. One way MLC reactions are achieved is in parent–F_1 combinations, or when one population has been irradiated. As in allograft reactions *in vivo,* the responding cells are various T-lymphocyte clones recognizing appropriate alloantigens on the stimulating cell membranes. Macrophages and dendritic cells provide good stimulation in an MLC, probably because of the presence on their surfaces of class II antigens and their ability to provide needed soluble factors.

The sequence of events in the responding cell at the biochemical and cellular levels is shown in Figure 14-8. Within an hour of mixing responding and stimulating cells together, there is a dramatic increase in RNA (principally rRNA) synthesis, followed very shortly by a rapid rise in the rate of protein synthesis. At about 15 hours the responding cells begin to enlarge in size as they make the transition from the typical resting T-cell diameter of 5 to 6 nm to the "blast" cell diameter of 10 to 12 nm or more. At about 18 hours, DNA synthesis can be detected, and the first mitotic figures are evident between 24 and 30 hours.

Proliferation of responding cells alone, of course, would seem an unlikely basis for allograft rejection. The observation mentioned in an earlier section of this chapter—that cytotoxic lymphocytes could be found in the lymph nodes draining the site of an allograft—stimulated a search for conditions under which cytotoxic lymphocytes could be generated *in vitro*. Ginsburg and his colleagues in Israel

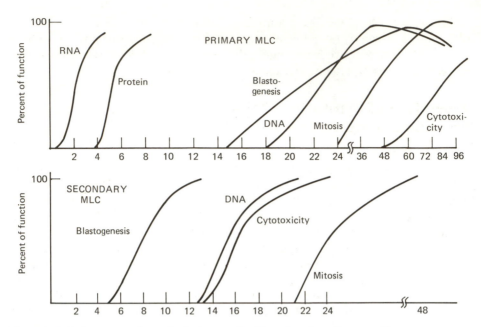

Figure 14-8 Sequence of events during a mixed lymphocyte culture reaction.

were among the first to describe the production of "killer" lymphocytes *in vitro,* using a system in which rat lymphocytes were sensitized by culture on mouse fibroblast monolayers. The cytotoxic cells generated in this manner were reasonably specific for the sensitizing mouse strain, and subsequent work showed that when such sensitized lymphocytes were injected back into a syngeneic rat, the rat would specifically reject skin grafts of the sensitizing mouse strain in an enhanced manner.

The first reports of successful generation of cytotoxicity in allogeneic mouse MLC reactions came from two labs in 1970. Both labs used ^{51}Cr release from allogeneic target cells to measure cytotoxicity and demonstrated a high degree of target cell discrimination: Only target cells bearing the class I product(s) of the sensitizing cells were killed by MLC-sensitized CTL. These results opened the way for a wide range of investigations into the nature of the generation of cytotoxicity against alloantigens *in vitro.* As in so many other areas of immunological investigation, these studies were greatly enhanced by the availability of large numbers of inbred congenic and recombinant strains of mice.

The relationship between proliferation and cytotoxicity in an MLC is shown in Figure 14-8. In most MLC systems, the appearance of cytotoxic lymphocytes in the cultures is preceded in time by a wave of DNA synthesis and cell division. A number of experiments have shown that the wave of cell proliferation is required for full development of cytotoxicity. If proliferation is prevented by appropriate drugs, or if the cells proliferating in the early stages of the MLC are killed by various treatments, the generation of cytotoxicity is drastically reduced. However, this reduction is antigen specific: Bach and his co-workers showed in both mice and humans that if the cell proliferating in response to one set of alloantigens is selectively killed with BUdr and light, both a proliferative and cytotoxic response can still be mounted by the surviving cells against another set of alloantigens, unrelated to the first.

As stated earlier, the responding cells in MLC reactions are T cells. With the report of distinct T-cell subpopulations in the mouse bearing different Ly antigens, it became of interest to determine whether Lyt-2$^-$ or Lyt-2$^+$ cells, or both, were responding to the alloantigens *in vitro*. It was found that in fact *both* T-cell popula- tions are involved in the development of a full MLC response. In the course of a normal, fully allogeneic mouse MLC reaction, the Lyt-2$^-$ T cell responds to class II MHC determinants present on macrophages and B lymphocytes, undergoes a pro- liferative response, but does not develop into a cytotoxic cell. The Lyt-2$^+$ cells respond to class I antigens and develop into cytotoxic effector cells. The way in which these two populations interact is shown in Figure 14-9.

The first step in activation involves the interaction of a resting T helper cell (Lyt-2$^-$ in the mouse; T4$^+$ in humans) with an allogeneic macrophage or dendritic cell. The T$_h$ cell recognizes the macrophage or dendritic stimulating cell through interaction of its T-cell receptor with the stimulating cell class II antigen. This step is very similar to the first step in T helper activation in the humoral response (p. 333). It seems likely, in fact, that the same pool of helper cells can function in both reactions. However in the case of allogeneic reaction, the T$_h$ cell recognizes the allogeneic class II molecule alone, without nominal antigen. As in the case of the humoral response, it seems likely that one result of this initial interaction is display by the T$_h$ cell of a receptor for IL-1. IL-1 must be supplied by the stimulating cell, and is necessary for T$_h$ cell activation. That is why only certain class II antigen- bearing cells can serve as stimulating cells in primary allogeneic reactions.

In parallel with activation of the T$_h$ cell by class II antigens and IL-1, the pre-CTL begins its activation sequence by interacting with a class I antigen. Pre-T helper cells can receive their class II signal only from cells that are also able to provide necessary factors such as IL-1. Pre-CTLs, on the other hand, can take their first signal from any cell bearing the class I antigen for which they are specific. That is because their second signal (IL-2) comes not from the class I-bearing cell, but from con- comitantly activated T helper cells. The sequence of events in pre-CTL activation has been studied particularly closely by many laboratories. Interaction of the pre- CTL with an appropriate class I signal alone is insufficient to cause expression of cytotoxic function. However, within four to six hours after receiving signal I, the pre-CTLs express the IL-2 receptor. If no IL-2 is available, the cells eventually revert to the resting, IL-2 receptorless state. If IL-2 is supplied, the pre-CTL proliferate and mature into fully functional CTL. At some point during the maturation procedure, the CTLs also make and secrete IL-2 as well as a spectrum of other lymphokines, notably the interferons.

In secondary CTL reactions, an oligatory role for Lyt-2$^-$ cells, responding to class II antigens, is less clear. Minami and Shreffler have reported that class II-

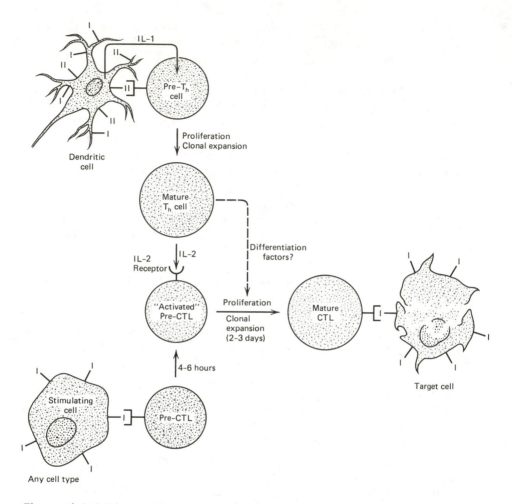

Figure 14-9 Cell interactions in the generation of cytotoxic T lymphocytes. A resting pre-CTL needs at least two signals to become functionally mature. Signal 1 is provided by the interaction of the pre-CTL's antigen receptor with a class I antigen on an allogeneic cell. As a result of this step, the pre-CTL becomes "activated," and expresses receptors for IL-2. However, the activated CTL is probably not cytotoxic at this stage, unless it is provided with a source of IL-2. This is normally provided by a nearby T helper cell, which is activated to produce IL-2 by interaction with a class II-bearing, IL-1 producing allogeneic cell, most likely a dendritic cell (cf. Figure 13-7). When the activated pre-CTL receives IL-2, it divides and matures into a fully cytotoxic cell, possibly under the influence of additional factors provided by the T_h cell. The mature CTL can then attack and destroy cells bearing the same class I antigens as the original stimulating cell.

bearing stimulator cells are not required in secondary MLC reactions. As we have seen, Lyt-2$^+$ CTL can be cloned and maintained as lines in the absence of Lyt-2$^-$ amplifier cells, provided that IL-2 is added to the cultures. IL-2 is thought normally to be provided by Lyt-2$^-$ cells, but it has been reported to be produced by Lyt-2$^+$ cells as well. It may be that in some instances primed Lyt-2$^+$ cells, on restimulation by appropriate class I MHC antigens, will produce sufficient IL-2 to promote their own growth. In most cases, however, even secondary responses will benefit from additional IL-2. Thus whereas Lyt-2$^-$ cells appear to be absolutely essential in primary MLC reactions, they are much less crucial, and in perhaps some cases superfluous, in secondary reactions.

The MLC reaction in other species seems to take place under much the same conditions, and with the same overall features, as the mouse reaction. In humans, the HLA-D locus provides the principal equivalent of I-region proliferation-stimulating loci in the mouse. The proteins coded for by the HLA-A, B, and C genes appear to be the major target antigens for cytotoxic effector cells.

The MLC reaction poses a fundamental and puzzling question related to clonal selection in the case of allograft reactions. Several investigators noted that the proportion of lymphocytes reacting to a given alloantigenic stimulus could be as high as 2 to 3 percent. This would imply that the repertoire of receptors involved in such reactions could accommodate no more than 30 to 50 or so different types of antigens. A similar observation was made many years ago by Simonsen in the GVH reaction. Given that these estimates were based on whole lymphocyte populations, only a fraction of which are T cells, and only a subfraction of which are immuno-logically virgin T cells of the appropriate phenotype, the fraction of responding cells is likely even higher.

A definitive solution of this paradox has not been developed, but it is a fact that certainly must be accounted for in any general theory of allograft immunity. The most likely explanation is that the CTL repertoire is a permutation of self-MHC recognition (Chapter 15). Thus it may not be surprising that 10 percent or so of CTL respond to a given allogeneic MHC, which as we saw in Chapter 9 is only a slightly altered form of self.

MHC Restriction of Cell-mediated Cytotoxicity (CMC)

In Chapter 13 we saw that the interaction of T_h cells with B cells and macrophages is MHC restricted. This same phenomenon is also seen in both the generation and expression of CTL function.

There have been two major systems used in the investigation of MHC re-strictions of cytotoxic interactions. In the first system, self-cells are altered by viral infection, which results in the expression of viral antigens on the surface of the infected cells. In the second system, self-cells are altered by direct chemical deri-vatization of existing cell surface molecules. In both cases, the altered cells are capable of triggering a reaction that leads to expansion of T helper cells, and

Table 14-1 Lysis of Normal and Virally Infected Target Cells by Immune Spleen Cells

Infected mouse strain used as effector cell source	Percent ^{51}Cr released from normal and infected target cells							
	H-2^k		H-2^d		(H-2^k × H-2^d) F$_1$		H-2^a	
	Infec.	Nor.	Infec.	Nor.	Infec.	Nor.	Infec.	Nor.
H-2^k	29.6	0.8	0	1.8	20.4	0.6	21.2	0
H-2^d	1.2	0.3	31.4	0	34.8	0	35.7	0
(H-2^k × H-2^d) F$_1$	23.0	0.5	36.6	2.1	37.3	0	—	—
H-2^a	21.5	1.2	24.0	0	24.2	2.1	37.3	0

Adapted from R. M. Zinkernagel and P. C. Doherty, H-2 compatibility requirement for T cell-mediated lysis of target cells infected with lymphocytic choriomeningitis virus. *J. Exp. Med. 141* (1975), p. 1427.

production of CTL specific for self class I antigens plus the nominal (viral or chemical) antigen.

Viral Modification of Self-Cells

The original observations in this system were made by Zinkernagel and Doherty, who were looking at the role of CMC in detection and destruction of virally infected self-cells. Their results are typified by the data in Table 14-1. Adult mice infected with lymphocytic choriomeningitis virus (LCV) develop cytotoxic T lymphocytes that will kill self- (or MHC syngeneic) target cells infected with the same virus.[1] The CTLs will not kill uninfected syngeneic cells, but more interestingly they also will not kill (or will kill only poorly) allogeneic target cells infected with and expressing antigens of the same sensitizing virus. On the other hand (data not shown here) they *will* kill virus-infected target cells from other inbred strains of mice bearing the same H-2 haplotype. Subsequent analysis using congenic and intra-H-2 recombinant strains showed that the regions of H-2 at which syngeneity was required are the K and/or D regions (Table 14-2). Syngeneity between sensitizing and target cells at I-region loci is neither necessary nor sufficient to allow cytolysis. We know from subsequent studies that the relevant K- and D-region gene products are the class I MHC proteins. The same phenomenon has been reproduced with other viruses and with a wide range of H-2 haplotypes.

Chemical Modification of Self-Cells

At about the time that Zinkernagel and Doherty were reporting their observations on cytolysis of virally infected cells, Shearer and his colleagues at NIH were

[1]This is, in fact, the cause of death in mice infected with LCV. Long before the virus itself can harm the host, nerve cells infected with T$_h$ virus are vigorously attacked and killed by the host's own immune system, resulting in death of the host.

Table 14-2 Effect of Various H-2 Region Compatibilities on Lysis of Infected Target Cell Monolayers

Virus systems	Immune spleen		Percent ^{51}Cr release from macrophages		
	Strain	H-2 type	SJL *sssss*	BALB/c *dddddd*	CBA/H *kkkkkk*
LCM	A.TL	*skkkkd*	25	64	1
	CBA/H	*kkkkkk*	2	1	34
	A/J	*kkkddd*	0	64	30
Ectromelia	A.TL	*skkkkd*	32	47	0
	CBA/H	*kkkkkk*	0	15	43
Sendai	A.TL	*skkkkd*	63	24	4
	A.TH	*sssssd*	63	59	3
	A/J	*kkkddd*	3	65	49

Taken from P. C. Doherty et al. Specificity of virus-immune effector T cells for H-2K or H-2D compatible interactions: implications for H-antigen diversity. *Transplant. Rev.* 29 (1976), pp. 89–124. Copyright © by P. C. Doherty (1976).

carrying out experiments in which they chemically attached defined haptens to the surface of cells. They tested whether these cells could be used to generate effector cells with some measure of specificity for hapten. Data typical of their original observations are shown in Table 14-3. Sensitization against TNP-modified syngeneic cells is carried out under more-or-less standard MLC conditions and results in the generation of effector cells that will lyse TNP-modified syngeneic target cells. These effectors will not lyse unmodified self-targets, or TNP-modified H-2 allogeneic targets, but they will lyse TNP-modified target cells syngeneic at H-2K. (Using other haptens, or other reacting haplotypes, the syngeneity required for target cytolysis may be at either K or D). As with virally modified syngeneic cells, syngeneity at H-2I is neither necessary nor sufficient for target cell lysis; the gene products involved are class I MHC proteins.

Dual Recognition or Modified Self?

The data from viral and hapten altered cell systems just described brought into focus an important fact about cytotoxic T cells. In order to interact with a foreign antigen on a cell surface, it is not sufficient for the T cell to "see" just the foreign antigens: it must also be able to interact with a surface-bound class I MHC molecule. These data have been interpreted as satisfying either of two possible models, as shown in Figure 14-10. In one model (modified self) the histocompatibility antigen is thought to be somehow modified by the viral antigen or chemical hapten, perhaps through simple physical association. The responding T cell now

Table 14-3 *In Vitro* Induction of Cytotoxicity of B10.BR Spleen Cells to TNP-modified Autologous Spleen Cells Assayed with TNP-modified Syngeneic, Congenic, Allogeneic, or Recombinant Spleen Target Cells

Responding cells	Stimulating cells	Target cells	Specific lysis (%) ± SE	Target cell H-2 region common to responding and stimulating cells
B10.BR *kkkkkk*	B10.BR–TNP *kkkkkk*	B10.BR *kkkkkk*	−4.0 ± 1.9	All of H-2
B10.BR *kkkkkk*	B10.BR–TNP *kkkkkk*	B10.BR–TNP *kkkkkk*	33.2 ± 3.0	All of H-2
B10.BR *kkkkkk*	B10.BR–TNP *kkkkkk*	B10.A–TNP *kkkddd*	31.5 ± 2.5	K,I-A,I-B
B10.BR *kkkkkk*	B10.BR–TNP *kkkkkk*	B10.A(2R)–TNP *kkkddb*	26.9 ± 2.2	K,I-A,I-B
B10.BR *kkkkkk*	B10.BR–TNP *kkkkkk*	C3H.OH–TNP *dddddk*	2.1 ± 2.1	D
B10.BR *kkkkkk*	B10.BR–TNP *kkkkkk*	A.TL–TNP *skkkkd*	−2.2 ± 2.2	I-A,I-B,I-C,S
B10.BR *kkkkkk*	B10.BR–TNP *kkkkkk*	A.TH–TNP *sssssd*	−0.4 ± 1.3	None
B10.BR *kkkkkk*	B10.BR–TNP *kkkkkk*	SJL–TNP *ssssss*	−0.7 ± 1.2	None
B10.BR *kkkkkk*	B10.BR–TNP *kkkkkk*	B10.D2–TNP *dddddd*	−2.2 ± 2.4	None

Taken from G. Shearer, T. Rehn, and C. Garbarino, Cell-mediated lysis of TNP-modified autologous lymphocytes. *J. Exp. Med. 141* (1975), p. 1348. Reproduced by permission of the Rockefeller University Press.

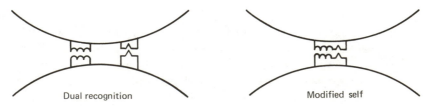

Figure 14-10 Dual recognition and modified self-models of MHC restriction of syngeneic CMC.

sees the originally syngeneic and ordinarily unrecognized (in terms of triggering a cytotoxic response) class I protein as nonself. A clone (or clones) of effector cell precursors is triggered, which has cell surface receptors recognizing the entire ligand–class I molecule complex. In the second model (dual recognition), the clone of effector cells elicited recognizes and attacks the target cells through two receptors: one recognizing self-class I antigens and facilitating cell–cell interaction but not triggering cytolysis and a second receptor specific for hapten or viral antigen, which cannot interact with the latter determinants in the absence of class I MHC syngeneity between effector and target, but which, once reacted with, permits cytolysis to proceed.

In the few years that have elapsed since the original data in the viral and hapten systems were reported, a large number of experiments have been carried out to distinguish between the dual recognition and modified self-models. Some of these experiments are ingenious in design, and taken by themselves would argue strongly in favor of one model or the other. Unfortunately, about an equal number of such experiments has been put forward on behalf of either model, and it is still not possible to decide between them. On a purely conceptual level, each has serious drawbacks. Dual recognition seems an exceptionally cumbersome mechanism and implies that at least the recognition phase in CMC of allogeneic and syngeneic target cells must proceed through separate mechanisms. (Obviously, recognition of a true self-MHC antigen does not occur in allogeneic CMC.) We also know that lymphocytes of the cytotoxic T-cell subclass do not per se make stable complexes with syngeneic target cells; thus a function for the putative "self"-receptor in dual recognition, as a stabilizer to allow interaction of the foreign ligand with its receptor, seems unlikely. The modified self-model is also troublesome. It is difficult to imagine how such a large array of different antigens—more than a dozen viral antigens so far, and a whole host of haptenic groups—could all be chemically linked to the same K or D protein. This is certainly the major weakness of the modified self-theory: How, in fact, is the modification carried out?

As was discussed in Chapter 12, and as will be discussed again in Chapter 15, current evidence suggests there is only a single T-cell receptor that recognizes self MHC plus nominal antigens. However, we still do not know how the structural information gleaned so far about the T-cell receptor relates to T-cell biology. Therefore, the question of just how CTLs and T helper cells perceive both MHC and nominal antigen must remain unresolved for now.

Natural Killer (NK) Cells

In the early 1970s researchers studying the cell-mediated immune response to syngeneic tumors in humans and in mice made a startling discovery. Lymphocytes from tumor-bearing patients or animals could often be shown to display modest levels of cytotoxicity toward their own tumor cells *in vitro*. As controls, investigators used lymphocytes from non-tumor-bearing individuals. In many cases the "control" lymphocytes displayed as much or more cytotoxicity toward the tumor targets as did lymphocytes from tumor-free individuals. Moreover, lymphocytes from a patient or mouse with one type of tumor were usually equally cytotoxic toward totally unrelated tumors, to which the original host had not been sensitized. There was an initial tendency to overlook some of these embarrassing controls, but soon the controls themselves became the primary object of study. It was quickly established that normal, healthy individuals have a special subpopulation of lymphocytes which, without any prior sensitization, will recognize, attack, and destroy a wide range of tumor cells. These cells have come to be called natural killer (NK) cells (see also Chapter 20). Because they seem to function efficiently with no prior exposure to their targets, and in the absence of antibody or complement, they are often categorized as a form of natural, as opposed to acquired, immunity.

The exact identity of the effector cell has been controversial since NK cell-mediated cytotoxicity (NKCC) was first described. NK cells are found principally in the peripheral circulation and in the spleen, are present in low levels in the lymph nodes and bone marrow, and are virtually absent from the thymus. NK cells are now thought to be lymphocytes, and have been estimated to be 1 to 2 percent of the total lymphocyte pool. They belong to the so-called null subclass of lymphocytes, displaying neither T- or B-cell antigens. They appear at about three weeks postpartum in the rat, and develop in the absence of a thymus.

Recently, a subset of null lymphocytes in humans, the so-called "large granular lymphocytes (LGL)" has been identified morphologically, and appears to contain, or to be identical with, the NK cell. The origins of LGL, and their relation to T cells, are unclear at present. However, Colin Brooks has recently shown that cloned CTL can be converted to NK-like cells by growing them in the presence of high concentrations of IL-2. There is a good deal of other indirect evidence for a lineal relationship between CTLs and NK cells. In mice, NK cells belong to the subclass of lymphocytes bearing the Ly-5 antigen, which can be used to positively select for NK effector cells. NK cell-specific antigens, termed NK-1 and NK-2, have also been described.

A useful animal model for the study of NK cells, and their relation to other immune functions and to virally and oncologically transformed cells, is the beige mouse. "Beige" is an autosomal recessive mutation (bg) such that bg/bg mice are phenotypically abnormal, whereas bg/+ mice are indistinguishable from normals. Bg/bg mice have normal T-cell, B-cell, macrophage, and granulocyte compartments but virtually no NK function. This condition mirrors almost exactly a rare condition in humans called Chediak-Higashi syndrome. Beige mice are more susceptible to viral infection, and to most transplantable syngeneic tumors, than are their normal counterparts. Interestingly, tumors that display resistance to attack by NK cells *in vitro* grow equally well in beige mice and normal mice. Studies in beige mice suggest that NK cells may also be important for limiting tumor metastases.

Different strains of inbred mice have different levels of NK activity, and can be grouped into high-responder and low-responder strains. Breeding studies show this trait linked to H-2, although how closely is not yet apparent. When bone marrow from a high- or low-responder strain is matured in an irradiated high- or low-responder mouse, the resultant chimera has the NK properties of the marrow donor, suggesting that NK status is genetically determined rather than environmentally conditioned.

There is now quite good evidence, based largely on the work of Wright and Bonavida, that NK cells kill their targets via a soluble mediator called NK cytotoxic factor (NKCF). NKCF is produced by NK cells on stimulation either by an NK-sensitive tumor target cell, or by appropriate lectins such as Con A or PHA. NKCF will attack exactly the same spectrum of tumor targets that NK cells attack, and is absorbed only by NK sensitive targets. Murine fibroblast interferon, which stimulates NK activity, also enhances the synthesis and release of NKCF. On the other hand, the same interferon renders at least some NK targets resistant to NK lysis. This has been correlated with an inability of interferon treated targets to stimulate NKCF release. However, IFN-treated target cells can be killed by exogenously generated NKCF. The relation of NKCF to other toxic factors such as lymphotoxin and tumor necrosis factor (see Chapter 20) is currently being investigated.

K Cells and Antibody-dependent, Cell-mediated Cytotoxicity (ADCC)

A wide range of cells of the immune system, including lymphocytes, granulocytes, and monocytes, have on their surfaces a structure called an Fc receptor. The existence of this structure is inferred from, and operationally defined by, the ability of certain subpopulations of these cells to bind immunoglobulin, complexed to antigen, via the Fc portion of the Ig molecule. The antibody is usually IgG, and the antigen may be soluble or cellular in form. Since not all cells of any class bear the Fc receptor, its distribution within a class is often a useful marker for functional subpopulations.

When an appropriate cell of the immune system bearing an Fc receptor comes in contact with a target cell coated with antibody, the target cell can be lysed in a fashion that is at least grossly similar to direct T-cell-mediated cytolysis (see Figure 14-11). Details of the mechanism(s) of cytolysis in either case are, however, lacking. For some reason, ADCC, at least as measured in *in vitro* systems, seems to be more effective against xenogeneic cells than allogeneic cells. However, in mice and especially in humans, substantial allogeneic killing via ADCC can be demonstrated. At present, we have no hard information on the role of ADCC *in vivo,* but we do know, for example, that in human patients undergoing allograft rejection, both cells and antibodies are present in the circulation that are capable of mounting a vigorous ADCC reaction against allograft cells in an *in vitro* assay. Thus it is at least possible, and perhaps likely, that antibodies may participate in this manner during the normal course of a graft rejection reaction.

Among lymphocytes, there is a "null" subclass displaying neither T-cell nor B-

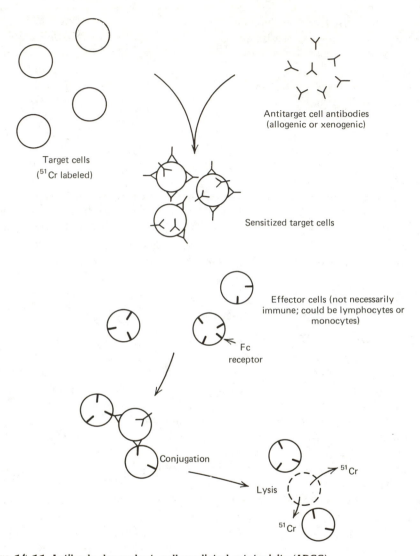

Figure 14-11 Antibody-dependent, cell-mediated cytotoxicity (ADCC).

cell surface markers (Thy-1 or sIg). Some of these are Fc receptor positive and very effective in mediating ADCC. These lymphocytes, which occur in all mammalian species examined, are called K cells. There is some evidence that they may be lineally related to T cells, in spite of the fact that they display no T-cell markers. It is also possible that they are related to NK cells. NK cells have Fc receptors but do not need antibody to kill their target cells. One interpretation of ADCC is that it represents antibody-facilitated killing by NK cells of otherwise NK-resistant targets. This hypothesis has not yet been rigorously tested.

Macrophages

Macrophages are not usually thought of as cytotoxic but, in fact, under some circumstances they can be. The mechanism of cytotoxicity involved in macrophage killing appears to be quite different from that used by CTLs and NK cells. However, because we know so little about the mechanism of killing in these latter cells, particularly CTLs, we cannot be sure that some degree of similarity does not exist.

The principal situation in which macrophages may be cytotoxic (as opposed to simply phagocytic) is in the defense against tumors (Chapter 20), and possibly in the defense against parasitically infected cells. One of the first to demonstrate macrophage cytotoxicity was John Hibbs and his colleagues. They observed that mice with chronic *Toxoplasma gondii* infections are unusually resistant to tumors. They later showed that macrophages from such mice are able to selectively attack and destroy tumor cells *in vitro* but do not harm normal cells. These observations opened a very active field of research—the study of "activated" macrophages. We now know that this altered state of the macrophage is the result of activation by T-cell lymphokines. Any immune episode resulting in the production of large quantities of lymphokines (particularly γ-interferon) may result in the activation of macrophages. Macrophages can also be activated directly by culturing in the presence of high levels of lymphokines. Precisely which lymphokines are involved is not clear, nor do we know at the molecular level what activation entails. It is also unknown how activated macrophages are able to distinguish tumor cells from normal cells.

Activated macrophages can kill target cells by two related mechanisms, one intracellular, the other extracellular. Intracellular killing is essentially the process of phagocytosis and intracellular lysosomal degradation reviewed in Chapter 16. Phagocytic damage to tumors has been demonstrated in many experimental situations, and there is good indirect evidence that such a mechanism is important *in vivo* as well. Phagocytic attack can be carried out by both activated and unactivated macrophages and is strongly promoted by opsonizing antibodies.

Killing tumor cells in the absence of phagocytosis (extracellular killing) probably proceeds at least in part through a process of exocytosis of lysosomes or their contents into the space between the macrophage and the tumor cell. Such exocytosis may be triggered by the inability of the macrophage to tear off or "swallow" tumor cells to which it is firmly bound, whether naturally or after opsonization. Lysosomal contents have been found deposited on the surface of artificial particles to which macrophages were induced to adhere. Lysosomal materials have also been found both on the surface of and in the cytoplasm of tumor cells undergoing macrophage attack both *in vivo* and *in vitro*. We know from a number of studies that purified lysosomal granules are highly toxic for almost any mammalian cell. Additional substances secreted by macrophages that may be involved in cytolysis, particularly of tumor cells, are discussed in Chapter 20.

Precisely how macrophage-secreted substances cause target cell death is unknown. Effects observed at the level of the target cell range from simple cytostasis and growth inhibition through nuclear disorganization and cell death. Whether any of the various steps in target cell degeneration that have been described in such great detail is a specific consequence of a particular macrophage product, or simply a manifestation of a generally sick cell about to die, is not really clear. However, a renewed interest in the possibility that CTLs may kill via a secretory mechanism is focusing renewed interest on the mechanism of extracellular killing by macrophages.

The Graft-versus-Host (GVH) Reaction

We have seen that when tissues such as skin are transplanted to an allogeneic, immunocompetent animal, rejection usually occurs within a short time, depending on the strength of the histocompatibility barrier. Lymphocytes injected into an allogeneic host will also be rejected in a vigorous manner. But suppose for a moment that the graft recipient is immunoincompetent. In the case of a skin graft, no particular complications will ensue: The graft vascularize, heal, and grow as though it were a normal component of self. But what if, in such a situation, the graft is of immunocompetent donor lymphoid cells? In this case, the cells will eventually find their way to the host lymphoid organs, where they will immediately find themselves surrounded by the largest graft they have ever encountered! Lymphoid cells, perhaps because of their high surface density of MHC antigens, present the allograft challenge in its most potent form, and this is the host milieu in which the vast majority of donor lymphocytes find themselves. The series of events following injection of competent allogeneic lymphocytes into an immunoincompetent recipient is called the graft-versus-host (GVH) reaction.

The GVH reaction has been studied in a number of experimental animal models, each of which has contributed something to our understanding of the GVH reaction itself, and quite often to our understanding of wider-ranging immunological questions. Yet little is known about the fundamental mechanisms underlying this extremely complex phenomenon. The complications arising from GVH reactions are a major barrier to bone marrow transplants in human patients (see section below), and thus a full elucidation of GVH mechanisms is of more than academic interest.

In the following sections, we first examine the various forms of GVH reactions studied in animal models and then try to piece together what is known about the cellular and molecular basis of this important and fascinating class of immunological reactions.

GVH Reactions in Newborn Mice

This form of the GVH reaction was one of the earliest to be studied, and takes advantage of the fact that newborn mice are immunologically incompetent for 24 to 48 hours after birth. Newborn mice are given a small intraperitoneal inoculum of allogeneic adult lymphocytes. A single litter forms the experimental unit; part of the litter is injected with syngeneic (host) lymphocytes as a control. A number of symptoms develop in the animals undergoing GVH, which distinguish them from the controls. One of the earliest symptoms is splenomegaly. The spleens of newborns injected with H-2 allogeneic lymphocytes undergo enlargement, which usually peaks at a week to 10 days. After this peak, spleen size (usually expressed as the spleen index: milligram spleen/gram body weight) may be highly variable and is not a good index of GVH disease. As we will discuss shortly, much of the spleen hypertrophy can be attributed to proliferation of host lymphoid elements. A similar sequence of events occurs in various regional lymph nodes, although quantitation is more difficult. Newborn mice undergoing GVH reactions will also develop diarrhea and fail to gain weight normally ("runt disease") or develop healthy fur. The time of appearance and severity of these symptoms depend on a number of factors, including the genetic disparity between graft and host, age of the host, and number of lymphocytes grafted. In a particularly strong reaction, all of the above symptoms develop in a compressed manner, and the hosts may die in two to three weeks.

GVH Reactions in Chickens

Symptoms similar to those produced in newborn mice may be produced in chickens, with the added advantage that the inoculating cells can be administered prior to hatching. Cells can be administered intravenously, through one of the many blood vessels associated with the extraembryonic membranes, or simply by placing the cells directly onto the chorioallantoic membrane itself. This latter method can be quantitated by scoring for nodules or "pocks," which develop on the membrane, producing a form of local (as opposed to systemic) GVH reaction. Using such a technique, Simonsen observed many years ago that a very high proportion of cells involved in GVH reactions (at least 2 percent) could respond to host alloantigens. This troublesome observation has been repeatedly confirmed, and must be accounted for in any model of T-cell-mediated cytotoxic reactions.

GVH Reactions in F_1 Hybrid Animals

GVH reactions can be induced by injection of parental lymphocytes into F_1 hybrids. Essentially the same consequences are observed as described above for newborn mice. However, since F_1 hybrids are effectively tolerant of lymphocytes from either parent throughout life, it is also possible to induce GVH reactions in postnatal and even adult F_1 animals. The symptoms are somewhat less severe with increasing age of the host, and extremely high doses of allogeneic cells are required to cause mortality beyond three to four weeks after birth. In fully mature recipients, it may be very difficult to induce a *severe* reaction by any criterion, although detailed pathological examination will almost always show some evidence of GVH disease. Because the grafted lymphocytes are not rejected, chronic low-grade GVH disease may develop.

GVH Reactions in Irradiated Allogeneic Adults

A rather severe form of GVH reaction can be induced in adult mice if the host is first given whole-body irradiation of at least 550 R. In most cases the irradiation alone may be lethal, especially above 600 R. If the hosts are inoculated intravenously with allogeneic lymphocytes, the mortality period may be significantly shortened. In this form of GVH reaction, host lymphoid cells are essentially depleted from the system within a few days by the irradiation alone. They persist long enough, however, to trigger an allograft reaction in the donor (graft) lymphocytes. The grafted lymphocytes can be found seeded throughout the host lymphoid system. This is of particular advantage in the spleen, where by four to six days after injection, the spleen will contain 95 to 98 percent donor cells. These cells can be readily recovered, and contain T cells highly cytotoxic toward target cells of host genotype *in vitro*. Radiation GVH reactions are thus often used as a system for generating cytotoxic lymphocytes.

Localized GVH Reactions

There are a number of GVH reactions that are localized to a single tissue or organ, usually because of the way the donor lymphocytes are introduced. The footpad GVH assay system is one such reaction. Donor lymphocytes are inoculated subcutaneously into the hind footpads of an adult allogeneic rat or mouse. The cells find their way to the popliteal lymph node (behind the knee), which is the primary draining node for the footpad, and are effectively trapped there. The lymph node undergoes a hypertrophic reaction that peaks at about seven days. The resultant increased weight of the popliteal node is a highly sensitive measure of the degree of GVH reaction induced.

If the donor lymphocytes are first irradiated, much less lymph node hypertrophy is evident, suggesting that the observed enlargement is not due to HVG activity. Yet the lymphocyte proliferation leading to hypertrophy is almost entirely among the host cells. Most of these cells are trapped from the lymph circulation as they pass through the node. These observations taken together suggest the following sequence of events. The reaction is initiated by donor cells in a true GVH reaction. Some local HVG reaction probably is occurring, but the number of donor lymphocytes is large compared to host lymph node cells, and the localized GVH reaction seems to suppress somewhat the localized HVG reaction. Host lymphocytes are "trapped" in the node as they pass through in the lymph circulation, and are stimulated to proliferate there, by factors liberated by the activated donor T cells.

Some evidence of systemic GVH can usually be detected accompanying the localized reaction; a few donor cells apparently do circulate beyond the regional node and lodge in other host lymphoid organs. However, the effective dilution by the host's body volume, plus loss of donor cells trapped in the regional node, greatly reduces the systemic reaction.

Cellular Basis of GVH Reactions

Role of Donor Lymphoid Cells in GVH Reactions

The graft-versus-host reaction is one of the most complex and least well understood of immune reactions. It is by definition dependent on viable donor *cells* for its initiation, and Gowans showed in the early 1960s that the crucial cell is a small, nondividing lymphocyte. In the mouse, lymph nodes and thoracic duct lymph are the best sources for reactive cells. The spleen is somewhat less good, whereas thymocytes and bone marrow are very poor sources of reactive cells. However, cortisone-resistant (medullary) thymocytes are highly reactive in GVH; the poor response of thymocytes as a whole simply reflects the fact that cortisone-resistant thymocytes comprise only 5 to 10 percent of total thymus cells. Similarly, although bone marrow per se is unreactive in GVH, it can be shown that there exist discrete subpopulations of bone marrow cells that can, on further maturation, cause a normal GVH reaction in an allogeneic host. These findings are all consistent with the reactive cell being a T lymphocyte, and this has indeed been shown to be the case. Lymphocytes from neonatally thymectomized adult donors, or lymphcytes from congenitally athymic (nude) mice are unable to elicit significant GVH disease. Lymphocyte populations highly enriched for B cells are similarly ineffective. Pretreatment of a lymphocyte population with anti-Thy-1 antiserum plus complement removes the GVH reactivity of the population.

Donor lymphocytes undergo a relatively limited period of proliferation in both systemic and local GVH reactions. This mitotic activity occurs early in the response, peaking at about three days. Proliferation of donor cells contributes only slightly to hypertrophic reactions in host lymphoid organs. Probably the most important role of donor T cells, on antigenic stimulation, is the secretion of a variety of soluble products referred to collectively as lymphokines. These factors are almost certainly involved in the proliferation of host cells in organs undergoing a GVH reaction, because in most cases a system has been selected such that host cells cannot recognize donor antigens as foreign. Lymphokines may also play a role in attracting host cells to the site of the GVH reaction and in localized destruction of host tissues. As discussed in the subsection on the radiation GVH, (Lyt-2$^+$) donor T cells may become highly cytotoxic toward host cells during the course of a GVH reaction, further contributing to the gradual degeneration of the host.

Role of Host Cells in GVH Reactions

Although host cells generally may be the ultimate target for damage in GVH reactions, host lymphoid cells actually play an active role in generating many of the symptoms associated with the GVH. First of all, since the donor lymphocytes tend to home in on host lymphoid organs, host lymphoid class II antigens provide the principal antigenic stimulus to reactive donor T cells. Other loci may also be capable of inducing GVH reactivity. The Mls locus in the mouse, for example, is located on chromosome 1, and is a potent stimulus for both T-cell proliferation *in vitro* and T-cell activation in GVH, in animals syngeneic at H-2. Second, in both systemic and local GVH reactions, where the host immune system has not been interfered with, host lymphoid cells proliferate in a rapid and nonspecific manner, presumably in response to various factors produced by donor T cells. As we will see, this may lead to polyclonal B-cell activation, including B cells reactive to self. Finally, host lymphoid cells may be particularly vulnerable to specific cytotoxic damage by sensitized donor T cells, because they bear the highest concentration of MHC-coded determinants and are at least *in vitro* particularly good targets for cell-mediated cytotoxic damage.

Pathology of GVH Disease

In addition to its usefulness for studying fundamental parameters of immune reactivity, the GVH reaction has important implications for human health. It is one of the principal complications in bone marrow transplantation, which might otherwise be the method of choice for dealing with aplastic anemia, severe combined immunodeficiency disease, and even certain forms of leukemia (after otherwise lethal levels of chemotherapy or whole-body irradiation).

The pathological manifestations of GVH disease in humans, as in other mammals, are very complex. The skin is one of the most sensitive targets for GVH disease, although probably the least life threatening in the immediate sense. Mice show a gradual loss of fur and drying out of the underlying skin. Humans undergoing even a mild GVH reaction develop a skin rash reminiscent of measles, accompanied by induration. In severe cases the foci may conjoin and become hemorrhagic and become infected. The sensitivity of skin to GVH attack may be related to the presence of Langerhan's cells, dendriticlike cells bearing high levels of class II antigens that are known to trigger T cells.

A more serious problem in all species is diarrhea due to degeneration of gastrointestinal tissues, particularly the mucosal glands. The liver is also affected. In humans, GVH may be accompanied by hepatomegaly as well as splenomegaly, with severe damage to the bile duct. Most key enzyme systems of the liver eventually become abnormal, and there is an increase in bilirubin production. As with a number of other diseases, GVH disease is also accompanied by a general immunosuppression of the host, increasing the chances for opportunistic infections.

Once GVH symptoms develop in patients after bone marrow transplantation (about three-fourths of all cases), very little can be done to treat them. It is fatal in roughly one-third of patients developing GVH symptoms. In a few cases the symptoms are sufficiently mild as to be nonthreatening, and in some cases the symptoms may disappear altogether or come under control with drugs such as hydrocortisone or methotrexate. The rate of success in terms of the original dysfunction (aplastic anemia, leukemia, etc.) with donors who are totally syngeneic (i.e., identical twins) is rather high, suggesting that GVH disease is a major contributor to failure of bone marrow transplants. Thus a great deal of effort has been expended in improving donor-recipient histocompatibility-matching techniques, so that allogeneic disparity can be reduced as much as possible. However, even when "perfect" matches are obtained, on the basis of currently identified HLA serotypes and known Lad loci, GVH symptoms will still develop in roughly one-half of grafted patients. As in the case of the failure of solid organ transplants to survive in similar situations, these failures underscore in a dramatic way the incompleteness of our knowledge of the structure of the major histocompatibility complex and of minor H loci.

Bibliography

General

Berke, G., Interaction of cytotoxic T lymphocytes and target cells. *Progress in Allergy 27,* 69 (1980).

Clark, W., and P. Golstein (eds.), Mechanisms in cell-mediated Cytotoxicity. *Advances in Experimental Biology and Medicine 146.* Plenum Press, New York (1982).

Golstein, P., Sensitivity of cytotoxic T cells in T cell-mediated cytotoxicity. *Nature 252,* 81 (1974).

Grebe, S. C., and J. W. Streilein, Graft-*versus*-host reactions: A review. *Adv. Immunol. 22,* 120 (1976).

Henkart, P. A., Mechanism of lymphocyte-mediated cytotoxicity. *Annual Review Immunol. 3,* 31 (1985).

Herberman, R., and J. Ortaldo, Natural killer cells: Their role in defenses against disease. *Science 214,* 24 (1981).

Research

Cerottini, J., and H. R. MacDonald, Lyt phenotype of cytolytic T lymphocyte precursors reactive against normal and mutant H-2 antigens. *J. Immunol. 126,* 490 (1981).

Dourmashkin, R. et al., Electron microscopic demonstration of lesions in target cell membranes associated with antibody-dependent cellular cytotoxicity. *Clin. Exp. Immunol. 42,* 554 (1980).

Eichwald, E. J., et al., Cell-mediated hyperacute rejection. IV. Lyt markers and adoptive transfer. *J. Immunol. 128,* 2373 (1982).

Gowans, J. L., The role of lymphocytes in the destruction of homografts. *Br. Med. Bull. 21,* 106 (1965).

Gowans, J. L., D. D. McGregor, D. M. Cowen, and C. E. Ford, Initiation of immune responses by small lymphocytes. *Nature 196,* 651 (1962).

Holmberg, L., B. Miller, and K. Ault, The effect of NK cells on development of syngeneic hematopoietic progeniton. *J. Immunol. 133,* 2933 (1984).

Jerne, N. K., The somatic generation of immune recognition. *Eur. J. Immunol 1,* 1 (1971).

Jooste, S. V., et al., The vascular bed as the primary target in the destruction of skin grafts by antiserum. *J. Exp. Med. 154,* 1319 (1981).

Loveland, B. E., and I. F. C. McKenzie, Which T cells cause graft rejection? *Transplantation 33,* 217 (1981).

Martz, E., Mechanisms of specific tumor cell lysis by alloimmune T lymphocytes: Resolution and characterization of discrete steps. *Contemp. Topics Immunobiol. 7,* 301 (1977).

Medawar, P. B., The behavior and fate of skin autografts and skin homografts in rabbits. *J. Anatomy 78,* 176 (1944).

Minami, M., and D. C. Shreffler, Ia-positive stimulator cells are required in primary, but not in secondary, mixed leukocyte reactions against H-2K and H-2D differences. *J. Immunol. 126,* 1774 (1981).

Mitchison, N. A., Passive transfer of transplantation immunity. *Nature 171,* 267 (1953).

Podack, E., and G. Dennert, Cytolysis by H-2 specific T killer cells: Assembly of tubular complexes during the lytic reaction. *J. Exp. Medicine 157,* 1483 (1983).

Rosenau, W., and H. Moon, Lysis of homologous cells by sensitized lymphocytes in tissue culture. *J. Nat. Canc. Inst. 27,* 471 (1961).

Shearer, G. M., T. G. Rehn, and C. A. Garbarino, "Cell-mediated lympholysis of trinitrophenyl-modified autologous lymphocytes. *J. Exp. Med. 141,* 1348 (1975).

Simonsen, M., The impact on the developing embryo and newborn animal of adult homologous cells. *Acta Pathol. Microbiol. Scand. 40,* 480 (1957).

Wilson, D. B., and R. E. Billingham, Lymphocytes and transplantation immunity. *Adv. Immunol. 7,* 189 (1967).

Wright, S., and B. Bonavida, Selective lysis of NK-sensitive target cells by a soluble mediator released from murine spleen cells and human peripheral blood lymphocytes. *J. Immunol. 126,* 1516 (1981).

Wright, S., and B. Bonavida, Studies of the mechanisms of natural killer cell-mediated cytotoxicity. IV. Interferon-induced inhibition of NK target cell susceptibility to lysis is due to a deficit in their ability to stimulate release of NKCF. *J. Immunol. 130,* 2965 (1983).

Zinkernagel, R. M., G. N. Callahan, A. Althage, S. Cooper, P. A. Klein, and J. Klein, On the thymus in the differentiation of "H-2 self-recognition" by T cells: Evidence for dual recognition? *J. Exp. Med. 147,* 882 (1978).

Zinkernagel, R. M., and P. C. Doherty, Restriction of in vitro T cell-mediated cytotoxicity in lymphocytic choriomeningitis within a syngeneic or semiallogeneic system. *Nature 248,* 701 (1974).

CHAPTER 15

The Role of the Thymus in Development of the T-Cell Receptor Repertoire

We saw in Chapters 13 and 14 that the initiation of both humoral and cell-mediated cytotoxicity reactions requires T-cell recognition of a self-MHC component, in addition to nominal antigen, on another cell surface. This recognition is presumably mediated by some form of the T-cell antigen receptor described in Chapter 12. The requirement for simultaneous recognition of self-MHC plus nominal antigen distinguishes the T-cell receptor recognition system from the B-cell/immunoglobulin system. A number of important questions have been posed concerning the development and expression of T-cell receptor function. What is the role of the thymus in this process? Is the thymus the only locus for development of this aspect of T-cell function? What is the relationship between recognition of MHC and nominal antigen? Are recognition of class I and class II MHC antigens under the same sort of developmental control? What is the connection between recognition of self-MHC plus nominal antigen and direct recognition of allogeneic MHC?

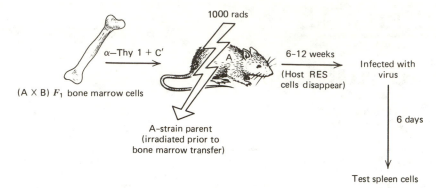

Figure 15-1 Construction and infection of a bone marrow radiation chimera.

A system for analyzing these and other questions about T-cell function became available with the development and careful characterization of bone marrow chimeras (Figure 15-1). To make a bone marrow chimera, marrow cells (containing T stem cells) from a normal healthy donor are injected into a lethally irradiated semiallogeneic or allogeneic recipient. The maturation of the T stem cells under the influence of the host thymus is then monitored. It is absolutely essential to achieve complete elimination of all host immune system cells prior to introduction of donor marrow cells. This usually requires at least 1000 R irradiation given in a single dose. Although the lymphoid elements of the thymus are totally eliminated by the radiation treatment, the epithelial elements of the thymus responsible for promoting T-cell differentiation are still intact. The marrow contains stem cells for the entire blood system, including all elements of the immune system, and normally infusion of bone marrow shortly after irradiation will rescue the animal from eventual death. Of course, great care must be taken to protect the animal from infection while newly formed immune system cells repopulate the lymphoid organs. In about two months the animals will be completely reconstituted and ready to use for experiments. Prior to use, however, it is necessary to test the lymphocytes of each animal with appropriate alloantisera to be certain that all host blood elements have been totally replaced by donor marrow-derived cells.

Acquisition of the CTL MHC-Recognition Repertoire

Radiation chimeras involving parental strains and F_1 progeny have been used to study MHC restriction of CTL-mediated cytotoxicity in virally infected cells. As we saw in Chapter 14, immune T cells from a virally infected $(A \times B)F_1$ hybrid animal will ordinarily be able to recognize and lyse virally infected cells from either the A or B strain parent (Table 14-1). However, if bone marrow cells from an $(A \times B)F_1$

mouse are injected into either irradiated parent, T cells subsequently isolated from that chimera, which still display the F_1 surface phenotype, will lyse only (or at least best) virally infected target cells from the chimeric parent (Table 15-1). On the other hand, a chimera produced using adult F_1 spleen cells in place of F_1 bone marrow cells behaves exactly as an F_1 animal in that it will display reactivity toward both parental cell types (Table 15-1, Experiments 3 and 4). The adult spleen cells have already matured in another thymus, and are not influenced by the new host thymus.

These observations suggested that the H-2 genotype of the thymus in which the stem T cells mature determines the perception of "self." This conclusion was strengthened by the results of experiments in which the irradiated bone marrow recipient was also thymectomized, and then transplanted with a different thymus prior to receiving bone marrow cells. As predicted, the H-2 halotype of the transplanted thymus determined the perception of self by the infused bone marrow cells (Table 15-2).

The experiments to this point are relatively straightforward in interpretation. T stem cells in bone marrow that have not yet been thymus influenced can be caused to alter the perception of self they would ordinarily develop if they mature in a nonself thymus. Since we imagine that the genetic and biochemical nature of T-cell receptors associated with individual cells does not change across relatively short periods of time, the simplest interpretation of these results would be that the T-cell precursors in bone marrow have a wider range of potential recognition than just self, and that some sort of selection process is taking place under thymic influence. Adult T cells, on the other hand (i.e., cells already thymus influenced), are unaffected by exposure to a non-self-thymus.

However, the story is not quite so simple. There are several observed exceptions

Table 15-1 CMC Specificity of Virus-infected Bone Marrow Radiation Chimeras

Experiment	Donor cell source	Chimera H-2 haplotype	Haplotype of virus-infected targets		
			d	b	k
1	Bone marrow	$(d \times b) \to d$	41	0	0
2	Bone marrow	$(d \times b) \to b$	0	25	0
3	Adult spleen	$(d \times k) \to k$	52	1	50
4	Adult spleen	$(d \times b) \to d$	49	38	0

Adapted from R. M. Zinkernagel et al., On the thymus in the differentiation of H-2 self-recognition by T cells: Evidence for dual recognition? *J. Exp. Med. 147* (1978), p. 882. Figures shown are percent destruction of virally infected target cell monolayers.

Table 15-2 Influence of Transplanted Thymus in Bone Marrow Chimeras

Bone marrow donor	Thymus donor	Thymectomized recipient	Haplotype of virally infected targets		
			d	*k*	*b*
d × *a*	—	*d* × *a*	0	9	0
d × *a*	*d*	*d* × *a*	50	10	0
b × *a*	*a*	*b* × *a*	40	50	0

The recipient was thymectomized, lethally irradiated and transplanted with the indicated thymus and reconstituted with syngeneic bone marrow cells. After a period of time, the chimera was infected with virus, and the specificity of its resultant effector T cells tested on the indicated target cells. Strain "a" is a k/d recombinant (Table 9-1)

that at first could not be explained by this hypothesis (Table 15-3). Parental bone marrow cells matured under the influence of an F_1 thymus would be expected to be able to interact with infected target cells from both parents; this was not observed. The same is true of F_1 bone marrow cells matured in a semiallogeneic F_1 host; only the shared parental haplotype is recognized in a subsequent virus-specific reaction.

The resolution of these apparent inconsistencies requires that we extend our understanding of the entire chimera-infection-cytolysis sequence. First, the pre-T cells as a population do "learn," by selection, an H-2 identity from the thymus in which they mature. This may be completely different from the H-2 haplotype they

Table 15-3 Lysis of Infected Targets by Virally Infected T Cells from Infected Chimeras of Various Construction

Bone marrow source	Recipient	Haplotype of infected target cell		
		A	B	C
A	(A × B) F_1	+	−	−
B	(A × B) F_1	−	+	−
(A × B) F_1	(A × C) F_1	+	−	−
(A × C) F_1	(A × B) F_1	+	−	−

themselves express (their H-2 phenotype). Second, in order for the matured T cells to perceive and interact with virally infected cells, the infected cells must display the MHC products the T cells were selected to recognize as self. As it turns out, the cells presenting virus to the helper T cell (the first cell to react) are themselves elements of the reticuloendothelial system (reticular cells, macrophages, dendritic cells, etc.), which in bone marrow chimeras derive from the marrow donor, not from the host. What is required is that the class II MHC molecules displayed by cells infected with virus match the class II preference learned by the T helper cells during thymic maturation. If donor T cells are selected for recognition of host class II antigens as self, but if no lymphoreticular cells displaying host class II products survive the radiation to present virus, then sensitization of T helper cells restricted to host-unique MHC products cannot take place.

Let us see how this hypothesis explains the observations in Table 15-3. A strain bone marrow cells matured in an $(A \times B)F_1$ hybrid can potentially perceive both A and B as self. However, the $A \rightarrow (A \times B)F_1$ chimera only contains A phenotype lymphoreticular cells; all $(A \times B)F_1$ lymphoreticular cells were destroyed by the supralethal radiation. Thus, the T cells in this chimera, which are phenotypically of the A haplotype, but which have the potential to recognize both A and B as self, are only presented with virus on A-strain lymphoreticular cells. Obviously, in a subsequent CMC reaction, they will only lyse A strain virally infected cells.

What about pre-CTLs? Let us assume for the moment that they too learn to recognize host class I MHC products (whether or not this occurs in the thymus will be discussed in the following section). Pre-CTL do need to "see" virus in the context of "learned" class I MHC molecules, but they do *not* need to see this activating signal on a special cell type (Figure 14-9). They should thus be able to be at least partially activated by virus on any cell in a bone marrow chimera, not just marrow-derived cells. But in order to be completely activated, they need T helper cell factors. The problem is thus one of simple geography (Figure 15-2): the T helper cells are only activated by certain infected marrow-derived cells, which display only half of the class II antigens that the T cells as a population have learned to recognize. Pre-CTL that recognize the class I antigens in these same cells will be activated very *efficiently* because there will be T helper factors in the immediate vicinity. Pre-CTL that react to class I antigens on other host cells will be partially activated, but will have difficulty in obtaining T helper factors. Thus although pre-CTLs capable of recognizing both sets of antigens in an F_1 are present, and even though both sets of CTLs can receive an appropriate first activating signal (virus plus class I protein), only the CTLs interacting with infected bone marrow-derived cells will be efficiently activated, since that is where activated helper T cells will be found. Thus the ability of T helper cells to be activated is rate limiting for the types of CTLs that ultimately mature.

In order to test this explanation of the observed discrepancies, Zinkernagel and his colleagues carried out so-called "chimeric transfer" experiments (Figure 15-3). In these studies, chimeras were prepared as described before, but after two to three months, instead of infecting the chimera itself, T cells were isolated from the

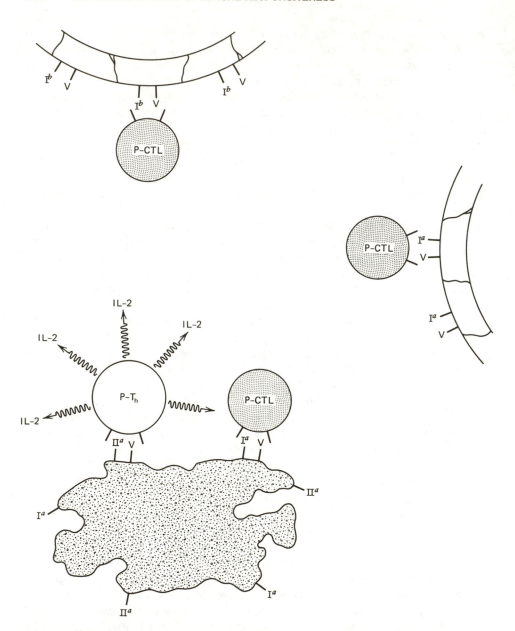

Figure 15-2 In this diagram, three pre-CTLs are each activated by an appropriate "signal 1" (self-class I + viral antigen). However, the pre-CTL getting its signal 1 from a bone marrow-derived macrophage or dendritic cell is in a better position to receive IL-2 from a neighboring activated T helper cell than are the other two pre-CTL, who must try to scavenge adventitious IL-2 diffusing out from some other reaction center.

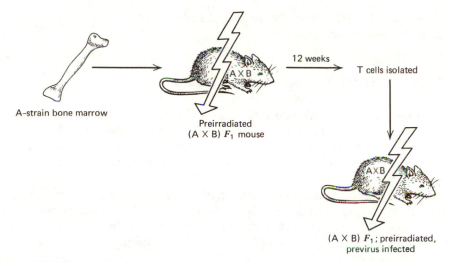

12 weeks

T cells isolated

A–strain bone marrow

Preirradiated
(A × B) F_1 mouse

(A × B) F_1; preirradiated,
previrus infected

Figure 15-3 Chimeric transfer experiment.

chimera and transferred to an irradiated, virus-infected F_1 mouse. Three things should be pointed out about this second recipient. First, it is irradiated so that no endogenous host antiviral reaction will take place; all subsequent cytotoxic activity will be from donor T cells. Second, a chimera is *not* being established in this second F_1; adult T cells, not bone marrow cells, are being transferred in. Third, since donor T cells are being transferred in immediately after radiation, the principal cells comprising the lymphoreticular compartments are still host (A × B) cells. Furthermore, infection occurred before donor cells were transferred in; thus, the principal presenting cell is an (A × B) cell. The fact that it is irradiated does not initially compromise its ability to present viral antigen. The results of these experiments are given in Table 15-4, and clearly show that the A stem cells that matured in

Table 15-4 Summary of Various Experiments Carried Out in Chimeric Transfer Studies

Bone marrow donor	Chimeric recipient	Second recipient	Lysis of virus-infected target cells	
			A	**B**
A	A × B	None	+	−
A	None	A × B	−	−
A	A × B	A × B	+	+

the chimeric $(A \times B)F_1$ thymus were indeed selected for recognition of both A and B MHC antigens as self.

_____

Extrathymic T-cell Maturation

In general, the conclusions concerning the influence of the thymus on development of the helper T-cell recognition repertoire *in bone marrow chimeras* have not been seriously challenged. Several observations in nude mice have, however, raised a serious challenge to the conclusions drawn in the chimeras with respect to CTL maturation.

In an experiment carried out by Kindred and Zinkernagel, a normal thymus, whose influence on T-cell development was to be studied, was transplanted into a nude mouse. The maturation of prethymocyte stem cells from the bone marrow of the nude mouse itself could then be studied in a very clean system—the question of residual mature T cells in the periphery of the bone marrow chimera, which always arose in the case of irradiation chimeras, was neatly canceled out. Lobes of fetal, neonatal, or irradiated adult thymus were transplanted under the kidney capsule of various nude mice, where they became readily vascularized and thus in systemic communication with the rest of the body. (Note that none of the donor thymic tissues contained mature T cells.) Between six and eight weeks later, the animals were either immunized directly with virus, or their spleen cells were passively transferred to a second, lethally irradiated mouse that was immediately immunized with virus. MHC restriction was then tested as before by assaying immune spleen cells on various infected and uninfected target cells.

When this was done, a picture of T-cell maturation somewhat different from that

Table 15-5 Restriction Maturation in Nude Mice

Nude strain used	Thymus donor[1]	MHC restriction observed[2]
A	A	*a* (only)
A	A × B	*a* (only)
A	B	NR
A × B	A	*a* (only)
A × B	B	*b* (only)
A × B	A + B	*a + b*

Condensed from information presented in R. Zinkernagel et al., *J. Exp. Med. 151,* 376 (1980).

[1]No mature T cells present.

[2]Tested in A × B environment.

obtained in the bone marrow chimeras emerged (Table 15-5). Although restriction of A × B phenotype T-cell precursors to the MHC of a transplanted parental thymus occurred in the nude mouse experiments just as in the chimera experiments, the "learning" of a new MHC specificity in the case of A or B nude precursors maturing in a transplanted (A × B)F$_1$ thymus could not be demonstrated.

A second observation with nude mice that challenged the idea of a primary role for the thymus in determination of the CTL repertoire was that nude mice supplied with an exogenous source of IL-2 could generate mature, fully competent CTLs. Since nude mice do not have a functional thymus, and none was introduced in the course of these experiments, it is clear that the pre-CTLs did not undergo any sort of MHC selection in thymus. And since IL-2 is the factor supplied by T helper cells, it seems quite likely that only T helper maturation is faulty in nude mice. These experiments suggested that pre-CTLs either have a pre-fixed MHC recognition repertoire, or that they might be selected for self-MHC recognition extrathymically.

That pre-CTL undergo at least part of their maturation in an extrathymic environment is also clear from the experiments of Duprez et al. (Figure 15-4). They removed the thymus from adult mice, and one week later gave them 940 R of

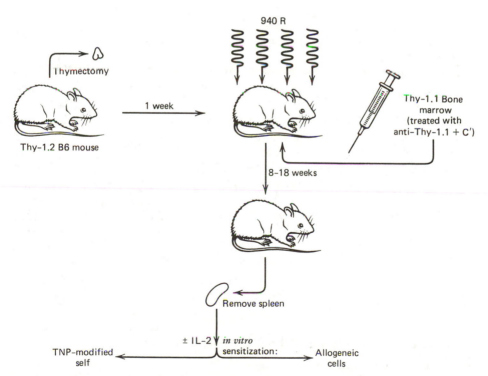

Figure 15-4 Experiment by Duprez et al. showing at least partial differentiation of pre-CTL in the absence of a thymus. CTL for both altered self and allogeneic targets can be generated if IL-2 is provided. See Table 15-6 for results.

Table 15-6 Results of Experiment Shown in Figure 15-4

Responder cells	Stimulator	IL-2	Target cells		
			D2	**B6–TNP**	**D2–TNP**
Experiment 1					
Unthymectomized chimera (B6)	D2	No	67	—	—
Unthymectomized chimera (B6)	D2	Yes	76	—	—
Thymectomized chimera (B6)	D2	No	4	—	—
Thymectomized chimera (B6)	D2	Yes	62	—	—
Experiment 2					
Unthymectomized chimera (B6)	B6–TNP	No	—	51	27
Unthymectomized chimera (B6)	B6–TNP	Yes	—	73	32
Thymectomized chimera (B6)	B6–TNP	No	—	0	0
Thymectomized chimera (B6)	B6–TNP	Yes	—	51	20

(—) means not tested. Note that MCH preference in haptenated-self-systems is not always as strong as in virus + self-systems. Data based on information presented in V. Duprez, B. Hamilton, and S. Burakoff, Generation of CTLs in thymectomized, irradiated, bone marrow-reconstituted mice. *J. Exp. Med. 156,* 844 (1982).

whole-body irradiation. The mice immediately received an infusion of anti-Thy-1 treated, MHC-syngeneic bone marrow cells. The donor marrow, although identical with the recipient at H-2, was from a strain congenic with the recipient for the Thy-1 allele; thus, in the adult chimera, the origin of any developing T cells could be unequivocally determined.

Spleen cells removed from these chimeras were unable to produce CTLs *in vitro* against allogeneic simulator cells, or against hapten-modified self-stimulator cells, *unless* supplied with exogenous IL-2. When IL-2 was provided, both types of CTL activity were readily obtained (Table 15-6). The function of these CTLs was indistinguishable either qualitatively or quantitatively from CTLs generated from spleen cells from normal adult mice. Moreover, pre-CTLs from the spleens of thymectomized chimeras showed the same degree of self-MHC restriction as spleen cells from unthymectomized chimeras. These results provide perhaps the strongest evidence that CTLs can mature outside the thymus, and do not need thymic interactions to learn self MHC preference. Whether CTL have a genetically restricted MHC recognition repertoire, or whether they have a repertoire equally broad as that of T helper cells, that is maturation-restricted elsewhere in the body, is not known.

Determination of MHC Preference in T Helper Cells

Bone marrow chimeras have also been used to study the acquisition of the MHC receptor repertoire of T cells that provide help for B cells. As with the studies on development of the CTL repertoire, most investigators utilized semiallogeneic chimeras of the type P1 or P2 → (P1 × P2), or of the type (P1 × P2) → P1 or P2.

Obviously, the best system in which to determine whether stem cells from an animal of one haplotype have the potential to produce T cells displaying preference for MHC products of a different haplotype would be a fully allogeneic chimera, for example, P1 → P2. For a number of years, attempts to produce such chimeras were unsuccessful. Finally, however, Singer et al. were able to obtain chimeras of this type and used them to examine development of helper T cell MHC preference. The system used by these investigators is shown in Figure 15-5. The main feature distinguishing their system from earlier ones is that they tested the competence of unprimed chimeric T cells in a primary *in vitro* system for generating PFC, rather than by directly challenging the chimera *in vivo*.

The competence of whole spleen cells taken from various chimeras to respond to TNP–KLH *in vitro* is shown in Table 15-7. Unfractionated spleen cells from semiallogeneic chimeras of any type are able to respond well to TNP–KLH *in vitro*. These experiments are simply positive controls; they do not in any way address the question of MHC preference of the chimeric cells. The important elements of these data are the results with the fully allogeneic chimeras. What is immediately obvious is that chimeras of the type P1 → P2 or P2 → P1 cannot mount a primary immune response to antigen *in vitro*, which agrees with numerous studies of such chimeras tested *in vivo*. On the other hand, a mixture of P1 and P2 bone marrow matured in a single parent type does produce spleen cells capable of responding to antigen. Most interesting of all, a combination of independently matured spleen cells from P1 → P2 and P2 → P1 chimeras also responds very well to antigen *in vitro*.

By analogy with the earlier experiments of Zinkernagel and his co-workers, a rather simple explanation of these experiments could be suggested. P1 bone mar-

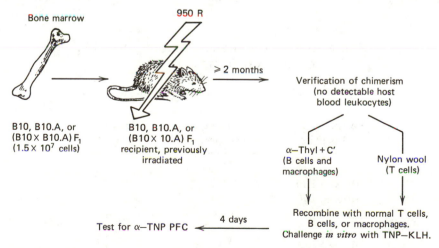

Figure 15-5 Allogeneic and semiallogeneic chimeras tested *in vitro* for ability to provide T-cell help in the response to the TNP–KLH.

Table 15-7 Semiallogeneic and Fully Allogeneic Chimeras Used by Singer et al.

	TNP PFC/culture	
Type of chimera	**+TNP–KLH**	**–TNP–KLH**
P1 → (P1 × P2)	102	0
P2 → (P1 × P2)	126	1
(P1 × P2) → P1	252	5
(P1 × P2) → P2	143	0
P1 → P2	1	1
P2 → P1	1	1
(P1 + P2) → P1	90	1
(P1 + P2) → P2	185	5
(P1 → P2) + (P2 → P1)	327	0

Unfractionated spleen cells from the indicated chimeras were tested for their ability to respond to TNP–KLH *in vitro*. P1 = B10; P2 = B10.A. Adapted from A. Singer et al., *J. Exp. Med. 153*, 1286 (1981).

row cells maturing in a P2 thymus will produce T helper cells that recognize P2 class II antigens as self. When harvested from the spleen of a P1 → P2 chimera, they are perfectly competent to react to antigen, but only in the context of P2 class II MHC products. These are obviously not present in the *in vitro* culture system, since all of the spleen cells are phenotypically P1. However, in both the (P1 + P2) → P1 (or P2) and the (P1 → P2) + (P2 → P1) situations represented in Table 15-7, each type of T cell (P1 or P2) will have available to it macrophages displaying the

Table 15-8 Demonstration That the Defect in Fully Allogeneic Chimeras Is Lack of Appropriate Antigen-presenting Cells

Source of chimeric T and B cells	**Source of macrophages**	**Anti-TNP PFC/culture**
B10.A → B10	None	5
B10.A → B10	B10.A	5
B10.A → B10	B10	94
B10 → B10.A	None	5
B10 → B10.A	B10.A	83
B10 → B10.A	B10	8

Adapted from J. Singer et al., *J. Exp. Med. 153*, 1286 (1981).

appropriate class II antigens; a positive response would be predicted, and is observed.

In order to test this hypothesis in a direct way, Singer et al. removed antigen-presenting cells (APC) from the spleen cells of P1 → P2 chimeras, and cultured the remaining T and B cells *in vitro* with TNP-KLH plus APC from either P1 or P2 normal spleens. The results in Table 15-8 show very clearly that T cells from a P1 → P2 chimera are able to help B cells when presented with antigen and APC from a normal P2 spleen but cannot respond to antigen using APC derived from a normal P1 parent. Thus in these experiments, which are among the clearest of this type carried out to date, there is no question that bone marrow helper T-cell precursors have the potential, as a population, to develop a preference for MHC antigens other than the ones they themselves are genetically programmed to display.

Diversity of the Mature T-Cell Recognition Repertoire

The foregoing experiments with radiation chimeras make it clear that bone marrow T-cell precursors are multipotent with respect to species MHC recognition. During thymic differentiation and selection, this MHC recognition repertoire is restricted such that mature T cells leaving the thymus show a marked preference for interaction with MHC products encountered in the thymic environment. We can now ask how strict this selected preference for MHC products is, and whether all mature T cells selected to recognize a given MHC product do so in the same way.

The first suggestion that the mature T-cell population is heterogeneous with respect to preference for individual learned MHC products came about some years ago in experiments with inbred strains of guinea pigs. It was observed that when (strain 2 × strain 13)F_1 guinea pig T cells were primed *in vitro* by antigen-pulsed APC of either parental strain, the resultant memory T cells would give a secondary reaction only with antigen bound to the parental APC used in priming. Subsequent experiments using T cells primed *in vivo* proved informative concerning a possible mechanism for the apparent MHC restriction observed with *in vitro* priming. Strain (2 × 13)F_1 guinea pigs were injected with a protein antigen such as OVA. T cells were isolated from the primed animals and challenged *in vitro* with OVA-pulsed strain 2 or strain 13 macrophages. As expected, it was found that macrophages from either parental strain could be used to present antigen to the primed F_1 T cells. However, the (at the time) rather startling observation was made that separate and probably nonoverlapping subpopulations of primed F_1 T cells were responding to each antigen-pulsed parental strain macrophage (Figure 15-6; Table 15-9). This finding implies that in the F_1, distinct subpopulations of T cells exist that display different sets of receptors specific for restriction antigens on macrophages contributed by one but not the other parent.

Given that such T-cell subpopulations exist in the F_1, the previous *in vitro*

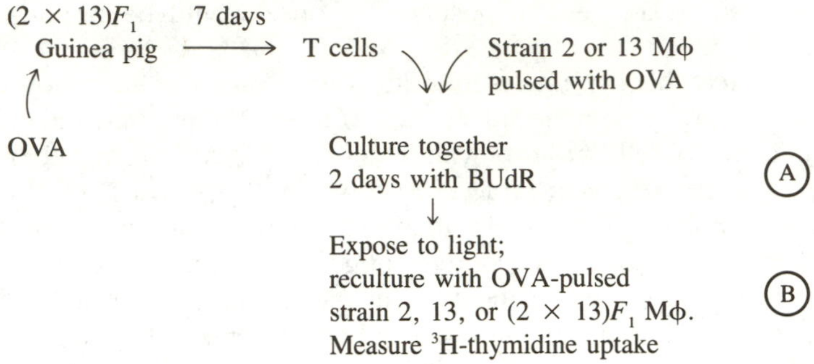

$(2 \times 13)F_1$ 7 days
Guinea pig $\longrightarrow$ T cells   Strain 2 or 13 Mϕ
pulsed with OVA

$\uparrow$

OVA

Culture together
2 days with BUdR   (A)
$\downarrow$
Expose to light;
reculture with OVA-pulsed
strain 2, 13, or $(2 \times 13)F_1$ Mϕ.   (B)
Measure ^{3}H-thymidine uptake

Figure 15-6 $(2 \times 13)F_1$ guinea pigs were immunized with OVA, and the primed T cells harvested. These were incubated with OVA-pulsed macrophages from either the strain 2 or strain 13 parent, in the presence of 5'-bromodeoxyuridine (BUdR). BUdR is incorporated into DNA in place of thymidine, and photosensitizes it; when subsequently exposed to light, BUdR-sensitized cells are killed. The data in Table 15-9 show that when F_1 T cells are stimulated with one strain of antigen-pulsed parental macrophages, then F_1 T cells capable of responding to those macrophages synthesize DNA and are ultimately eliminated, but T cells capable of responding to macrophages of the other parental type are still represented in the remaining population. The use of PPD as an unrelated antigen at step A shows that the response is antigen specific. The numbers shown in Table 15-9 are cpm $\times 10^{-3}$ ^{3}H-TdR incorporated. [Based on data presented in W. E. Paul et al., Independent populations of primed F_1 guinea pig T lymphocytes respond to antigen-pulsed parental peritoneal exudate cells. *J. Exp. Med.* 145, 618 (1977).]

priming results in the guinea pig system are readily understood. In the total population of F_1 T cells primed *in vitro* with antigen on antigen-presenting cells (APC) from one parental strain, only that subpopulation of F_1 T cells bearing the appropriate surface receptor allowing interaction with the priming parental strain APC would be activated. When this primed population of F_1 T cells is secondarily challenged with antigen on APC of each parental type, only that subpopulation of F_1 T cells expanded in the primary reaction is capable of reacting now in a secondary

Table 15-9 Results of the Experiment Shown in Figure 15-6

Macrophages used at A	Antigen used at A	OVA-pulsed Mϕ used at B		
		Strain 2	Strain 13	$(2 \times 13)F_1$
2	None	1.0	4.9	3.4
	PPD[a]	86.8	55.9	90.1
	OVA	1.9	25.4	19.1
13	None	26.8	22.4	22.3
	PPD[a]	95.3	67.7	102.7
	OVA	102.7	4.5	65.9

[a]The response to PPD is not MHC restricted in this system.

Table 15-10 Transcomplementation in IA of Hybrid Antigen-presenting Determinants

Experiment	Filler cells	MHC region								Medium	GAT
		K	A	B	J	E	C	S	D		
1	A/J	k	k	k	k	k	d	d	d	178	340
	B6	b	b	b	b	b	b	b	b	309	767
	A/J + B6	k/b	k/b	k/b	k/b	k/b	d/b	d/b	d/b	377	896
	(B6 × A)F$_1$	k/b	k/b	k/b	k/b	k/b	d/b	d/b	d/b	361	16,878
	B10.A(4R)	k	k	b	b	b	b	b	b	436	955
	[B10.A(4R) × B6]F$_1$	k/b	k/b	b/b	b/b	b/b	b/b	b/b	b/b	370	13,146
2	(B6A)F$_1$	k/b	k/b	k/b	k/b	k/b	d/b	d/b	d/b	1,547	35,350
	[B10.MBR × A.AL]F$_1$	b/k	k/k	k/k	k/k	k/k	k/k	k/k	q/d	788	1,055

Subclone 12-5-a-2 was assayed on filler cells from various strains and hybrid mice. The MHC region of these mice has been included for clarity of presentation. Data are presented as the proliferative response assayed on day 2 by [^{3}H]TdR uptake. Taken from M. Kimoto and C. G. Fathman, *J. Exp. Med. 152*, 759 (1980). By permission.

The filler cells act as APC. At the time this work was carried out, B and C were still considered valid subregions of I.

fashion, and obviously only with parental APC from the original stimulating parental strain. F_1 T cells capable of reacting with APC from the opposite parent will only give a primary response, which has magnitude and kinetics different from a secondary reaction.

The diversity of the mature T-cell receptor repertoire has been further explored in an elegant series of studies by Fathman and co-wokers using a variation of the T-cell cloning technique described in Chapter 14 for CTL. T helper cells from (A × B)F_1 mice previously immunized with the synthetic antigen GAT were cloned and the various clones obtained were tested for MHC preference. GAT was presented on APC of A, B, or (A × B)F_1 origin. It was found that some T-cell clones responded to GAT only on A (and F_1) strain APC; some clones responded only to strain B (and F_1) GAT-pulsed APC; and some clones responded to GAT on F_1 APC, but not on either parental strain APC. The response to GAT in intact F_1 spleen cell populations is obviously a composite of these various clonally defined specificities. One could surmise that T helper cells from a clone recognizing GAT on F_1 APC, but not on APC from either parent, must be restricted to responding to GAT in the context of an F_1-unique MHC determinant, such as might be generated by transcomplementation of IA or IE subregion-encoded subunits. The data in Table 15-10 shows this to be the case. T-helper cell clones were generated from the spleen cells of a GAT-primed (B6 × A/J)F_1 hybrid mouse. One of the clones thus generated (12-5-a2) responded to GAT on F_1 APC but not on APC derived from either parent, or a mixture of APC from both parents. The cloned cells also responded to GAT on (B10.A4R × B6)F_1 APC, but not on APC from B10.A4R mice. This suggested that the cloned T_h cells were responding to GAT in the context of determinants in the K-IA region of the hybrid mouse. Experiment 2 of this table shows that the crucial subregion is IA, which must be of the H-2$^{k/b}$ genotype. Thus this clone is recognizing a determinant unique to the $A_\beta^k A_\alpha^b$ or the $A_\alpha^k A_\beta^b$ molecule, that is not found on the $A_\beta^k A_\alpha^k$ molecule. (There is, of course, no $E_\beta^b E_\alpha^b$ molecule; see p. 247.) These studies have been recently extended even further, using the same cloning technique, together with mutant strains and hybridoma antibodies, to show that different T_h subpopulations exist that recognize different domains of the same class II β chain. These and similar studies suggest that mature, postthymic T cells are quite heterogeneous with respect to self-MHC recognition.

The Nature of MHC Restriction

At the level of individual T cells, all evidence suggests that only a single receptor, for a single nominal antigen-MHC complex, is present on a given T cell (whether helper, suppressor, or CTL). Thus a particular T cell is in fact *a priori* restricted and does not change its MHC or nominal antigen specificity throughout its (and its progeny's) history. *Populations* of T cells, on the other hand, are quite heterogeneous with respect to MHC plus nominal antigen preference. In terms of the MHC portion of this preference, heterogeneity can be restricted at two points. First of all, the available evidence suggests that bone marrow T-cell precursors are much more pluripotent in terms of specieswide MHC recognition than are mature T cells. We can therefore infer the existence of an antigen-independent step in the restriction of the T-cell MHC repertoire, which occurs during thymic maturation. But it is clear that even after this first restriction occurs, from species MHC to a particular self-MHC, the mature, postthymic T-cell population is still relatively heterogeneous, particularly in heterozygotic animals. In the latter, there will be separate populations of T cells recognizing as self each parental version of each MHC molecule, plus (in the case of class II antigens) populations of T cells recognizing hybrid-unique molecules arising as a result of transcomplementation between parental chromosomes. Moreover, it now appears from the work of Fathman and others that within each of the above categories there are likely to be subpopulations of T cells recognizing different determinants on each of the defined MHC molecules.

When a particular nominal antigen enters the system it will be perceived by the immune system in the context of a limited number of the total available MHC products. Thus we can infer the existence of a second, antigen-dependent step in MHC restriction. As a result of the primary immunizing event, only those T cells capable of responding to the immunizing antigen, in the context of a particular MHC product or portion thereof, will be clonally expanded. The antigen itself thus plays a role in determining which populations and subpopulations of self-MHC-specific T cells are activated. In a secondary reaction, obviously only those T cells selected and expanded in the primary event will be capable of responding in a secondary fashion; the MHC receptors they display will determine with which APC and B cells they can cooperate. This is the basis for the MHC restrictions seen in this and the previous chapter.

We are left with the following questions. If T cells do not recognize MHC alone, but a complex formed by MHC plus nominal antigen, how can MHC preference be selected for in the thymus in the absence of nominal antigen? Are there separate receptors for MHC and for nominal antigen? If a single receptor is reacting with both MHC and nominal antigen, how is the MHC-nominal antigen complex formed? Is a stable complex made on the presenting cell surface, which then fits into the T-cell receptor, or are the two component antigens simply "trapped" together through independent interactions with receptor subsites?

These are all major questions with which immunologists are still grappling. At present the evidence from molecular genetics indicates that only a single receptor molecule is expressed on each T cell, although this could conceivably be modified as more information is gathered. But assuming for the moment a single receptor, can we even imagine the answers to some of the questions just posed?

There are a few experiments in the literature that bear on the nature of antigenic complexes perceived by T cells. One of the questions just posed was whether stable MHC-nominal antigen complexes form on antigen presenting cells. An inherent, *a priori* sort of problem this notion imposes is that in humoral responses, in particular, the number of soluble antigens responded to in a T-cell-dependent fashion is quite large. On the other hand, even in heterozygous mice bearing a full complement of functional IA and IE region-encoded class II peptides, the maximal number of unique Ia proteins for one individual is only eight. In Chapter 10, preliminary structural evidence was presented suggesting that the "variable" portions of class II molecules will probably be limited to a restricted portion of the β subunit. How could limited regions of only eight peptide chains be capable of associating in a meaningful way with the soluble antigenic universe, when upward of several thousands of Ig V-region genes are required to do the same thing for antibody molecules? A similar argument could be made for the association of a large number of viral antigens with class I MHC proteins. Nevertheless, because the requirement for some sort of association or interaction of MHC and foreign antigen is suggested by single receptor models, numerous experiments have been carried out to look for such complexes.

One approach used by a number of laboratories has been to attempt to identify such complexes using antibody specific for either MHC or nominal antigen. For example, antibody against class I MHC antigens has been used in an attempt to cocap viral antigens on infected cell surfaces, and vice versa. With only a few exceptions, such experiments have failed. Similarly, attempts to immunoprecipitate viral antigens from detergent-solubilized, infected cell membranes using antibody against class I antigens have also generally failed. Although one cannot rule out completely interactions between class I and foreign antigens on this basis, it is certainly possible to rule out stable, high-affinity interactions between the two. It is generally agreed that in both humoral and cellular T-cell reactions, the association of MHC and foreign antigens, if it occurs at all, must be a fairly weak one.

A second approach to analyzing associations of class II antigens and foreign antigens on antigen presenting cells is shown in Figure 15-7. T_h-cell hybridomas were produced by fusing T_h cells with an appropriate T-cell tumor, and selecting and propagating resultant hybrid cells that retained the functional properties of the T_h-cell partner. Among the properties retained was the original MHC restriction for antigen-presenting cells of the T_h-partner cell haplotype. One such hybridoma was itself fused with normal T_h cells of a different specificity and MHC restriction, to create a second-order hybridoma. In the example shown in Figure 15-7, a hybridoma specific for OVA presented on H-2^a antigen-presenting cells was fused with T_h cells specific for KLH presented on H-2^{m}APC. The resultant hybridoma was able to respond to either an OVA/H-2^a *stimulus, or a KLH/H-2^m* stimulus. However, it was unable to respond to OVA presented on H-2^m APC, or to KLH on H-2^a APC. This experiment strongly suggests that either recognition of MHC antigens and of nominal antigens are not entirely independent of one another, or that MHC and nominal antigen are somehow physically linked on the APC surface. For example, if the T-cell receptors for MHC and nominal antigen are completely independent, then if MHC and nominal antigen moved independently on the APC surface, the hybridoma should be able to engage both receptors and respond. Since the parental restrictions were retained in the second-order hybridoma, one or the other of these two systems

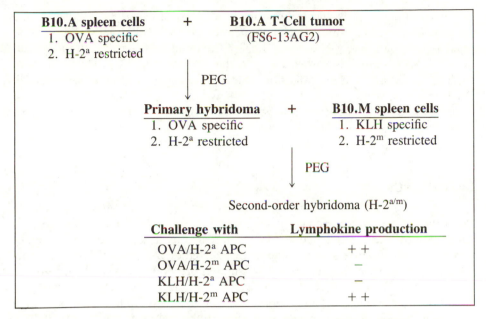

Figure 15-7 Based on data presented in J. W. Kappler, B. Skidmore, J. White, and P. Marrack, Antigen-inducible, H-2-restricted, interleukin-2-producing T cell hybridomas. *J. Exp. Med. 153* (1981), p. 1198. The ability of hybridomas to provide T-cell help was measured by their ability to produce IL-2 upon presentation of antigen on various cells. OVA/H-2ª APC, for example, means the hybridoma was presented with OVA on H-2ª antigen-presenting cells.

(T-cell receptor or APC surface antigens) must be linked. Because of the failure to demonstrate convincingly an association of MHC and nominal antigen on APC in either humoral or cytotoxic reactions, the conclusion at the time was that most likely it is recognition that is linked, rather than presentation. This is certainly consistent with current evidence pointing to only a single antigen receptor on T cells.

A single receptor model would also explain the high frequency of alloreactive T cells. If all T cell receptors recognize self-MHC plus some non-self-determinant, one could imagine that some of these receptors might cross-react with allogeneic MHC products ("altered self") with sufficiently high affinity to cause T-cell triggering.

The main difficulty with the idea of a single receptor for MHC plus nominal antigen is thus the bone marrow chimera experiments. Data from these experiments show that the MHC context in which a nominal antigen must be perceived can be altered by the thymic environment in which a particular population of bone marrow cells matures. What this must imply for single receptor models is that pre-T cells have encoded in their DNA a replicate set of receptor genes for the universe of nominal antigen as it would be seen in the context of each type of MHC in the species. This seems an unusually cumbersome genetic burden, and in fact no one really believes it is likely to be true. Thus for the moment we really cannot explain how self-MHC perception is changed in the thymus. Usually when we cannot explain something, it is an indication of incomplete information at our disposal. Doubtless that is the case here, and we may hope to see some new piece of information emerge in the not-too-distant future that will help make more sense of this intriguing problem.

Summary

All of the information presented in the preceding sections ultimately highlights a single point about T-cell-dependent immune reactions. T cells, like B cells, cannot respond directly to free, soluble antigen for which they are specific. T cells can only perceive antigen on the surface of an antigen-presenting cell and only in the context of an appropriate MHC product. This is the phenomenon of MHC restriction, and it applies to both humoral and cell-mediated cytotoxic responses. If a particular antigen cannot associate properly with the APC MHC products, or if the T cells as a population do not have an appropriate receptor system for recognizing a particular foreign antigen in the context of a self-MHC product, then the help needed for a response to that foreign antigen will not develop.

Thus an enormous amount of immunological research, in a variety of experimental systems that seemed at times to yield conflicting or unconnected data, appears at present to be resolving into a picture that can be summarized in a single paragraph. But understanding the biological implications of this system of immune responsiveness poses a whole new series of questions. What, for example, is the biological advantage of being able to perceive antigen only in the context of an MHC protein? What is the significance of seeing antigen in the context of self? Self as opposed to what? MHC restriction would seem to add another level of complexity, increasing the chances of something going wrong. And yet it is a system that is absolutely conserved throughout higher vertebrates. We can be sure that there are advantages that outweigh the disadvantages; we simply have not yet perceived them.

Another intriguing question about this system is the difference in distribution and function of class I and class II MHC products. Both serve as restricting elements in antigen presentation. Why then are class I antigens found on all cells in the body, whereas class II antigens are restricted almost entirely to antigen-presenting cells and B cells? And why are soluble antigens presented (and perceived) only in the context of class II antigens, and viral antigens only in the context of class I antigens? How would foreign antigens know with which MHC antigen to associate? These questions and others related to MHC regulation of immune responsiveness will likely occupy the attention of immunobiologists for several years to come.

Bibliography

General

Möller, G. (Ed.), Acquisition of the T cell repertoire. *Immunol. Rev. (Transplant. Rev.) 42* (1978).

Research

Duprez, V., B. Hamilton and S. Burakoff. Generation of CTLs in thymectomized, irradiated, bone marrow-reconstituted mice. *J. Exp. Med. 156,* 844 (1982).

Katz, D. H., B. Skidmore, L. Katz, and C. Bogowitz, Adaptive differentiation of murine lymphocytes. I. Both T and B lymphocytes differentiating in F_1 → parental chimeras manifest preferential cooperative activity for partner lymphocytes from the same parental type corresponding to the chimeric host. *J. Exp. Med. 148,* 727 (1978).

Kimoto, M., and C. G. Fathman, Antigen-reactive T cell clones. I. Transcomplementing hybrid IA-region gene products function effectively in antigen complementation. *J. Exp. Med. 152,* 729 (1980).

Paul, W. E., E. M. Shevach, S. Pickeral, D. W. Thomas, and A. S. Rosenthal, Independent populations of primed F_1 guinea pig lymphocytes respond to antigen-pulsed parental peritoneal exudate cells. *J. Exp. Med. 145,* 618 (1977).

Sprent, J., H. Von Boehmer, and M. Habholz, Association of immunity and tolerance to host H-2 determinants in irradiated F_1 hybrid mice reconstituted with bone marrow cells from one parental strain. *J. Exp. Med. 142,* 321 (1975).

Von Boehmer, H., W. Haas, and N. K. Jerne, Major histocompatibility complex-linked immune-responsiveness is acquired by lymphocytes of low-responder mice differentiating in thymus of high-responder mice. *Proc. Natl. Acad. Sci. USA. 75,* 2439 (1978).

Wagner, H. et al. T cell-derived helper factor allows *in vivo* induction of cytotoxic T Cells in nu/nu Mice. *Nature 284,* 278 (1980).

Zinkernagel, R. M., G. N. Callahan, A. Althage, S. Cooper, J. W. Streilein, and J. Klein, The lymphoreticular system in triggering virus plus self-specific cytotoxic T cells: Evidence for T help. *J. Exp. Med. 147,* 897 (1978).

V

Immunology and Human Health

Immunology has been regarded for most of the present century as primarily a clinical discipline, although at this point in your immunology course, or in your reading of this textbook, you may understandably have lost sight of any such connection. Nevertheless, during all of the years that immunology has come into its own as a strong basic science discipline, the number of human pathologies found to have an immunological component has continued to grow at a steady pace. To the long list of infectious diseases that were the wellspring of early immunological research, we now must add allergy, cancer, congenital and acquired immune deficiencies, and a seemingly ever-expanding list of autoimmune diseases as areas of clinical medicine in which the immune system plays an important role. Manipulation of the immune system to facilitate cell, tissue and organ transplantation must also be included.

Although at one time or another research in each of these categories of clinical immunology led to a corresponding burst of new activity in basic research, the situation has now reversed. With few exceptions the human follows the mouse about the laboratory as a system for original investigation. Probably 90 percent or more of the information presented so far in this text was first generated in inbred strains of mice. With few and relatively insignificant exceptions, the information thus generated has been directly applicable to humans. The major effort in almost every area of human immunology at present is applying the enormous store of information we have obtained in the mouse to the various clinical problems seen in humans that have an immunological basis or component. Thus if your future career is in medicine, a course of the type you are now taking is probably the best preparation you could get for understanding the immunological basis of a wide range of human diseases.

CHAPTER 16

Immunity to Infection

Without question, the immune system evolved in vertebrates to meet the challenge of eliminating a wide spectrum of pathogenic microorganisms that invade both intracellular and interstitial spaces of the host. The need to understand the details of just how this challenge is met was certainly a major force in the early development of immunology as a science. Indeed, exploring the relationship between immunity and infection was the very definition of immunology up until the 1950s. The student who finishes a modern course in immunology, based on a textbook such as this one, will be only dimly aware of the enormous amount of research and intellectual excitement that accompanied the unraveling of this relationship, although he or she will doubtless be a willing and grateful recipient of the fruits of this research.

Nevertheless, it is a fact that research into immunity to infection occupies only a small proportion of contemporary immunological inquiry; time and technology have taken immunologists to other frontiers and to questions having little if anything to do with host survival in a world of hostile and predatory microflora. A detailed consideration of these subjects is of obvious importance to those who continue on into the study of medicine or the study of parasitic and infectious

411

diseases from a public health point of view; presumably they will be exposed to such detail at an appropriate stage in their future careers. But some level of knowledge and appreciation of these subjects is appropriate even for those who view immunology principally as a way of approaching fundamental problems of cellular and molecular biology. As we have already seen, the most esoteric and sophisticated experiments in immunology very often bring us right back to fundamental questions about the relationship of the immune system and intra- or extracellular pathogenic microorganisms. What follows is a brief presentation of "classical" immunology, which will introduce some of you to what may later be your major interaction with immunology, and to provide for the rest of you at least a rudimentary insight into this enormously important field.

We will first survey the repertoire of bodily defenses against infection by microorganisms, and then examine how these defenses operate in various types of infectious diseases.

Nonimmunological Defenses against Microorganisms

Although the immune system certainly provides the most sophisticated host defense against foreign intrusions, there exists a remarkable array of nonimmunological barriers to infection that confer a considerable degree of protection in their own right. These barriers exist independently of exposure to any particular antigen and are often referred to collectively as *innate* or *natural immunity,* although the use of the term *immunity* in this context may be misleading. Immunity per se is best used to refer to the specific array of immune system-related defenses that are characteristic of acquired immunity, that is, those responses arising only after, and in direct response to, exposure to antigen.

Nonimmunological defense mechanisms may be either anatomical or systemic in nature. The skin itself, when completely healthy, is an effective barrier to entry of environment pathogens. Its generally low surface pH (except in the axillary and groin regions) is inhibitory to bacterial growth, as is its general dryness. Many oils produced by the skin are highly fungicidal; most fungal infections occur on skin areas not protected by sebaceous glands. On the other hand, internal epithelial linings exposed to the environment are more susceptible to penetration by foreign organisms and even inert materials because of their generally moist and sticky surface. This property, while preventing the microbe from entering more deeply into the body itself, may allow it to adhere long enough to utilize whatever specific mechanisms it may possess to penetrate the epithelial cell membrane. These usually involve the binding of bacterial coat lectinlike proteins to epithelial cell surface sugar molecules. This attachment may then trigger some sort of endocytotic action by the cell, although in some cases disease damage may occur at the cell surface, without penetration. Bacteria may also penetrate beyond the epithelium and spread systemically through blood or lymph. The main barrier to penetration of epithelial surfaces is immunological (see following). However, a variety of nonspecific mechanisms are also involved: routine sloughing of epithelial cells; coughing followed by expectoration or swallowing: ciliary "sweeping" of microorganisms, which keeps them moving and hinders attachment; more or less constant washing of exposed surfaces by various secretions; and bodily elimination by defecation, sneezing, crying, etc.

Nonimmunological mechanisms are particularly important in limiting infections of the upper respiratory tract. Many inhaled inert particles, as well as potentially infectious microbes, stick to the mucus bathing the walls of the tract. They are swept by cilia, which also line these walls back into the throat, where they are either expectorated or swallowed. Those that are swallowed face a perilous sojourn through acid, digestive enzymes, and hostile indigenous flora. Smaller microbes (less than ca. 0.5 μm) often escape ciliary sweeping and enter the lungs, where they are dealt with by alveolar macrophages (see next section). However, the importance of the ciliary system can be seen in patients who have ciliary defects. These individuals experience a vastly increased incidence of infections of the ears, sinuses, and bronchial systems, as well as of the lungs proper.

A variety of secreted and circulating nonimmunological substances can be particularly effective in limiting bacterial growth and function (Table 16-1). They may do so by relatively nonspecific means (pH, ionic strength, or ionic content) or by

Table 16-1 Soluble Substances Involved in Nonimmunological Host Defenses against Microbial Infection

Substance	Biochemical nature	Occurrence	Action
Lysozyme	Enzyme, ca. 15,000 MW	All body fluids except sweat and spinal fluid; cytoplasmic granules of macrophages	Attacks bacterial cell walls (principally gram positive). Works particularly well in combination with antibody
β-Lysin	Cationic protein	Platelets and whole serum (not plasma)	Attacks gram-positive bacteria
Spermine	Polyamine	Semen	Gram-positive bactericide
Leukin	Basic polypeptide	PMNs	General bactericide
Plakin	Basic polypeptide	Platelets	General bactericide
Interferon	Low molecular weight proteins	Virally infected cells	Prevent translation of viral (but not host) proteins

highly specific molecular activities. The alternate complement pathway discussed in Chapter 9, which leads to the generation of opsonins and anaphylotoxins, is a highly efficient, albeit immunologically nonspecific, defense against microbial infection.

Saliva contains glycolipids that compete with bacterial cell wall products for attachment to epithelial surface receptors, thus physically blocking attachment and entry into the cell. Lysozymes occur in many secretions (tears, urine, nasal mucus) and are a fairly potent hydrolyzer of bacterial wall mucopeptides. Lysozyme is a small (ca. 15,000-dalton) basic peptide that hydrolyzes the β-1,4-glycoside bond between muramic acid and *N*-acetylglucosamine (NAG). Because the muramic-NAG unit is a major constituent of bacterial cell walls, lysozyme is a potent, if nonspecific, bactericide. In the digestive tract, some secretions (produced at least in part by host flora) contain fatty acids that may destabilize the membranes of nonresident microorganisms.

The normal colonization of various external portions of the body (surface and alimentary canal) by nonpathogenic bacteria can impede invasion and growth by potential bacterial pathogens. There are numerous examples of this phenomenon. Salmonella and Shigella are discouraged from establishing residence in the digestive tract and bowel by products (principally fatty acids) secreted by local gut flora. Harmless pharyngeal streptococci discourage invasion by the more troublesome pneumococci. There are other examples affecting bacterial growth on the skin. Such relationships are usually detected by the consequences of natural or induced elimination of the indigenous bacteria.

Nutritional factors such as vitamins and minerals can also affect nonspecific host defense mechanisms. A decrease of vitamin A in the diet of mice leads to increased bacterial, viral, and parasitic infections, while above-normal levels of this vitamin lead to enhanced protection. Vitamin A appears not to affect microbial agents directly but rather to enhance host defense mechanisms leading to their elimination. The mechanism of this effect is unknown, and it has not yet been demonstrated in humans. A similar effect of vitamin E has been noted in chicks. The effects of vitamin C have been the subject of a public debate since Pauling published his book, *Vitamin C and the Common Cold,* in 1970. Since that time numerous well-controlled clinical trials have been conducted to determine the validity of some of his claims. Most of these trials show that vitamin C taken prophylactically has no effect on the incidence of upper respiratory infections but that the severity of the symptoms may be reduced. In animal studies, vitamin C appeared to have an effect similar to vitamins A and E, enhancing nonspecific host resistance to disease. At present there is no known mechanism for the effects of vitamin C, although it is known to generally stimulate the activity of PMNs and perhaps macrophages. Robert Good and his co-workers have carried out intensive investigations into the role of zinc in immune function. T cells are particularly compromised by the absence of zinc in the diet, probably because one of the thymic hormones (*facteur thymique serique;* FTS) requires zinc for appropriate molecular conformation and function.

Finally, in most species examined, one can identify a genetically based pattern of innate or natural resistance to specific diseases. This is seen in the highly variable patterns of disease susceptibility among various species, and between sexes within a species. One species may be highly susceptible to a particular disease, while another species in the same or a nearby ecological niche may be completely resistant. Such patterns exist in all members of a species, independent of antigen exposure. There are some indications of human racial differences in susceptibility to individual pathogens—blacks, for example, are more susceptible to tuberculosis than are whites. Such differences, however, are usually difficult to discern because of differences in life-style and socioeconomic factors. The assumption of a genetic basis for these variations is based mostly on observations made in breeding experiments in animals. Although the exact mechanisms of species-related natural resistance are not really known, it is presumed that they involve such things as variations in body temperature; the presence, absence, or relative amounts of certain enzymes; or the presence of specific nucleotide sequences in host DNA allowing insertion of viral genomes, etc.

The above mechanisms of natural immunity are all very distinct from the components of the immune system described in previous chapters. However, one mechanism of host protection that must be included under the heading of natural immunity, but which may indeed be closely related to mechanisms normally defined as part of the acquired immunity armory, are the so-called "natural killer" or NK cells. These cells will attack and destroy many tumor cells directly and without previous sensitization to them. NK cells appear to be lymphocytes, and in humans are particularly associated with large granular lymphocytes (LGL). NK cells and the mechanisms by which they recognize and destroy tumor cells will be discussed more fully in Chapter 20.

Immunological Defenses against Disease

The Role of Lymphocyte in Disease

The role of lymphocyte in disease is no different than the role we have already studied for these cells in other immune reactions. B cells of course make antibody. In the case of bacterial cell wall antigens, many of the B cell responses appear to be relatively T cell independent (see Chapter 12). T helper cells are involved in helping B cells make antibody to a wide range of soluble toxins produced by microorganisms. T helper cells also initiate inflammatory reactions at the site of infections, attracting macrophages and PMNs. Factors produced by T helper cells also activate macrophages. These factors may be used by the macrophages to more actively phagocytize cells in their environment. The T cells themselves are probably activated by microbial antigens displayed on the macrophage surface. In the case of viral infections, cytotoxic T lymphocytes appear to play a major role in eliminating infected cells. The assumption is that this is by a direct, cell-mediated cytotoxic mechanism (Chapter 14), but a role for CTL (particularly previously primed CTL) in initiating inflammatory reactions cannot be discounted.

Role of Circulating and Secretory Antibody in Resistance to Infection

Although lysis of gram-negative bacteria by antibody plus complement can be demonstrated *in vitro,* complement-mediated bacteriolysis may only be a minor factor in immune defenses against bacteria *in vivo.* Gram-positive bacteria are highly resistant to complement lysis even *in vitro.* The plasma membranes of both gram-positive and gram-negative bacteria appear to be as susceptible to complement-mediated lysis as those of animal cells; however, the presence of a thick, lipid-poor cell wall confers a substantial degree of protection against complement cytolysis. The ability of antibodies to agglutinate cells and bacteria in *in vitro* assays also probably plays no significant role per se in immunity to infection *in vivo.* Although some bacteria clearly can be killed directly by antibody and complement *in vivo,* it seems likely that the major role of IgM and IgG antibody in the elimination of bacteria is opsonization for phagocytosis.

On the other hand, antibody (particularly secretory antibody) plays a key role early in the course of microbial invasions by preventing the establishment of both bacterial and viral infections. Most mucosal and epithelial linings contain substantial numbers of IgA antibody-producing cells. IgA antibodies seem to function chiefly by neutralizing bacteria and viruses before they attach to and penetrate epithelial cells, since they neither bind complement nor promote phagocytosis. The presence of IgA-producing lymphocytes is particularly important throughout the gut, where they are involved in extravascular local immune reactions. Immunity to an invading organism is developed essentially *in situ,* with neither the IgA nor the cells that produce it entering either the blood or lymph circulation. In the lower digestive tract, IgA antibodies secreted directly into the bowel (coproantibodies) play a key role in preventing establishment of a number of pathogenic organisms (*Vibrio cholerae, Shigella, Salmonella,* etc.) IgG antibodies can also be highly effective in neutralizing viruses that circulate in the bloodstream during the course of an infection (e.g., polio virus).

The principal targets of antibodies involved in resistance to infection are microbial cell surface antigens, including endotoxins. Although these antigens are relatively immutable in most bacterial strains, they can change periodically in viruses, and routinely during infection by many multicelled parasites. The influenza virus, for example, produces new strains several times each century, with wide-ranging and often devastating effects during the period required for human populations to develop immune resistance to the new antigens.

Antibodies also play a crucial role in the neutralization of bacterial exotoxins, such as those produced in tetanus, botulism, or diphtheria. Exotoxins are highly immunogenic, but in primary infections the delay between toxin production and antibody production may allow toxin levels to build to a point too great to be dealt with immunologically. In such cases, passive immunization with an immune serum is often highly effective. Active immunization can be induced with molecularly altered, nonpathogenic forms of individual toxins (toxoids).

There are often low levels of antibodies to many pathogenic microbes in the sera of healthy animals, prior to infection episodes. These so-called "natural anti-bodies" are probably produced to cross-reacting antigenic determinants in food, on nonpathogenic microbes, or by exposure to subinfective levels of pathogen itself. They can provide some measure of protection during the two to three days required to trigger a primary immune response.

Phagocytosis—The Role of Macrophages and PMNs in Disease

By far the most important element in host resistance to infectious disease is phago-cytosis (literally "eating of cells"). The process of phagocytosis is also one of the most primitive of host defense mechanisms, having its counterpart in most species of metazoa examined. In lower species, it is a fairly simple, relatively mechanical process, probably evolving directly from the feeding processes of free-living uni-cellular organisms such as amoebas. In the higher vertebrates, it begins to interact with, and be enhanced by, elements of the humoral immune system.

Phagocytosis, as a specialized host defense form of the more general pinocytic process, can be mediated by a variety of cells associated with the blood system, but the most important of these are polymorphonuclear cells (PMNs) and macrophages (both fixed and circulating). Both types of cells are attracted to sites of infection or tissue damage by a variety of soluble chemotactic factors.

Macrophages (and monocytes) are phylogenetically the more primitive; gran-ulocytic phagocytes are not found until the appearance of animals with closed circulatory systems. Granulocytic phagocytes are fully differentiated as they leave the bone marrow, whereas macrophages must mature from monocytes, which have a limited phagocytic capacity and no cytoplasmic specialization for killing and digesting bacteria. On the other hand, macrophages can continue to divide at the site of an infection, whereas PMNs are a truly terminal, fully mature cell type. Macrophages are also much longer lived than PMNs, particularly in humans where the lifetime of the PMN is only a few hours. PMNs rarely participate in more than one round of killing, whereas macrophages can participate in several temporally spaced phagocytic cycles. Although there are some differences in the processes by which these two cell types ingest and destroy foreign particulate matter, the sim-ilarities are more striking. We will thus discuss the process of phagocytosis in general terms, referring where appropriate to elements unique to one or the other cell type.

The first step in the phagocytic process is the formation of stable contact with the

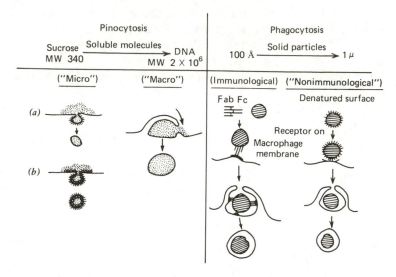

Figure 16-1 Endocytic activities of the macrophage. A schematic representation of the uptake of both soluble and particulate substances by macrophages. The determinants of "micro" pinocytosis of soluble antigens are unclear but are morphologically similar to the process as seen in endothelial and mesothelial cells. The "macro" form is the most prominent in macrophages and results in vesicles that may reach 0.8 microns in diameter. Solutes that bind to the plasma membrane are taken up at rates that may be 1000 times greater than unbound molecules. The nature and topography of phagocytic receptors is poorly understood, and the term receptor is used in an operational sense. [From Z. A. Cohn, Properties of macrophages. *Phagocytic Mechanisms in Health and Disease,* R. C. Williams and H. H. Fudenburg (eds.), Intercontinental Medical Book Corporation, New York (1972). Copyright by the Intercontinental Medical Book Corp., New York, 1972.]

particle to be ingested (Figure 16-1). This need not be a biological particle—inert, inorganic particles will be ingested as well. (In fact, a frequently used method for isolation of macrophages involves feeding them minute iron particles, and then separating them from other cells with a magnet.) Formation of a stable contact can occur mechanically, if the particle is large enough or dense enough not to move when contacted by a phagocyte, or if the particle is physically "trapped" between the phagocyte and some fixed tissue element, or between two phagocytes. This is often referred to as "contact" or "surface" phagocytosis. The second way in which a stable contact can be formed is by a process called *opsonization,* wherein the particle is bound to the phagocyte through the mediation of bifunctional macromolecules called *opsonins.* Although the existence of a variety of nonspecific, "serum factor" opsonins has often been postulated, the most important and effective opsonins are various classes of immunoglobulin molecules, and certain components of complement (see Chapters 4 and 7). If antibodies combine with microorganisms via interaction of their antigen combining sites with cell surface antigens, and the antibodies are of an appropriate type (usually one or more subclasses of IgG), the opsonized particle will then bind firmly to the surface of either a PMN or a macrophage. This is accomplished by interaction of the Fc region of the Ig molecule with an Fc receptor on the cell surface (see Figure 16-1). If this Ig, or any other Ig bound to the cell surface (including IgM, which does not interact with Fc receptors) binds and activates complement, additional opsonization may occur through liberation of C3b fragments. These contain one site that allows them to bind firmly to the cell surface, and a second site that can interact with a specific C3b receptor present on the membrane of most phagocytes. (The Mac-1 antigen in macrophages is associated with the C3b receptor.) Both IgG and C3b, as opsonins, greatly facilitate the process of phagocytosis through stabilizing the initial contact between the phagocytic cell and its target.

The second step in phagocytosis is ingestion of the foreign particle. Both PMNs and macrophages are highly motile. The phagocytic process is distinct from pinocytosis, where the engulfed material more or less "sinks" in the membrane, a vesicle forming when the membrane closes over the material as it enters the cell. In phagocytosis, the temporary immobilization of a part of the plasma membrane through stable attachment of a particle, with uninterrupted flow of adjacent portions of the membrane, results in outward movement of portions of the membrane and the formation of a phagocytic vacuole or phagosome (Figure 16-2). The pro-

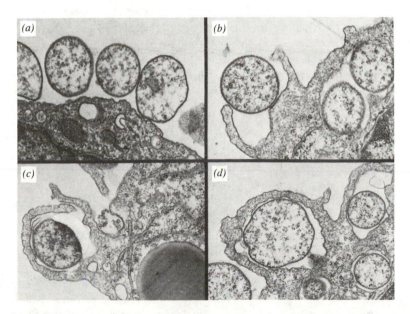

Figure 16-2 Electron micrographs illustrating the phagocytosis of *Mycoplasma pulmonis* by mouse macrophages upon addition of antimycoplasma antibody, × 21,000. [From J. G. Hirsch, The digestive tract of phagocytic cells. *Phagocytic Mechanisms in Health and Disease*, R. C. Williams and H. H. Fudenberg (eds.), Intercontinental Medical Book Corporation, New York (1972). Copyright by the Intercontinental Medical Book Corp., New York, 1972.]

cess of encapsulization can be interfered with by substances that disrupt cytoskel-etal structures, but not selectively, that is, not without concomitant disruption of general membrane motility. However, the presence of the particle at one site on the membrane, whether fixed by opsonization or not, must confer some unique transient properties on surrounding membrane. Although encapsulation of the particle could be accounted for by simple flow of the membrane, fusion of mem-brane to close the capsule and form the phagosome cannot. For example, one does not see random fusion of membrane segments with self-membranes or with adja-cent identical phagosomes.

After the phagosome (secondary granule) detaches from the plasma membrane, it moves rapidly to the interior of the cell, where it fuses with cytoplasmic granules (primary granules) containing substances that degrade the included particle. These substances include peroxides and peroxidases, degradative enzymes such as lysozyme, and lipophilic membrane-perturbing molecules.

The membrane distortions involved in particle ingestion apparently trigger a series of metabolic changes in phagocytes that are connected with the killing and digestion of phagocytized microorganisms. In the PMN these include increased glycolysis, increased oxygen consumption (the "respiratory burst"), and increased hexose monophosphate shunt activity. These activities lead to increased energy production and to generation of hydrogen peroxide and superoxide radicals. Al-though the ingestion process itself can occur anaerobically, oxidative mechanisms are very important in bacterial killing. Hydrogen peroxide and superoxide (O_2), in an undefined reaction involving myeloperoxidase (MPO) and halide ions, particu-larly free or bound iodine, are involved in chemical degradation of bacterial cell walls. MPO is present in the lysosomal granules of PMNs in very high concentration, constituting as much as 5 percent by dry weight of the total cell content in humans. The importance of both MPO and H_2O_2 in microbicidal action can be seen in certain hematological disorders. In chronic granulomatosus disease, MPO is pre-sent in PMNs in normal amounts, but for some reason the cells fail to generate H_2O_2 during the respiratory burst following ingestion. Microbicidal action in such cells is greatly reduced. In genetically inherited MPO deficiency diseases, where the H_2O_2-generating apparatus functions normally but intracellular MPO is very low or absent, there is also a greatly impaired microbicidal activity (somewhat compensated for by higher levels of free H_2O_2).

PMNs also can employ a number of nonoxidative bactericidal mechanisms, although these are probably less important than oxidative mechanisms when oxy-gen is available. The pH within the phagocytic vesicle is very low, which favors peroxidase reactions, and which will at least inhibit replication of most bacteria. Primary granules fusing with the phagocytic vacuole release cationic proteins that damage bacterial cell walls and a variety of hydrolytic enzymes, including lysozyme, that function in digestion.

Like the PMN, most macrophages can also phagocytize particles under anaerobic conditions, but require oxygen for efficient killing. (An exception is the alveolar macrophage, which also requires oxygen for the phagocytic process.) Macrophages apparently utilize catalase rather than myeloperoxidase in H_2O_2-dependent degradative reactions. Bactericidal proteins such as those found in PMNs are absent in macrophages, although the latter contain a wide range of hydrolytic enzymes stored in cytoplasmic granules. These enzymes appear to be involved in digestion rather than killing per se.

Phagocytosis is an extremely important defense against microbial invasion and infection, far exceeding many of the more sophisticated elements of the immune system that we have considered elsewhere in this text.

Immune Responses to Specific Pathogens

Bacterial Diseases

The number of diseases in humans caused by bacteria is very large, and a comprehensive (or even cursory) description of them is beyond the scope or intent of this text. However, a few selected examples will be discussed here in order to give an impression of the way the immune system responds to bacterial infection.

Diseases Caused by Bacterial Toxins

Numerous bacteria produce disease in humans through release of soluble protein factors called toxins. Bacterial toxins are nearly always highly immunogenic, and the principal immune defense against disease in such cases involves neutralization of the toxins by antibody. Antibody may also be involved in opsonization of the bacterium itself for phagocytosis. Examples of such bacteria include *Staphlococcus aureus,* which can cause problems ranging from skin disease to food poisoning and toxic shock syndrome; *Clostridium botulinum,* whose toxin is a potent disruptor of neuromuscular transmission; and *Vibrio cholera.*

Pyogenic Bacteria

The role of antibody in facilitating complement lysis of bacteria is probably of relatively limited importance *in vivo.* All gram-positive, and many gram-negative, bacteria appear to be completely refractory to complement-mediated lysis due to properties of the bacterial cell wall covering the otherwise complement-sensitive plasma membrane. Thus the major immune defense against many such bacteria is phagocytosis, potentiated by antibody and certain of the complement components. Infections by these organisms attract large quantities of macrophages and PMNs. However, many of them are also relatively resistant to phagocytosis, and thus loci of infections can accumulate large quantities of pus. Bacteria of this type are thus called pyogenic (pus generating), and include most of the streptococci, which causes diseases ranging from meningitis to scarlet fever; *Hemophilus influenzae,* which is a major agent in meningitis; and *Neisseria gonorrhoeae.*

Intracellular Bacterial Infections

The most common example of bacteria that live inside cells is *Mycobacterium tuberculosis*. These organisms induce a normal antibody response, one result of which is that they are readily phagocytized by macrophages. However, once engulfed, they are able to avoid interaction with the bactericidal lysosomal granules and survive quite well as intracellular parasites. The principal immune defense in such cases may be T-cell-mediated inflammation. T cells, responding perhaps to bacterial antigens on the surface of infected macrophages, produce a number of lymphokines that may aid the macrophages in overcoming their intracellular infections. One undesirable side effect of this process, however, is the local tissue damage often associated with tuberculosis. The bacterium causing leprosy (*M. leprae*) has a similar life history to *M. tuberculosis,* living intracellularly, producing no toxin, and inducing T-cell immunity.

Another group of intracellular bacterial parasites are the *Chlamydiae*. These microorganisms are endocytosed by a number of cell types and ultimately destroy the host cells. However, if the bacteria are appropriately opsonized, destruction by phagocytes is quite efficient.

Resistance to Viral Infection

The term "virus" is an ancient one, and for many centuries was used to give some sort of identity to imagined pathogens that could not be seen. Even into the present century the distinction between bacteria and viruses was not always clear. For many years viruses were distinguished from bacteria solely on the basis of their ability to pass through very fine filters.

Viruses can be of the RNA type, or the DNA type, and either single or double stranded. They may multiply very rapidly, totally destroying the cell they grow in, or they may take up long-term residence in a cell, integrating into the host genome and in many cases causing no harm whatsoever to the host. A partial list of common viral diseases is given in Table 16-2.

There are several stages of viral infection where host defense mechanisms come into play. If the host has been actively immunized, either by previous infection or clinical exposure to attenuated virus, circulating or secretory antibodies may neutralize incoming viruses prior to their attachment to and penetration of host cells. If the virus does succeed in establishing an infection, and viral antigens are expressed at the infected cell surface, then cellular immune mechanisms come into play. T cells detect the viral antigens and react to the cell as if it were foreign. After a period of three to five days required for sensitization and full mobilization of the T-cell response, the CTL subset of T cells can attack and destroy the virally infected cells.

Table 16-2 Common Human Diseases Caused by Viruses

DNA viruses	Disease(s)
Adenoviruses	Respiratory infections
Herpes viruses	
H. simplex 1	Cold sores
H. simplex 2	Genital blisters
H. varicella	Chicken pox
H. zoster	Shingles
Epstein-Barr virus	Mononucleosis
Papova viruses	Warts (cervical cancer?)
Vaccinia (pox) viruses	Smallpox (probably extinct)

RNA viruses	
Myxoviruses	Influenza
Paramyxoviruses	Measles; mumps; parainfluenza
Picornaviruses	Common cold; poliomyelitis
Rhabdoviruses	Rabies
T-cell leukemia virus III	AIDS (Acquired Immune Deficiency Syndrome)
Togaviruses	German measles; yellow fever; myelitis

This involves direct contact between the effector T cell and the target cell, but the mechanism by which the target cell is destroyed is not known. T helper cells activated by virally infected cells may also initiate inflammatory reactions at the site of the infection. Details of the T-cell response to virally infected cells were presented in Chapter 14.

Although many human diseases caused by bacteria and fungi have been brought under control (in some parts of the world) by immunization, this is much less true for a number of viral diseases, such as influenza. One major reason for this is that some viruses seem periodically to alter their antigenic makeup, presumably by changing their coat or capsid protein structure. This is represented at the epidemiological level by massive outbreaks of flu. The Hong Kong flu epidemic of 1969 represented a new substrain of type A virus; persons with immunity developed against previous type A viral infections were defenseless against the new substrain. Although antibodies developed against one substrain will usually cross-react with a new substrain, this is of only marginal value to the host, since the principal host defense to virally infected cells is cellular, not humoral. Cellular immune "memory" developed in an infection by one viral substrain may not be reactivated by a slightly different substrain, and even if it were, the reactivated T cells would likely not recognize cells infected by the altered virus (Chapter 14).

Even in those cases where antibodies could be effective in controlling viral diseases, immunization against specific viruses may be ineffectual, because many viral diseases involve several viruses. Colds, for example, can be caused by at least 100 antigenically distinct viruses, making immunization for the common cold impractical.

A very important host defense against viral infection involves interferon. Interferon (or, more appropriately, interferons) were discovered in 1957 by Isaacs and Lindenmann. They treated isolated chick chorioallantoic membrane (CAM) with inactivated influenza virus, washed the membranes free of nonassociated virus particles, and then reincubated the treated membranes in fresh culture medium. After a period of incubation, they were able to demonstrate a factor in the culture medium that interfered with the growth of active virus on untreated CAM. They called this factor interferon.

Interferons have been the subject of intense investigation during the past two decades. They are produced by a variety of cell types in all vertebrates tested in response to viral infection. They can also be induced both *in vivo* and *in vitro* by a variety of nonviral substances such as polyanions, polynucleotides, polysaccharides, etc. Interferons are induced very rapidly in infected cells, but usually do not have any effect on viral maturation in the producer cell. Rather, they are secreted and act in a prophylactic fashion to prevent infection of healthy neighboring cells. Moreover, it now seems clear that interferons themselves do not have any direct antiviral activity but rather induce production of host factors that interfere with various stages of the viral infectivity cycle.

Interferons have been grouped into three broad classes. Alpha-interferons (IFN-α), previously called leukocyte interferon, are produced principally by leukocytes but also by fibroblasts under some conditions. There are at least three distinct IFN-α species in humans. All are about 20,000 daltons and stable at pH 2. Beta-interferon (IFN-β; also called fibroblast interferon) is the principal interferon produced by fibroblasts infected with virus or stimulated with synthetic double-stranded RNA. IFN-β in humans, like IFN-α, is acid stable. Its molecular weight is about 23,000. Gamma-interferons (IFN-γ; immune interferon) are larger than IFN-α or IFN-β (40,000–60,000 daltons) and are acid labile. They are produced by T cells that have been stimulated by antigen or by mitogens and by some T-cell lines. All three classes of interferons are structurally and antigenically distinct.

The mechanisms by which interferons confer protection against viral infection are still the subject of intense investigation. Cellular RNA and protein synthesis are required, after binding of interferon to the plasma membrane, in order for viral resistance to be developed. Whether or not IFN *must* enter the cell is unclear, since apparently as few as 10 molecules of IFN per cell can confer complete protection and it is difficult to determine whether so few molecules have actually entered the cell. Chromosome 21 in humans appears to be involved with interferon action, although whether it codes for an interferon receptor, or is a target for interferon induction of host synthetic activities, is not yet known.

Several points in the reproductive cycle of viruses have been suggested as the target for host activities induced by interferon. These include specific inhibition of transcription of the viral genome, specific inhibition of translation of viral mRNA, and inhibition of viral assembly. Excellent experimental evidence has been gathered to support an action at each of these loci and given the heterogeneity of interferons, it is possible that all of these points are susceptible.

Interferons have been proposed to have a number of effects in addition to inhibition of viral infection/replication. These include inhibition of cell division, general enhancement of cellular functions, alteration of plasma membrane properties, and either an inhibition or enhancement of immune function, depending on how it is used. Given the impurity of most interferons, it is possible that some of these activities are caused by materials isolated with interferons, rather than by the interferons themselves. Recently there has been considerable interest in the purported antitumor properties of interferons; a great deal of money is currently being spent to produce interferons in large quantities for rigorously controlled clinical tests. It will be some years before a definitive statement can be made about the effects of interferons on tumor growth in humans. Such studies, as well as studies on the activities and fundamental mechanisms of interferon activity, are being substantially aided by the large-scale cloning of interferon genes, and production of various of the interferons in the cloning vectors.

The Immune Response to Parasitic Infections

Parasitic infections are a major health problem in most parts of the world. Although largely controlled in the major industrialized nations by indirect public health measures, prevention by vaccination has not yet been achieved. For the most part this is because the immune response to many parasites is complex and not well understood. The lack of a source of purified antigens for most parasites also remains a problem. The World Health Organization has begun a major effort to bring parasitic diseases under control worldwide; developing a better understanding of the immunology of parasitic infections is a major component of this effort.

The major parasite-induced diseases in humans are listed in Table 16-3. Host resistance to these diseases is complex, and may involve important nonimmunological mechanisms. We survey here briefly what is known about the involvement of the immune system in the course of infection by these organisms.

Amebiasis (*Entamoeba histolytica*) Infections.   These infections, which are among the few pathogenic amoebic infections, occur by oral ingestion of amoebic cysts, which, once past the acidic milieu of the stomach, germinate and produce trophozoites. The latter attach to the mucosal lining of the lower gut and feed on local flora and residual food digested by the host. In many cases the mucosa is not penetrated, and the pathology may be relatively benign (low-grade fever, diarrhea). If penetration does occur, local ulcers may form, with accompanying symptoms of dysentery and colitis. The parasite may also spread to the liver, and even in some cases to the lung or brain, with more severe consequences.

Amebiasis is an example of a protozoan parasitic infection that provokes an

Table 16-3 Parasitic Infections in Humans

Protozoan	Metazoan (Helminthic)
Amebiasis	Ascariasis (N)
Leishmaniasis	Echinococcosis (C)
Malaria	Schistosomiasis (T)
Toxoplasmosis	Filariasis (N)
Trypanosomiasis	Trichinosis (N)

(N) = nematodes; (C) = cestodes; (T) = trematodes.

immune response, but in which immunological mechanisms play little or no role in the course of the disease caused by the parasite. Both humoral (IgM and IgG) and cellular (delayed and immediate hypersensitivity) responses can be detected. However, neither the magnitude nor quality of these responses can be correlated with the state of the disease, and to date attempts to transfer immunological protection passively have failed. *In vitro,* serum from patients can be shown to interact and interfere with trophozoite function. However, antibodies isolated from such sera have absolutely no protective effect, and previously infected hosts are generally as susceptible to subsequent infection as are naive hosts.

Leishmaniasis (*Leishmania sp.*).   Leishmaniasis (*Leishmania sp.*) is spread by sand flies, and the parasite enters the host with the insect's bite. Resultant disease presents in several different forms, each caused by a different species of *Leishmania* parasite. In all cases the parasites infect macrophages. In visceral leishmaniasis the host responds by producing large quantities of antibody indiscriminately, that is, antibody of many different specificities besides antibody directed against parasite antigens. Some cellular response (delayed-type hypersensitivity) may be apparent toward the end of the infection. Chemotherapy used to cure the disease results in reduced antibody production and increased delayed hypersensitivity, suggesting the latter may be involved in overcoming the infection. Cutaneous leishmaniasis, on the other hand, induces principally a cell-mediated immune response. Little or no antibody is produced. Delayed-type hypersensitivity is apparent during early stages of the infection and appears to be the major agent in recovery of the host. Whether the response is directed against the parasite itself, or against parasite-infected macrophages, is unclear. Individuals who recover from cutaneous leishmaniasis usually have permanent resistance to further infection, and cellular immunity appears to be the crucial immune agent in this protection.

Malaria (*Plasomodium sp.*)   *Plasmodium* organisms exist principally in the bloodstream, but in erythrocytes rather than macrophages. The parasites are transmitted to their vertebrate hosts through the bite of an anopheles mosquito. The parasites migrate to the liver where they enter hepatocytes and undergo asexual reproduction. After leaving the hepatocytes, the resulting merozoites infect red cells or, in some instances, reenter hepatocytes. Young children are particularly susceptible, although infants of mothers who have experienced the disease are protected for up to six months by maternal antibody. Infections can persist for many years, depending on the type of *Plasmodium* involved. The mechanism of persistence in the face of a host immune response is unclear. Since red blood cells turn over rapidly, the parasites cannot efficiently "hide" themselves from immune mechanisms by remaining within erythrocytes. Antigenic variation of the type seen in *Trypanosomes* (see below) is possible, but little convincing evidence has been put forward in support of this hypothesis.

The principal defense against malaria in humans is humoral. As in *Leishmania* infections, there is a polyclonal switch-on of antibody, such that large quantities of immunoglobulins of varying classes and antigenic specificities are produced. One danger of this polyclonal switch-on is that autoantibodies may be produced. In fact, anti-DNA and anti-smooth muscle antibodies have been detected; these may contribute to the severity of the disease. However, protective antibody is produced as part of this general activation process, and passively transferred antibody can reduce disease symptoms in infected patients. For some reason, long-term memory to malaria does not seem to be induced. Delayed hypersensitivity responses can be detected, but as with amoebic infections there is no correlation between the magnitude of the hypersensitivity response and state of the disease. Merozoites seem to be readily phagocytosed by macrophages as they leave hepatocytes; this is thought to be a part of natural immunity to malaria.

Toxoplasmosis (*Toxoplasma gondii*)   This is an intracellular parasite usually found in cats. Humans become infected by ingesting sporocysts shed by cats. The parasite initially goes through a rapidly dividing phase which, like *Plasmodium,* infects a cell, reproduces, and then leaves the cell. The parasite can spread to and infect many different tissues in the body. The parasite then enters a more slowly growing stage and remains for a longer time in an infected cell, and may even become encysted there. Both cellular and humoral defenses are active against *Toxoplasma,* and it is usually kept under control. Since some parasites usually remain in the host, drugs that compromise the immune system may allow a controlled infection to flare up and cause severe diseases. Toxoplasmosis may also be a danger to the fetus if a pregnant woman becomes infected for the first time during pregnancy, because the parasite can invade the fetus before the maternal immune response brings it under control. Spontaneous abortion or severe tissue damage can result. On the other hand, a controlled infection in the mother usually presents no problem to the fetus.

Trypanosomiasis (*Trypanosoma sp.*)   Trypanosomes cause African sleeping sickness (*T. brucei*) and Chagas' disease (*T. cruzi*). *Trypanosoma brucei* is injected into the vertebrate host through the bite of a tsetse fly. The parasite lives in the host's bloodstream; eventually it enters the nervous system (including the CNS), causing the sleepiness that usually presages coma and death. The host mounts a humoral response against the parasite, which decreases the number of parasites in the system. Recent evidence also suggests that host macrophages may be important in clearing various parasitic forms. However, trypanosomes have evolved an extremely effective defense against immunological attack called antigenic variation. Binding of antibodies to the surface of the parasites induces them to shed those antigens and to begin expressing new surface antigens toward which the host has not yet developed an immune defense. This allows the parasites to escape destruction by the immune system for a short period until antibodies against the new antigens begin to appear in the bloodstream, when the cycle is repeated. These antigenic variations appear to be genetically programmed (rather than being the product of random somatic events), and the number of variations has to date only been limited by the life span of the host. These parasites also cause polyclonal B-cell activation; autoimmune complications (see Chapter 18) are a serious concomitant of the disease. It may also be due to destruction of host cells which have parasite antigens bound to them.

The parasite *Trypanosoma cruzi* is spread by reduviid bugs. It is passed in the feces of the bug and enters the wound made by the bug when it feeds. *T. cruzi* has both an intracellular dividing form and a blood form. The cellular form prefers nervous and cardiac tissue, and death of the host is usually due to heart failure or nervous disruption. *T. cruzi* cannot change its surface antigens as can *T. brucei.* Antibody-dependent cell-mediated cytotoxicity (see Chapter 14) seems to be the major host defense against this parasite.

Ascariasis (*Ascaris lumbricoidies*).   Humans become infected with *Ascaris* by ingestion of embryonated *Ascaris* eggs. After hatching, the larva penetrates the intestinal wall and enters the circulation. It migrates through the lungs and the bronchial tree to the trachea, where it is coughed up, swallowed, and resumes its life in the intestine. While in the circulation and in the lungs the worms may cause an allergic reaction, particularly if the individual has been infected before. Elevated IgE and eosinophil levels are seen at this time, and T cells are also involved. However, treatment of experimental animals (mice) with Thy-1.2 antibodies results in a decrease in the number of larvae reaching the lungs, suggesting that the T cells involved may be suppressor T cells (see Chapter 13). No immune response is mounted against the adult worms, as they are free in the intestinal lumen and are inaccessible to the host immune system. (However, the adult worms do migrate, and sometimes leave the GI tract on their own, via the anus or mouth.)

Hydatidosis (*Echinococcus granulosis*).   *Echinococcus* is a small tapeworm that infects canines. Humans become infected with the larvae by ingesting the eggs. After hatching, the larvae penetrate the intestinal wall, and lodge somewhere in the body, usually in the peritoneal cavity. They grow into a large hydatid cyst that contains many larvae. The cysts have been known to contain up to 15 quarts of liquid; at this stage they crowd out other organs and have to be surgically removed. The fluid in them is very high in protein; rupture of the cyst can result in anaphylactic shock and death in a sensitized individual. *Echinococcus multiocularis* is a similar worm, whose cysts are found only rarely in humans. It has many small cysts that may break off and be carried away to infect other parts of the body, much in the manner of a cancer. Immunologic studies done on this species show that specific antibodies, both IgM and IgG, are produced. Interaction of antibody-coated parasites with complement or with lymphoid cells may help to prevent parasite proliferation. The cyst is composed of two layers, the outer one being very tough, and therefore resistant to destruction; this may explain the apparent lack of lysis of the cysts by antibody plus complement.

Filariasis (family *Onchocercidae*). Filarial worms are transmitted by various flies and mosquitos, including anopheles. Adult worms settle in the lymphatic vessels of their host, usually in the lower half of the body. Some species also inhabit subcutaneous or deep connective tissues. The females release larvae called microfilariae, which enter the bloodstream; these are highly antigenic but for some reason do not provoke a response. As the females mature they elicit an acute inflammatory response mediated by IgG_4, attracting polymorphonuclear cells, plasma cells, and eosinophils to the area and causing abscesses around the killed worms. Eventually the area becomes filled in with scar tissue. After many infections over a period of years, enough scar tissue builds up to block the lymphatics, and the disease known as elephantiasis results. Worms of the genus *Onchocerca* often infiltrate the eyes; the resulting immune response causes a disease known as River Blindness (because of the habitat of the vector). The role of the immune response in the development of disease is suggested by a good correlation between the cellular response to adult and larval antigens, and the course of the disease. Adult worm antigens elicit secondary responses in patients who have elephantiasis, but not in patients with any other stage of the disease. A cellular response to microfilarial antigens is seen only in the patients with no microfilariae present, indicating that the cellular response may be responsible for clearing the larvae from the bloodstream. Interestingly, people who are first exposed to the worms as adults rarely exhibit microfilaremia, while people who live in endemic areas and were exposed as children have high levels of circulating microfilariae. This suggests the presence of some tolerance, developing either over an extended period of time, or while the patients are infants.

Schistosomiasis (*S. monsoni, S. japonicum, S. haematobium*) *Schistosome cercariae* are released from their snail intermediate hosts and penetrate the skin of people walking in water where the snails reside. The larval worms migrate through the lungs and settle in the veins surrounding the urinary bladder or small intestine. They often cause hepatomegaly, because a large proportion of the eggs are unable to penetrate the bladder or intestinal wall and are carried up the portal vein to the liver, where they stimulate granuloma formation. About 60 percent of the entering cercariae are killed before they reach the lungs, by specific antibody and complement, or by IgG or IgE antibody and macrophages, neutrophils, or eosinophils through antibody-dependent cell-mediated cytotoxicity (Chapter 14). They have also been shown to activate complement by the alternative pathway in the absence of specific antibody, which in fact may kill a large number before the specific immune response is activated. As the worms mature, however, fewer and fewer are destroyed by the immune response. Stimulation with antigen shows that the immune response is not suppressed; the secondary response is fully functional. The worms are known to bind host blood group antigens, immunoglobulin via its Fc portion, and MHC antigens from cell surfaces. Masquerading as host tissue may allow the worms to avoid detection and destruction by the immune system. Recently it has been shown that young worms from the lungs are not killed by antibody or by cells, even though both agents have been shown to bind to the worms. This may be due to a change in the outer membrane covering the worm; soon after entering the host the membrane changes from a normal double lipid layer to a heptalaminate structure composed of two lipid bilayers.

Trichinosis (*Trichinella spiralis*)   These larvae reside in the muscle tissue of their hosts and are passed on to the next host when the meat is eaten. Humans generally contract trichinosis by consuming undercooked pork. (The larvae are killed by heat.) The larvae mature quickly in the intestine, mate, and the females burrow into the submucosa or lymphatic ducts and release new larvae. Any worms left in the intestine after two weeks are expelled by an allergic response that involves IgE and eosinophils. A delayed hypersensitivity response, initiated by the infiltration of T-cell lymphoblasts, is also seen. The larvae migrate from the intestine to other tissues, preferring skeletal muscle. They invade individual muscle cells and encyst, ultimately killing the cell by consuming its cytoplasm for nutrients and excreting metabolic wastes. The encysted larvae are protected from the immune response, and destruction of host tissue results in muscle weakness, which may lead to death if muscles of the diaphragm (a preferred spot) are heavily infested.

Bibliography

General

Cudkowicz, G., M. Landy, and G. Shearer (eds.), *Natural Resistance Systems Against Foreign Cells, Tumors and Microbes,* Academic Press, New York (1978).

Dick, G. (ed.), *Immunological Aspects of Infectious Diseases,* University Park Press, Baltimore (1979).

Friedman, R. M., *Interferons: A Primer,* Academic Press, New York (1981).

Mitchell, G. F., Responses to infection with metazoan and protozoan parasites in mice. *Adv. Immunol. 28,* 451 (1979).

Research

Anwar, A. R. E., J. R. McKean, S. R. Smithers, and A. B. Kay, Human eosinophil-and neutrophil-mediated killing of schistosomula of *Schistosoma mansoni in vitro.* I. Enhancement of complement-dependent damage by mast cell-derived mediators and formyl methionyl peptides. *J. Immunol. 124,* 1122 (1980).

Clark, R. A., and S. Szot, The myeloperoxidase-hydrogen peroxide-halide system as effector of neutrophil-mediated tumor cell cytotoxicity. *J. Immunol. 126,* 1295 (1981).

Villalta, F., and F. Kierszenbaum, Role of inflammatory cells in Chagas' disease. *J. Immunol. 133,* 3338 (1984).

CHAPTER 17

Reactions of Immunological Injury: Hypersensitivity and Inflammation

Hypersensitivity Reactions and Inflammation

During the development of immunology as a science, it was observed in a variety of situations that exposure to a particular antigen would in some instances lead not to protective immunity, nor to tolerance, but to a state in which subsequent exposure to the same antigen elicited a complex set of responses that were in fact harmful, and sometimes fatal, to the host. Inasmuch as the responses were antigen specific, they were included in the group of reactions regarded as immunological in nature.

Subsequent work demonstrating the involvement of lymphocytes and antibodies in these phenomena proved the correctness of this early conclusion.

These reactions are termed collectively *hypersensitivity reactions*. The tissue damage resulting from them is due largely to a process termed *inflammation*. The classic clinical manifestations of inflammation are an increase in blood vessel diameter and blood flow at the affected site, an increase in vascular permeability permitting escape of various leukocytes into surrounding tissue spaces, and local pain. Inflammation can be triggered by physical wounding and subsequent microbial infection, by hypersensitive responses to a variety of foreign antigens, or it may be the byproduct of an immune reaction against altered self components. In any event, as the offending antigen is removed from the site, these symptoms are reversed, and tissue regeneration is initiated. Although all of these aspects are readily observed when the inflammatory locus is at the surface of the body, it may be more difficult to diagnose inflammation at internal body sites. Often this can be inferred only indirectly, for example by impairment of organ function or the appearance in the circulation of molecules associated with inflammation, or tissue degradation products. If not reversed, inflammatory damage can be quite severe.

Hypersensitivity reactions fall into two principal categories, reflecting the two major subdivisions of the immune system itself. The first category includes those reactions initiated by antibody, principally IgE; these are termed *immediate hypersensitivity reactions,* because the accompanying inflammatory symptoms are manifested almost immediately after administration of antigen to a sensitized animal. The second category of reactions, initiated by T lymphocytes, is referred to as *delayed hypersensitivity.* Damage from these reactions is usually not obvious for a number of hours, or even days, after challenge of the sensitized host.

In terms of initial cellular and molecular mechanisms, there is little indeed to distinguish between immunity and hypersensitivity. If a distinction is to be made at all, it must be a quantitative rather than a qualitative one. Immune responses often involve components of both, and the ultimate effect in the host is determined by the balance between the two. This balance can be shifted by relatively trivial means, such as the form, amounts, timing, or route of administration of antigen.

Immediate Hypersensitivity (IH) Reactions

IH reactions occur as an indirect result of antibody–antigen reactions under certain special circumstances. Actually, neither antibody nor antigen play a direct role in the development of the pathological symptoms associated with IH. Substances released or activated as a result of the formation of antigen–antibody complexes, either in solution or on the membrane of certain cells, actually cause the tissue damage reactions characteristic of inflammation. There are basically two categories of IH reactions: those initiated by IgE plus antigen at the surface of mast cells or basophils (anaphylaxis), and those initiated by the formation of antibody–antigen complexes that subsequently bind and activate components of complement involved in inflammatory reactions (immune complex disorders).

Anaphylactic Reactions

Anaphylaxis means literally "reverse protection." This term was first used by Richet, who received the Nobel prize in medicine in 1913, to describe the rapid, often lethal sequence of events occurring in certain instances on the secondary administration of antigen. He studied anaphylaxis as a model for human allergy, a connection that proved to be valid.

Anaphylaxis has been studied most intensively in the guinea pig. A wide variety of antigens, administered in the proper dosage and form, and with an appropriate interval between the initial and challenging injections, will elicit a systemic anaphylactic reaction. Timing is critical, because in many species the hypersensitive state does not persist long after the initial exposure to antigen and cannot be "boosted" with repeated exposures. Within minutes after a challenging dose, the recipient may experience breathing difficulties, vomiting, convulsions, lowered blood pressure, and in some cases, unless rescued by drugs, death. The principal causes of death are severe shock and respiratory failure. The same sequence of events may occur in humans (e.g., in penicillin or bee venom hypersensitivity), except that the symptoms often occur in an even more accelerated fashion. The hypersensitive state also may persist over a longer time in humans.

The hypersensitive state can be transferred from a sensitized animal to an unsensitized animal by serum, but not by lymphoid cells. This was first demonstrated in humans in 1921 by Prauznitz and Küstner, who transferred serum from an allergic patient to a normal individual. When the latter was skin tested with the original allergen 24 hours later, definite allergic sensitivity was demonstrable. On the basis of the specificity of the reaction, the serum factors responsible for the allergic reaction were assumed to be antibodies. Serum factors were known to be heat sensitive but in humans at least they could not be identified with any known antibody class and were referred to simply as P–K or reaginic antibodies. In the 1960s, the Ishizakas in Japan showed that reaginic antibodies in humans belong to the then-novel IgE antibody class.

Depending on the particular animal, both IgG and IgE (or its electrophoretically identified counterpart in species where the existence of IgE has not been otherwise established) may initiate systemic anaphylactic reactions. In those species where IgE has been conclusively identified, it usually is the more potent of the two in initiating such reactions. Only rarely are IgM and IgA involved.

IgE-mediated hypersensitivity activity in serum can be distinguished from that mediated by other Ig classes in that the former can be destroyed by heating (60°C for three hours). Moreover, IgE antibody does not form precipitating complexes with its antigen, although antigen binding per se seems to be indistinguishable from other Ig classes. Because IgE does not cross the placenta in humans, newborn infants of allergic mothers face no immediate threat from hypersensitivity to environmental antigens. There may, however, be a genetically linked predisposition to the development of IgE-mediated allergies in the offspring of allergic patients. Such allergies are termed "atopic."

Mechanisms of Anaphylaxis

During the initial exposure to antigens, IgE antibodies may be produced in addition to other Ig classes. In normal individuals, IgE is produced only in response to parasitic infection. Which characteristics of the widely varying parasites lead to a common IgE immunogeneic pathway is unknown. Nor is it known at what level control of IgE production is lost in allergic individuals.

IgE antibodies are cytophilic for mast cells and basophils and seek out and bind to these cells around the capillary beds in various tissue spaces. Binding IgE to the cell surface occurs through interaction of the Fc region of the molecule with a plasma membrane Fc receptor, leaving the antigen-binding sites of the molecule facing outward from the cell. Upon reexposure to the antigen (allergen), IgE molecules on the surface of the target cells become cross-linked by the antigen, leading to a distortion of the IgE molecules. This activates a series of enzymatic reactions leading to the ultimate release of granules stored in the cell (Figure 17-1). These granules contain a variety of pharmacological agents that actually mediate the accompanying inflammatory symptoms (see the following).

Degranulation can also be initiated by antibodies directed against the exposed portions of IgE on the mast cell or basophil surface. This reaction is independent of complement and presumably results from the cross-linking of surface IgE by the second antibody. In this sense, the second antibody is simply mimicking the antigen. Sensitization and degranulation of mast cells can be prevented by pretreating target cells with the Fc portion of IgE, which blocks binding of intact IgE to the cell surface.

Anaphylactic reactions are modulated by a series of complex interactions with various nervous system agonists, including both catecholamines and acetylcholine. The prostaglandins also exert some influence on the course of allergic reactions.

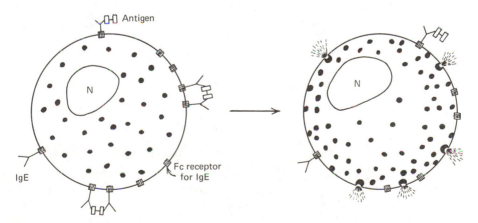

Figure 17-1 Release of histamine from mast cells triggered by antigen-cross-linked IgE bound to cell surface Fc receptors.

These interactions are not yet very well understood but modify both release of pharmacological agents from mast cells and basophils and the effect of these agents on target tissues. Thus, factors in the body that influence agonists of the sympathetic and parasympathetic nervous systems can also influence the course of an allergic attack.

The pharmacological agents that mediate inflammatory reactions are listed in Table 17-1. Histamine, which is formed by the enzymatic decarboxylation of histidine, is stored in secretory granules in mast cells, basophils, and, in some species, platelets. Histamine in platelets normally plays a role in the initiation of inflammatory reactions at the site of wounds or infections. It increases capillary size and permeability, thus facilitating the infiltration of the white blood cells that ultimately cause inflammation. Histamine also causes constriction of smooth muscle around blood vessels and bronchioles, narrowing their lumena. Both of these effects may be greatly exaggerated during an allergic attack. Mast cells are particularly abun-

TABLE 17-1 Pharmacological Agents Involved in Immediate Hypersensitivity Reactions

Agent	Found in	Action	Structure
Histamine	Mast cells, basophils, and platelets	Causes smooth muscle to contract; increases vascular permeability	H_2N—$(CH_2)_2$—C—N group with imidazole ring (H, N, CH CH)
Serotonin	Mast cells, basophils, and platelets	Causes smooth muscle to contract	HO … indole ring … NH … $CH_2CH_2NH_2$
SRS-A	Lung tissue	Causes smooth muscle to contract	Leukotriene
ECF-A	Mast cells?	Attracts eosinophils	Two tetrapeptides (molecular weight ca. 500)
Bradykinin	Serum (α-2-globulin)	Smooth muscle contraction; increases vascular permeability)	(H_2N)Arg-pro-pro-gly | phe | $(COOH)$arg-phe-pro-ser

dant in lung tissue; when histamine is released into local tissue spaces, the resultant constriction of the bronchioles impedes the passage of air in and out of the lungs, which is a major factor in the respiratory failure seen in systemic anaphylaxis or allergy.

Serotonin, a tryptophan derivative, also causes increased permeability of capillaries and smooth muscle contraction. In animals, although not in humans, it is stored in granular form in mast cells and platelets, and is released by IgE-antigen complexes at the cell surface. Recent evidence suggests that the serotonin stored in platelets is probably synthesized elsewhere. In rodents, it is a more active anaphylactic agent than histamine, but seems to play little, if any, role in human systemic anaphylaxis. Both serotonin and histamine are rapidly degraded by serum enzymes, which probably prevent the tissue-damaging effects of these otherwise useful agents from getting out of hand.

SRS-A (slow-reacting substance of anaphylaxis) has recently become the focus of intense study. It is located principally in lung tissue, but its precise cellular location is unknown in most species. In the rat, it is probably produced in monocytes. Lung tissue from a hypersensitive individual cultured with the sensitizing allergen releases SRS-A, which can cause prolonged constriction of smooth muscle in unsensitized individuals. In the guinea pig, release of SRS-A depends on the presence in the sensitized tissue of IgG_1 antibodies, although whether they act via a cell surface receptor is unknown. IgG_1 in the guinea pig does not bind complement. SRS-A is thought to be more important in asthma through its constrictive action on bronchioles. The structure of SRS-A was recently established; it is a leukotriene, a member of the ubiquitous prostaglandin group (Table 17-1). The same team that elucidated the structure of SRS-A also worked out a scheme for its synthesis. The biology of this molecule, which is present only in trace quantities in even the most active tissue, can now be studied in detail.

Eosinophil chemotactic factor of anaphylaxis (ECF-A) is a mixture of two tetrapeptides produced in IgE-mediated hypersensitivity reactions and is thus presumed to come from mast cells or basophils. The significance of ECF-A in hypersensitivity reactions is obscured by the general uncertainty about the role of eosinophils themselves. Because the latter contain large quantities of aryl sulfatase, which degrades SRS-A, it may be that ECF-A is elaborated to prevent SRS-A-mediated reactions from getting out of hand.

Regulation of IgE Production

A number of investigators have reported significant variations among inbred mouse strains in the ability to produce IgE, and hence in their tendency to develop anaphylactic responses. Since all members of a given strain exhibit the same ability to produce IgE, it seemed likely that IgE production is under some sort of genetic regulation. The amount of IgE produced by members of a mouse strain is independent of the antigen used, and the magnitude of the IgE response is unrelated to the magnitude of response in other Ig classes of the same strain. However, IgE production in low-response strains can be modulated. Katz and his colleagues showed that low-level radiation treatment, or administration of the drug cyclophosphamide, could elevate the IgE response in low-responder strains to levels comparable to high-response strains. This suggested that low-responder strains are not inherently defective in their ability to produce IgE, but rather are subject to some sort of immunological regulatory mechanism that selectively suppresses the IgE response to antigens.

Further analysis of the suppressor theory of IgE regulation has led to the description of two separate suppression mechanisms. Several research groups have shown that certain subclasses of T cells, called suppressor T cells (see Chapter 13), may be involved in the regulation of IgE production. This conclusion came from experiments in which the radiation or drug-induced elevation of the overall IgE response could be partially reversed by the passive transfer into the treated mouse of T lymphocytes from an untreated mouse of the same strain. A second mechanism for altering the ability to produce IgE in an antigen-unrelated fashion involves soluble factors present in the serum of low- and high-responder strains of mice. Two factors have been identified by Katz and his co-workers. A soluble factor present in the serum of low-responder strain mice, when passively transferred from untreated mice into radiation- or drug-treated mice, is very effective in suppressing the consequent increase in IgE production against a wide range of immunogens. A factor with opposite (enhancing) activity has been identified in both high- and low-responder strains. It seems likely that at least in mice the production of IgE in response to a particular immunogen may be regulated in part by the relative concentrations of these two factors in the system. More recently, Marcelletti and Katz have shown that a complex cascade mechanism involving the induction by IgE itself of Fc receptors for IgE on T cells, regulates production of IgE. These T cells produce enhancing and suppressive factors that modulate B-cell production of IgE.

The presence of IgE-modulating factors in the serum of animals with low IgE responsivity may have important implications for human allergy. It may be the case that persons with low or absent allergy reactions are actively suppressing IgE production when exposed to common allergens (or any other immunogen). If the nature of the suppressive factor or its method of production can be understood, it may be possible to either passively administer the factor to, or induce actively its production in, patients suffering from IgE-based allergic reactions.

IgE-mediated Anaphylactic Reactions in Humans

Hypersensitivity reactions in humans initiated by interaction of allergens with cell-bound IgE are summarized in Table 17-2. They may be localized or systemic in nature.

Local Allergic Reactions.   *Hay fever* (allergic rhinitis) affects about 10 percent of the population in the United States. It is caused principally by production of IgE antibodies to a variety of plant pollens, industrial chemicals, microbial spores, or microscopic insect parts associated with common household dust. Although the

Table 17-2 Common IgE-mediated Allergic Reactions in Humans

Disorder	Common allergens	Symptoms
Hay fever	Pollens, spores, dust	Sneezing; excessive mucosal secretions
Asthma	As in hay fever; may also be psychosomatic element in some cases	Breathing difficulties; chest discomfort, coughing
Allergic dermatitis	(May be secondary to hay fever or asthma)	Eczemalike eruptions on skin and face
Anaphylaxis	Foods, drugs, insect venoms	Breathing difficulties; shock (vascular collapse)

IgE is produced and disseminated systemically, the symptoms of the reaction are usually localized to the initial points of body contact with the allergen where IgE is fixed to mast cells or basophils—nose and mouth passages, the eyes, and, occasionally, the skin.

The nasal passages are particularly sensitive to airborne allergens. The nose is very rich in small blood vessels and secretory glands, in connection with its role in warming and moistening incoming air. It also functions to trap airborne particles before they reach the lungs, and thus is a natural trap for allergens. Enzymes in the nasal mucus partially degrade pollens and spores, exposing additional allergenic determinants. To make the nasal passages even better targets for allergic attacks, they contain not only mast cells but also IgE-producing plasma cells just under the mucosal lining. Histamine release from the mast cells causes local blood vessels to dilate, leading to swelling of the surrounding tissues, and at the same time directly or indirectly triggers secretion and sneezing. ECF-A attracts eosinophils to the affected area, which may lead to inflammation of local tissues, although the role of eosinophils in inflammatory reactions is not clear.

Asthma is a very complex condition that in only some cases (perhaps half) has an immunological or allergic basis. The component of asthmas that has an allergic basis is also initiated by IgE-allergen interactions at the surface of mast cells or basophils, in both of which the lung is particularly rich. The severe difficulty in breathing (dyspnea) experienced during an allergy attack is the result of three principal abnormalities: constriction of the bronchi and alveoli, mucosal blockage of bronchi and alveoli, and pulmonary edema. Bronchial constriction can readily be understood in terms of the known activities of histamine and SRS-A. The way in which these agents might act to trigger secretion of mucus is less clear, but production of a highly viscous mucus is characteristic of an asthmatic lung and can lead to continued blockage of airways long after the clearance of allergen from the system.

An unfortunate side effect of allergic asthma is that the patient develops an increased sensitivity to the mediators of the disease, especially histamine. Asthmatics may develop strong symptoms of the disease at levels of histamine 100 times less than that required to induce moderate symptoms in normal healthy individuals.

Systemic IgE-mediated Anaphylaxis in Humans. The allergic reactions generated in hay fever and asthma tend to remain fairly localized because the allergen is trapped in compartments that are effectively at the surface of the body (oral and nasal cavities, esophagus, lungs). In those cases where the allergen reaches the blood or lymph circulations, the resultant reaction can be widespread and involve several organs. Common substances that may trigger systemic reactions are insect venoms, drugs, or even certain foods.

In a venom-sensitive individual, the results can be quite severe and even fatal. One of the most serious consequences that may develop is irreversible shock, which results from the vasodilation and increased vascular permeability caused by histamine and other mediators, and the consequent drop in blood pressure. Pulmonary edema may also develop, making breathing difficult.

Food allergies can also result in systemic reactions, although occasionally the symptoms may be expressed in the skin as well (urticaria, hives). Mast cells residing in the intestinal wall can bind IgE, and when activated by specific food allergens release their pharmacological agents causing vomiting, cramps, and diarrhea. Allergic reactions to drugs may take several forms. The type of severe generalized reaction described above may occur for some drugs, such as penicillin. Other drugs may provoke immune complex reactions or delayed hypersensitivity reactions (see following sections).

Immune Complex Disorders

Immune complex disorders, another class of immediate hypersensitivity reactions, are initiated by antigen–antibody complexes that form freely in solution (in the plasma) rather than at a cell surface. Normally, the concentration of any antigen in the system is sufficiently low, or the antigen is present for a sufficiently brief time, that antigen–antibody complexes are quickly and safely removed by the phagocytic machinery of the immune system. However, under a variety of special conditions, antigen–antibody complexes may persist in high concentrations for prolonged periods, and in such cases significant damage to host tissues may result. These reactions must be considered separately from systemic anaphylaxis.

Antigen–antibody complexes often stick to the walls of capillary vessels and may actually pass between the endothelial cells and settle on the underlying basement membrane. The complexes bind complement, and release C3a and C5a fragments. These then attract polymorphonuclear leukocytes to the area, which phagocytize the complexes. In the course of doing so, they release hydrolytic enzymes (principally cathepsins D and E) into the surrounding space, causing inflammation and destruction of local tissues, including capillary walls, which may lead to local hemorrhage.

The complexes may also bind to and activate platelets and basophils attracted to the area by activated complement components. These reactions are probably not mediated by surface Fc receptors since they can be effected by F(ab)$_2$ fragments. Nevertheless, the end result is the release of additional pharmacological agents stored in these cells, which can further exacerbate inflammation.

These reactions can be induced with virtually any antigen given in large and repeated doses, whether locally or systemically. They are an important natural side effect in a wide range of diseases, ranging from autoimmune disorders to parasitic and microbial infections. If the complexes are cleared by the reticuloendothelial system, the accompanying inflammation may be acute, and heal rapidly. If the complexes are not phagocytized, or if antigen is constantly generated *in situ,* chronic inflammatory disease may set in. One of the most common organ sites for immune complex disease is the kidney. The resulting glomerulonephritis can seriously impair the normal sieving function of the kidneys, resulting in excretion of valuable blood products. Immune complexes may also settle in capillaries in the skin, causing a rash (Arthus reaction).

Before 1940, immune complex disorders were a common side effect in persons passively immunized with serum raised in animals (horses, cows, goats, etc.). The serum itself serves as a potent and broad-spectrum antigen, inducing a correspondingly broad spectrum of antibodies in the host. With continued administration of the heterologous serum, antigen-antibody complexes begin to deposit in various sites throughout the body, with the consequences noted above. This particular syndrome was referred to as serum sickness. It is now rarely seen, since programs of active, prophylactic immunizations have replaced the practice of passive immunization with heterologous antiserum. It is, however, often a problem in transplant patients receiving heterologous antilymphocyte serum (ALS) or globulin (ALG) an an immunosuppressive reagent.

Immune complex disorders that arise endogenously still remain a serious clinical problem. Any persistent infection (bacterial, viral, parasitic) can lead to sustained presence in the system of foreign antigens, with consequent formation and deposition of antigen–antibody complexes. Chronic immune complex symptoms are a frequent side disorder in cancer patients, with complexes formed between antibody and freely circulating tumor antigens. And finally, as we will see in Chapter 18, immune complex deposition and the resultant inflammation is a common consequence of autoimmune disease.

Delayed Hypersensitivity Reactions

The second major class of hypersensitivity reactions are those initiated by lymphocytes rather than antibody. Classically they are observed by injection of antigen into the skin of a sensitized individual. The symptoms are then observed *in situ* some 24 to 48 hours later—hence the name "delayed hypersensitivity." Such reactions were described as early as 1890, although their dependence on lymphocytes, as shown by passive transfer experiments, was not clear until the work of Landsteiner and Chase in the 1940s.

The prototypical delayed-type hypersensitivity (DTH) reaction is the tuberculin reaction and, again, the animal model most commonly used is the guinea pig. In a guinea pig previously sensitized to tubercle bacilli, intradermal injection of either the bacilli or antigenic proteins derived therefrom (tuberculin or purified protein derivative, PPD), will cause a DTH reaction. About 8 to 10 hours after the injection, lymphocytes and macrophages (and a lesser number of granulocytes) begin to infiltrate the injection site. This infiltration continues, reaching a peak 24 to 48 hours later. At the peak of the infiltration, many of the lymphocytes are blastoid and synthesizing DNA. Two things are clear about this phage of the reaction. First of all, there must be intact lymphatic drainage from the site of the injection in order for the reaction to be initiated. If drainage is ablated or otherwise circumvented, cellular infiltration and subsequent events will not occur. On the other hand, the infiltrating cells clearly arrive at the site via blood vessels, not via the lymphatic circulation. Thus the reaction is apparently not initiated *in situ,* but in nearby draining lymph node(s). Activated lymphocytes leaving the draining node eventually enter the bloodstream and then arrive at the reaction site.

The second important factor known about the infiltration stage of the reaction is that the vast majority of the lymphocytes are attracted to the site nonspecifically, that is, they themselves have no specificity for the sensitizing antigen. In passive transfer experiments where cells from a sensitized donor are labeled with tritiated thymidine, only about 5 percent or so of the cells infiltrating the site of the reaction are labeled. Conversely, if unlabeled sensitized cells are transferred to an unsensitized host whose own cells were previously labeled by chronic exposure to ^{3}H-TdR, greater than 90 percent of the infiltrating cells are labeled. Thus it is clear that the sensitized cells have as at least one of their functions the recruitment of other cells to the reaction site. We may presume this occurs through the release of lymphokines by antigen-specific T cells at the injection site.

Twelve to 24 hours after injection of antigen into a sensitized animal, the injection site shows visible signs of a DTH reaction. The area around the site becomes reddened (erythema), due to capillary dilation, in a manner typical of a localized inflammatory reaction. It usually becomes thickened and hard to the touch (induration), due to a dense accumulation of leukocytes just below the skin. In severe cases, there may be visible necrosis of tissue at the center of the lesion. Depending on the amount of antigen injected, the reaction usually subsides between 48 to 96 hours.

Delayed reactions can also be produced systemically. If a sensitized guinea pig is given tuberculin or PPD intravenously or intraperitoneally, it can go into shock as early as 5 to 8 hours later. This reaction peaks at about 24 hours, and can be fatal. The basis of the systemic reaction is unknown. Animals are usually sensitized for DTH reactions by injection of antigen, in combination with Freund's adjuvant, into multiple subcutaneous sites around the body. Humoral responses and DTH reactions usually proceed in parallel. The responding cells in DTH are known to be T lymphocytes and include both Lyt-2$^-$ and Lyt-2$^+$ subsets. T cells from sensitized individuals can be used to pass the hypersensitive state and will proliferate vigorously when exposed to the sensitizing antigen *in vitro*.

In DTH reactions, T cells themselves probably do not cause tissue damage directly. Rather, on contact with sensitizing antigen they secrete a variety of soluble factors (lymphokines), which trigger a complex series of cellular and molecular events. These lymphokines seem to be identical to those secreted during the proliferative response of sensitized T cells to antigen *in vitro*. Some of these lymphokines attract other lymphocytes, or monocytes and granulocytes, to the reaction site *in vivo;* these cells release a variety of enzymes and other factors that lead to a localized state of inflammation and tissue damage characteristic of the DH state. Damaged cells are cleared from the site by phagocytes.

In the sections that follow, we examine each of the principal lymphokines involved in DTH reactions and their known or postulated modes of action. These factors were defined some years ago on the basis of their cellular activities *in vivo* and *in vitro.* Many of these same factors have doubtless been "rediscovered" and renamed by immunologists studying soluble factors released by sensitized T lymphocytes *in vitro* (Chapters 13 and 14). Unfortunately, we do not know in most cases which "classical" hypersensitivity factors correspond to which of the more currently defined lymphokines, so for now we shall have to retain the older terminology.

Factors Affecting Cell Traffic Patterns

One of the earliest factors to be identified and isolated is the macrophage *migration inhibition factor* (MIF). The effects of this factor were described as early as 1932. Rich observed that when spleen fragments from normal guinea pigs are cultured *in vitro,* lymphocytes and macrophages will slowly migrate out of the fragments and settle on the surrounding tissue culture dish. This same phenomenon can be observed using spleen fragments from guinea pigs sensitized to tuberculin. However, if tuberculin is added to the tissue culture medium in which the sensitized spleen fragments are cultured, only lymphocytes migrate into the surrounding medium. Macrophage migration is inhibited. Nothing in the serum of a tuberculin-sensitized guinea pig affects macrophage migration of either normal or sensitized animals; the phenomenon seems to involve one or more cell types resident in the spleen itself. The same phenomenon is observed using antigens other than tuberculin, as long as the sensitizing protocol induces delayed hypersensitivity. No such effect can be observed in guinea pigs undergoing a normal humoral immune response, or an immediate hypersensitivity reaction.

Continued analysis of the inhibition effect suggested that lymphocytes might be the key cell involved, and that macrophages played a more or less passive "target cell" role. A major step forward in these investigations was made possible by the development of the capillary tube migration assay for MIF (Figure 17-2) by George and Vaughan in 1962. This introduced a degree of precision and sensitivity into analysis of this effect that had been previously lacking. The relationship between macrophages and lymphocytes was finally resolved in 1966 when it was shown more or less simultaneously by two different labs that sensitized lymphocytes, on

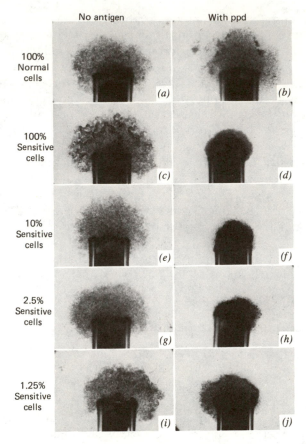

Figure 17-2 Mixed populations of normal and sensitive peritoneal exudate cells with and without antigen. Note that 15 μg/ml PPD in the media inhibits the populations when the sensitive cells make up 100 percent (*d*), 10 percent (*f*), or 2.5 percent (*h*) of the total population. [Taken from J. R. David, H. S. Lawrence, and L. Thomas, Delayed hypersensitivity in vitro. *J. Immunol. 93,* 274 (1964). Copyriht by the Williams and Wilkins Co. and the author (J. R. David), 1964.]

contact with the specific sensitizing antigen, produce a soluble factor that strongly inhibits the migration of macrophages. This factor was promptly named macrophage migration inhibition factor (MIF). MIF produced by sensitized lymphocytes in response to antigen can inhibit the migration of either normal or sensitized macrophages. Thus both immunological specificity and MIF production are lymphocyte functions, and macrophages do indeed play a more or less nonspecific role as target cells for MIF. The production of MIF has been shown in a wide range of DH-sensitized animals, including humans, and is used as one of several routine assays to detect the hypersensitive state.

MIF in guinea pigs is composed of at least two species, one of which has a pI of 3 to 4 and a molecular weight of 65,000, and the other of which has a pI of 5 and a molecular weight of 25,000 to 40,000. Human MIF contains three distinct species. One appears early after T-cell stimulation and has a pI of 4 to 5 with a molecular weight of about 23,000. After more prolonged stimulation *in vitro,* two additional species can be detected, with PIs of 2.4 to 3.3 and 4.3 to 5.6, and molecular weights of 65,000 and 23,000 to 43,000, respectively. Murine MIF is also molecularly heterogeneous.

The supernates from activated lymphocyte cultures that contain MIF activity have been analyzed by a number of laboratories for other factors which might play a role in DTH-associated phenomena. One of the first to be defined was a factor that has a seemingly opposite effect of that exerted by MIF—it *attracts* macrophages. This factor, called *macrophage chemotactic factor* (MCF), although similar in a number of its properties to MIF, is clearly a distinct molecule. It only exerts an effect on macrophages (or monocytes) across a concentration gradient; if macrophages are exposed to a uniform concentration of MCF, no effect on the behavior of the cells can be observed. MCF is produced only by sensitized T lymphocytes, and only on contact with the specific sensitizing antigen. Unlike MIF, MCF is not strictly species specific; whereas guinea pig MIF will not inhibit rabbit macrophages, guinea pig MCF attracts both guinea pig and rabbit macrophages.

There is also a set of factors that exert chemotactic and migration inhibitory effects on leukocytes. *Leukocyte inhibitory factor* (LIF), which is distinct from MIF, has been studied mostly in humans. It is tested for in a capillary migration assay in the same way as MIF, except that the capillary tube is usually loaded with neutrophilic PMNs. Whether or not it directly inhibits the migration of eosinophils or basophils is less clear, because of the difficulty in getting large quantities of pure populations of these cells for study. LIF has absolutely no effect on macrophages or monocytes. The *leukocyte chemotactic factor* (LCF) also exists and is specific for leukocytes.

Factors that Affect Cellular Activity

It was originally observed that preparations containing MIF activity, in addition to affecting the movement of macrophages and monocytes, also alter their level of activation. At one time it was thought that this activity was distinct from MIF, and it was accordingly given a separate name, MAF (macrophage activation factor). However, it now seems likely that both activities reside in the same molecule. MIF causes macrophages to become generally more "sticky" in that they adhere more tightly to glass and plastic substrates; they also phagocytize bacteria and inert particles more rapidly than do unstimulated macrophages. These enhanced activities are not directed exclusively toward the original stimulating antigen; the macrophages become more reactive and phagocytic to a wide variety of antigens and cell types, including in some cases syngeneic tumor cells. These activities require at least 72 hours incubation of the macrophages in the presence of MIF to be affected, whereas the migration inhibitory properties of MIF are obvious within 12 hours. Another delayed effect of MIF on macrophages is an increase in glucose oxidative metabolism, which also is not observed until three days of culture with MIF. This extensive lag period seen *in vitro* may be an artifact, since macrophages found at the site of a DTH reaction *in vivo* after 12 to 24 hours are highly activated. Recently, several laboratories have reported that many of the activities of MAF are mimicked by γ-interferon; this is a possibility that will certainly be followed up in the next year or so.

A factor distinct from MIF that stimulates blastogenesis, DNA synthesis and proliferation in unsensitized lymphocytes has been identified. It is usually referred to as blastogenic factor (BF). Like the other factors described above, BF is produced by sensitized lymphocytes on interaction with antigen. However, once produced, it also acts on cells in a completely antigen-independent manner. Its effect is usually monitored by uptake of ^{3}H thymidine into the lymphocytes, a process that, depending on the species, may reach a maximum in three to five days. BF is a protein, with a molecular weight of about 30,000. It apparently functions by recruiting lymphocytes arriving at the site of the DH reaction. Whether BF acts on T cells or B cells, or both, is not clear. It may be identical with IL-2 (Chapter 13). If it reacted with and activated T cells in a nonspecific way, it is possible that they might produce more soluble factors that could, in effect, amplify the response. On the other hand, this could then create a problem in ultimately controlling or "damping" the reaction. Thus, at present, the precise role of BF is still uncertain.

The way in which these factors work *in vivo* is difficult to test. It is clear, however, that they do affect the course of DTH reactions *in vivo*. If the supernatant medium from a culture of sensitized lymphocytes plus antigen is concentrated and injected subcutaneously into an unsensitized animal, typical symptoms of a DTH reaction, including appropriate cell infiltrates, erythema, and induration, can all be observed. This occurs within six to eight hours, reflecting the short circuiting of the antigen encounter and lymphocytes activation step that was carried out *in vitro*.

A reasonable picture of the sequence of events for an experimentally induced local DH reaction might be something like the following. Circulating, sensitized T cells encounter the antigen at the site of injection. Given the requirement for an intact lymphatic drainage, it seems unlikely that these initially reacting lymphocytes remain at the site, but rather proceed to and are trapped in the local draining lymph node. Alternatively, antigen could move from the site into the draining node, initiating the reaction there. In either case, the presence of activated lymphocytes in the primary node likely results in a marked reduction in its efferent drainage (see Chapter 2). Thus more lymphocytes may reach the reaction site via the bloodstream, but lymphatic drainage from the site to the primary lymph node will slow down somewhat as a result of its blocked drainage. This would lead to a gradual buildup of white cells at the reaction site. Sensitized T cells, on interaction with antigen at the site, will begin to produce and release the various soluble factors just described. More macrophages and monocytes will be attracted to the site and be trapped there by CF and MIF, respectively. The macrophages will be activated by the MAF activity of MIF. Leukocytes will also be attracted to the site and trapped there by LCF and LIF. So far, the increased number of lymphocytes infiltrating DH lesions has not been explained in terms of a specific factor; altered lymphatic flow may be sufficient to account for this effect. At any rate, lymphocytes arriving at the site may be acted on by BF, which, in view of the action of nonspecific mitogens generally in relation to DH (see following), seems likely to lead to the production of still more of the factors mentioned previously.

Studies by Gershon and his colleagues on delayed hypersensitivity in mice suggest that some of the mediators traditionally associated with immediate hypersensitivity reactions may also, at least in the mouse and perhaps in other species as well, play a role in DTH reactions. Mice have no basophils, and their mast cells contain predominantly serotonin rather than histamine; although some histamine is present in the mouse, it has no effect on mouse blood vessels. The serotonin can be displaced from mast cell granules by reserpine. The displaced serotonin is eventually secreted and then rapidly degraded by extracellular enzymes. The unexpected observation was made that reserpine-treated mice display no DTH reactivity, unless the extracellular breakdown of serotonin is inhibited. Furthermore, DTH cannot be passively transferred into reserpine-treated mice with sensitized lymphocytes. However, DTH can be transferred with lymphocytes *from* a reserpine-treated mouse *to* an unsensitized mouse, even though the donor in this case was not exhibiting any DTH symptoms. Thus, in mice it would appear that serotonin, a mediator classically associated with IH, may be important in DTH reactions as well.

Bibliography

General

Cochrane, C. G., and D. Koffler, Immune-complex disease in experimental animals and man. *Adv. Immunol. 16,* 185 (1973).

Freedman, S. O., and P. Gold (eds.), *Clinical Immunology,* Second Edition, Harper & Row, New York (1976).

Fudenberg, H. H., D. P. Stites, J. L. Caldwell, and J. V. Wells, *Basic Clinical Immunology,* Lange Medical Publications, Los Altos, California (1976).

Ishizaka, K., and T. Ishizaka, Mechanisms of reaginic hypersensitivity and IgE antibody response. *Immunol. Rev. 41,* 109 (1978).

Rocklin, R. E., K. Bendtzen, and D. Greineder, Mediators of immunity: Lymphokines and monokines. *Adv. Immunol. 29,* 56 (1980).

Tung, A. S., N. Chiorazzi, and D. H. Katz, Regulation of IgE antibody production by serum molecules. *J. Immunol. 120,* 2050 (1978).

Research

David, J. R., Lymphocyte mediators and delayed-type hypersensitivity. *N. Engl. J. Med. 288,* 143 (1973).

Goetze, J., and K. Austen, Structural determinants of eosinophil chemotactic factor of anaphylaxis. *J. Exp. Med. 144,* 1424 (1976).

Jardieu, P., T. Uede, and K. Ishizaka, IgE-binding factors from mouse T lymphocytes. *J. Immunol. 133,* 3266 (1984).

Katz, D. H., R. F. Bargatze, C. A. Bogowitz, and L. R. Katz, Regulation of IgE antibody production by serum molecules. VII. The IgE-selective damping activity of suppressive factor of allergy (SFA) is exerted across both strain and species restriction barriers. *J. Immunol. 124,* 819 (1980).

Leonard, E., and M. Meltzer, Characterization of mouse lymphocyte-derived chemotactic factor. *Cell. Immunol. 26,* 200 (1976).

Marcelletti, J., and D. Katz, FcRe+ lymphocytes and regulation of the IgE antibody system (I–IV). *J. Immunol. 133,* 2821, 2829, 2837, 2845 (1984).

Murray, H., G. Spitalny, and C. Nathan, Activation of mouse peritoneal macrophages in vitro and in vivo by interferon-γ. *J. Immunol. 134,* 1619 (1985).

Newman, W., S. Gordon, U. Hammerling, A. Senik, and B. R. Bloom, Production of MIF and an inducer of plasminogen activator by subsets of T cells in MLC. *J. Immunol. 120,* 927 (1978).

Pick, E., Effect of migration inhibitory factor (MIF) on macrophage c-AMP and on responsiveness to adenylate cyclase stimulators. *Cell. Immunol. 32,* 329 (1977).

CHAPTER **18**

Autoimmunity

The subject of autoimmunity brings into focus one of the central questions of immunology: How does an individual organism distinguish self from nonself? The molecules of which self is constructed are qualitatively the same as those used in the construction of any other living organism, yet the immune system remains completely inert to components of self while vigorously attacking and destroying anything regarded as nonself. This principle was noted in the early 1900s by Paul Ehrlich, who labeled this aversion to self-reactivity *"horror autotoxicus."*

There are a number of parameters that seem to be true of autoimmune diseases generally. (1) Females experience such diseases more frequently than males, the ratio in some cases being as high as four or more to one. This may be related to the

Table 18-1 HLA Allele Associations with Specific Diseases

Disease	HLA[a] allele	Relative risk[b]
Hodgkin's disease	A1	1.4
Acute lymphocytic leukemia	A2	1.4
Hemochromatosis	A3	8.2
Bechet's disease	B5	6.3
Allergic rhinitis	B7	9.0
Chronic autoimmune hepatitis[c]	B8	9.0
Myasthenia gravis[c]	B8	3.7
Tuberculosis	B8	5.1
Ankylosing spondylitis	B27	87.4[d]
Reiter's syndrome	B27	37.0
Salmonella arthritis	B27	30.0
Psoriasis vulgaris[c]	Cw6	13.3
Multiple sclerosis[c]	DR2	4.4[d]
Goodpasture's syndrome	DR2	14.2
Tubercular leprosy	DR2	8.1
Systemic lupus erythematosus[c]	DR2	4.0
	DR3	4.1
Grave's disease[c]	DR3	3.9
Type 1 diabetes[c]	DR3	4.5[d]
	DR4	4.6[d]
Addison's disease[c]	Dw3	6.3
Celiac disease	DR3	54.0
Dermatitis herpetiformis[c]	DR3	56.4
Myasthenia gravis[c]	DR3	3.9
Chronic active hepatitis	Dw3	6.9
Sjogren's syndrome	DR3	9.7
Pemphigus vulgaris	DR4	14.4
Rheumatoid arthritis[c]	DR4	6.0[d]
Hashimoto's disease[c]	DR5	3.5
Juvenile arthritis[c]	DR5	6.6
Scleroderma pigmentosum[c]	DR5	5.0

[a]The assignment to HLA DR specificities was made before development of our recent and more detailed knowledge of the HLA-D region based on molecular genetics. It is likely that more than just the DR locus class II molecules are involved.

[b]Relative risk is determined by dividing the frequency of the disease in individuals with the allele by the frequency of the disease in individuals without the allele.

[c]Diseases with definite autoimmune component.

[d]The relative risk for these diseases may vary considerably in different ethnic groups. For example, the relative risk of Japanese with HLA-B27 for ankylosing spondylitis is over 300.

fact that females generally have more vigorous immune responses than do males. (2) Although some indication of antiself reactivity is evident in most elderly individuals, they do not seem to suffer particularly from overt symptoms of autoimmune disease; debilitating forms of autoimmune disease usually appear during the breeding years. (3) Tissue damage in autoimmune pathologies is nearly always inflammatory in nature, usually related to deposition of antibody–antigen complexes in various tissue compartments.

The causes of autoimmune disease are rarely understood. In most cases it is doubtful that antiself reactivity is the primary dysfunction; more often, it seems likely that autoimmunity developed secondarily to some other problem, such as viral infection, or some natural or imposed disordering of immune components or other physiological systems.

A discussion of autoimmunity necessarily intersects closely and often with the study of tolerance (Chapter 13). There is also a significant association of many autoimmune diseases with specific HLA alleles (Table 18-1). The reason for an association between a particular disease and a particular HLA antigen is unclear. One possible explanation is that different HLA molecules may act as points of attachment or entry into the cell for different pathogenic organisms. Another possibility is that some microbes may have major antigens that "mimic" certain MHC antigens, such that the host views the microbe as self, allowing it to flourish. Yet a third hypothesis is that the combination of some microbial antigens with some HLA molecules fails to create an antigenic complex reacted against by the host, either because of a "hole" in the T-cell receptor repertoire for the resulting complex, or because the complex preferentially activates a suppressor rather than a helper pathway.

Autoimmunity is obviously important to study from a clinical point of view, since so many humans are afflicted with primary or secondary autoimmune disorders. But it also provides, in effect, an interesting natural experiment, the results of which, when properly interpreted, will doubtless tell us a great deal about how the immune system functions.

Autoimmune Diseases in Humans

Systemic Lupus Erythematosus (SLE)

SLE is a generalized, systemic inflammatory disorder, and is perhaps the most prominent example of an autoimmune disease in which autoreactivity is directed toward a wide spectrum of self-tissues and antigens. This suggests that the defect may be at the level of control over self-reactivity generally, rather than escape or *de novo* generation of an individual antiself clone. It is thus of considerable theoretical interest as well as being important clinically.

SLE, like many autoimmune diseases, is seen most frequently in females, most often between the teen years and middle life. It seems to have a genetic element in that family members of someone with SLE show a higher incidence of SLE and other autoimmune disorders than does the population at large. There is a high association with HLA-DR3. The most prominent symptoms are a generalized fever and weakness and erythematous lesions that are prominent on the face, particularly the nose. These lesions are highly sensitive to ultraviolet light, including sunlight. Other symptoms include pleurisy and kidney dysfunction. Hypergammaglobulinemia and low levels of serum complement are also common companion symptoms, as are antibodies to T lymphocytes. These latter tend to be specific for T8$^+$ suppressor cells, and there is thus a shift to higher T4/T8 ratios in SLE patients.

A diagnostic feature of SLE is the presence in the blood of so-called LE cells. These are granulocytes that have ingested large quantities of Ag-Ab complexes, particularly those involving nucleic acids. These cells, found in bone marrow as well as blood, typically have a dense, amorphous cytoplasmic mass that displaces the cell's own polymorphic nucleus to the cell periphery. A second characteristic of SLE is a high level of antibodies in the serum reactive with nucleic acids. These will react with single- and double-stranded DNA, RNA, and poly A. Antibodies may also be produced that react with nucleic acid-associated proteins such as histones. In addition to nucleic acid antibodies, many individuals also have serum antibodies specific for their own T lymphocytes. T-cell activity is generally depressed in SLE patients, with a normal or elevated B-cell function.

The pathological concomitants of SLE result mainly from the deposition of Ag-Ab complexes in blood vessels (vasculitis) and renal glomeruli (glomerulonephritis). Seventy-five percent of patients have nephritis at autopsy. The specific damage in these cases is inflammatory, involving phagocytic cells attracted to the site by complement fragments. However, a role for antibodies in the mediation of complement-dependent cytotoxicity and in antibody-dependent cell-mediated cytotoxicity (Chapter 14) cannot be ruled out.

The etiology of SLE, as of most autoimmune diseases, is not well understood. It is not known whether development of antiself reactivity is the primary dysfunction, or whether it is a secondary consequence of some other pathological condition. As noted previously, there does seem to be a genetic predisposition to autoimmune dysfunctions in the families of SLE patients. A high level of myxovirus particles in renal biopsy material, plus the presence of antibodies specific for double-stranded DNA, has led to the postulation of a viral infection as the primary disorder, which could lead to exposure of self-DNA from lysed cells as well as alteration of cell surface self-antigens. However, this must remain simply only one of a number of reasonable possibilities.

Rheumatoid Arthritis (RA)

RA is a systemic inflammatory disease of the connective tissue, although it affects primarily the synovial membranes of bone joints. These membranes become heavily infiltrated with lymphocytes and monocytes and often have the appearance of localized delayed hypersensitivity reactions. In some advanced cases, the infiltration of lymphocytes (principally T4$^+$) may become so heavy that nodules form, with well-organized lymphoid follicles. If unchecked, the inflammation process can cause nearly complete (and irreversible) destruction of joint tissues.

RA is two to three times more common in women than men, and usually affects women in their middle to late years. Patients with RA have a much higher than expected frequency of the class II antigen HLA-DR4.

The majority of patients with RA have a form of antibody in their serum and synovial fluid called rheumatoid factor (RF). These antibodies are usually of the IgM class, and react with the Fc portion of self-IgG molecules. RF can be produced by isolated synovial tissue from RA patients. One possibility is that an unusual IgG is produced as part of the etiology of the disease, and that the sudden high levels of these molecules induce the production of RF by synovial B cells. It has also been suggested that the reactivity of RF with IgG, which is of a rather low affinity, is a secondary specificity, a cross-reaction with a more relevant disease-associated antigen. RF also reacts with certain nuclear proteins, for example. Activation of complement by the RF-IgG complexes is thought to be a major source of the inflammatory damage in RA. However, low levels of RF also occur in normal individuals, and substantial amounts of RF injected into normal subjects fail to induce noticeable RA symptoms. Thus the exact role of rheumatoid factor in RA is unclear. RA patients also have autoantibodies directed against connective tissue and nucleic acids, although the main damage appears to be from Arthus-like lesions in the synovial membranes and small arteries. However, various T-cell lymphokines have been identified in synovial fluid in RA patients, suggesting a possible involvement of DH injury as well.

The etiology of rheumatoid arthritis is uncertain. The pathological correlates of the disease, as it progresses, definitely have an immune basis, but it is uncertain whether a breakdown in self-tolerance is what actually initiates RA. Loss of self-tolerance, or alterations in self-antigens, may be secondary to some other disease process. For example, a high percentage of juvenile RA patients have high levels of serum antibodies to rubella virus. However, juvenile RA is in many ways distinct from adult RA and no general agreement exists on how the latter originates.

Autoimmune Thyroiditis (AT)

There are two commonly seen forms of AT: Hashimoto's thyroiditis and Grave's disease. These diseases are examples of autoimmunity directed toward a highly restricted set of autoantigens, that is, those associated with the thyroid gland. AT is seen most frequently in women over 30 years of age, and there is a linkage of at least some forms of AT with HLA-DR5 and HLA-B8.

AT is characterized by the presence in the serum of high levels of antibodies to thyroglobulin and thyroid cells. This is more pronounced in Hashimoto's thyroiditis than in Grave's disease, and low levels of thyroid autoantibody can also be detected in normal individuals, especially older women. In severe cases, renal deposition of Ag–Ab complexes may be seen, resulting in varying degrees of kidney damage. In Grave's disease, the IgG fraction of serum contains factors (presumably autoantibodies) that stimulate hyperplasia of thyroid epithelial cells.

Cell-mediated immunity is also important in AT. T cells directly cytotoxic for thyroid cells have been found in patients with Hashimoto's thyroiditis. T cells displaying DTH reactivity to thyroglobulin have been found in inflammatory exudates of patients with both Hashimoto's and Grave's syndrome. The thyroid gland is usually enlarged and infiltrated with lymphocytes. Organized germinal centers may even be apparent. There is evidence throughout the gland of inflammatory reactions, although whether these are triggered by cell-lymphokines or by complement is less clear.

There is a definite genetic linkage in AT. Usually half of the siblings in an affected family will have covert or overt disease symptoms, with a significantly higher incidence in females. Identical twins display almost identical onset and progression of AT, which provides the strongest evidence that AT is not secondary to some environmentally induced event. Simultaneous AT is seen six times more frequently in both indentical twins than in both fraternal twins.

Autoimmune Hemolytic Anemias (AHA)

The autolytic anemias are a group of anemias characterized by the presence of cytolytic autoantibodies to self red blood cell antigens. This is another instance of an autoimmune disorder with a fairly restricted antigenic target. The majority of patients with AHA are afflicted with a form called idiopathic AHA, reflecting the fact that the autoimmune dysfunction is probably primary rather than secondary to another disease. However, some forms of AHA are almost certainly secondary to other disorders; the frequency of these types of AHA higher in older people.

The erythrocyte autoantibodies may be of two types—warm or cold—reflecting the optimal temperature at which agglutination of red cells occurs in the presence of the patient's own serum. Persons with "cold" autoantibodies may experience agglutination of red cells in blood vessels near the surface of the skin when exposed to the cold. This condition reverses itself upon warming of the affected parts.

Myasthenia Gravis (MG)

MG is a disease characterized by extreme muscular weakness, usually beginning in the head and throat, but in most cases eventually spreading to the entire body. Prior to 1934, the disease was not well diagnosed and was largely untreated, and patients usually died from respiratory failure within a year or so after diagnosis. In 1934 it was discovered that anticholinesterase drugs had a marked palliative effect on MG, and together with the advent of mechanically assisted respirators in 1939, the mortality rate began to drop radically. Currently, MG is acutely fatal in only about 10 percent of those afflicted, although it is never completely curable. It is more frequent in women than in men (about 2:1) and is seen earlier in women (average

age of onset = 28 years) than in men (average age of onset = 42 years). In men (more rarely in women) the symptoms may be limited to the extraocular muscles. There is a higher frequency of HLA-DR3 in MG patients than in the population as a whole.

The primary defect is an impairment in neuromuscular transmission, specifically in the interaction of acetylcholine with its postsynaptic receptor. There is compelling evidence in animal models that this is due to antibody-induced down-regulation of the acetylcholine receptor (AChR) and, to some extent, to complement-mediated focal lysis of the neuromuscular endplate. Most human MG patients have high levels of AChR antibodies in their serum, and biopsies of muscle tissue show decreased AChR; half or more of the remaining AChR may be complexed with antibody. Serum from MG patients can induce MG symptoms in animals. Some relief of symptoms can be obtained by inhibitors of acetylcholinesterase, which increases the effective concentration of acetylcholine in the vicinity of the motor endplates and makes up somewhat for the lower number of acetylcholine receptors. Delayed hypersensitivity to neural components has also been demonstrated in MG patients, who exhibit a high degree of autoimmune disorders generally.

Most MG patients have thymic hyperplasia, and in some this will progress to a thymoma. Instead of involuting and atrophying with age, the thymus become increasingly lymphoid in character, developing lymphoid follicles and even germinal centers in the thymic medulla reminiscent of the situation in autoimmune thyroiditis. In some cases, the thymus may become neoplastic. In the majority of patients, removal of the thymus has some, and in some cases a marked, palliatory effect. This has led to the proposal that a soluble thymic substance may be a factor in MG. Of particular interest is the thymic hormone thymopoietin, which can be shown to block neuromuscular transmission.

Multiple Sclerosis (MS)

MS is a chronic, demyelinating disease of the central nervous system. Onset of symptoms usually occurs in the late twenties and early thirties. Symptoms during the early course of the disease are often vague and relatively benign, making prompt and accurate diagnosis difficult. The disease is characterized by temporary (but recurring) disruptions of nervous function, particularly in those pathways concerned with vision, kinesis, and tactile sensation. Intervals between episodes may be months or even years. Usually the severity of dysfunction during these episodes increases as the disease progresses, but occasionally may remain relatively mild or disappear.

Nervous tissue of MS patients is characterized by plaques of demyelination. These plaques contain high levels of IgG, although whether it is specific for neural antigens is unclear. On the other hand, antibodies in the circulation of MS patients can readily be shown to promote complement-mediated damage to myelinated nerve cells. B lymphocytes found in the cerebrospinal fluid also secrete CNS-specific antibodies.

MS lesions are usually infiltrated by mononuclear cells (lymphocytes and mono-cytes). T cells from MS patients respond strongly to nerve tissue *in vitro* by produc-ing MIF. This activity is particularly evident just prior to and during the early phases of an MS attack.

Considerable evidence has accumulated that MS may be associated with low-grade, persistent viral infections, particularly measles virus. A high proportion of MS patients show elevated measles virus antibody titers both in the serum and in the cerebrospinal fluid. MS patients usually have impaired immune responses to paramyxoviruses, and particularly to measles viruses. Measles virus has been identi-fied as the causative factor in at least one other encephalitic disease. However, at present a role for measles virus in MS must remain only a highly intriguing speculation.

Summary

The disorders just described are a representative, and by no means complete, sampling of human disorders with a strongly suspected autoimmune basis. The evidence that onset of immunity to self is what is actually pathogenic for the disease is strong in disorders such as autoimmune thyroiditis and certain of the autoim-mune hemolytic anemias, suggestive in SLE and arthritis and only indirect in my-asthenia gravis. These diseases also span the spectrum of target specificities seen in autoimmune disorders, from the highly restricted damage seen in AHA and thy-roiditis to the generalized inflammatory tissue damage seen in SLE.

Attempts in the laboratory to discover the basis for these various autoimmune disorders, and perhaps to identify an underlying common defect, have occupied a number of researchers in recent years. In the following sections we explore some of the animal models used to study autoimmune disease, and examine current hypotheses proposed to explain the development of reactivity to self-antigens.

Possible Mechanisms Underlying the Development of Autoimmune Disease

The development of immunity to self, where previously there was at least opera-tional tolerance, could conceivably be the result of one of three mechanisms, each of which has been seriously entertained at one time or another.

Generation of Antiself Clones. It might be that clones of T cells and/or B cells reactive to self ("forbidden clones") have been eliminated during ontogeny of the immune system, and that autoimmunity represents an aberrant generation of new antiself clones. This might occur through the unscheduled operation of a postnatal somatic mutation–generation event, in the absence of a program for selectively removing clones with potential reactivity to self-components. This concept was first proposed by Burnet in connection with his clonal selection theory.

Derepression of Existing Antiself Clones. Alternatively, T- and/or B-cell clones with potential antiself activity may exist normally in the body but are kept in check by some sort of immunoregulatory apparatus. Autoimmune disease would then represent a failure of this system to suppress the functional *expression* of these antiself clones. Expression of such clones could be brought about as a failure in the regulatory mechanism itself, or through stimulation of the immune system by a pathogen that fortuitously cross-reacts with some self-component.

Modification of Self. The two foregoing hypotheses both operate at the level of effector function, requiring some change in the status of the immune system itself as an explanation for the development of autoimmunity. It is equally conceivable that what changes is the nature of "self" itself. We know, for example, that both viruses and chemicals can alter the immunological properties of self-components (Chapter 14). Any alteration occurring in cell surface or serum components may make them appear as foreign to an otherwise unaltered immune system. Such changes could come about as the result of interaction with environmental factors (i.e., viruses and chemicals) or changes occurring entirely within the body (age- or disease-related breakdown or alteration of self-components).

The first of these possibilities seems, on the basis of currently available evidence, to be a rather unlikely explanation for autoimmune disease. The latter two, and especially the second, each have a substantial amount of experimental and clinical evidence to sustain them. We now examine in detail the experimental findings leading to this conclusion.

Experimental Animal Models in Autoimmune Disease

New Zealand Black (NZB) and White (NZW) Mice: Models for Spontaneous Systemic Autoimmune Disease

New Zealand Black (NZB) and New Zealand White (NZW) mice are probably the most intensely studied animal models for autoimmune disease. They are made particularly attractive for study by virtue of the fact that the disease symptoms develop spontaneously with age, and are virtually identical to the syndromes accompanying human disorders such as SLE and certain of the autoimmune hemolytic anemias (AHA).

The NZB mouse is an excellent model for the idiopathic AHA seen in humans. AHA is the primary cause of death in this strain, particularly among females. Anti-erythrocyte autoantibodies appear early in life, between two to four months and persist in high levels in the serum in most individuals until death. Lower levels of other autoantibodies, such as antinuclear and antinucleic acid antibodies, and anti-T–lymphocyte antibodies, are also observed. The development of AHA in NZB mice is under the control of perhaps one, but no more than a few, genes although their location is not yet known.

NZB mice exhibit a number of immunological aberrations in addition to AHA, and it is these aberrations that may provide a clue to the underlying dysfunctions that can lead to autoimmune disease. They exhibit a relative resistance to induction of tolerance to a number of antigens. Whereas most mouse strains have low levels of B lymphocytes capable of binding certain erythrocyte autoantigens, NZB mice have very high levels of both T and B cells capable of binding such antigens. Furthermore, unlike other mouse strains, the autoantigen-binding B cells of NZB mice mature and secrete autoantibodies. Young and "middle-aged" mice often display hyperreactivity to a number of antigens; heightened antibody as well as T-cell-mediated responses can be observed. On the other hand, older NZB mice exhibit abnormalities in a wide range of T-cell-associated functions. These include decreased responses to T-cell mitogens, decreased GVH reactivity, and difficulty in rejecting allogeneic skin grafts. These functions can be at least partially restored by injections of lymphocytes from younger NZB mice. Older NZB mice also contain higher than normal numbers of Ly-1$^+$ B cells, which secrete high levels of IgM antibody. The antigenic specificity of this antibody is unknown.

A particularly intriguing T-cell dysfunction in NZB mice is the loss in suppressor T cell (T_s) activity that occurs as the autoimmune state develops. This loss of suppressor activity is general, that is, it is directed at a wide range of soluble and cellular antigens. As we saw in Chapter 13, suppressor T cells are responsible for preventing T helper cells from cooperating with B cells in the production of antibody. If thymocytes from young (less than three months of age) NZB mice are injected into older mice with evidence of autoimmune disease, there is a transient reappearance of generalized suppressor T-cell activity, and at the same time a temporary decrease in levels of erythrocyte autoantibody. On the other hand, if spleen cells from older NZB mice are injected into asymptomatic young mice, production of erythrocyte autoantibody by the donor cells is rapidly shut off (Figure 18-1). These experiments, together with others of a similar nature, strongly suggest that development of autoimmune disease in NZB mice may be directly related to loss of suppressor T-cell function. If, in fact, precursor B cells with potential antiself reactivity do exist, development of autoimmune disease may represent a "derepression" and maturation of these normally suppressed clones through a generalized loss of T-cell suppression. The resistance to tolerance induction, and the more or less generalized hyperactivity to a wide range of antigens noted earlier, may also be reflections of a defective suppressor T-cell system.

Experiments in NZB mice by Cantor and Gershon and their colleagues suggested

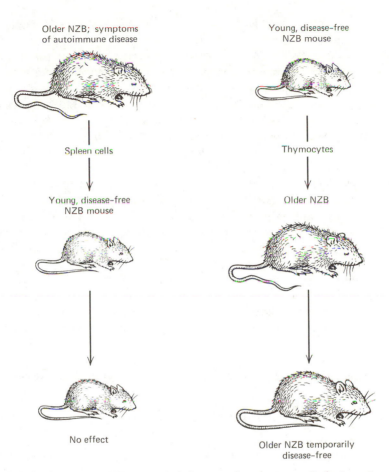

Older NZB; symptoms
of autoimmune disease

Young, disease-free
NZB mouse

Spleen cells

Thymocytes

Young, disease-free
NZB mouse

Older NZB

No effect

Older NZB temporarily
disease-free

Figure 18-1 Experiments suggesting the existence of suppressor cells in the spleens of young NZB mice, and the absence of such cells in older NZBs (see text).

that young NZB mice are deficient in a particular subset of T cells (Lyt-1,2,3$^+$; Qa1$^+$) that either are themselves, or give rise to, suppressor T cells, including T_s cells preventing antiself reactivity. If NZB mice are provided with a source of Lyt-1,2,3$^+$; Qa1$^+$ cells, the development of disease symptoms can be halted and even reversed.

When NZB mice are crossed with NZW mice, the resulting (NZB × NZW)F$_1$ mice (B/W mice), particularly the females, have a markedly different autoimmune syndrome, typical of the more generalized autoimmunity seen in SLE in humans. The major diagnostic feature is the presence of antibody to nucleic acids, particularly double-stranded DNA. These antibodies are present in B/W mice as early as two weeks of age. As the disease progresses, immune complexes involving nucleic acids deposit in the kidneys, leading to glomerulonephritis. B/W mice also have typical LE cells. As with the AHA condition of NZB mice, there is now good evidence that development of the SLE-like syndrome in B/W mice is related to a failure of T-cell suppression to prevent autoantibody production.

Studies in NZB and NZW mice have also shed some insight into the consistently higher frequency of autoimmune disease seen in female mammals generally. It has been observed that prepubertal castration of male mice results in earlier and more severe autoimmune disease. In a study carried out by Talal and his associates, both male and female (NZB × NZW)F$_1$ mice were castrated prior to puberty, and then treated with either androgens or estrogens. Mice of both sexes treated with estrogens showed early and severe development of autoimmune disease, whereas mice of both sexes treated with androgens showed a delayed onset and much reduced incidence and severity of disease compared with untreated controls. Furthermore, uncastrated female adults treated with androgens also showed reduced severity of disease and prolonged survival compared to untreated adult females. Similar results were seen in adult male mice treated with androgens at eight months of age, a time when autoimmune symptoms are developing in an accelerated manner (Figure 18-2).

Thus it seems clear that sex hormones play an important and direct role in regulating autoimmune responses. This may also be related to the fact that (at least in mice) females mount more vigorous immune responses generally. Male hormones administered under a variety of experimental situations have been observed to decrease both humoral and cellular immune responsiveness. Talal has shown that this effect of androgens is dependent on intact thymic function, suggesting that these hormones may be affecting maturation or function of T suppressor cells.

Experimental Autoimmune Thyroiditis

A condition mimicking the symptoms seen in humans in Hashimoto's or Grave's disease can be induced experimentally in animals by several means. The most common method is to inject an animal with autogeneic or syngeneic thyroid tissue that has been emulsified in Freund's adjuvant. Alternatively, purified thyroglobulin, emulsified in adjuvant, can be administered. Another approach is to introduce slight chemical modification into the syngeneic thyroglobulin, or to inject allogeneic thyroglobulin. All of these methods result in the production of varying degrees of autoreactive antithyroglobulin antibodies. More importantly, perhaps, they induce a state of autoreactive thyroid inflammatory disease.

For a long while it has been assumed that thyroglobulin is restricted to the thyroid, which might act as an immunologically privileged site. According to this theory, true tolerance to self-thyroglobulin never develops, since thyroglobulin is not available to interact with the immune system during ontogeny. Thus introduction of thyroglobulin in adult life could induce an immune response, the B-cell clones capable of producing antithyroid antibody having never been eliminated. However, we now know this is not true. Thyroglobulin in fact circulates in both the lymph and the blood stream of normal, healthy animals, albeit in low levels. The

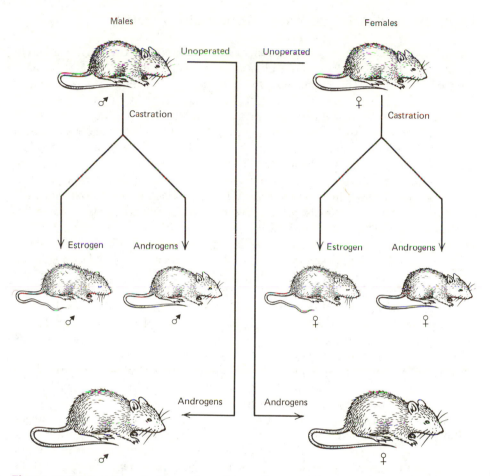

Figure 18-2 Effect of castration and sex hormones on autoimmune disease in (NZB ×
NZW)F$_1$ mice.

rapidity with which an immune response to self-thyroglobulin can be induced by
the means mentioned above suggests that potentially autoreactive T- and B-cell
clones are also present and capable of functioning. B cells binding radioactive self-
thyroglobulin are readily demonstrable. Yet ordinarily no immune response to
circulating thyroglobulin develops. Clearly, some sort of regulatory function must
exist that normally prevents an autothyroglobulin reaction from developing; autoimmune thyroiditis represents a breakdown of this function. The nature of this
regulatory mechanism is the subject of intense investigation in several laboratories.
Some evidence has, in fact, been obtained for a defective thymus-dependent suppressor function in a chicken model for spontaneous autoimmune thyroiditis.

Experimental Allergic Encephalomyelitis (EAE)

The groundwork for an experimental model for multiple sclerosis (MS) was laid in the last century when Pasteur developed his vaccine for treatment of humans infected with rabies. The attenuated rabies virus was injected into patients together with variable amounts of homogenized brain tissue. Some of the patients treated with vaccine developed neurological problems, including temporary paralysis. It was initially thought that these problems were caused by incompletely attenuated rabies virus, but this was eventually disproved. In the early 1930s, the first production of an acute, disseminated encephalomyelitis, after injection with nervous tissue extracts, was reported in monkeys. In 1947, several laboratories reported that emulsion of CNS tissue in complete Freund's adjuvant yielded a material which, on injection into various animals, gave a severe and reproducible disseminated encephalomyelitis. The histopathological concomitants of experimental allergic encephalomyelitis (EAE), as it came to be called, were intriguingly similar to those seen in MS, and for the past 30 years or so EAE has been intensively studied in an attempt to understand the genetic, pathological, and histological parameters of MS.

The study of EAE was aided considerably by the identification and thorough characterization of a protein component of CNS white matter, called myelin basic protein (MBP), that can induce many of the symptoms of EAE. MBP, with a molecular weight of about 20,000, appears to contain the antigenic sequences responsible for the immunopathology of EAE. The complete amino acid sequence is known and is quite similar from species to species. Biologically active portions of the molecule have been identified, and somewhat surprisingly encephalitogenic portions of the molecule are different in different species.

EAE is one of the clearest cases in which T cells are the principal agent causing an autoimmune inflammatory disease. EAE can be transferred by lymphocytes but not by serum. The specific cells involved are Lyt-2$^-$ in mice, and the potency of transfer can be greatly increased by incubating the cells *in vitro* for two to three days with MBP. Treatment of mice with anti-Lyt-1 serum after MBP induction of EAE greatly reduces the symptoms. Cloned MBP-specific, Lyt-2$^-$ T-cell lines are highly potent in causing EAE. MBP-reactive, EAE-inducing Lyt-2$^-$ T cells can be recovered from the spinal columns of mice with EAE.

It has been observed that class II antigens on CNS vascular epithelium increases after immunization with MBP prior to the onset of inflammatory symptoms. It is possible that these cells are crucial in presenting MBP to T helper cells and that they may serve as an initial focus for inflammatory damage.

When whole CNS tissue extract is injected into test animals, specific antibodies are produced in addition to the DTH symptoms just described. Although most of these react with MBP, a significant proportion do not, and these can be shown (in the presence of complement) to demyelinate brain cells *in vitro*. However, it is unclear whether such antibodies play any role in the pathogenesis of EAE, since although clearly produced in response to injected tissue or MBP they would not normally cross the blood–brain barrier. As noted previously, EAE symptoms cannot

Table 18-2 Comparative Immunologic
Responses in EAE and MS

Immunologic event	EAE	MS
CNS lesions		
IgG deposits	±	+
Complement deposits	± or 0	0
CSF compartment		
Elevated IgG	+	+
Oligoclonal IgG	ND[a]	+
Altered κ/λ ratio of IgG	ND	+
Ig-secreting mononuclear cells	ND	+
Vascular compartment		
Gel-ppt or C-fix antibodies	+	0
Antiglial-demyelinating antibodies	+	+
Cutaneous reactivity (DH)	+	0
MIF production	+	+ or 0

Taken from N. Talal, *Autoimmunity,* Academic Press, New York
(1977), p. 673. Copyright © 1977 by Academic Press, Inc. Reprinted
by permission.
[a]ND: not determined.

be transferred with immune serum. The CNS lesions seen in MS patients do often
contain IgG, although whether such IgG is specific for neuroantigens is unclear.

The crucial question, of course, is how valid a model EAE in animals is for MS in
humans. A comparison of the features of EAE and MS is shown in Table 18-2, and
indicates a number of important reservations discussed at length in the reference
from which the table was taken. In addition, as noted earlier, MS is a chronic
condition characterized by alternating periods of expression and remission of
overt symptoms. EAE is an acute, monophasic condition. Demyelination is extensive in MS, and only mild in EAE. The differences between MS and EAE are particularly marked when highly purified or synthetic MBP is used to induce EAE, suggesting that other CNS antigens may be important in the immunopathology of demyelinating disease. There is also increasing evidence that the onset and continuing
immunopathology of MS may include a chronic viral component.

Whether or not EAE is an exact reflection of MS in humans remains to be seen.
Nevertheless, the numerous similarities between the two continue to make this a
valuable model for the study of autoimmune neurodegenerative diseases generally.

Experimental Autoimmune Myasthenia Gravis

That MG might be an autoimmune disease, in which neuromuscular transmission is inhibited by elements of the immune system, was suggested as early as 1960.
This idea was not put on a firm experimental basis until 1973, however, when

Lindstrom and his colleagues in San Diego were able to produce MG in the laboratory, first in rabbits and now, more routinely, in rats. Purified acetylcholine receptor (AChR) prepared from the main electric organ of *Torpedo californica* or from mammalian muscle tissue is emulsified in Freund's adjuvant and injected subcutaneously into the test animals. The subunits of AChR are also effective, particularly α and β chains, but intact AChR induces the most severe symptoms. About 10 days after immunization, the animals pass through an acute phase of MG and begin a chronic MG phase at about 30 days. The acute phase, the analog of which in human MG is not well defined, is characterized by infiltration of neuromuscular junctions by phagocytes, which causes extensive damage to endplate regions, This results in muscular weakness, particularly in the forelimbs. Complement component C3 is also a critical factor in the acute phase. For reasons that are yet unknown, the acute, phagocytic phase is self-limiting, and the clinical symptoms of MG may temporarily disappear.

The chronic phase, beginning at about 30 days and proceeding to death (or in a few cases, recovery after about 90 days), is more similar to the MG seen in humans. Few, if any, phagocytes are seen in this stage, and there is little evidence for T-cell-mediated, delayed hypersensitivity reactions. (However, T cells that proliferate in an MHC-restricted fashion in response to isolated AChR can be recovered from animals with experimental MG.) Instead, there is a high level of serum antibody to AChR, and a greatly reduced level of AChR in muscle tissue. HIgh levels of AChR-antibody complexes are also found in the serum. The antibody response is both T cell and macrophage dependent. There is obvious complement-mediated lysis of postsynaptic membrane, and the remaining intact membrane is often completely cleared of AChR, presumably by antibody-mediated down-regulation. The loss of AChR is directly correlated with a loss of ACh sensitivity and neuromuscular transmission, and the rapid onset of muscular weakness.

Experiments using inbred mice have suggested that class II molecules are involved in the immune response to AChR, and in the development of experimental MG. Alteration of host class II molecules, or treatment of the host with anti-class II antibodies, strongly affects the course of disease induced by purified AChR or its subunits. Whether the critical events occur on antigen presenting cells, or on suppressor T cells, is uncertain. However, the clear involvement of class II antigens in the experimentally induced disease is intriguing in light of the known association of MG with specific class II allotypes in humans (Table 18-1).

The cellular and molecular events in experimental and human MG are so similar that there can be little doubt that human MG results from an autoimmune attack on ACh receptors. However, as with many diseases with autoimmune effector mechanisms, it is unclear in human MG what triggers the initial perception of the self-AChR as foreign.

Autoimmunity and Graft-versus-Host Disease

The graft-versus-host (GVH) reaction, and the accompanying pathological symptoms (GVH disease), were described in detail in Chapter 14. Briefly, they result from the introduction of immunocompetent adult T lymphocytes into an allogeneic host. The graft (T lymphocytes) perceives the host as foreign and mounts an immunological attack against it. Depending on the immune status of the host, the graft itself may be rejected almost immediately, in which case GVH disease may be absent or mild; or, if the host is immunoincompetent, the graft may not be rejected at all, in which case GVH disease will be severe and perhaps fatal.

One of the consequences of a GVH reaction is that *host* lymphocytes are triggered to proliferate quite vigorously. This is presumed to be in response to factors produced as a consequence of donor T-cell activation. This proliferation takes place in host lymphoid organs, principally the spleen, and appears to involve mostly B lymphocytes.

A chronic form of GVH disease can be induced in adult F_1 mice by injection of parental T lymphocytes. The injected parental T cells recognize antigens of the other parent on the F_1 host cells, and begin to proliferate and release a spectrum of T-cell lymphokines. Some of these attract host immune cells and stimulate them to proliferate as well. Proliferation of host lymphocytes in the spleen continues for many months after a few initial injections. Eventually, the spleen becomes histologically disorganized, and in many cases lymphoid malignancies develop. These may be reticulum cell sarcomas, or B-cell lymphomas. The neoplasms are always of host, never of donor, cell origin.

Mice with chronic GVH disease have a high incidence of autoimmune disease, particularly autoimmune hemolytic anemia. Antibodies to host red cell antigens appear in the serum and lymph, as do antinucleic acid antibodies. Glomerulonephritis caused by antibody–autoantigen complexes is quite common. The antibodies are of host, not donor, origin, marking this as a true autoimmune phenomenon. The most likely interpretation of these phenomena is that the activated donor T cells can induce host B cells, including clones with antiself potential, to not only proliferate but to mature to the antibody producing stage. Ordinarily, T-cell help would not be available for activation of these clones, either because the appropriate T_h clones are absent, or because they are under specific T_s suppression. Activation of donor T cells by host MHC antigens may bypass the need for antigen-specific host T_h cells. Since the donor T cells are not rejected by the host, because of the parental-F_1 relationship, the donor T cells can persist over long periods of time, leading to chronic manifestation of autoimmune symptoms.

Activation of Antiself B-Cell Clones with Polyclonal B-Cell Activators

A great deal of the theoretical and experimental evidence presented so far has suggested that B cells capable of producing antibodies to self-antigens probably exist freely in the body. If this is true, then indiscriminant activation of B cells in the body ought to activate antiself B cells and lead to the production of autoantibodies. A variety of agents are capable of promoting the differentiation of B lymphocytes to plasma cells. One of the most potent is bacterial lipopolysaccharide (LPS), described in Chapter 13. A number of investigators have injected LPS into mice, and looked for the appearance of antiself antibodies. All such experiments have been positive, and antibodies to a wide range of self-antigens have been found, including erythrocytes, lymphocytes, and nucleic acids (including poly A). These studies provide strong support for the notion that antiself B cells do exist in normal, asymptomatic adult animals, but are somehow prevented from maturing to autoantibody producing plasma cells.

Summary

In the preceding sections we have explored a number of experimental animal models for autoimmune disease. As with human patients, the principal form of tissue damage is inflammatory. In most cases this can be attributed more readily to immune complex deposition and activation of complement. Only in EAE is there a strong indication of T-cell involvement in initiating inflammation. On the other hand, reactive T helper cells can be shown to be present at the sites of most autoimmune inflammatory reactions, so it is difficult to exclude a role for them in most autoimmune diseases. The end point is the same for both complement-induced and T cell-induced reactions: attraction of macrophages and PMNs to the reaction site. In most cases, both initiating mechanisms probably contribute to autoimmune tissue damage.

The demonstration of a wide range of autoreactive B and even T lymphocytes in normal, healthy humans and animals has made the concept of ontogenic elimination of self-reactive clones essentially untenable as an explanation for self-tolerance. Immune recognition of self as the result of alteration of autologous macromolecules is difficult to analyze. Immune responses to self are often accompanied by the presence of a viral infection and a concommitant antiviral immune response, and viruses can alter the immunological perception of self (Chapter 14). However, in such cases the subsequent immune response is directed to a combination of self plus virus, and not to self alone. Thus unless the virus persists there should not be chronic, ongoing antiself reactivity. When all the evidence is weighed, a direct connection between viral alteration of self-components and autoimmune disease, although attractive, cannot yet be made.

The body will also mount an immune response against self-macromolecules or cells modified by combination with drugs or chemicals. When the chemical is very small, it may form essentially a hapten–carrier complex with a self-component. When this new complex induces a DTH reaction, a component of the reactivity may be directed toward self. This is the basis of contact hypersensitivity, for example. However, in the absence of the haptenating chemical, no appreciable antiself reaction seems to remain.

Modification of self-molecules by processes associated with age and deterioration could also conceivably play a role in the development of autoimmunity, although such processes, if they exist at all, are not well understood. Of some interest in this respect is the observation that suppressor T-cell activity is considerably reduced in older humans. We do know that when the primary structure of thyroglobulin is chemically altered, it can then be used to induce a general immune reaction to unaltered thyroglobulin. It is conceivable that self-components altered by endogenous means might likewise induce a generalized reactivity toward themselves or other closely related self-components.

The best available current evidence is pointing increasingly to a defect in regulation of antiself reactivity as the cause for a large number of autoimmune disorders. This interpretation assumes the existence of antiself clones as part of the immune repertoire of normal individuals. These clones may not be directed to self per se, but may cross react with self heteroclitically. It may be that loss of reactivity toward the primary antigen would present too much of a risk for survival. These clones, including probably helper T cell as well as B-cell precursors, would ordinarily be prevented from expressing their potential by an appropriate regulatory mechanism. An attractive possibility would be self-specific suppressor T cells that could function to prevent T helper cells reactive to self from activating antiself B cells. Both the GVH- and B-cell mitogen data just presented strongly suggest that antiself B cells are themselves not suppressed *in vivo*. Both of these systems bypass the need for T-cell help, and the fact that in both cases antiself B cells are subsequently activated suggests that nonfuctioning antiself T_h cells are what prevent development of autoimmunity in normal individuals. Whether the antiself T_h cells are missing altogether or simply suppressed in normal human individuals remains to be determined, but the evidence accumulating in animal models makes the latter possibility seem most likely.

Bibliography

General

Autologous immune reactions as regulatory mechanisms. *Fed. Proc. 37*/10, 2360 et seq. (1978).

Burnet, F. M., *Autoimmunity and Autoimmune Disease,* F. A. Davis, Philadelphia (1972).

Cruse, J. M., D. Whitcomb, and R. E. Lewis, Jr., Autoimmunity—Historical perspective. *Concepts in Immunopathol. 1,* 32 (1985).

Cunningham, A. J., Self-tolerance maintained by active suppressor mechanisms. *Transplant. Rev. 31,* 23 (1976).

Freedman, S. O., and P. Gold (eds.), *Clinical Immunology,* Second Edition, Harper & Row, New York (1976).

Fudenberg, H. H., D. P. Stites, J. L. Caldwell, and J. V. Wells, *Basic Clinical Immunology,* Lange Medical Publications, Los Altos, California (1976).

Ishizaka, K., and T. Ishizaka, Mechanisms of reaginic hypersensitivity and IgE antibody response. *Immunol. Rev. 41,* 109 (1978).

Kolb, H., and K. Toyka, Autoimmune tissue damage: Humor or cellular effector mechanisms. *Immunol. Today 4,* 331 (1983).

Kunkel, H. G. (ed.), Rheumatoid arthritis. *Springer Seminars in Immunopathology,* Volume 4, No. 2 (1981).

Lindstrom, J., Immunobiology of myasthenia gravis, experimental autoimmune myasthenia gravis, and Lambert-Eaton syndrome. *Ann. Rev. Immunol. 3,* 109 (1985).

Louis, J. A., and W. O. Weigle, A model of immunologic unresponsiveness and its relevance to autoimmunity. *Pathobiol. Ann. 6,* 259 (1976).

Möller, G. (Ed.)., Autoimmunity and self-nonself discrimination. *Transplant. Rev. 31,* (1976).

Rocklin, R. E., K. Bendtzen, and D. Greineder, Mediators of immunity: Lymphokines and monokines. *Adv. Immunol. 29,* 56 (1980).

Talal, N. (ed.), *Autoimmunity: Genetic, Virologic and Clinical Aspects,* Academic Press, New York (1978).

Research

Brostoff, S., and D. Mason, Experimental allergic encephalomyelitis. Successful treatment *in vivo* with a MAb that recognizes T helper cells. *J. Immunol., 133,* 1938 (1984).

Burns, J. et al., Recovery of MBP-reactive T cells from spinal cords of Lewis rats with EAE. *J. Immunol. 132,* 2690 (1984).

Christadoss, P., J. Lindstrom, and N. Talal, Cellular immune response to acetylcholine receptors in murine experimental autoimmune myasthenia gravis. Inhibition with anti-I_a antibodies. *Cellular Immunol. 81,* 1 (1983).

Cooke, A., P. Hutchings, and J. Playfair, Suppressor T cells in experimental autoimmune hemolytic anemia. *Nature 273* 154 (1978).

DeBaets, M. et al., Lymphocyte Activation in Experimental Autoimmune Myasthenia Gravis, *J. Immunol., 128:* 2228 (1982).

Hayakawa, K., R. Handy, D. Parks, and L. Herzenberg, The Ly-1 B cell subpopulation in normal, immunodefective and autoimmune mice. *J. Exp. Med. 157,* 202 (1983).

Katz, D. H., R. F. Bargatze, C. A. Bogowitz, and L. R. Katz, Regulation of IgE antibody production by serum molecules. VII. The IgE-selective damping activity of suppressive factor of allergy (SFA) is exerted across both strain and species restriction barriers. *J. Immunol. 124,* 819 (1980).

Kishimoto, S., S. Tomino, H. Mitsuya, and H. Fugiwara, Age-related changes in suppressor functions of human T cells. *J. Immunol. 123,* 1586 (1979).

Primi, D., C. Smith, and L. Hammarstrom, Role of suppressor T cells in autoimmune responses induced by polyclonal B cell activators. *Scand. J. Immunol. 7,* 121 (1978).

Sobel, R. A. et al., The immunopathology of EAE. II. Endothelial increases prior to inflammatory cell infiltration. *J. Immunol. 132,* 2402 (1984).

CHAPTER **19**

Clinical Organ Transplantation

It seems that humans have been fascinated with the possibility of transplantation to restore broken or worn-out body parts for quite some time. Some of the very earliest medical texts we know of describe attempts at replacing at least external tissues of the body. As early as several hundred years B.C., Hindu surgeons described a technique for constructing noses from tissue obtained elsewhere on the body. This was necessitated by a fairly common punishment for a number of crimes in ancient India—cutting off the nose! Tagliacozzi, a sixteenth-century Italian surgeon, described a procedure for using tissue taken from the arm to rebuild a partially destroyed nose. With only minor modifications, this technique is still used today and is even called the "Tagliacozzi flap" procedure. But from the beginning everyone who dabbled in tissue transplantation seems to have noticed one important fact: shuffling tissues around from one part of the same body to another can work if you know what you are doing. Exchanging tissues between two different individuals is another story altogether—it just does not work.

As surgical techniques advanced, so did the temptation to try increasingly heroic and dramatic transplants—even, in 1908, the transplantation of an intact head from one dog to another! Most attempts were restricted to transplants in animals that could be of potential benefit to human health—kidney, heart, liver, and lung. Although brief function could be detected in some instances, all attempts at exchanging body parts between other than genetically identical individuals (identical twins in humans; members of completely inbred strains in animals) failed after a matter of a few days or at best a week or two.

Experimental Tissue Transplantation

Clinical organ transplantation as we know it today began with the efforts of Peter Medawar to understand skin graft rejection in badly burned patients during World War II. His observations in these patients, coupled with his own laboratory investigations in animals, convinced him that graft rejection was an immunological phenomenon. Once he convinced the rest of the scientific world of this fact, transplantation became not a surgical problem, but an immunological problem. The focus then shifted to the laboratory, and over the next 10 years intense research into ways of circumventing immunological rejection led to the first attempts to transplant a major organ (a kidney) in a human patient in Boston in 1954. Before we consider the current status of organ transplantation in humans, we will briefly review the experimental work in animals that provided the basic understanding of the rejection process necessary to begin such work.

Establishment of Transplant Rejection as an Immunological Problem

Two important experimental approaches contributed to our understanding of transplant rejection as an immunological phenomenon. The earlier and perhaps more germinal approach was an outgrowth of an attempt to define the genetic rules of the growth or rejection of transplanted tumors. It had been observed that transplanted tumors grew well in certain stocks of mice whose breeding was restricted to other members of that stock, if, and only if, the tumor transplant was between members of that stock. If tumors of other mice were transplanted to members of the inbred stock, they were rapidly rejected, as were tumors carried successfully in the inbred stock when transplanted to other mice. This observation led to a rapid burst of activity among geneticists, who soon established that susceptibility to such strain-restricted tumors was under the control of varying numbers of dominant genes. In the course of doing so, they developed a number of truly inbred strains of mice, which survive today and still provide the foundation for not only investigations of tissue transplantation phenomena, but for all areas of immunological research where genetics is important.

The first suggestion that acceptance or rejection of these tumor grafts might have an immunological basis was made by J. B. S. Haldane in 1933. The first well-formulated experiments to test this hypothesis were carried out by Peter Gorer in the following years. Using inbred strains of mice, Gorer showed that the genes regulating tumor growth coded for antigens found on the surface of the tumor cells and that these antigens were also found on the surface of normal cells (Chapter 8). This provided an important link between the rapidly growing literatures on tumor genetics and on transplantation of tissues and organs. Furthermore, since the surface antigens were capable of inducing specific antibodies, the possibility that tumor (and graft) rejection had an immunological basis now had to be considered seriously.

The second major development in the history of transplantation immunology derived from experiments carried out by Peter Medawar during World War II, which demonstrated conclusively that the rejection of normal tissue transplants is an immunological phenomenon (Figure 19-1). In a series of remarkably incisive experiments, he established two important facts about graft rejection that led to general acceptance of the idea that such reactions are immunological. First, graft rejection, like the host response to bacteria or molecular antigens, results in a state of antigen-specific memory. That is, if individual A receives and rejects a graft from B, then a subsequent graft from B will be rejected much more quickly than was the primary graft. On the other hand, the rate at which A rejects a graft from C is the same whether or not A has previously rejected a graft from B. Second, the subsequent graft from B will be rejected in an accelerated manner even if grafted onto a site on the body totally different from the primary graft. Thus, the development of rejection, and the resultant memory state, were shown to be systemic in nature and not controlled by physiological or biochemical events restricted to the site of the graft.

The Allograft Reaction

The rules of allograft transplantation are simple and are diagrammed in Figure 19-2. Transplants of cells, tissues, or organs from one animal to another will be uniformly rejected if the two partners in the exchange differ by one or more histocompatibility genes. As discussed in Chapters 8 and 9, these genes code for cell surface histocompatibility antigens, which are detected and responded to principally by the T-cell compartment of immune system of the recipient. The most intensely studied form of this "host-versus-graft" reaction is the allograft reaction, which occurs when grafts are exchanged between two members of the same species displaying different allelic forms of one or more histocompatibility antigens. In fact, histocompatibility genes and antigens per se are actually defined only in terms of exchanges between allogeneic partners (see Table 19-1 for terminology).

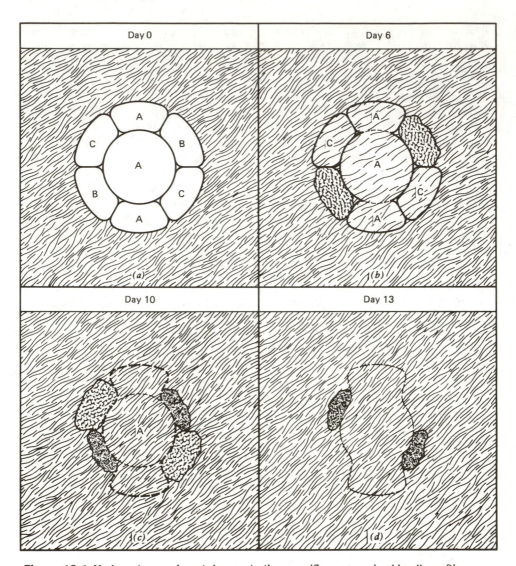

Figure 19-1 Medawar's experiment demonstrating specific memory in skin allografting. (a) A rabbit that had previously rejected a strain B graft is regrafted with skin from itself (A), skin from strain B, and a third party skin graft (C). The grafts are placed in a shaved area on the back. (b) Six days later, the strain B graft starts to degenerate. Grafts from A and C look normal and even begin to show a little fur growth. (c) By day 10, the strain B graft has dropped off, leaving a small red scar that heals rapidly. The A strain skin begins to move into the area from both the A strain graft and from the surrounding host skin. The various A strain grafts merge at this point. The strain C grafts begin to degenerate. (d) At day 13, the B-strain grafts have completely disappeared. The strain C grafts look like the strain B grafts several days earlier. The A strain grafts have merged with each other and with the host skin and have developed fur.

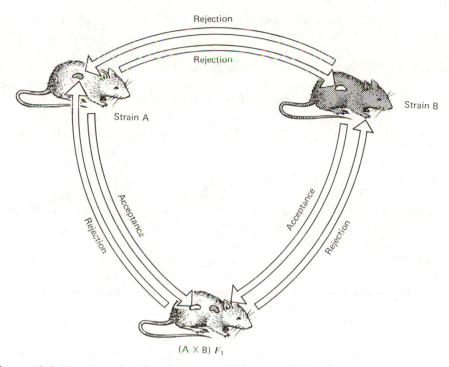

Figure 19-2 The rules of graft exchange among completely homozygous inbred animal strains and their F_1 progeny.

Exchange of grafts in either direction between two allogeneic individuals leads to rejection, whether or not either or both are homozygous or heterozygous for the histocompatibility (H) loci distinguishing the two. In the case of two individuals completely homozygous for all H loci, the first generation (F_1) progeny, which are uniformly heterozygous for the distinguishing H loci, will permanently accept a graft from either parent. However, either parent will perceive a graft from the F_1 as

Table 19-1 Terminology Used in Discussing Transplantation Immunology

Graft exchanged between	Graft designation	Antigens involved
Self/self	Autograft	None
Identical twins; two members of an inbred strain	Syngeneic graft	None
Two nonidentical members of the same species	Allograft	Alloantigens
Members of different species	Xenograft	Xenoantigens

foreign, due to the presence on the F_1 cells of H antigens coded for by the other parent. This illustrates the general point that in order for graft acceptance to occur, it is not necessary that the host and donor have identical alleles for all H genes present in the species; it is only necessary that all of the H antigen alleles present on donor cells be perceived as self by the recipient, even though the latter may have additional surface H antigens on its own cells. If the parents are each heterozygous for one or more H loci (which is generally the case in outbred populations, including humans), then the first-generation progeny will, in nearly all cases, reject parental grafts, due to the presence on parental cells of H antigens coded for by the noninherited H allele(s).

Both in the mouse and in humans, rejection is most rapid if donor and recipient differ by genes in the major histocompatibility complex (MHC). Skin grafts exchanged between individuals allogeneic at this complex will ordinarily be rejected in 10 days to two weeks. Differences at minor H loci have only been well studied in the mouse. If donor and recipient are identical at the MHC (H-2), but differ at one or more minor H loci, skin graft rejection may occur anywhere between two weeks and several months. Just what a "strong" versus a "weak" histocompatibility difference means at the mechanistic level is uncertain. One likely possibility is that it may reflect the frequency of recipient lymphocytes responsive to the donor surface H antigens. We know, for example, that the frequency of lymphocytes responding to differences at the MHC is quite high. The frequency of lymphocytes responding to other H loci may be considerably lower, and it may require more time for enough cells to be triggered and/or to be clonally expanded in order to inflict irreversible damage to the graft. Consistent with this notion is the observation that the time of first onset of rejection symptoms is greatly prolonged in weak H differences, which could well reflect time required for clonal expansion of responding cells.

As mentioned earlier, a second graft from the same donor (or one genetically identical) will be rejected much more quickly than the first graft. The basis for this accelerated "second-set" rejection has been the source of some debate, but the most likely explanation is that in cell-mediated allograft rejection, as in the humoral immune response, initial immunization both increases the frequency of responding cells, and qualitatively alters them in the direction of more promptly responding to antigenic challenge.

Skin transplants have been used extensively as a model system to study allograft rejection in laboratory animals. In standard skin transplant studies in the mouse, a small piece of skin (ca. 1 cm) is removed from the donor, and transplanted to a site on the recipient (usually on the back) where a piece of skin of similar size and shape has been removed. The graft is held in place by a piece of Vaseline-impregnated gauze, and secured with a wraparound bandage containing plaster. Within two days the blood vessels of donor and recipient establish initial connections, and the graft takes on a healthy pink color. There is rapid proliferation of both donor and recipient epithelial cells around the edges of the wound, leading to fairly firm attachment of the graft in about five days. In syngeneic transplants the grafting process continues until the transplanted skin is indistinguishable from surrounding skin, with all skin functions (hair growth and color, sweat production, oil secretion, etc.) fully operational.

If the donor and recipient are allogeneic, the first stages of the process are much the same. Vascularization is accomplished, the graft becomes pinkish in color, and mitotic activity around the sides of the wound associated with healing can be observed. However, once circulation of host blood elements through the donor tissue is initiated, there is a rapid infiltration and concentration of host immune cells in the graft. This is not seen in the case of syngeneic grafts. The cell infiltrate includes cells of most lymphoid classes, including lymphocytes, macrophages, and granulocytes. The sequence of events leading to this infiltration unclear. It may be that host lymphocytes enter the graft, become triggered by donor antigens, and attract other cells to the graft site. Alternatively, donor cells or transplantation antigens may leave the graft and be trapped in the draining lymph node, initiating the immune response in the node. Sensitized lymphocytes would then leave the node and eventually make their way back to the graft site where they are trapped, or alternatively, recognize donor antigens and liberate factors that attract other cell types to the area. Evidence has been put forward to support either model; the truth may in fact be some combination of both.

In about 7 days the graft begins to show the first signs of rejection. Sensitized host lymphocytes begin to attack graft cells. Graft blood vessels are particularly vulnerable, and gradually the connections between donor and host vessels degenerate. The graft darkens from congested blood, becomes indurated and finally separates from the graft bed. This occurs in about 10 to 14 days when donor and recipient differ across H-2, and up to several months if they differ at a minor H locus.

A number of reactions can be observed in host lymphoid organs in concert with the events in the graft itself. The first signs of activity are seen in the T-dependent regions of the draining lymph node (paracortical regions; see Chapter 2). Proliferative activity can be seen as early as 2 to 3 days after grafting. This activity peaks at about 5 to 6 days and then gradually subsides. Germinal centers and follicular activity are not usually seen until 5 to 7 days after grafting, and peak later than paracortical activity. There is also an increase during this period of phagocytic activity in the medullary portions of the node.

The Role of Lymphocytes in Allograft Rejection

N. A. Mitchison originally showed that allograft immunity can be passively transferred from one animal to another by lymphoid cells, but not by serum. This provided the first suggestion that graft rejection, unlike other forms of immunity known at the time, might be mediated directly by lymphoid cells rather than by antibodies. The next major contributions came from the work of Gowans, who showed that immunity is specifically transferred by small, nondividing, circulating lymphocytes. However, Gowans also showed that the lymphocytes infiltrating a graft site are mostly large, rapidly dividing lymphocytes, and furthermore, in the case of passively transferred cells, that the majority of cells infiltrating the graft site are of host, not donor, origin. Most of the infiltrating cells are actually not lymphocytes, but granulocytes and monocytes or macrophages. The picture that has emerged from these and other studies is that allograft memory resides in small, resting lymphocytes, which, when rechallenged with antigen are triggered to divide, become blastoid, and mature to a more active state. Some of them may attack the graft directly (CTL); others (Th cells) produce lymphokines that attract macrophages and granulocytes. The mechanisms by which lymphocytes, and particularly cytotoxic T lymphocytes (CTLs), attack and destroy target cells was discussed in detail in Chapter 14.

A great deal of attention has been focused during the past 10 years on Lyt-2$^+$ cytotoxic T lymphocytes as effector cells in allograft rejection. The notion of an effector cell attacking and destroying a foreign cell on a direct, cell-to-cell basis is an attractive one. Investigation of this phenomenon has certainly been aided by the availability of a simple, clean, and highly quantitative *in vitro* assay system (the ^{51}Cr release assay) for measuring CTL function. Unquestionably, sensitized CTLs are found in lymph nodes draining graft sites, and they can destroy graft cells *in vitro*. But it has been more difficult to demonstrate a role for these cells in graft rejection *in vivo*. In fact some experiments have shown that passively transferred immune Lyt-2$^-$ cells may be more effective in provoking graft rejection than are Lyt-2$^+$ CTLs. As just noted, the site of a rejecting allograft is infiltrated with a large number of cells, only a relatively few of which are lymphocytes. Careful analysis of passive transfer studies has shown that only a fraction of the lymphocytes attracted to a graft site are donor cells specifically immune to graft antigens. Most of the cells found in graft rejection sites are host monocytes and granulocytes. It is entirely conceivable that these cells, associated with the inflammatory stages of delayed hypersensitivity, play an important and perhaps a major role in graft rejection. A rejecting tissue graft looks histologically quite similar to the site of a delayed hypersensitivity reaction. As discussed in Chapter 17, the enzymes produced by cells infiltrating a DH reaction are capable of causing considerable tissue damage. Both Lyt-2$^-$ and Lyt-2$^+$ cells, but particularly the former, produce lymphokines that can mobilize the cells and cellular events involved in DH reactions. Lyt-2$^-$ cells respond to class II antigens, which in skin are associated mostly with Langerhan's cells scattered throughout the dermis, and which in other grafts may be associated principally with the blood vessels. In the latter cases, in particular, survival of the graft could be seriously compromised by a delayed hypersensitivity reaction. As frustration with the failure to determine the lytic mechanism of CTL increases, and with continued difficulty in demonstrating a role for systemically administered CTL in graft rejection *in vivo,* transplantation immunologists may develop a renewed interest in the role of delayed hypersensitivity in graft rejection.

The Role of Donor ("Passenger") Leukocytes in Triggering Graft Rejection

As we saw in Chapter 14, the host T-cell response to foreign MHC antigens (alloantigens) involves two T-cell subsets—T helper cells and cytotoxic T cells (CTLs). Each subset has its own requirements for being triggered. T helper cells must see class II alloantigens (signal 1), and need soluble factors, such as IL-1 (signal 2), produced by certain class II bearing cells. CTLs, on the other hand, must see class I alloantigens as signal I, and need second signals such as IL-2 that are produced by activated T helper cells. Once activated, CTLs can attack just about any graft cell displaying the sensitizing class I antigen—essentially every every cell in the graft— in the absence of IL-2. However, CTLs cannot be activated *unless* T helper cells are also activated, and the latter are much more restricted in terms of the types of graft cells that can cause their activation. Only class II antigen bearing cells can activate them, and such cells are only a minor portion of any grafted tissue. Moreover, probably only a limited subset of class II bearing graft cells can actually activate the host T helper subset.

Once graft rejection reactions began to be studied *in vitro,* and it became evident that leucocytes were the most strongly stimulatory cells (e.g., in mixed leucocyte culture reactions; see Chapter 14), the notion of a role for "passenger leucocytes" in transplanted tissue was put forward. As MLC reactions were studied in more detail, and it became apparent that among leucocytes macrophages and dendritic cells have the most potent stimulatory properties, the passenger leucocyte hypothesis was further refined. Whereas originally most proponents imagined that circulating leucocytes trapped in the blood volume of transplanted tissues and organs provided a principal triggering stimulus for host T cells, more recent attention has been focused on fixed cells such as histiocytes, dendritic cells, and possibly certain cells of the vascular endothelium. The latter have been shown, under some circumstances at least, to be able to present antigen to T cells.

This general line of thinking has led some investigators to explore a new approach to circumventing transplant rejection. Although all cells in a transplant are potential targets for activated CTLs, CTL activation per se may be initiated by only a few cells in the transplant. Can these cells be removed prior to transplantation?

Although attractive on theoretical grounds, so far no one has come up with a practical way of putting this idea into effect for most transplants. Lafferty found in mice that allogeneic fetal thyroid tissue, if cultured for 10 to 14 days *in vitro* prior to transplantation, lost its immunogenicity. It has been speculated that this loss of immunogenicity was related to a selective "dying off" of passenger leukocytes during the culture period. The thyroid parenchymal cells maintained their functional and histological integrity. Other investigators showed that pancreatic islet cells treated with class II antibodies and complement survive much longer than control islets when transplanted into allogeneic mice. This too would be consistent with elimination of immunoprovocative passengers cells. However, although this approach is still being pursued for the transplantion of small pieces of tissue, it is not clear how passenger cells could ever be effectively eliminated from larger donor organs such as heart, kidney, liver, etc. Dendritic cells and histiocytes are widely spread throughout every compartment of these organs, usually intimately intercalated with other cell types. Major organs are normally transplanted into the recipient immediately upon removal from the donor, with little or no time for intervening manipulation. Thus, although our present understanding of T cell activation and transplant rejection suggests that passenger leukocytes are probably a major element in provoking the rejection reaction, at present there is no obvious means for eliminating them.

The Role of Antibodies in Allograft Rejection

The role of antibodies in transplant rejection is still controversial. Certainly lymphocytes, particularly T lymphocytes, are both necessary, and probably sufficient, to cause rejection of a primary skin allograft in most species. However, the apparent absence of a role for antibody in this situation could conceivably be related to the absence of good vascular connection in the first day or two of skin engraftment, since if the graft is allowed to heal in (using a specifically tolerant host), passive administration of antigraft antiserum will lead to rapid graft rejection. As mentioned earlier, antibody seems to play a major role in secondary skin allografting situations. Kidney transplantation is an example of a situation in which participation of antibody in primary graft rejection is suspected. Direct, immediate establishment of full donor–host circulation is accomplished surgically at the time of transplantation. In both humans and animals, rejection of a primary kidney allograft is accompanied by deposition of antigen–antibody complexes in the glomerular blood vessels. These complexes bind C1q and C3, and appear to lead to vascular lesions that some think may be a major factor in the loss of kidney function associated with rejection. The degree of buildup of these complexes in the glomeruli, and the severity of the accompanying vasculitis, correlate well with the rate of rejection. The vasculitis might be caused directly by complement, or it may be related to the high local concentration of PMNs which are most likely attracted by the C3a and C5a released from the antibody–antigen–complement complexes. Complement components may also activate platelets, leading to localized intravascular coagulation. It is usually assumed that the complexes involve antigen embedded in the donor cell surface, but it cannot be ruled out that soluble donor antigen of some form is actually involved.

To complicate the picture further, there is also good evidence that antibodies may in fact *protect* an allograft from detection and/or destruction by the immune system. Nearly 40 years ago, in some of the early attempts to define the basic mechanisms of transplant rejection, it was observed that antiserum raised against donor transplantation antigens, when passively transferred into a prospective recipient prior to transplantation antigens, would in some cases actually increase the length of time required for rejection to occur. This phenomenon is usually referred to as enhancement. More recent experiments have shown that antibody against the histocompatibility antigens of donor tissue can block the access of specifically sensitized cytotoxic T cells to donor target cells *in vitro*. Such antibodies, called blocking antibodies, may be the analog of enhancing antibodies *in vivo*. However, the situation is made even more confusing by the finding that not only antibody but antigen and antibody–antigen complexes can also interfere with cell-mediated immune reactions both *in vivo* and *in vitro*.

Detailed study of allografting in experimental animals has made us aware of an impressive repertoire of defenses against transplanted tissues. T cells seem to object particularly strongly to this procedure, probably as a spinoff of their aversion to virally and oncologically transformed self-cells. Antibody plays a variety of roles in transplantation, but on balance is probably a negative factor as well. The particular way in which each of these agencies is involved in rejection varies considerably in different transplant situations. But a thorough understanding of how each works has led to strategies for managing them, at least to some degree. In the remainder of this chapter, we briefly review the current status of transplantation of major organs in humans.

Clinical Organ Transplantation

Kidney

By far the organ with which the most success has been achieved in terms of human allografting has been the kidney. Nearly 50,000 transplants have been carried out since 1963. A number of factors have contributed to the success of kidney allografts. The most important factor is undoubtedly the greater potential for obtaining a good histocompatibility match between donor and recipient. Because it is possible for an individual to live and function normally with a single healthy kidney, it has been possible to secure organs from living donors. Such donors are ordinarily close family members, particularly siblings, ensuring much better histocompatibility matches than can be obtained from cadavers. As shown in Figure 19-3, kidneys obtained from HLA-identical siblings have an excellent prospect for survival. In such cases, the five-year survival rate is better than for untransplanted patients kept on hemodialysis. Parent-to-child transplants, which represent at least a 50 percent mismatch, fared less well. Cadaver transplants survived least well of all. On the other hand, the *rate* of graft and patient survival beyond five years is not very different for any of the donor sources. Apparently, if a kidney survives that long, the immune system has made whatever adjustments are necessary for long-term survival.

Interestingly, in the case of cadaver donors, only a marginal correlation could be found between the degree of matching of known class I HLA antigens and transplant survival (Figure 19-4). Perfect matching at the A, B, and C loci offers at best a 15 percent improvement in survival rate. The effect is only noticeable in the first 12

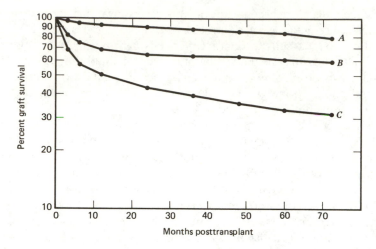

Figure 19-3 Kidney graft survival rates for indentical twin donors (A), parent donors (B), and randomly selected cadaver donors (C). Data from a Scandinavian study carried out between 1969 and 1980.

months after transplant; after that, the rejection *rate* is essentially the same regardless of the degree of HLA-A,B,C incompatibility, The same phenomenon has also been observed in the transplantation of other organs. It thus appears that factors other than class I MHC antigen compatibility can influence survival of kidney transplants. It has become increasingly clear that matching at the D locus,

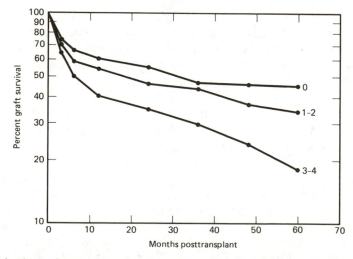

Figure 19-4 Kidney first-graft survival rates with cadaveric donors, as a function of the number of class I locus mismatches. Determined retrospectively; A and B locus only. Data from 1970 to 1982.

either serologically (Figure 19-5) or by MLC matching (Figure 19-6), is of major significance in kidney graft survival. Improved tests for HLA-D and DR typing, and increasing use of these tests in conjunction with transplantation, is one of the most important factors in the improvement of transplant success in the past decade.

Until recently, in the case of cadaveric donors, most serotyping, and all MLC typing, could only be done retrospectively. For the majority of organ transplants involving random cadaveric donors, retrospective tissue typing could suggest what measures might be required to keep a transplant functioning, or why it failed, but was of no value for matching donors and recipients. Cadaveric transplants had to (and in some cases still must) be done very quickly, with little or no forewarning, and the typing tests require hours or days to perform. However, steadily improving techniques for preserving kidneys from donors with recent brain death are changing this situation. Freshly removed kidneys that are in good physiological condition can be perfused with cold electrolyte solutions and stored in ice for up to 24 hours with no negative consequences. Renal viability and function adequate for transplantation can be maintained up to 72 hours by keeping the organ cooled and on the equivalent of a heart–lung machine. As these techniques become more widely applied, prospective tissue matching and physical transport to bring appropriate recipients and donor organs together may considerably improve the survival of cadaveric organ transplants.

A related factor that we can infer must be of great importance in human transplantation immunology is minor histocompatibility antigens. As discussed in Chapter 9, these have been well defined in mice but, aside from the H-Y antigen, are virtually undescribed in humans. The most perfectly (if retrospectively) MHC-

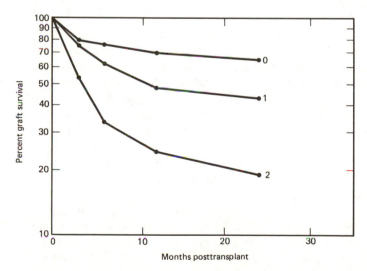

Figure 19-5 Kidney first-graft survival rates with cadaveric donors, as a function of the number of serologically detected class II antigen differences (based on an earlier scheme where only one class II locus was recognized). Data from 1977 to 1982.

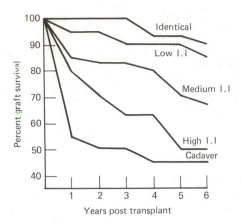

Figure 19-6 Comparison of graft survival among 20 MLC-identical, 17 low I.I. (Incompatibility Index), 17 medium I.I., 10 high I.I., and 125 cadaver recipients. I.I. scoring is for living related donors. [Taken from D. T. Uehling, J. L. Hussey, F. O. Belzer, C. Kan, and F. H. Bach, MLC incompatibility index for donor-recipient matching. *Transplant Proc. 9*, 103–105 (1977). (By permission of Grune and Stratton, Inc.).]

matched cadaver organs are still rejected in over half the cases, and much more rapidly than sibling or parent kidneys. Minor histocompatibility antigens are the likely explanation for greater survival of HLA-matched sibling transplants compared with equally well-matched cadaver transplants. Siblings could be expected to differ at fewer minor H loci than randomly selected, HLA identical members of the population at large. At present there is little hope for matching minor loci in the case of cadaveric donors.

A number of other factors affecting kidney transplant survival are known, or at least suspected, and they seem to apply to other organ transplants as well. One major problem is presensitization. As many as one-third of transplant patients have cytotoxic antibodies in their serum for 50 percent of the known HLA specificities. Fifteen percent of these patients may have antibodies cytotoxic for 90 percent of the known specificities. The existence of high levels of such antibodies, even though they may not be specifically directed toward donor antigens, generally bodes ill for survival of a transplant. The causes of presensitization are unclear.

Another important factor that can affect survival statistics is pre- and postoperative management of the patient. Particularly in the early years of kidney transplantation (1963 or so), patient management protocols varied considerably from institution to institution around the world. This undoubtedly influenced survival of the graft and of the patient, and thus introduced considerable variation into interpretation of survival versus HLA phenotype. As procedures become increasingly standardized at major transplantation centers, histocompatibility correlations will doubtless become more statistically meaningful.

Some transplant centers now encourage repeated kidney transplants when necessary. Patients are closely monitored, and at the first signs of a rejection crisis that cannot be managed easily with drugs, the kidney is removed and the patient returned to hemodialysis until another suitable donor organ can be procured. Although subsequent kidneys may survive somewhat less well, especially if the original transplant was from a cadaver, aggressive management protocols of this type have improved patient survival statistics markedly in the past 10 years.

Organ transplant patients are at high risk for a variety of infectious diseases, presumably as a result of the chronic inimmunosuppression they must undergo in order to control rejection. Cytomegalovirus infections are a particular problem, and other infections of the lungs and liver are also common. On the other hand, long-term hemodialysis places the patient at high risk for neurologic and vascular disease, and in view of the current rate of success with at least HLA-identical sibling organs, kidney transplantation certainly seems preferable to long-term dialysis.

Another risk factor faced by transplant patients generally is the development of cancer. Malignancies of cells and tissues of the immune system are particularly high—the rate of occurrence of reticulum cell sarcoma in transplant patients is 300 times that in the normal population, while lymphomas occur 35 times more frequently. This has led to the suspicion that the immunosuppressive drug used, all of which act directly on the immune system, might be directly or indirectly carcinogenic. However, many nonimmune system tumors, such as skin cancer, also occur more frequently in transplant patients and may result from impaired immune surveillance caused by the immunosuppression.

Survival statistics for kidney allografts are still continuing to improve. Two major factors have contributed to this in recent years. One was the realization that transplant patients who had been multiply transfused prior to transplantation had a markedly lower rejection rate than patients who had not been transfused at all. The reasons for this are not clear, but speculation has centered on the possibility that exposure to class I antigens in the absence of class II (e.g., on red blood cells and platelets) may induce tolerance to the class I antigens. There is some support for this notion based on studies in animals. Whatever the reason, the effect is real, and it is now routine procedure in most kidney transplant centers to give transplant recipients multiple blood transfusions prior to surgery.

The second major factor in improved kidney transplant success in recent years is development of the drug cyclosporine A (CyA). We will discuss CyA in more detail at the end of this chapter. It has had a remarkable effect on preventing rejection not only of kidneys (Figure 19-7), but almost every other organ as well.

Bone Marrow

Transplantation of bone marrow has increased markedly in recent years. The current rate of transplantation is nearly 200 per year, compared with only a dozen or so per year 10 years ago.

The three clinical situations in which a bone marrow transplant may be beneficial are aplastic anemia, leukemia, and severe combined immunodeficiency disease. In the latter disease which, although invariably fatal if untreated, is actually

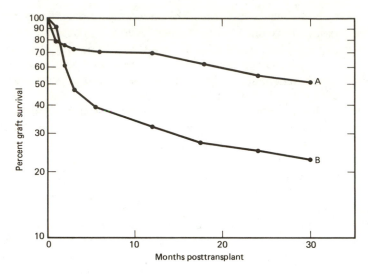

Figure 19-7 Kidney allograft survival with (a) low-dose steroid plus cyclosporin A; (b) standard azathioprine-based treatment.

quite rare, bone marrow transplantation (BMT) serves the fairly straightforward function of replenishment of the recipient's hemopoietic stem cell compartments. Because the recipient has no immune defense, the success of the grafts in terms of "take" is usually better than 90 percent, even when nonidentical, nonsibling marrow is used. However, graft-versus-host disease (GVHD; see Chapter 14) is a serious problem, even in the case of well-matched donor–recipient combinations. Seventy percent of HLA-identical sibling bone marrow grafts result in GVHD in the recipient, although the symptoms are usually milder than when the marrow is from a nonsibling donor. Current statistics for patients receiving HLA-matched sibling marrow transplants are encouraging. Although the number of cases being followed is small, it appears that the five-year survival figure may be close to 50 percent. Most efforts to improve these statistics focus on reducing GVHD. Reduction of the total number of grafted cells, and separation of stem cells from more immunologically mature (and aggressive) marrow cells seem particularly promising techniques.

In aplastic anemia and leukemia, problems other than GVHD complicate the picture. In the case of leukemia, incomplete eradication of the disease prior to BMT is still a major problem, leading to a high rate of recurrence of the primary disease. Many transplant centers are using increased levels of chemotherapy or whole-body irradiation, and sometimes a combination of both, in attempts to eradicate all traces of malignant cells prior to BMT. The levels of such treatment tolerated by patients seem to vary with age. Younger patients can sustain significantly higher levels of both chemotherapy and irradiation, which has led to a correspondingly high remission rate in patients under 18 years of age. More vigorous therapy to remove the leukemia has the beneficial side effect of preventing recipient rejection of the grafted marrow cells. However, it adds the unwelcome complication of placing the patient at extremely high risk for infectious disease; this remains a major cause of death after BMT.

Because of the rapidly changing approaches to BMT and leukemia, it is difficult to draw conclusions or make projections about the impact of BMT on remission. Current overall prospects for prolonged remission are in the range of 20 percent; this will almost certainly be higher for younger patients, especially those first treated for their disease after 1976–1977.

Aplastic anemia patients can be helped significantly by BMT if the diagnosis of the disease is made early and an MHC-identical sibling donor is available. Rejection of the graft is a major problem and is dealt with in much the same way as in leukemia patients—by intensive chemotherapy and/or whole-body irradiation. GVHD is also a major cause of failure. However, patients surviving one year after BMT have a better than 90 percent chance of permanent, or at least very long-term, recovery (Figure 19-8). An interesting recent finding is that patients transplanted with marrow from a male donor have a higher engraftment rate, less problems with GVHD, and higher survival rates. The basis for this finding is unclear at present, but it emerged from a well-coordinated international study involving 144 patients treated in 24 different transplant centers. Bone marrow transplant teams are now being urged to use male donor marrow whenever possible.

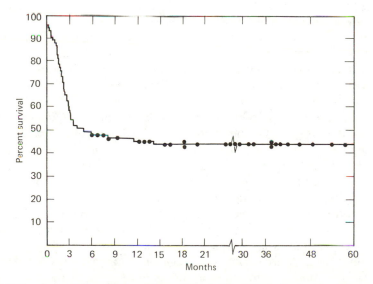

Figure 19-8 Survival of 73 patients with severe aplastic anemia treated by marrow transplantation from HLA-identical siblings. [From R. Storb, P. L. Weiden, R. Prentice, C. D. Buckner, R. A. Clift, A. B. Einstein, A. Fefer, F. L. Johnson, K. G. Lerner, P. E. Neiman, J. E. Sanders, and E. D. Thomas, Aplastic anemia (AA) treated by allogeneic marrow transplantation: The Seattle experience. *Transplant. Proc.* **9**, 181–185 (1977). (By permission of Grune and Stratton, Inc.).]

Heart

Transplantation of bone marrow and kidneys has one very important advantage over other organs—the possibility of obtaining transplantable material from a living donor. Not only will the donor material be in much better condition at the time of transplant, but the possibility also exists of obtaining a good MHC match from a sibling donor.

A healthy, transplantable heart is only obtainable on the unplanned death of an unselected donor. Given the high incidence of heart disease in this country, and the consequently large number of potential heart transplant recipients, it is obvious that the number of organs available as the result of accidents, strokes, etc., involving otherwise healthy donors can never be sufficient to meet the need. A heart, like any other organ, must be transplanted very shortly after removal from the donor. Little time is available for more than ABO matching of donor and recipient. Furthermore, the high mortality rate among patients with advanced heart disease obviates formation of large pools of typed recipients to whom well-matched donor organs could be delivered. The possibility of transplatning animal hearts into humans has been tested on numerous occasions and simply does not work.

Nevertheless, since the first heart transplant in 1967, the success of this technique has steadily improved. Well over 500 patients suffering from end stage heart disease have received transplants, of which more than 130 are still alive. Patients receiving transplants since 1974 have fared better than those transplanted in the preceding years at all centers. This improvement can be attributed to a number of factors. Experience from the early years showed that certain patients are very poor risks for both the surgery and the subsequent chronic immunosuppression involved in heart transplantation. These include patients with pulmonary vascular disease, diabetics, persons over 50 years of age, or individuals with systemic or latent infections. Another factor, considered to be paramount by Shumway at Stanford, is better preservation of the heart between the time it is removed from the donor until it is implanted in the recipient. Although it is seldom possible to carry out a complete tissue typing of the donor, it is now routine in most centers to test for the presence of the specificity of HLA-A2. For reasons that are unclear at present, mismatches for HLA-A2 show a high incidence of allograft coronary atherosclerosis.

Other areas in which continued improvements have been made are earlier diagnosis and better management of rejection episodes, more careful control of infections in immunosuppressed patients, and better immunosuppressive drugs and drug regimens. As with kidney transplantation, the introduction of CyA has greatly improved graft acceptance rates. One year survival rates are now over 80 percent at most centers, with five-year rates at 50 percent or more.

There still remain formidable barriers to widespread adoption of heart transplantation. Ninety percent of patients diagnosed as having end-stage heart disease, but otherwise certified as suitable for a coronary transplant, die within three months. Thus the pool of such patients is small at any given time. The scarcity of organs suited for transplantation has already been mentioned. The cost of such treatment is staggering at present. Preservation of hearts after removal from the donor is still not as successful as with kidneys, further complicating the problems if tissue matching and getting the proper organ to the best recipient.

Although survival statistics for the few who can receive heart transplants is now good and steadily improving, the supply-and-demand problem suggests that the future of heart replacement may be with mechanical pumps. Although the technology for doing this is crude at present, we may expect to see rapid progress in this area over the next few years. Live organ transplantation, however, may not be entirely displaced, but may become one of several alternatives for at least the foreseeable future.

Liver

Although liver transplantation has proved to be both surgically feasible and manageable from a rejection standpoint, the number of transplants performed is still fairly modest. Patients with chronic and incurable liver disease, children with certain inborn errors of metabolism, and patients with certain localized, primary liver tumors, have constituted the bulk of recipients so far (over 300 recorded worldwide since this procedure was introduced in 1963). Most of the complications are technical rather than immunological in nature and include advanced deterioration of the recipient at the time of transplantation (often due to unavailability of a donor organ, which, like the heart, must come from an otherwise healthy, recently expired donor) and improper function of the biliary drainage system after transplantation. The latter problem accounts for nearly one-half of all liver transplant failures. The general metabolic integrity of most transplanted livers is still excellent at the time of overall transplant failure. Immunological rejection as a cause of dysfunction accounts for only about 10 percent of all liver transplant failures. This may be due to the low density of MHC antigen on liver cells. Liver cells are notoriously resistant to immune damage in *in vitro* assays.

Despite the overall fairly high failure rate, patients who survive beyond three to four months do reasonably well. The longest surviving patient with a liver transplant has survived more than 12 years. The apparent low immunogenicity of the liver may make it a more attractive candidate for transplantation once some of the technical difficulties have been resolved. However, as some of the technical problems are overcome, the percentage of failures due to immunological rejection is beginning to rise.

Lung

Transplantation of lungs in humans has now come to a virtual halt. The technical problems are enormous. Lungs deteriorate extremely rapidly after removal, making organ exchange even between closely situated institutions risky. There is also a fairly critical requirement for size matching between donor and recipient if the transplanted lung is to function properly. The surgical reconnection of bronchial passages has proved extremely difficult, and failure of bronchial anastomoses accounts for nearly all transplant failures in patients surviving beyond the first few days. To date, too few patients have survived long enough for a meaningful evaluation of immunological rejection. Almost no lung transplants have been performed in this country in the past seven to eight years; however, lung transplantation in animals continues to be an active area of experimentation.

Pancreas

Pancreas transplantation has been perhaps the least successful of all the major organ transplant attempts. A major problem is that it is usually only attempted in advanced stages of diabetic disease, when the patient's status is already so seriously compromised that almost any major surgery is risky at best. Beyond that, the complicated and delicate surgical techniques required have discouraged all but a few centers from even attempting this procedure. Anything short of perfection in the transplantation procedure almost always leads to malfunction of the exocrine portion of the pancreas. Uncontrolled exocrine secretions into the transplant site are a major cause of failure.

Recently, attention has been focused on transplantation of isolated endocrine elements of the pancreas as an approach to managing diabetes. Islets of Langerhans, freed of most of the associated exocrine tissue, have been used successfully in both animal and human studies. Another approach, pioneered by Brown and his colleagues at UCLA, involves the use of cryopreserved ($-196°C$) fetal pancreases to reverse diabetes in adult animals. This has worked successfully in rats and may be scaled up for human application within the next few years. Although the problem of transplant rejection must still be dealt with, the ability to freeze-store fetal pancreases will allow the development of a large bank of prospectively typed donor organs, and increases the likelihood of good donor–recipient histocompatibility matches.

A potential major advantage of transplanting islets or fetal pancreas fragments is that these elements can be maintained in tissue culture for up to two weeks prior to transplantation. Recent studies have shown that cells bearing class II antigens can be selectively eliminated during culture, greatly reducing the immunogenicity of the tissues upon transplantation.

Future Directions

With only a few exceptions, one or two of which we have noted, the surgical and physiological barriers to transplantation of most organs have been dealt with successfully. In many instances, transplantation may never be a particularly useful approach to treatment of organ-localized disease because of the general unavailability of donor organs. The future of organ replacement in some of these cases may rest on the development by biomedical engineers of mechanical replacement parts. But in other instances, such as kidney, bone marrow, and, perhaps ultimately, fetal pancreas transplantation, both surgical problems and problems related to availability of donor organs have been essentially overcome, and the major barrier to transplantation in disease management is immunological. The future of clinical transplantation in these latter instances thus depends on advances in research being carried out in animal models in laboratories throughout the world.

There are several directions in which transplantation research seems to be moving. One is a continued exploration of the genetic and immunological factors involved in histoincompatibility. At present, even when almost all of the known histocompatibility factors are matched between nonconsanguinous donors and recipients, survival of the transplant is not much enhanced over a more or less random match. Yet when the same degree of match is obtained between siblings, the success rate is very high. Clearly, there are a number of histocompatibility factors of which scientists are not yet aware. By analogy with other mammals, we may expect humans to have a series of non-MHC histocompatibility loci, although few have yet been unambiguously identified. If the number of such loci turns out to be large, then the possibility of obtaining a good match may be very small. On the other hand, studies with animals have shown repeatedly that when the MHC is well matched, rejection problems are reduced manyfold. Recent advances in direct molecular mapping of the human MHC, together with the development of highly specific monoclonal antibodies, may be expected to greatly increase the accuracy of donor–recipient matching.

Another important area of research in organ transplantation is the continued identification and testing of new immunosuppressive agents. Drugs currently used to immunosuppress transplant recipients are highly effective, but often have wide-ranging harmful effects to the patient both related and unrelated to the need to prevent rejection. Ideally, one would like to be able to suppress just those T cells involved in the response to histocompatibility antigens present on the donor organ. However, traditionally used immunosuppressive drugs such as steroids, azathioprine, and antilymphocyte or antithymocyte antibodies cause widespread, nonspecific suppression of immune responsiveness. Thus the number one complication of organ transplantation is not rejection, but placing the recipient at risk for infection from otherwise innocuous microorganisms. In addition to nonspecific suppressive effects on the immune system, most of these drugs have harmful effects on other metabolic systems. Corticosteroids such as prednisolone, for example, which are given in doses ranging from 20 to 100 mg/day, can cause diabetes, peptic ulceration, weight gain, hypertension, osteoporosis and osteonecrosis, deep-vein thrombosis, cataracts, hyperlipidemia, and psychological disturbances. Many of these complications can be managed with appropriate secondary treatment, but the risks involved are only justifiable in the context of end-stage organ failure.

In the early 1970s, Jean Borel noticed that a neutral decapeptide found in the fermentation broth of the fungus *Trichoderma polysporum* had potent immunosuppressive properties. He spent a number of years following up this observation, and ultimately developed a drug, Cyclosporin A (CyA), that has revolutionized immunosuppression in transplant patients. Although its specific mechanism of action is unknown, it appears to prevent activation of T helper and T cytotoxic cells, but not T suppressors or any other cells of the immune system. The major defect in CyA-treated animals appears to be lack of production of IL-2 by T helper cells, and an impaired ability of pre-CTL to utilize IL-2. The function of B cells, macrophages, and granulocytes is unimpaired. Such effects have been seen both *in vivo* and *in vitro,* in both animals and humans.

The effects on specific T-cell functions are rapidly reversible. However, rabbits given an appropriate regimen of CyA have been reported to retain an allografted kidney even after withdrawal of the drug, suggesting a state of tolerance may have been induced. This point is still controversial and has not been documented in humans. As with many other experimental protocols in the early stages, there are still considerable variations in timing, dose, and route of administration used by different research groups that make comparisons difficult.

Like other immunosuppressive drugs, CyA is not without harmful side effects. These include variable degrees of hepatotoxicity and nephrotoxicity, and an increased incidence of viral infections and perhaps lymphomas. There is a distressing increase in body hair in patients treated with CyA. On the other hand, bone marrow toxicity is less than for other drugs.

CyA is now being evaluated worldwide in every currently used transplantation procedure. Preliminary results are very encouraging. It is as potent an immunosuppressive drug as anything currently in use, and the undesirable side effects are overall less severe than other currently used regimens. In the Stanford heart transplant program, the use of CyA has not only improved graft survival markedly but has reduced the average postoperative hospital stay from 72 to 42 days, making the procedure less expensive. The reduced hospital stay is made possible because patients treated with CyA (and reduced steroids) have fewer negative side effects and are better able to fight off opportunistic infections.

A third strategy under intensive study at the present time is to create a situation in which immunological tolerance can develop toward the donor organ. In a limited number of cases, such as the transplantation of fetal pancreas or pancreatic islets, this may be possible by selective elimination of class II antigen-bearing cells prior to transplantation. There is increasing experimental evidence that class I antigens by themselves may be tolergenic in the absence of an accompanying class II stimulus. Another approach currently being tested is thus to expose the recipient to donor class I antigens alone prior to transplantation. This is probably the basis for the transfusion effect alluded to earlier. The effect could possibly be enhanced, for example, by pretreating with isolated donor platelets, or with donor blood cells treated with class II antibodies plus complement to remove class II antigen-bearing white cells.

A variation of this general strategy is to treat the *host* in such a way that tolerance toward donor tissues will develop. One promising approach in this direction is a technique called total lymphoid irradiation (TLI). TLI was originally developed for treatment of patients with Hodgkin's disease, a type of lymphoma particularly common in young people. Small doses of radiation (ca. 100 R) are given sequentially to selected lymphoid tissues over a period of several weeks until a cumulative dose somewhere in the vicinity of 2000 R is reached. This will usually completely eradicate the lymphoma. It was noticed by Henry Kaplan and his associates at Stanford, who pioneered this technique, that Hodgkin's patients at the end of treatment and for several months to several years afterward had depressed T-cell functions. The potential significance of this for transplantation was explored by Strober and Slavin at Stanford. They found that rats treated with a course of TLI had a generalized depression of the ability to reject skin grafts for about two months after the end of treatment. This was shown to be due to antigen nonspecific suppressor T cells. If the rats were injected with donor bone marrow at the end of TLI and before skin grafting, long-term donor-specific tolerance could be established. GVH disease did not develop in the rats, perhaps because host Ia-bearing cells were eliminated by the radiation treatment. The rats completing such therapy were mixed lymphoid chimeras; that is, lymphocytes of both donor and host origin were present.

Experiments in medium-sized animals, transplanted with hearts or kidneys, have generally confirmed the results using TLI in rats, although the question of chimerism with marrow infusion is still unsettled. However, in nearly all cases a state of generalized tolerance, lasting up to six months after cessation of treatment, can be achieved with TLI alone. In the past several years, TLI has been used in humans as an adjunct to other forms of drug immunosuppression. The results are highly encouraging. Survival of transplants is as good or better than with drugs alone, but most importantly the dose of steroids needed to achieve graft acceptance can be greatly reduced. At the time of this writing it is still too early to tell if long-term tolerance of the grafts will develop in humans.

Bibliography

General

Brynger, J. (ed.), Clinical kidney transplantation. *Transplant Proc. 14* (1982).

Calne, R. Y., Recent advances in clinical transplantation of the liver and pancreas. *Transplant. Proc. 15,* 1263 (1983).

Kahan, B., and J. Borel, Proceedings of the First International Congress on cyclosporine. *Transplant. Proc.* Vol. XV, No. 4, suppl. 1 and 2 (1983).

Kaplan, H., Selective effects of total lymphoid irradiation on the immune response. *Transplant. Proc. 13,* 425 (1981).

Monaco, A., and M. Wood (eds.), Proceedings of the 8th International Congress of the Transplantation Society. *Transplant. Proc. 13* (1981).

Sutherland, D. E., Current status of pancreas transplantation. Registry statistics and an overview. *Transplant. Proc. 15,* 1303 (1983).

Research

Albrechtson, D., T. Moen, and E. Thorsby, HLA matching in clinical transplantation. *Transplant. Proc. 15,* 1120 (1983).

Batchelor, J. et al., Transplantation antigens *per se* are poor immunogens within a species. *Nature 273,* 54 (1978).

Billingham, R. E., L. Brent, and P. B. Medawar, Quantitative studies on tissue transplantation immunity II: The origin, strength, and duration of actively and adoptively acquired immunity. *Proc. Roy. Soc. Lond. 143,* 58 (1954).

Eichwald, E. J., et al., Cell-mediated hyperacute rejection. IV. Lyt markers and adoptive transfer. *J. Immunol. 128,* 2373 (1982).

Gowans, J. L., The role of lymphocytes in the destruction of homografts. *Br. Med. Bull. 21,* 106 (1965).

Gowans, J. L., D. D. McGregor, D. M. Cowen, and C. E. Ford, Initiation of immune responses by small lymphocytes. *Nature 196,* 651 (1962).

Jooste, S. V. et al., The vascular bed as the primary target in the destruction of skin grafts by antiserum. *J. Exp. Med. 154,* 1319 (1981).

Loveland, B. E., and I. F. C. McKenzie, Which T cells cause graft rejection? *Transplantation 33,* 217 (1981).

Medawar, P. B., The behavior and fate of skin autografts and skin homografts in rabbits. *J. Anatomy 78,* 176 (1944).

Mitchison, N. A., Passive transfer of transplantation immunity. *Nature 171,* 267 (1953).

Slavin, S., B. Reitz, C. P. Bieber, H. S. Kaplan, and S. Strober, Transplantation tolerance in adult rats using total lymphoid irradiation: Permanent survival of skin, heart, and marrow allografts. *J. Exp. Med. 147,* 700 (1978).

Wilson, D. B., and R. E. Billingham, Lymphocytes and transplantation immunity? *Adv. Immunol. 7,* 189 (1967).

CHAPTER 20

Immunity and Cancer

What is Cancer?

Tumors Can Provoke Specific Immune Responses

Immune Responses to Tumors

The Role of Antibody in Tumor Immunity
Cytotoxic T Lymphocytes
The Role of Macrophages in Tumor Control
NK Cells

Immunotherapy

The Use of Monoclonal Antibodies in the Diagnosis and
Treatment of Cancer
*Diagnostic Applications of Tumor-specific Monoclonal
Antibodies*
*"Magic Bullets": The Use of Monoclonal Antibodies to
Destroy Tumor Cells*
Biological Response Modifiers

Not long after microbiologists began to describe the body's ability to overcome infectious disease by immune mechanisms, others began to speculate that similar mechanisms might be involved in other types of diseases, particularly cancer. And indeed, when biologists isolated cells or tissue fragments from a tumor taken from one animal and attempted to grow them in a second animal, the transplanted tumor tissue was rapidly rejected. For some reason, this observation seemed to attract geneticists more than immunologists. The latter had an almost endless variety of infectious diseases still to be worked on. Geneticists spent a good deal of energy trying to define the genetic factors involved in the rejection of transplanted tumors, with little result.

The nascent field of tumor immunology was dealt a nearly lethal blow by Peter Gorer in the 1930s, when he demonstrated convincingly that rejection of transplanted tumors was simply a manifestation of the general phenomenon of rejection of foreign tissues. Tumors from animal B, when transplanted to animal A, are rejected not because they are tumors, but because they display the same B-type antigens on their surface that trigger rejection of any of B's tissues by animal A. As we saw in Chapters 8 and 14, this seminal observation gave rise to the study of major histocompatibility complexes, provided a rational basis for the transplantation of tissues and organs, and eventually led to the discovery of cell-mediated cytotoxicity. But it discouraged serious attempts to find an immunological basis for tumor resistance for nearly 20 years.

What Is Cancer?

Cancer is a disease characterized by chronically unregulated cell growth. Over the years, in an attempt to elucidate the mechanisms underlying oncological transformation, a number of properties of tumor cells have been described that were thought to distinguish them from the normal cells from which they arose. These properties included a more rapid growth rate, a higher metabolic rate and a concomitant need for more oxygen (or alternatively a higher production of lactic acid), abnormal or at least altered cell membranes, a higher than normal DNA content, and a tendency to invade surrounding tissues or to metastasize (via blood or lymph) to distant tissues.

When we realize that many (perhaps a great majority) of tumors arise from developmentally immature, even stemlike, cells, many of these distinctions drop away. In such cases, comparison of the tumor cell with its fully differentiated counterpart is not valid; the comparison must be made with the equivalent stage of cell development in the tissue of origin. There is in fact little evidence, for example, that tumor cells are different from normal immature cells in terms of cell cycle time and general metabolism.

Two properties, however, are likely to be altered in all tumor cells. There appear to be qualitative alterations in the genomic DNA that are responsible for the loss of growth control; and, probably as a direct consequence of this, there are almost always alterations in the plasma membranes of tumor cells that distinguish them even from the primitive cells from which they arose.

Genetic changes in growth regulation are obviously at the heart of the oncological process, and the nature of these changes has been the subject of intense investigation for half a century or more. In recent years, the discovery of oncogenes has shed a great deal of light on the nature of oncological transformation and has perhaps provided a common thread that will eventually allow the grouping of cancers into subsets of related disorders. Until now, oncologists have despairingly viewed cancer as a collection of a seemingly limitless number of distinct diseases. A full discussion of oncogenes is beyond the scope or intent of this text; for an introduction to the subject, the student is referred to the excellent review by Michael Bishop cited at the end of this chapter. The current state of affairs is exemplified by the papers that appear in most current issues of *Cell, Nature,* and *PNAS.* In brief, oncogenes are altered forms of genes that, in their normal state, participate in regulated cellular proliferation. (In their normal state in the cell, oncogenes are referred to collectively as protooncogenes.) They often code for growth or differentiation factors or for their receptors or for associated regulatory elements. Some are kinases that appear to be involved in the initial steps of cell proliferation. Although by no means have all cancers been linked to oncogenes, the number that can be is increasing almost daily. This will clearly be a major field of cancer research for some decades to come.

The changes in membrane properties of normal cells when they become oncologically transformed are generally accepted as being responsible for such properties as invasion of surrounding tissues (malignancy) and migration to distant sites in the body (metastasis). These alterations may be the direct result of alterations in structural elements encoded by oncogenes, or they may result from expression of new structures encoded by genes derepressed as a result of oncogene activation. At any rate, in many instances these membrane alterations result in immunologically detectable changes in the surface membranes of tumor cells. The ability to detect these changes was what finally rescued the field of tumor immunology from the difficulties imposed by Gorer's findings in the 1930s.

Tumors Can Provoke Specific Immune Responses

Renewed interest in tumor immunology arose from the work first of E. J. Foley in 1953, and then (and perhaps more forcefully) by Prehn and Main in 1957. Immunologists had attempted to get around the problem of tumor rejection due to allogeneic differences by transplanting tumors between members of the same inbred strain. On occasion, it appeared that rejection of H-2-identical tumors was occurring, suggesting the existence of tumor-specific antigens. However, the possibility lingered in the minds of many that tumor rejection between members of the same inbred strain could still be due to low levels of genetic heterogeneity within the strain, especially in strains that had not been inbred under controlled conditions for long periods of time.

Prehn and Main tried to meet these objections by designing a rigorous, well-controlled experiment (Figure 20-1). Fibrosarcomas were induced in inbred mice by injecting a small amount of the chemical carcinogen methylcholanthrene (MCA) subcutaneously. When a tumor developed, it was removed and divided into small fragments. These fragments were then implanted subcutaneously into fresh mice of the same inbred strain. When the tumor fragments began to grow, indicating vascularization and resumption of tumor development, they were surgically removed. These mice were then examined for evidence of having mounted an immune response to their tumor by reimplanting a new fragment of the same tumor. In 12 of 14 initial tests, positive responses (rejection or delayed growth of the tumor) were seen.

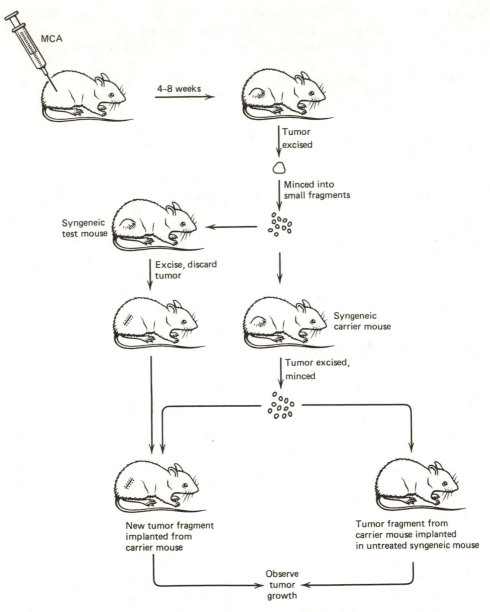

MCA

4–8 weeks

Tumor excised

Minced into small fragments

Syngeneic test mouse

Excise, discard tumor

Syngeneic carrier mouse

Tumor excised, minced

New tumor fragment implanted from carrier mouse

Tumor fragment from carrier mouse implanted in untreated syngeneic mouse

Observe tumor growth

Figure 20-1 The Prehn-Main experiment to demonstrate an immune response to a syngeneic tumor. (See text for details.)

A follow-up to this experiment, carried out by George Klein and his collaborators a few years later, provided the final evidence to persuade the scientific community that immune responsiveness to tumors is real. This was done by demonstrating immunity to a tumor in a single animal (Figure 20-2).

Sarcomas were induced in the thighs of mice by subcutaneous injection of methylcholanthrene. When the tumor had grown to 1 cm or so, the entire limb carrying the tumor was amputated. Portions of the removed tumor were irradiated and used to provide several "booster" immunizations of tumor cells. The amputated mice were then given varying doses of live cells saved from the original tumor. The susceptibility of these mice to cancer induction by these tumor cells was compared to untreated syngeneic mice, and to syngeneic mice given injections of irradiated tumor cells on the same schedule as the booster immunizations given to the amputated experimental group. Both the immunized/amputated/boosted mice, and the syngeneic mice given booster shots only, showed increased resistance to live tumor cells, compared to untreated mice.

Variations of these experiments carried out over the next decade or so supported the general notion that tumors can provoke a tumor-specific immune response but also provided some additional qualifications. For example, although this general type of experiment can show immunity to both chemically and virally induced experimental tumors, it has been very difficult to demonstrate specific immunity, whether cellular or humoral, to spontaneously arising tumors. Moreover, even with induced tumors, immunity is only readily demonstrable after excision of relatively small experimental tumors. If the tumor grows to a centimeter or more in diameter before removal, in most cases secondary implants grow as well as in untreated mice. And even in "successfully" immunized mice, immunity may not be demonstrable until a week or more after excision, and only then to relatively small innocula of tumor cells.

The failure to demonstrate immunity to spontaneous tumors probably reflects the fact, as we will discuss below, that such tumors display low or absent levels of tumor antigens. This may be one reason they escaped detection by the immune system and became established tumors. The immunosuppressive effects of large tumors (whether spontaneous or experimental) may be related to the development of suppressor T cells since, as we will also see below, treatments that would inhibit T_s cell development or function tend to reveal hidden tumor immune responsiveness. The refractory period seen after tumor excision may thus be required for decay of T_s function.

The experiments of Prehn and Main, and of Klein and his colleagues, strongly suggested that tumor cells must have unique antigens on their surface that can be recognized by the immune system as nonself. These tumor-specific antigens (TSA) act in a sense like transplantation antigens and are sometimes also referred to as tumor-specific transplantation antigens (TSTA). In the 1960s and 1970s, a great deal of research was devoted to identifying the properties of these antigens, and the nature of the immune responses they provoke.

One of the first things noticed by investigators working with the immune re-

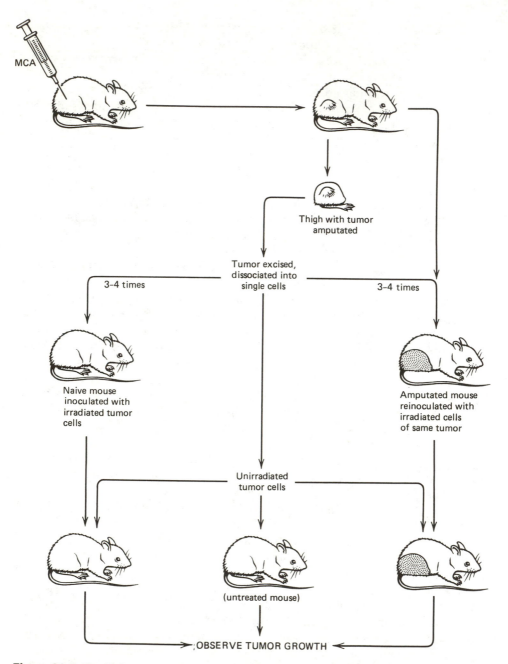

Figure 20-2 The Klein experiment showing an immune response to an autochthonous tumor. (See text for details.)

sponse to tumors induced by chemicals such as MCA, benzpyrene, or other chemical carcinogens was a lack of cross-reactivity among tumors induced by the same chemical. For example, a mouse immunized repeatedly with irradiated cells from one tumor induced by MCA would, as Klein showed, be relatively resistant to live cells taken from that same tumor. However, such a mouse would not be resistant to an MCA-induced tumor induced in another, syngeneic animal.

The reason for this is apparent when one isolates antibodies against MCA-induced tumor cells. Antibodies produced against one MCA-induced tumor cross-react very poorly or not at all against cells from other MCA-induced tumors. It quickly became apparent that different tumors induced by the very same chemical display completely unrelated TSA. In fact, we now know that even when two tumors are induced by the same chemical carcinogen at two different sites on the same animal, the two tumors will display unrelated TSA. Although the lack of cross-reactivity in such cases was detected by antibodies, we also know that T cells fail to cross-react as well. Whether NK cell tumor recognition is affected by serologically detected tumor antigens is unknown.

The molecular nature of antigens induced by chemical or physical carcinogens is unknown in most cases. Since a principal target for such carcinogens is the DNA, it may be that the resultant antigens are mutated versions of normal membrane proteins. It is also possible that in some cases the action of chemical or physical carcinogens may cause expression of latent viruses or at least viral antigens. This question is particularly obscure in humans, where tumors with a proved chemical or physical origin are rare.

A wide range of viruses, both DNA and RNA, can cause cancer in animals. In contrast with tumors caused by chemical or physical carcinogens, tumors caused by viruses express antigens that are characteristic of the inducing virus, regardless of the host. Even animals of completely different species may develop tumors with cross-reacting antigens, if they are caused by the same oncogenic virus. These antigens are usually encoded in the viral genome. They can be detected by antibodies and by T cells. As we saw in Chapter 14, the T-cell response to viral antigens generally is MHC restricted, and as far as can be determined, oncogenic virus-associated antigens are no exception.

In addition to the widely cross-reactive tumor antigens associated with the virus itself, cell transformation by an oncogenic virus may also result in expression of new host-encoded antigens. These are presumed to arise as a result of altered regulation of portions of the host genome resulting from the viral infection.

The nature of antigens on spontaneously arising tumors is often unclear. Many spontaneous tumors that develop into detectable malignancies do so because they are poorly immunogenic; that may have been one of the reasons they escaped detection and destruction by the immune system. In a number of cases, the antigens they do express are antigens found on the embryonic counterpart of the tissue in which the tumor arises. Some have taken this as an indication that oncological transformation causes cellular dedifferentiation. A more likely explanation is that tumors arise most easily from stem cells or primitive progenitor cells that are present at a low level in nearly all tissue. These cells and their antigens are present at a much higher level in embryonic tissues and not normally detectable in adults. These cells may be dividing continually, or at least may exist in a state more closely associated with rapid growth than are most fully differentiated, essentially terminal cells. Once these become oncologically transformed and growth regulation is lost, these cells and the "fetal" antigens they bear will rapidly become detectable. Examples of fetal antigens include the carcinoembryonic antigen associated with cancer of the gut tissues; alpha-fetoprotein, an embryonic liver protein found in liver cancer; and the TL antigen in mice, associated with ontologically immature thymocytes but found also on certain thymomas.

Immune Responses to Tumors

The repertoire of immune defenses used by the body in defending against tumors is no different from those we have seen in other immune responses. There are no special immune mechanisms for dealing with tumors. In a sense, immune reactions against spontaneous tumors are a form of autoimmunity, since the tumors are always derived from self. Thus tumor immunity is quite similar to both autoimmune disease and the response to viral infection; all three situations involve the mobilization of the immune system to attack self tissues. And as with both autoimmune disease and viral infection, inflammatory damage is a major component of the immune response to tumors.

The Role of Antibody in Tumor Immunity

In both experimental animals and in humans, it is possible to demonstrate serum antibodies reactive with tumor antigens. Often these antibodies will bind complement, and it is thus at least theoretically possible that these antibodies may facilitate complement-mediated lysis of tumor cells *in vivo*. In fact, complement-mediated lysis of tumor cells by serum antibodies can often be demonstrated *in vitro*. However, these is scant evidence that this is a significant defense mechanism *in vivo*. It may be that the generation of complement fragments 3a and 5a, both of which are potent attractants for granulocytes and macrophages, is a more important role for complement-binding antibodies. Antibodies (and complement fragments) that bind to tumor cells might also opsonize them for phagocytosis by macrophages or granulocytes, or facilitate cytolytic macrophage attacks on tumor cells (see below).

Antibodies may also *interfere* with the host immune response to tumors. Such a phenomenon was demonstrated originally with noncancerous allogeneic transplants. It was observed that passively infused antibodies specific for transplant surface antigens (principally class I MHC antigens) could significantly prolong rejection of the transplanted organ or tissue. Among the first to demonstrate a similar phenomenon in tumors were the Hellstroms. They found that serum from both experimentally induced and spontaneous murine tumors could block *in vitro* cell-mediated destruction of tumor cells. This serum was most effective when taken from animals with progressing tumors. Serum taken from animals with regressing tumors, or from animals one to two weeks after surgical removal of a tumor, had little or no blocking ability. Blocking serum has also been found in human cancer patients bearing a wide range of tumor types.

It is not at all clear that antibodies are actually the sole or even principal blocking factor in serum from tumor bearing animals or patients. Antibodies specific for tumor antigens could conceivably block access of CTLs or NK cells to tumor cells. However, at least some classes of tumor-specific antibodies might be expected to facilitate complement-mediated killing or ADCC. (Only IgG1 and IgG3 mediate macrophage ADCC.) On the other hand, shed tumor antigen present in serum (particularly in the form of membrane microvesicles) could also possibly block CTL or NK killing. At present, the mechanism of the blocking activity of serum from tumor-bearing individuals is still uncertain. There is some suggestion that complexes of tumor antigens and the corresponding antibodies may be the most effective blocking agent.

Cytotoxic T Lymphocytes

Cytotoxic T lymphocytes (CTLs), almost from the moment of their first description, provided immunologists with a major riddle. Why should a system exist whose sole purpose seemed to be to cause rejection of transplanted cells and tissues with exquisite specificity? In casting about for a biological rationale for the existence of CTLs, immunologists, under the influence largely of Burnett, decided on immune surveillance against cancer. This was not entirely a shot in the dark. In general, animals with impaired thymic function show an increase in the incidence of cancer (although, as we will see, this correlation is not absolute). Very old and very young animals, in which thymic function is thought to be less than optimal, have higher cancer rates than members of the same species in the middle (breeding) years. In fact, cancer is currently the number one disease cause of death in children under 10, although this is certainly in part because other causes of death have been brought under control. Transplant patients receiving drugs that suppress CTL function show increased rates of many kinds of cancer. There is a bit of a problem interpreting this latter fact, however, since the greatest increases occur in cancers of the immune system itself, and it is difficult to dissociate the potential carcinogenic effects of the drugs from their immunosuppressive function.

Many tumors show infiltration by T cells, and when these can be recovered and tested *in vitro,* they are often able to attack and destroy tumor cells of the type from which they were recovered. Lymphocytes from inbred animals bearing a particular tumor can also be used to transfer tumor-specific immunity to members of the same strain, and it can be shown that the cell in which this immunity resides is a T cell.

It is also relatively easy to demonstrate a protective, antitumor effect of CTLs in

the so-called Winn assay (Figure 20-3). CTLs are harvested from an animal undergoing successful tumor rejection. These are mixed together with a dose of tumor cells
large enough to cause a tumor and are injected into a suitable site in a recipient
animal. In experiments of this type, CTLs raised against a syngeneic tumor can be
shown to inhibit the development of that tumor in a transplanted animal. There are
several difficulties, however, in extrapolating from such results a major role for
CTLs in tumor control *in vivo*. First of all, the local concentration of CTLs, and the

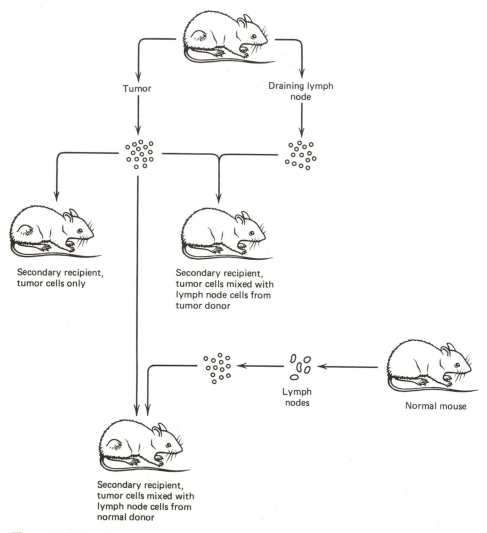

Figure 20-3 The Winn assay measuring anti-tumor reactivity in a lymphocyte population.
(See text for details.)

effective CTL:tumor cell ratio, is very high in a Winn assay. It is not clear that such ratios could obtain *in vivo*. Second, in the Winn assay all the CTLs and tumor cells are in immediate and direct contact. In real situations *in vivo,* circulating CTLs must cross over the vascular endothelium to reach the tumor; the tumor itself may be many cell layers deep around any given capillary.

Immune surveillance theories of cancer control based on the CTL as the principal effector began to lose support in the mid-1970s for two reasons. The first was a simple conceptual one. Zinkernagel and Doherty showed that a major biological function of CTLs is in surveillance of virally infected self cells. This relieved a great deal of the need to have to define a biological role for CTLs. In light of this new understanding, CTLs could be imagined to play a role in the elimination of tumors caused by viruses, but the existence of CTLs did not have to be explained solely on the basis of immunity to cancer.

The second challenge to the idea of a prime role of CTLs in cancer control was a more serious one, and consisted of two separate observations. The first was that nude mice, which do not have a functional T-cell system, do not have a higher incidence of cancer than do their normal counterparts. In fact, some strains of nude mice have if anything a lower incidence of at least some types of tumors. The second observation came about during a search for cell-mediated cytotoxicity in human cancer patients. Such cytotoxicity is, in fact, relatively easy to demonstrate, and at first seemed to point to a possible major role for CTLs in tumor immunity. The problem arose in trying to demonstrate target specificity for the cellular cytotoxicity. CTLs are always exquisitely specific for target cells of the type used to induce them. But when cytotoxic lymphocytes taken from a patient with a particular turnover were tested against a panel of various types of tumors taken from different patients, they usually killed them all. Moreover, when lymphocytes from individuals without cancer were used as controls, the level of cytotoxicity against the same panel of targets was often just as high as when cancer patient lymphocytes were used. (One can just imagine junior researchers being sent back to the bench to repeat their experiments over and over and over. . . .) These results led to the discovery of NK cells, which we will discuss below (see also Chapter 14).

Thus, during the past decade, there has been a declining interest in CTLs as an effector element in tumor immunity. It seems clear that they are not the sole cellular defense element, and perhaps not a major one. But it would probably be a mistake to dismiss them out of hand. Recent evidence has created new interest in a role for CTLs in tumor defenses. For example, one of the principal arguments put forward by those eager to jump on the anti-CTL bandwagon was that tumor specific CTLs infused into animals bearing the target tumor rarely cause any damage to the tumor. But in recent years it has been observed that if the animals are first rendered immunodeficient, particularly in their T-cell compartments, the efficacy of infused antitumor CTLs is greatly increased. This has led to the notion that established tumors may trigger T suppression that somehow counteracts CTL function. This may even have been a factor in the initial establishment of the tumor. In general, it has been found that CTLs are more effective against tumor cells in the first few days after tumor innoculation, and essentially ineffective later on. However, we cannot extrapolate this to how CTLs might behave in the case of spontaneously arising tumors. In such situations, if the tumor cells are appropriately antigenic, CTLs may be very effective in eliminating a tumor before it becomes established. It must always be remembered that the tumors we see developing are only the ones that have successfully evaded all the body's defense mechanisms. That does not mean that the mechanisms are faulty.

Renewed interest in CTLs as an element in tumor defense has also been stimulated by the definition of lymphocyte-derived tumor necrosis factors, or lymphotoxins. These molecules were studied for many years by Granger and his associates and were defined as molecules derived from T cells that had cytostatic and under some circumstances cytotoxic properties. Recently the gene for human T cell lymphotoxin has been cloned and sequenced. It is a glycoprotein with a molecular weight of 25,000 or so that has potent antitumor effects both *in vivo* and *in vitro* while causing little or no damage to nontransformed cells. It is currently being explored for potential human clinical application.

So the wheel turns. Having gone from a situation in which everyone thought that CTLs were the only cellular defense against cancer that mattered to a situation in which practically no one thought they were important, we are beinning to see renewed interest in them as at least one element in the cellular response to tumors. How important CTLs are in comparison to NK cells and macrophages in the overall response is difficult to assess at present, but clearly they are not an element to be dismissed.

The Role of Macrophages in Tumor Control

There is a great deal of direct and indirect evidence suggesting that macrophages are an important element in host defenses against tumors. As mentioned in Chapter 14, activated macrophages are selectively cytotoxic toward tumor cells *in vitro*. Macrophages are activated by T-cell lymphokines and can destroy target cells either by phagocytosis or, more commonly in the case of tumor cells, by a direct cell-killing mechanism. Macrophages are often found in high concentrations in tumors, particularly in those undergoing regression. Macrophages isolated from regressing tumors are always highly cytotoxic to tumor cells *in vitro*, while those from progressively growing tumors may or may not be cytotoxic. Moreover, cells taken from progressively growing tumors are often resistant to killing by macrophages isolated from regressing tumors.

Macrophages may use several mechanisms to kill tumor cells by direct contact, For the most part, this appears to involve secretion of toxic substances into the space formed between the macrophage and the tumor cell after the binding event. Even more than CTLs, macrophages form a complex, interdigitating interface with their target cells, creating many membrane-limited pockets into which toxic molecules could be secreted, and in which they could reach quite high concentration.

One must still explain, as in the case of CTLs, how the macrophage itself would escape damage by the purported toxic molecules.

One toxic molecule that has been studied by Dolph Adams and his co-workers is called cytolytic protease (CP). CP is a neutral serine protease of about 40,000 daltons. The ability of macrophages to kill tumor cells correlates well with their ability to produce and secrete CP. Macrophages that do not secrete CP do not kill tumor cells. Macrophage supernates that have been enriched for CP kill the same spectrum of tumor targets as do activated macrophages. CP is able to kill tumor cells at concentrations of 10^{-9} M.

Another molecule that is being intensely studied at the moment is macrophage-derived tumor necrosis factor (TNF). The gene for TNF has been isolated and studied by the same group that is working on lymphotoxin (T cell-derived tumor necrosis factor). The two molecules may be evolutionarily related in that they share about 30 percent sequence homology. Macrophage TNF is a glycoprotein of about 24,000 daltons. When molecularly cloned TNF is infused into tumor-bearing animals it causes extensive haemorrhagic necrosis of the tumor, with no apparent damage to normal tissues. Similarly, *in vitro,* TNF will selectively kill transformed cell lines but has little or no activity against untransformed cells.

There have also been reports that macrophages may kill tumors by secreting oxidatively active products such as hydrogen peroxide into intercellular spaces. In fact, this probably does go on during macrophage-mediated tumor killing, but since tumor cells have varying sensitivities to peroxide this is probably not a major factor. Why CP and TNF should selectively kill tumor cells is unknown.

NK Cells

As discussed above and in Chapter 14, natural killer (NK) cells were discovered almost accidentally in the course of looking for cytotoxic cells in tumor immunity. It was found that in many cases lymphocytes from normal, healthy donors displayed as much cytotoxicity toward a particular tumor *in vitro* as did cells taken from a patient carrying that tumor. At about the same time, other investigators noted that nude mice and neonatally thymectomized mice, kept in germ-free environments, did not have appreciably different cancer rates than did normal mice. These observations marked a change in focus from the CTL to the newly defined NK cell as the principal mediator of immune surveillance against cancer.

It has been postulated that the principal function of NK cells is in surveillance against spontaneously arising tumors. Although difficult to prove, this is an attractive hypothesis. Because NK cells require no period of activation, they can function immediately on contact with a transformed cell, giving the host at least several days' headstart before T- and B-cell compartments are brought into play. Tumor cells that are resistant to NKCC *in vitro* grow best *in vivo*. Interferons, which enhance NK cell activity, also confer protection in animals against transplanted syngeneic tumors.

The evidence that NK cells are important in tumor immunity is substantial, but mostly indirect. NK cells are quite effective in killing tumor cells *in vitro*. When mice or rats are given innoculations of tumor cells, there is at least a transient rise in the level of NK cells in the spleen and blood. Mice infused with purified NK cells resist transplanted tumors much more effectively than untreated mice. Humans with Chediak-Higashi syndrome, and mice with the "beige" mutation, are both deficient in NK cells and experience a higher frequency of spontaneous tumors.

Although defined originally in terms of the ability to recognize and destroy a wide range of tumor target cells, it is now clear that NK cells also attack other types of cells. Two additional classes of NK-sensitive cells are stem cells or immature cells generally, and certain virus and mycoplasma infected cells. Since many tumor cells often share a number of features in common with virally infected or developmentally immature cells, a common sensitivity of these two cell types to NK lysis may not be surprising. The surface structures of these various cell types recognized by NK cells is not known.

NK cells are found in the highest concentration in rodents in the spleen, and in humans the peripheral blood lymphocytes are a good source of NK activity. There is a high degree of correlation between NK cells and large granular lymphocytes (LGL) in both rodents and humans. LGL are devoid of T- and B-cell surface markers but display the Fc receptor. However, antibody is not required for NK killing, and NK cells are not phagocytic, so the relevance of the Fc receptor is unclear. It may be that NK cells are capable both of NK killing and ADCC under different circumstances.

NK cells in humans display the M1 marker (Mac-1 in mice) and the T-10 marker. Mouse LGL with NK activity display the Ly5 and the NK-1 and NK-2 antigens. In most species, NK cells are low during infancy, high during the breeding years, and decline again in old age. This is the reciprocal of the age-related pattern of cancer incidence.

Given the wide range of target specificities of NK cells as a population, the question naturally arises as to whether individual NK cells have the same broad range of specificities, or whether the population is composed of multiple clones with more restricted specificities. This question would be easier to approach if we knew the nature of the target cell antigenic structure recognized by NK cells, but unfortunately this remains a major unknown. The one thing that is clear is that NK cells do not recognize MHC antigens on target cells; blocking of MHC antigens has no effect on NK killing, and MHC-deficient tumors make perfectly good NK target cells. When LGL cells with NK activity are cloned, the individual clones show a variety of target cell recognition patterns. Some are very widely specific, lysing nearly the full range of NK-sensitive target cells. Other clones show a more restricted target cell specificity, and some will kill only one or two of the target cell test panel. Of course, the test panels in these experiments are not exhaustive, so it would seem safe to say that most NK cells are multispecific. However, the wide range of target specificities displayed by individual NK cells is something of a puzzle at present. We do not know, for example, whether this indicates that NK cells display a spectrum of different receptors on different cells.

Immunotherapy

The various elements of the immune system provide our innate defenses against cancer. Can these elements be manipulated to any advantage in the treatment of cancers that "sneak through"? This question defines the field of immunotherapy. There are two distinct components of immunotherapy. In one, elements of the immune system (principally antibodies) are removed from the body (or, more frequently, are generated in another animal) and either concentrated or chemically modified, and then reintroduced into the body in attempts to locate and/or destroy tumor cells. In the second approach, various manipulations are carried out in attempts to alter the function of components of the immune system within the body itself, in order to potentiate destruction of the tumor.

The Use of Monoclonal Antibodies in the Diagnosis and Treatment of Cancer

As discussed earlier, many spontaneously arising tumors seem to be minimally immunogenic to the host. Thus it has been difficult in human cancer patients to identify and isolate, in useful quantities, antibodies specific for tumor antigens. However, with the advent of techniques for producing monoclonal antibodies (mAbs) outside the body, an increasing armamentarium of tumor specific mAbs has been produced and characterized. In some cases these antibodies are specific only for the individual tumor used to induce their formation. But in an increasing number of cases, mAbs have been produced that are reactive with tumor cells of the same histological type in nearly all patients with that tumor type.

The strategy for producing tumor-specific mAbs is basically the same as for any other monoclonal antibody (see pp. 74–77). Human tumor cells are isolated and injected into mice. Where practical, the mice receive multiple injections of the same tumor, spaced one to two weeks apart. A week or so after the final injection, the spleen is removed from the mouse and the spleen cells are fused with an appropriate B-cell tumor to produce hybridomas (Figure 4-7). The monoclonal antibodies produced by these hybridomas are screened for their ability to react with the original tumor, but not with the normal tissue counterpart of that tumor, or with tumors of other histological origins. These tumor-specific mAbs are then tested against the same histological type of tumor cells from other patients. Those mAbs capable of reacting with the same type of tumor in many different patients are then selected for further use.

Diagnostic Applications of Tumor-specific Monoclonal Antibodies

Monoclonal antibodies have been used in several ways to aid in the detection of cancer. One strategy is to "tag" the mAb with a radionuclide that can be detected by an external radioactive scanner. The tagged antibody is injected into the patient's bloodstream and hopefully finds its way selectively to the tumor. The patient is then examined with a whole-body radiation scanner, and tumor deposits are visualized on X-ray film.

A number of problems were encountered with this technique during its developmental stage in animal models, such as (1) nonspecific sequestration of the antibody in noncancerous tissue spaces (particularly kidneys), (2) too-rapid clearance of the antibody from the bloodstream, before it can concentrate in the tumor, (3) dissociation, or (4) degradation of the radioactive tag. However, many of these problems have been overcome with experience, and recently this technique has proved a valuable adjunct in the imaging of certain tumors in humans. It is not used as a means for primary tumor detection but has had some success in spotting previously unsuspected metastases.

A second application of mAbs is in the detection of circulating tumor antigens or tumor-associated macromolecules. A number of such products have been identified. Certain hepatomas (liver tumors) and other tumors secrete a molecule called α-fetoprotein (AFP), so-called because it is a serum protein normally found only in fetuses. The presence of AFP in the circulation of adults can be an indication of an active liver tumor. Similarly, certain tumors of the alimentary canal secrete carcinoembryonic antigen (CEA), another protein normally associated with embryonic cells. Testicular tumors often secrete a form of human chorionic gonadotrophin (HCG), and on occasion even AFP. Yet other tumors may shed some form of surface antigenic products into the general circulation. With appropriate monoclonal antibodies, all of these products can be monitored by ELISA assays (Figure 6-16). While again not particularly useful for primary tumor detection, these analyses have proved valuable in gauging the effectiveness of cancer treatments. For example, in the case of a testicular tumor that was secreting HCG prior to surgical removal or drug treatment, reappearance of HCG in the circulation at some point after treatment is usually an early warning that the tumor has returned.

"Magic Bullets": The Use of Monoclonal Antibodies to Destroy Tumor Cells

One of the principal limitations in the use of chemotherapeutic drugs is that they must be delivered systemically. Although the drugs have some degree of selectivity for cancer cells, they are always toxic at some limiting dosage for normal cells as well. Bone marrow is by far the most sensitive tissue compartment. Opportunistic infections and anemia are the most common—and most dangerous—side effects of chemotherapy. Both problems are directly related to bone marrow toxicity. The experiments using radiolabeled mAbs to seek out tumors demonstrate that these antibodies can, when properly produced and screened, circulate throughout the body and lodge only within the tumor itself. Such antibodies should be ideal vehicles for delivering anticancer drugs directly to a tumor.

Tumor-specific mAbs have been conjugated with a variety of biological toxins for use as antitumor reagents. Such conjugates are called immunotoxins or "magic bullets." The most common toxins used are ricin and diphtheria toxin, which are both potent inhibitors of protein synthesis. Each of these toxins has the ability to kill a cell if even one, or at best a few, molecules succeeds in entering the cell. As shown in Figure 20-4, both ricin and diphtheria toxin are composed of two chains, A and B. In both cases, the B chain functions to bind the dimer to the cell surface, and to facilitate entry of the A chain into the cell. The A chain is the actual toxic molecule. The B chains for both toxins bind to galactose, allowing these toxins to bind to virtually any cell in the body. Magic bullets are usually constructed by conjugating only the A chain to the tumor-specific mAb, so that random contacts with cells during circulation of the immunotoxin in blood or lymph will not result in the death of healthy cells. However, A chain-only conjugates are usually less effective than conjugates made using the intact toxin. This is presumably due to loss of the entry-facilitating properties of the B chain. Various approaches to this dilemma are under investigation. The most promising in the long run are those that seek to modify the B chain (or, by site-specific mutagenesis, the B-chain gene) such that it no longer binds to galactose but retains its entry–facilitation function.

The major barrier to the use of magic bullets *in vivo,* of course, is the extreme potency of the toxin portion of the molecules. In order to avoid damage to normal cells, the tumor specificity of the mAb portion must be absolute. This is difficult to achieve. As we have seen, most antibodies are, to some extent, cross-reactive with related, and sometimes even with totally unrelated, molecules. Morever, although a given tumor antigen may not be detectable on normal cells in the tissue of origin, it may be present on a very small proportion of immature, stemlike cells within the tissue, since these are often the cells from which the tumor arises. The elimination of such cells along with the tumor could have serious consequences.

Another problem arises from nonspecific clearance of immunotoxins in the kidneys or by circulating or fixed macrophages and other phagocytic cells. Severe damage to cells or tissues entrapping immunotoxins is bound to occur. This problem may be exacerbated by formation of complexes of immunotoxin with circulating tumor antigen. Such complexes are deposited more efficiently in the kidneys and are more likely to be taken up by phagocytes. This problem could likely be greatly reduced by using $(Fab)_2$ or Fab fragments instead of intact mAb.

Aside from specificity, stability of the immunotoxin is also a concern. On one hand, the linkage of the toxin and the mAb must be as stable as possible in the circulation, so that toxic molecules are not released indiscriminately in normal tissue. Although isolated A chains have only a fraction of the potency of intact-toxin molecules, no one wants large quantities of A chain circulating throughout the body. On the other hand, the nature of the bond between the mAb and the toxin must be such that it can be dissociated once the conjugate is endocytosed, so that free A chain can make its way to ribosomes, where it exerts its protein synthesis inhibiting effect.

Despite these limitations and qualifications in the use of immunotoxins *in vivo,* research is continuing. The limitations of chemotherapy, particularly against solid tumors, have already been realized. Impressive results have been obtained in a few

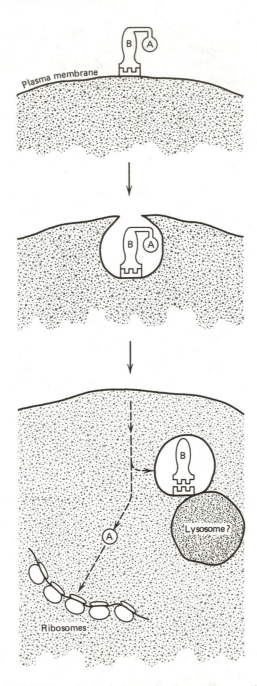

Figure 20-4 "Magic bullets" (immunotoxins) may be the next generation of chemotherapeutic drugs. Toxins of the type most commonly used to make magic bullets have two subunits. The A subunit is an extremely potent inhibitor of protein synthesis and

animal systems, providing hope that magic bullets may ultimately find use in humans. The promise of greatly improved target specificity and incredible potency makes these efforts well worth pursuing.

Another use of toxin-conjugated mAbs, that may see clinical application even sooner, is in the purging of tumor cells from leukemic bone marrow prior to autochthonous reimplantation. Many leukemia patients, especially those with acute lymphoblastoid leukemia (ALL), respond well to chemotherapy; early stage ALL patients can often be cured by chemotherapy alone. However, a certain fraction of these patients will relapse, and during the second course of their disease will usually respond less well to normal levels of chemotherapy. One possible approach to treating such patients is to give them much higher, in effect, lethal, doses of chemotherapy, thus ensuring destruction of the tumor, and then to rescue them from fatal anemia and leukopenia with a bone marrow transplant.

Transplantation of allogeneic bone marrow of course carries with it the complication of graft-versus-host (GVH) disease (see Chapters 14 and 19), something a person in relapse with leukemia does not need. One way to avoid GVH would be to use autochthonous (self) bone marrow. Bone marrow could be removed from patients during remission, that is, after treatment results in the disappearance of clinically detectable disease. A number of mAbs specific for ALL-associated antigens are available. These could be conjugated with toxins, and used to purge the marrow of any remaining tumor cells. The purged marrow could then be stored in liquid nitrogen and used to restore marrow function if the patient subsequently relapses and must be treated with toxic levels of chemotherapy. In a recent laboratory study in which normal marrow was purposely contaminated with ALL cells *in vitro*, a combination of four different anti-ALL "magic bullets" were used for purging. The ALL cells were reduced by at least six logs without damage to marrow stem cells. This method will likely be used in controlled clinical trials in the near future.

Biological Response Modifiers

A second approach to applying our knowledge of how the immune system works in the treatment of cancer patients consists of manipulating various immune elements *in vivo*. A number of agents capable of doing this, called biological resonse modifiers (BRMs) have been tested in experimental animals, and a few have been used clinically.

---

can cause rapid cell death. The B subunit binds the toxin to the cell and, in some way not yet clear, accelerates endocytosis of the A subunit into the cell. Once inside the cell, the A chain is released at some step from either the endocytic vesicle, or a subsequent processing vesicle, and finds its way to the ribosome where it exerts its inhibitory effect.

In the case of magic bullets, mABs recognizing tumor surface antigens are conjugated with the A subunit of toxin. The mAb binds specifically to the tumor cells and are presumably endocytosed in a fashion similar to the intact toxin, although the efficiency of entry of A into the cell is generally lower than when it is attached to the B chain.

Two major classes of BRMs have been examined to date. One class consists of selected microbial products, such as BCG (Bacillus Calmette-Guerin, an attenuated form of tubercular bacillus that is an active ingredient of complete Freund's adjuvant). Attenuated forms of *B. persussis* or *C. parvum* have also been used. These materials have been applied with some success in the treatment of certain types of cancer. For example, BCG injected directly into early stage malignant melanomas (a deadly form of skin cancer) has proved to be beneficial in triggering regression of the tumor. BCG may also be of some benefit as an adjunct form of therapy in breast cancer as well, although in general a positive effect of BCG on solid tumors deep in the body (or even advanced-stage melanoma) has been difficult to demonstrate unequivocally. Microbial agents used as BRMs appear to function principally by stimulating macrophage activity. As discussed elsewhere in this chapter and in Chapter 14, "activated" macrophages are one of the body's principal defenses against cancer.

The second class of BRMs, one that is still very much in an experimental stage with respect to use in cancer therapy, is the lymphokines. Most attention has been focused on the interferons, although very recently the interleukins have stimulated considerable interest. As discussed in Chapter 16, the interferons (IFNs) are a group of glycoproteins related by their production in response to viral infection, and by their suppressive effect on the spread of viral infection within the body. The precise mode of action of the various interferons is not known in every case (there are three major groups of interferons—alpha, beta, and gamma—and each group may have several subtypes, depending on the species). Some of the properties of interferons would seem to be of potential benefit in treating cancer. Alpha-IFN, and to some extent Gamma-IFN, enhance NK cell activity. Gamma-IFN has a pronounced stimulatory effect on macrophage activity; recent studies using recombinant Gamma-IFN suggest this substance may be identical with MAF (see Chapter 17). Numerous animal model studies using whole interferons suggested that these agents may indeed have a powerful antitumor effect.

The availability of most IFNs in cloned recombinant form has allowed clinical trials of their effectiveness in treating cancer. Previously, not enough material for clinical use could be generated, using the existing lengthy isolation and purification protocols. Recombinant IFN has the advantage of providing large quantities of absolutely pure material, but may suffer as a clinical reagent in that antiviral or antitumor effects seen in animal models may have resulted from the combined action of multiple IFN subtypes.

Clinical tests with IFNs are still in the very early stages, and few tests have proceeded beyond phase I (testing of a new drug to determine toxicities and dosage limitations). Alpha IFN showed some benefit when in phase I studies in patients with lymphoma, breast cancer, kidney cancer, melanoma, and AIDS (Kaposi's sarcoma). Clinical trials using recombinant beta and gamma IFNs are still too preliminary to yield any meaningful data. Because of its potent immunomodulatory effects *in vitro* and in animal systems, the results of current phase I trials with gamma IFN are awaited with particular interest. No trials at all with combinations of

IFNs, which will likely be more effective than individual IFNs, have yet been initiated.

The immunomodulatory effects of IL-2 have been discussed in several chapters of this text. T helper cells play pivotal roles in both humoral and T-cell-mediated cytotoxicity reactions, and one of the key modulatory factors in both types of reactions is IL-2. Cancer patients quite often display a markedly decreased function of their $T4^+$ (T helper) subset of lymphocytes. This may explain the fact that many cancer patients appear to be immunosuppressed, not only with respect to their tumor, but generally. An immune defect related to inadequate T helper cell function could conceivably be redressed by supplying exogenous IL-2. Again, the availability of recombinant IL-2 has made direct laboratory and clinical tests possible. Phase I trials with advanced cancer patients unresponsive to other forms of treatment have recently begun. It is too early yet to know whether IL-2 has any effect on advanced oncological disease. One problem encountered using large quantities of IL-2 is excessive water retention—weight gains of 10 kg or more are not uncommon.

As with immunotoxins, exploration of BRMs as cancer chemotherapeutic agents is still in a very early stage. It is too soon to say how effective any of the approaches described here will be. All of them have the attraction of using "natural" substances to help fight disease, instead of chemical poisons. But simply because something is natural does not mean it is not dangerous—toxic side effects have been noted with all of these reagents. Nevertheless, given the practical limitations discussed earlier with standard chemotherapy, it is safe to predict that research into magic bullets and BRMs will continue at a brisk pace in the years ahead.

Bibliography

General

Bishop, J. Michael, Cellualr Oncogenes and retroviruses. *Annual Review of Biochemistry, 52,* 301 (1983).

Doherty, P. C., B. Knowles, and P. Wettstein, Immune surveillance of tumors in the context of MHC restriction of T cell function. *Advances in Cancer Research 42,* 1 (1984).

Granger, G. A., A. L. Orr, and R. Yamamoto, Lymphotoxins, macrophage cytotoxins and tumor necrosis factors. An interrelated family of antitumor effector molecules. *J. Clinical Immunol. 5,* 217 (1985).

Hellstrom, K. E., and I. Hellstrom, Immunological enhancement of tumor growth. In I. Green, et al. (eds.), *Mechanisms of Tumor Immunity.* Wiley, New York (1971), p. 147.

Levine, A. Transformation-associated tumor antigens. *Advances in Cancer Research 37,* 75 (1982).

Mihich, E., Biological response modifiers: Their potential and limitations in cancer therapeutics. *Cancer Investigation 3,* 71 (1985).

North, R. J. Models of adoptive T-cell mediated regression of established tumors. *Contemp. Topics Immunobiol. 13,* 243 (1984).

Oldham, R. K., Biologicals and biological resonse modifiers: New approaches to cancer treatment. *Cancer Investigation 3,* 53 (1985).

Ortaldo, J., and R. Herberman, Heterogeneity of natural killer cells. *Annual Review of Immunology 2,* 359 (1984).

Vitetta, E., and J. Urh, Immunotoxins. *Ann. Rev. Immunol. 3,* 197 (1985).

Research

Brunner, K. T. et al., Quantitation and clonal isolation of CTL precursors selectively infiltrating sarcoma virus-induced tumors. *J. Exp. Med. 154,* 362 (1981).

Foley, E. J., Antigenic properties of methylcholanthrene-induced tumors in mice of the strain of origin. *Cancer Research 13,* 835 (1953).

Gray, P. et al., Cloning and Expression of cDNA for Human Lymphotoxin, a Lymphokine with Tumor Necrosis Activity. *Nature 312,* 721 (1984).

Klein, G. et al., Demonstration of resistance against methylcholanthrene-induced sarcomas in the primary autochthonous host. *Cancer Research 20,* 1561 (1960).

Krolick, K. et al., In vivo therapy of a murine B cell tumor using antibody-ricin A chain immunotoxin. *J. Exp. Med. 155* 1797 (1982).

Pennica, D. et al., Human tumor necrosis factor: Precursor structure, expression and homology to lymphotoxin. *Nature 312,* 724 (1984).

Prehn, R. T., and J. M. Main, Immunity to methylcholanthrene-induced sarcomas. *J. Nat. Cancer Inst. 18,* 769 (1957).

APPENDIX I

Production and Testing of Congenic Resistant Mouse Strains

Because of the importance of congenic resistant (CR) strains of mice to many phases of contemporary immunological research, it is very important for the student to have a solid understanding of how CR strains are produced, and of the usages and limitations of such strains. The standard procedure for the production of strains congenic for histocompatibility loci is shown in Figure A-1. The object of this procedure is to get one or at best a very few tightly linked histocompatibility genes from inbred strain B onto the genome of inbred strain A, as free as possible from contamination by other B genes.

In the first mating, A males are bred to B females. (Together with appropriate matings later on, this eliminates the introduction of Y-chromosome-linked histocompatibility genes, which by appropriate breeding experiments can be introduced separately.) The resultant F_1 hybrids will be uniformly heterozygous for all histocompatibility loci at which A and B differ. A number of such matings of A and B mice may be utilized to initiate the procedure, since by definition the F_1 progeny from all such matings will be genetically identical. If skin grafts from the F_1 hybrids are grafted back to parent A, they will be rejected, since all carry one b allele for each histocompatibility locus.

The next step in the procedure is to backcross male F_1 mice to female A-strain mice. Those loci that can segregate will do so, generating a new distribution of a and b alleles for each of the histocompatibility loci. Theoretically, in some number of offspring, all of the H genes could be homozygous for the a allele. If the total number of H genes is more than a few (which is certainly the case in mice) the likelihood of this occurring at the first backcross generation is extremely small. Most offspring will be a mixture of a/a homozygous and a/b heterozygous for the various alleles.

In practice, several successive backcross generations are produced before any further new steps are introduced into the procedure. Obviously, each backcross generation reduces the total number of b alleles among the total pool of offspring, the result of which is that any particular member of say the fourth or fifth backcross

515

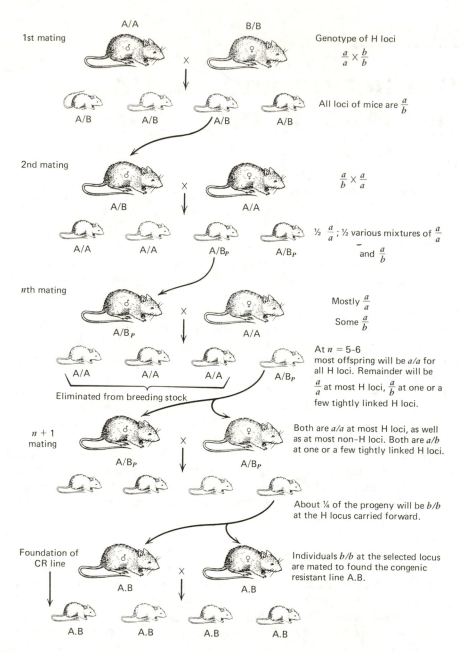

Figure A-1 Production of inbred strains congenic for a histocompatibility locus. A/B indicates a mouse some of whose H loci are *a/b*.

generation will be *mostly a/a* for the various H genes, and *a/b* for only a few. A fair number now may in fact be homozygous *a/a* for *all* the H genes. These can be detected, and subsequently eliminated from the breeding pool, by monitoring the ability of a graft of their skin to survive on an A-strain (*a/a*) recipient. The progeny whose skin grafts are rejected by the A parent by definition have one or more *b* alleles of some H gene in their genome. Those progeny whose skin grafts are accepted by the A-strain parent are by definition *a/a* homozygous at all H loci, and can be removed from the breeding stock. The backcross matings are continued for a minimum of 10 generations, with progeny homozygous *a/a* for *all* H loci being culled at each generation after detection by grafting to the A parent. Early on in the procedure, the *b* H genes will be present as part of an initial chromosome. As more crosses are carried out, crossovers will occur such that parts of the *b* chromosome are lost. Constant screening however keeps the selected *b* H gene in the breeding line.

After a dozen or so generations, relatively few of the progeny retain *b* alleles for H genes; but of those that do, simple mathematical analysis indicates that the likelihood that any one is heterozygous *a/b* for more than one H allele is quite small. And, of course, the number of *b* alleles for other, non-H loci is also extremely small, being in sum no more than 2^{-n}, where n is the total number of backcross generations.

The next step in the procedure is to produce animals that are homozygous *b/b* for the various selected H genes (Figure A-1). This is accomplished by beginning brother-sister matings within the litters produced from the last backcross mating, using those littermates still retaining the *b* alleles in question (as detected by skin grafting to the A parent). If the *b* allele for a single H gene has been retained and is freely segregating, then roughly one-quarter of the progeny from the mating will be *b/b* for the H gene in question. These can readily be detected by a reversal of the previous grafting technique. If a particular mouse is, in fact, *b/b* for a particular H gene, then it will reject an A-strain skin graft, which is *a/a* for that gene. (Remember, the mouse under study is itself *a/a* at all other H loci.) Mice that are now found to be *b/b* at the H locus in question can be used to start an inbred strain of mice, as previously described. This strain of mice will have the B-strain genotype for the selected H locus, superimposed on an A-strain genetic background. The standard notation for such a strain is that it is A.B for that locus. Throughout this phase of the procedure, more and more non-H (unselected) *b* material continues to be lost from either side of the H locus.

At this point, of course, an H locus has been selected for, but its identity is not known. The simplest first step in identifying or at least defining the various loci is to determine the total number of *different* loci existing among the pool of A.B CR strains. This can be done most efficiently using something called the "F_1 test" (Figure A-2). The theory underlying this test is the following. Consider two A.B CR strains, A.B1 and A.B2, whose relationship to one another is not known. Either they carry the same H gene from B, or different H genes from B. To distinguish these two possibilities, the two strains are mated to produce (A.B1 $\times$ A.B2) F_1 hybrids,

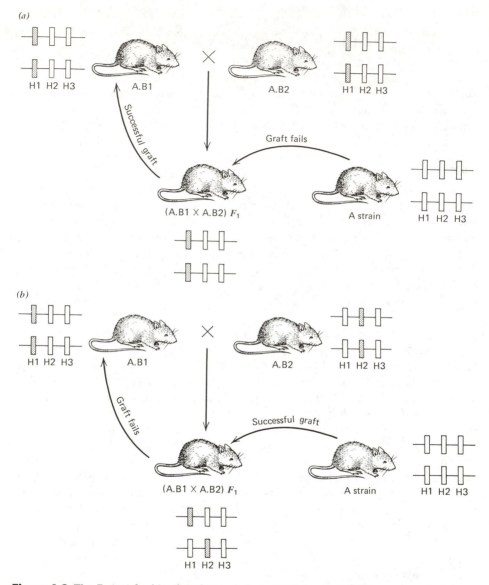

Figure A-2 The F_1 test for identity of genetic loci. (*a*) Histocompatibility gene carried over from B is the same in A.B1 and A.B2. (*b*) Histocompatibility gene carried over from B is different in A.B1 and A.B2.

which are then grafted with an A-strain skin graft. If A.B1 and A.B2 are homozygous (*b/b*) at different H loci, then the F_1 will be *a/b* heterozygous at both loci, and the A graft (which is *a/a* at both loci) will be accepted. If, on the other hand, A.B1 and A.B2 are in fact carrying the same B-strain H gene, both will be homozygous (*b/b*) at that particular locus, and so will the F_1 hybrid. In this case, the A-strain skin graft will be rejected. By repeating this test with the various A.B CR strains produced from the original procedure, it will be possible to sort them into groups based on the identity or nonidentity of their H loci.

The groups may be further analyzed by studying the pattern of segregation of the individual H loci with other known (mapped) genetic traits. Remember that CR strains, although selected for on the basis of acquired histocompatibility genes, almost always have other genetic material transferred in from the donor strain. This is often grossly observable in the CR phenotype, which may have the fur type or color of the H-gene donor, or its tail structure, or other physical traits. Since it is mathematically unlikely that these genes are far removed from the selected H gene, the two are thus inferred to be closely linked. When two H loci deduced to be different by the F_1 test are assignable to different, freely segregating linkage groups, the case for distinctness is considerably strengthened.

The value of CR strains in immunogenetic research depends entirely on the degree of certainty about just how much of a chromosomal segment has been "grafted in" by the procedures just described. If a particular locus is transferred onto a given genetic background, its boundaries are operationally the next detectable loci on the centromeric and telomeric portions of the recipient chromosome, and any portions of genetic material lying within these regions from the donor chromosome may be transferred undetected with the marker locus. This is an important caveat to bear in mind when using CR strains, or when interpreting experiments in which such strains are used, for example in the production of specific antisera or in assigning genes to specific chromosomal loci. For an example of the problems that can arise when the boundaries of a transferred locus are uncertain, see the account of the IJ locus presented on page 208.

APPENDIX II

MHC Gene Complexes in Other Species

For theoretical and practical reasons, the mouse and human MHC systems have been examined in greatest detail. However, equivalent gene systems have been detected in virtually every vertebrate species where an appropriate search has been made. Phylogenetic analyses are useful in that they can provide insights into the evolution of MHC gene complexes, particularly if pushed into the lower vertebrate orders; the origin of MHC genes, both structurally and functionally, is still something of a mystery. Traces of genes—or at least DNA sequences—related to Ig, MHC, and Thy-1 molecules have been found in a variety of invertebrates, particularly in the protochordates and colonial tunicates. Vertebrate organisms, measured against most other life forms, are rather large and have long generation times. This gives the more rapidly reproducing parasites that live in vertebrates an evolutionary adaptive advantage. The vertebrate answer to this challenge may well have been the development of mechanisms to allow rapid diversification of key defensive molecules such as immunoglobulins, T-cell receptors and MHC molecules. The genes and proteins of the vertebrate immune system, including the MHC, may in a sense contain the fossil evidence of over 500 million years of host–parasite coevolution.

A comparison of structure and function of MHC complexes among vertebrates may also indicate which features are rigorously conserved throughout evolution and are therefore likely to be most important biologically. For example, in at least five other species besides mouse and humans, one or more components of complement map within or very close to the MHC. This could suggest some as yet undetected genetic regulatory relationship between these complement components and class I or class II MHC genes. On the other hand if, as has been suggested, genes for these complement components were accidentally "trapped" within the MHC, then this event must have occurred long ago in evolution, since one of the species having MHC-associated complement genes is the chicken (Table A-1).

In the following sections, we will examine briefly the main features of MHC genes and gene products in those vertebrate species that have been studied in addition to mice and humans. A limited number of references for these species is given at the end of this chapter. The author will be happy to supply a more complete list upon request.

Table A-1 Some Characteristics of the MHC Gene Products of Various Vertebrate Species

| Species (locus) | Class I loci | | Class II loci | | Complement genes in MHC |
	Number of loci	Number of serological specificities	Number of loci	Ir gene function	
Cat (FeLA)	?	0?	?	?	?
Chicken (B)	1	29	1	Yes	Yes
Chimpanzee (ChLA)	2				
Cow (BoLA)	1	12	1		
Dog (DLA)	3	18	1		Yes
Frog	≥1	?	≥1	?	
Goat (GLA)	2	12		Yes	Yes
Guinea pig (GPLA)	2	4	3	Yes	Yes
Horse (ELA)	2	18	≥1		
Humans (HLA)	3	>100	3–4	Yes	Yes
Marmoset (MaLA)			≥1		
Mouse (H-2)	3	>100	2	Yes	Yes
Pig (SLA)	2 (3)	22	≥1	Yes	Yes
Rabbit (RLA)	1	10	≥1		
Rat (Rt-1)	2	39	2	Yes	
Rhesus monkey (RhLA)	2	25	≥1		Yes
Sheep (OLA)	2	9			
Syrian hamster (Hm-1)	2	0	≥1		

Cat (FeLA). Little information exists in the literature regarding the feline MHC. Attempts to produce lymphocyte-specific antibodies, which usually detect different alleles of class I MHC gene products, have failed for the most part. Grafts exchanged between randomly selected domestic cats show prolonged rejection times (two to three weeks) characteristic of differences at minor rather than major histocompatibility loci. Cats also seem not to develop cytotoxic T cells during viral infections, a process linked to class I MHC antigens. Mixed leucocyte cultures are almost always negative, although there is a good response to the T-cell mitogen Con A. The information gathered so far would suggest very limited polymorphism of both class I and class II genes. This could possibly be tied to the observation that some of the larger wild cats show little polymorphism at other genetic loci. Nevertheless, the situation with the MHC in cats may suggest that extensive polymorphism of MHC products is not absolutely required for a species to be successful. (see also the Syrian hamster).

Chicken (B). A great deal of work has been done on the MHC of the chicken. The BF locus codes for a 43,000-dalton peptide that associates with β2-microglobulin on the surface of most somatic cells and seems to be directly homologous to human and mouse class I proteins. It is highly polymorphic, with nearly 30 serologically defined antigens. A class II-like molecule of 30,000 daltons is coded for by a gene or genes in the BL locus; these antigens are found only on B cells and monocytes. A third locus, BG, is unlike anything found in H-2 or HLA. It codes for a class I-like molecule that is highly polymorphic but found only on red blood cells. (It may be useful to bear in mind that bird erythrocytes are nucleated.)

Inasmuch as birds and mammals diverged at different times and from different reptilian stem lines, some 1.5 to 2.0 × 10⁸ years ago, the similarities in avian and mammalian MHC systems indicates an impressive conservation of the basic features of major histocompatibility complexes.

Chimpanzee (ChLA). Interest in the possible use of organs from higher primates for transplantation into humans spurred a great deal of interest in the early 1970s in the MHC complexes of species like the chimpanzee and the Rhesus monkey. When initial transplants failed completely, interest in the accompanying MHC research waned. The animals are expensive to buy and maintain, and because there do not appear to be any fundamental differences between subhuman primate and human MHCs, attention now has focused almost exclusively on the latter.

Cow (BoLA). So far at least one class I-like locus (A) has been defined in the cow, with 16 alleles and associated serological determinants. The corresponding peptide (or peptides) has not been isolated and studied. A second, closely linked locus (BoLA-D) stimulates mixed leukocyte reactions, which is usually a class II gene function. The arrangement of the BoLA genes, and their chromosomal location, are not known at present.

Dog (DLA). The MHC locus of dogs has been fairly closely studied because of the use of these animals in experimental transplantation. The dog has three class I genes (A, B, and C), and one class II-like locus that has Ir gene function and can stimulate in an MLC. Canine class I genes, of which a total of 12 alleles have been identified, code for a 40-kd protein associated in the plasma membrane with β-2m. It seems very likely that at least C4 maps to DLA.

Frog. The existence of an MHC-like locus in frogs was inferred about 10 years ago, first as the locus for genes coding for erythrocyte antigens, and later as the locus for genes controlling lymphocyte antigens, as well as MLR and graft rejection. The breeding properties of frogs can be manipulated to give large numbers of genetically identical individuals and these have been used to carry out lymphocyte immunization programs. This has allowed the production of a number of different alloantisera, defining a series of MHC alleles. These antisera have been used to immunoprecipitate material from spleen cell extracts, resulting in the isolation of 40 to 44-kd molecules that map to the MHC. These molecules are always found in association with a 13,000-dalton peptide very similar to β-2m. The larger molecule appears almost certain to be the amphibian analog of a class I protein. Class II antigens mapping to the MHC locus have also been isolated. These consist of α and β chains with molecular weights of 30 to 35 kd; both chains appear to be highly polymorphic. Thus, the appearance of an MHC with features strikingly similar to mice and humans can be placed at least as early as the amphibians.

Goat (GLA). The MHC of the goat contains genes for both class I and class II antigens and encodes complement genes as well. The extent of polymorphism of class I genes has not been fully determined, but at least a dozen alleles have been defined at two class I loci. The class II loci have been characterized both by immune response function and by MLC typing.

Guinea Pig (GPLA). So far, two class I loci, designated GPLA-B and GPLA-S, have been described. Four alleles of the GPLA-B locus have been characterized, and only one genotype of GPLA-S is known. The products of the B and S loci are 40,000-dalton peptides (slightly smaller than mouse or human) that associate on the cell surface with β-2 microglobulin.

The I region of guinea pigs, which appears to lie outside of the B and S loci, contains at least three subregions, each coding for unique peptides. Two of the loci each code for peptides of 33,000 and 25,000 daltons, whereas the third locus codes for a single peptide of 27,000 daltons.

Guinea pigs were brought from South America to Europe by the Spanish in the sixteenth century; currently used American guinea pig strains were derived from a limited number of breeding pairs of the European stock. This history may explain the apparent low degree of polymorphism of the guinea pig MHC genes.

Horse (ELA). Little work has been done on the horse MHC system. At present, it appears that there are two class I-like loci, with 20 or so associated serologically defined antigenic specificities. These loci are closely linked to an MLR locus, which in mice and humans would indicate a class II gene.

Marmoset (MaLA). Interest in the MHC of this New World primate stems from the fact that the multiple fetuses are normally hematopoietic chimeras and thus mutually tolerant after birth. This would provide an opportunity to study the role of MHC antigens in the development of immunological tolerance.

The existence of at least one class II locus has been inferred by use of HLA-D antibodies to isolate a dimeric molecule with subunits of 28 kd and 33 kd. This dimer is biochemically similar to numerous other mammalian class II molecules. The fact that it can be immunoprecipitated by an antibody to human class II proteins exemplifies the high degree of structural conservation among vertebrate MHC genes and gene products. Class I genes or gene products have not yet been identified in the marmoset, but almost certainly exist.

Pig (SLA).   Pigs have three class I loci, with more than 20 serologically defined specificities. The class I gene products are 42,000-dalton peptides associated with β-2 microglobulin. Class II gene products include peptides of 31,000 and 25,000 daltons, but the number of coding loci involved is unclear. Several inbred lines of pigs are currently being developed by David Sachs at the National Institutes of Health for use in studying the immunological parameters of organ transplantation in mammals larger than mice.

Rabbit (RLA).   Although the rabbit was one of the earlier models for studying transplantation, serious study of the rabbit MHC was begun only recently. The rabbit has class I molecules similar to those found in other species, but it appears at present that these are encoded by a single locus with limited polymorphism. Some of these may be expressed at the cell surface unassociated with β-2 microglobulin. There is also evidence for at least one class II locus in the RLA.

Rat (Rt-1).   The structure of the rat MHC, Rt-1, is, as might be expected, very similar to the mouse H-2 complex. Two class I loci (Rt-1A and Rt-1D) flank two sets of genes coding for class II MHC proteins. This arrangement is typical only of rat and mouse; most other species seem to have the arrangement typical of the human HLA, in which a cluster of class II genes is located centromerically to a cluster of class I genes.

A limited amount of structural information suggests that rat MHC products are very similar to those of mice and humans. Rat class II genes have Ir function. So far, complement components have not been mapped to Rt-1, but it would be very surprising if they were not ultimately found there.

Rhesus Monkey (RhLA).   Not surprisingly, the MHC region of the Rhesus monkey shows a great deal of homology with HLA. Two class I loci, A and B, code for a 44,000-dalton peptide found on the surface of virtually all cells in association with β-2 microblobulin. A DR locus contains one or more pairs of class II α and β genes that code for peptides biochemically very similar to their HLA counterparts. The gene coding for complement factor B (B$_f$) also maps to RhLA. An interesting locus called "48" may code for class I molecules analogous to Tla antigens in mice.

Syrian Hamster (Hm-1).   The Syrian hamster is one of the most interesting of animals from the point of view of MHC study. Mutual immunization between randomly selected hamsters produces antibodies that are directed only against class II antigens. The antigens thus defined consist of a fairly orthodox α (39 kd) and β (29 kd) chain. These molecules appear to function in antigen presentation and can induce both MLC and GVH reactions. Although of fairly limited polymorphism, a number of distinct alleles of hamster class II genes have been identified.

The surprising fact, of course, is that no class I antigens are detected by cross immunization of one animal with spleen cells of another. Streilein and his associates have now shown convincingly that there exists but a single, monomorphic class I gene at each of two class I loci in Syrian hamsters. The gene products are 47-kd peptides that associate in the membrane with β-2m. Preliminary amino acid sequence data suggests normal homology (70 percent or so) with mouse and human class I MHC proteins. But no polymorphisms have ever been detected.

The implications of this striking finding are currently the subject of much discussion among immunologists. As we have seen in Chapter 14, one of the principal functions of class I MHC proteins is thought to be the facilitation of recognition by cytotoxic T lymphocytes (CTL) of virally infected cells within the body. Many immunologists believe this may require some sort of physical interaction between the virus and the class I protein. According to this view, the value of polymorphism of class I genes within a species is that if viruses evolve a way to escape interacting with the class I proteins of some members of the species, they will still be trapped by other members, and the species will survive. The existence of an evolutionarily successful species with monomorphic class I genes certainly challenges this idea.

Bibliography

Balner, H. et al., The major histocompatibility complex of chimpanzees. Identification of several new antigens controlled by the A and B loci of ChLA. *Tissue Antigens 12,* 1 (1978).

Briles, W., and R. W. Briles, Identification of haplotypes of the chicken major histocompatibility complex (B). *Immunogenetics 15,* 449 (1982).

Darden, A. G., and J. W. Streilein, Syrian hamsters express two monomorphic class I MHC molecules. *Immunogenetics 20,* 603 (1984).

Flajnik, M. et al., Identification of class I MHC-encoded molecules in the amphibian Xenopus. *Immunogenetics 20,* 433 (1984).

Gill, T. J. *et al.,* Orientation of loci in the MHC of the rat, and comparison to man and the mouse, J. Immunogen. 9, 281 (1982).

Goujet-Zalc, C. et al., Molecular characterization of two Ia-like antigens in marmosets. *Immunogenetics 19,* 155 (1984).

Jonker, M. et al., Typing for RhLA-D in Rhesus monkeys: Genetics of the D antigens and their association with DR antigens in a population of unrelated animals. *Tissue Antigens 19,* 69 (1982).

Lazary, S. et al., Equine leukocyte antigen system. II. Serological and MLR studies in families. *Transplantation 30,* 210 (1980).

Millot, P., Comparison of the segregation of sheep histocompatibility genes OLA-A1, A8, B7, B9 and OLX-5 in eighteen hamster × sheep fibroblast hybrid lines. *J. Immunogen. 9,* 185 (1982).

Nizetic, D. et al., The major histocompatibility of the mole rat. *Immunogenetics 20,* 443 (1984).

Parham, P., and H. Ploegh, Molecular characterization of HLA-A,B homologues in owl monkeys and other non-human primates. *Immunogenetics 11,* 131 (1980).

Pollack, M. S. et al, Preliminary studies of the feline histocompatibility system. *Immunogenetics 16,* 339 (1982).

Proceedings of the second international bovine lymphocyte antigen (BoLA) Workshop. In *Animal Blood Groups and Biochem. Genetics 13,* 33 (1982).

Raff, R. F. et al., The canine MHC. Population study of DLA-D alleles using a panel of homozygous typing cells. *Tissue Antigens 21,* 360 (1983).

Tykocinski, M. et al., Rabbit class l MHC genes: cDNA clones of an expressed gene and a putative pseudogene. *J. Immunol. 133,* 2261 (1984).

Vaiman, M. et al., Genetic organization of the pig SLA complex. Studies on nine recombinants and biochemical and lysostrip analysis. *Immunogenetics 9,* 353 (1979).

Van Dam, R. H. Definition and biological significance of the major histocompatibility system (MHS) in man and animals. *Vet. Immunol. Immunopathol. 2,* 517 (1981).

Van Dam, R. H. et al., Phenotyping by the mixed lymphocyte reaction in goats (LD typing). *Vet. Immunol. Immunopathol. 2,* 321 (1981).

Wilkinson, J. M. et al., Rabbit MHC antigens: Occurrence of non-β2-microglobulin-associated class I molecules. *Molec. Immunol. 19,* 1441 (1982).

GLOSSARY

Many of the terms defined in this glossary may have broader definitions when applied to biology generally. The definitions listed here give only the meaning of the particular term when applied to immunological systems and phenomena.

Acquired Immunity Immunological resistance to disease developed after birth. Cf. *Innate immunity.*

Active Immunization The induction of a state of immunity in an animal by exposing it to a specific antigen. In this case, the state of immunity is produced by the animal's own immune system. Cf. *Passive immunization.*

ADCC Antigen-dependent, cell-mediated cytotoxicity. See *CMC.*

Adenopathy Swelling or enlargement of glands, particularly the lymph nodes.

Adjuvant As used in immunology, a substance mixed with antigen in order to elicit a stronger or more sustained response. The most commonly used is Freund's adjuvant, which is a mixture of mineral oil, lanolin, and killed mycobacteria. When mixed thoroughly with aqueous antigen, an oil-in-water emulsion is formed, from which antigen is released over a prolonged time after subcutaneous inoculation. The killed mycobacteria, and to some extent the mineral oil itself, seem to intensify macrophage activity at the site of the injection, which may account in part for the enhanced immune response to the included antigen.

Adoptive Transfer The transfer of previously sensitized immune elements to a nonimmune recipient.

Afferent (Nerve, Blood Vessel, Lymphatic Vessel) Leading toward a structure.

Agglutination The clumping together of cells (including bacteria) via a multivalent molecule or agglutinin (q.v.).

Agglutinin Any multivalent molecule capable of cross-linking cells or bacteria. IgM is a particularly potent agglutinin, as are most lectins.

Alexin Name originally used to describe complement activity in normal and immune serum.

ALL Acute lymphoblastic leukemia.

Allele An alternate form of a gene. Only one allele for any given gene is expressed per haploid genome, although any number of alleles of the same gene can be present in a species as a whole.

Allergen A substance capable of inducing an allergic reaction.

Allergy An immune reaction resulting in damage to self-tissues and cells, usually through inflammatory reactions.

527

Alloantiserum   Antiserum raised in one member of a species against allelic molecules (usually cell-surface antigens) of another member of the same species.

Allogeneic   Immunogenetic term defining the relationship between two members of the same species, whether blood related or not (excluding identical twins or members of the same inbred strain).

Allogeneic Effect   Nonspecific activation of B cells by factors from T cells activated in an allogeneic reaction (i.e., against cell-surface alloantigens).

Allograft   Graft exchanged between two nonidentical (genetically) members of the same species.

Allotype   Protein end product of the expression of an allelic gene. Among immunoglobulins, where the term is most commonly used, it refers to the particular allelic variant of an isotypic light or heavy chain gene expressed in a particular individual.

Anamnestic Response   Positive form of immunological memory, that is, an enhanced response as a result of previous exposure to an antigen.

Anaphylaxis   A state of hypersensitivity caused by release of vasoactive amines and other agents from mast cells or basophils. Release of these substances is triggered by the interaction of cell-bound antibody (usually IgE) with antigen (allergen).

Anaphylotoxin   Pharmacological agent released during an anaphylactic reaction. Histamine and serotonin are major anaphylotoxins.

Antibody   Any immunoglogulin binding a defined antigen at its antigen-combining site (paired V_H–V_L domains, or F_V region).

Antigen   Any molecule capable of interacting in a stable way with the antigen-combining site of an immunoglobulin molecule. An antigen molecule can be free in solution or occur as part of a cellular membrane.

Antigenic Determinant   That portion of an antigenic molecule that interacts directly, by molecular complementarity, with the antigen-combining site of an immunoglobulin molecule.

Aplastic   Not expanding in cell number by mitosis.

Ascites   Serous fluids accumulating in the peritoneal cavity. Tumor cells growing in the peritoneal cavity usually induce accumulation of ascites fluid.

Atopy   IgE-mediated allergic hypersensitivity in humans. The term formally means "out of place" and reflects the fact that allergies were once thought to be aberrant reactions to rare or unidentified antigens.

Atrophic   Wasted; reduced in size by cell death or degeneration.

Autoantibody   Antibody directed against self-antigens (autoantigens), whether or not the antibody was originally produced in response to self-antigens.

Autoantigen   An antigen or antigenic determinant present on self-tissues. A true autoantigen is one that is present naturally and not generated secondarily by drug-induced tissue alterations or by viral infection.

Autochthonous   Coming from self.

Autograft   A graft from one part of the body to another in the same individual.

Bacteriolysin   A term used earlier in this century to describe that property of immune serum that, together with alexin (complement), induces the lysis of bacteria. Now known to be appropriate classes of immunoglobulin.

BCG   *Bacillus Calmette-Guerin*. An attenuated form of *Mycobacterium bovis*. Can be used as a specific vaccine or in an adjuvant as a nonspecific immune stimulator.

Bence-Jones Protein   Monoclonally derived immunoglobulin light chains present (often in dimeric form) in the urine of certain myeloma patients.

Benign   With regard to tumors, lacking the capacity to invade surrounding normal tissues. Benign tumors may grow rapidly or slowly. Cf. *Malignant*.

Blast Cell   A cell shortly before, during, or shortly after cell division. Has a higher cytoplasm: nucleus ratio than in the resting state.

Blastogenesis   The production of blast cells. Usually in association with cell activation caused by antigen or mitogen.

Blocking Antibody   Antibody that blocks access to a particular antigen by other cells or molecules with antigen-specific receptors.

Bovine   Deriving from a cow, ox, or other closely related species.

Bursa of Fabricius   Saclike projection from the gut near the proctadeum in birds. The bursa influences the maturation of B lymphocytes.

Capping   Phenomenon wherein plasma membrane molecules, physically cross-linked by an extracellular ligand, aggregate at a restricted region of the cell surface.

Carcinogen   A substance capable of causing cancer. Carcinogens may be physical (e.g., electromagnetic radiation), chemical (e.g., methylcholanthrene, various other coal tar products), or biological (e.g., certain viruses).

Carcinoma   Tumor originating in epithelial cells.

Carrier   An immunogenic molecule used to "carry" or present a small nonimmunogenic molecule in such a way that it (the small molecule) can induce an immune response.

CEA   Carcinoembryonic antigen, an antigen found on embryonic gut cells and also on certain tumors, particularly of the alimentary canal.

Chemotaxis   Movement of a cell from one location to another under the influence of a chemical gradient. For example, phagocytes can be attracted to the site of an infection by complement fragments diffusing out from the site of an infection.

Chemotherapy   Treatment of cancer using drugs (as opposed to radiation therapy or surgery).

Chimera   An animal or tissue derived from multiple genetic sources, by other than a normal reproductive process.

Clone   A group of cells all derived from a single cell progenitor.

Clonotype   A particular gene product produced by members of a single clone.

CMC   Cell-mediated cytotoxicity; the process of destruction of one cell (the target cell) by another cell (the effector cell). The common types of CMC in immunology are direct, cytotoxic T lymphocyte-mediated CMC, in which target-cell recognition is through a membrane-bound T-cell receptor; ADCC, mediated by most leukocytes with an Fc receptor against an antibody-coated target cell; LDCC, mediated by various leukocytes against a target cell coated with an appropriate lectin; and NKCC, mediated by NK (natural killer) cells against tumors.

CML   Cell-mediated lympholysis. See CMC.

Coisogenic (Conisogenic)   Identical in genetic composition except at a single genetic locus, where an alternate form (mutant or allelic) of a specific gene is present. In mice, for example, coisogenic strains have been derived as the result of a mutation in one of the genes coding for an MHC protein. Cf. Congenic.

Colostrum   The first milk secreted after giving birth.

Con A   Concanavalin A, a lectin extracted from jack beans. Binds to the surface of most cells. Depending on the species of animal involved, and the form in which it is utilized, Con A may completely activate T cells or B cells or both.

Congenic Identical in genetic composition except at a defined chromosomal segment, where alternate allelic gene forms are present. In mice, congenic strains usually have identical genetic backgrounds and differ only at a defined chromosomal segment such as a portion of the MHC, or some other histocompatibility locus. Cf. Coisogenic.

Conjugate When used as a noun in immunology, the term *conjugate* may refer to a complex of a cytotoxic effector cell bound to its target, or to a complex of a toxin molecule bound to an antibody.

Consanguinous Sharing the same blood; in a less strict sense, any closely related family members.

Coproantibody Antibodies (principally IgA) present in the lumen of the lower digestive tract and/or in feces.

Cortex The outer, peripheral region of a defined anatomical structure.

CTL Cytotoxic T lymphocyte.

Cytophilic Cell loving. Commonly used to refer to antibodies that bind to cell surfaces by interaction of their Fc regions with a membrane-bound Fc receptor.

Cytotoxic Destructive of cells.

Determinant See antigenic determinant.

Domain Structural unit of about 110 amino acids, occurring in immunoglobulin light and heavy chains. Each domain has one internal disulfide loop. There is a considerable degree of sequence homology among Ig domains, and they are thought to be duplications of an ancestral prototypical gene that gave rise to all of the known Ig polypeptides. Recent studies suggest a domainlike structure for MHC proteins as well.

Edema Abnormal accumulation of serous fluid in tissue spaces. Usually due to a failure of the lymphatic system to drain off leakage occurring normally (or after trauma) in capillary networks.

Effector Cell The cell actually carrying out a specific function, such as cell-mediated cytotoxicity.

Efferent (Nerve, Blood Vessel, Lymphatic Vessel) Leading away from a structure.

ELISA *E*nzyme-*l*inked *i*mmuno*s*orbent *a*ssay.

Endocytosis Internalization of extracellular materials.

Endotoxin Lipopolysaccharides localized in the cell walls of gram-negative bacteria. Responsible for most of the pathogenic effects of these organisms. Their effect is exerted while they are still embedded in the intact cell wall.

Enhancement Refers to the prolonged survival of a transplant occasionally observed when the recipient has been preexposed to the donor's tissues. Presumed to be due to antibodies or antigen-antibody complexes that interfere with the afferent or efferent phase of the cell-mediated cytotoxic response.

Epitope Antigenic determinant (q.v.).

Erythema Redness due to localized capillary enlargement or rupture. Common in localized inflammatory reactions.

Erythropoiesis Generation of red blood cells.

Etiology Study of the origins of disease.

Exotoxin Diffusible proteins secreted by both gram-positive and gram-negative bacteria that are responsible for the pathogenic effects associated with the producing bacterium.

Fc Receptor Receptor found on a wide range of cells in the immune system that is specific for the Fc portion of a specific immunoglobulin molecule.

Follicle Roughly spherical aggregation of cells. In lymph tissue, cells interacting during the production of antibody are often collected into follicles, at the center of which may be a germinal center (q.v.).

Freund's Adjuvant See *Adjuvant.*

Genotype The combined genetic material received from both parents.

Germinal Center A histologically discernible region of lymph nodes and spleens; populated mostly by B lymphocytes. During immune reactions leading to antibody production, cells within the germinal centers undergo extensive proliferation.

Germ-Line The genetic material actually transmitted from one generation to the next. Germ-line DNA does not display any of the gene rearrangements seen in fully differentiated B cells, for example.

Granulocyte Any one of the granular leukocyte blood cells; eosinophils, neutrophils, or basophils.

H-2 The major histocompatibility gene complex of the mouse.

Haplotype When used with reference to the MHC, a haplotype is defined as the particular collection of alleles of MHC genes present on one parental chromosome. In a more general sense, defined as the sum total of genetic material inherited from one parent.

Hapten A low molecular weight compound that cannot by itself induce an immune response, although it can combine with antibody (cf. *Immunogen*).

Hemagglutinin Any molecule capable of agglutinating red blood cells (antibodies to red cell antigens, various plant lectins, etc.)

Hemolysin An historical term, still occasionally used to describe that property of anti-erythrocyte serum which, together with complement, induces the direct and rapid lysis of red blood cells. It is now known to be anti-red cell IgM.

Hemopoiesis Generation of the various blood cells. Usually implies lymphopoiesis (q.v.) but sometimes used to mean only erythropoiesis.

Heteroclitic An antibody induced by one antigenic determinant that reacts more strongly with a different antigenic determinant.

Heterograft Graft from a genetically disparate individual; it is preferable to use the terms "allograft" or "xenograft" (q.v.).

Heterologous Not the same as the original (antigen; cell; antibody).

Histocompatibility Antigen Any cell-surface antigen capable of provoking graft rejection.

HLA The human major histocompatibility gene complex.

Humoral In solution or suspension; refers particularly to the antibody and complement immune mechanism, in contrast to cell-mediated immunity.

Hybridoma A cell derived by fusion of a normal cell with a tumor cell. Most hybridomas are selected to retain the functional properties of the normal parent cell and the continuous proliferation characteristic of the tumor parent cell.

Hyperplasia   Faster-then-normal increase in the size of an anatomical compartment as a result of increased cellular proliferation.

Idiopathic   Primary disease; pathological state arising as such and not as a result of previous or other disease.

Idiotype   An antigenic determinant associated with the antigen-combining site of an immunoglobulin molecule.

Imaging   In cancer diagnosis, the visualization of an internal tumor by means such as X ray, CT scan, NMR scan, etc.

Immunity   From the Latin *immunitas,* meaning roughly "freed from having to pay taxes." In the general sense, refers simply to resistance to extraneous, nonself (foreign) matter. As used by contemporary biologists, refers specifically to those mechanisms of resistance involving the immune system.

Immunogen   A substance capable of provoking an immune response. All immunogens are antigens (q.v.) but not all antigens are necessarily immunogens (most haptens, for example, are not immunogens).

Immunoglobulin   A globular serum glycoprotein with antibody activity. All immunoglobulins are variants of the basic H_2L_2 tetrapeptide structure.

Induration   The process of becoming hardened. During a cutaneous delayed hypersensitivity reaction, the skin becomes hardened to the touch in the area of the reaction.

Inflammation   A complex set of tissue responses to injury or other trauma, characterized by altered patterns of blood flow; destruction of damaged cells; removal of cellular debris; and healing of damaged tissues.

Innate Immunity   The repertoire of defenses, both immunological and nonimmunological, that exist prior to and independently of exposure to specific environmental antigens.

Interferon(s)   A group of mostly low molecular weight, acid stable proteins secreted by virus-infected cells that can protect noninfected cells from virus infection.

In Vitro   Literally "in glass." Used to refer to experiments involving living cells or tissues carried out outside the body.

In Vivo   Refers to experiments or procedures carried out in a living animal.

Isotype   A product of a gene, some form of which is carried by and expressed in the genome of each member of the species. For example, the γ_1 gene is carried by each human, although the particular *allele* of γ_1 that is carried can differ among individuals.

K Cells   Also called null cells. Nonphagocytic cells of unknown lineage, similar to lymphocytes but with neither T- nor B-cell surface markers. K (for "killer") cells can destroy antibody coated target cells by ADCC (q.v.).

Karyotype   The chromosomal profile of a given cell.

Kinins   Peptides released during anaphylaxis that induce contraction of smooth muscle and dilation of blood vessels.

LD Antigens (also Lad; Lymphocyte-determined Antigens)   Cell surface antigens that provoke a proliferative response in allogeneic T cells.

LDCC   Lectin-dependent cell-mediated cytotoxicity. See CMC.

Lectins   A group of proteins, usually plant-derived, capable of binding to the surfaces of animal cells. (see *Con A, PHA.*)

Leukemia   Cancer originating in any of the defined classes of hemopoietic cells.

Leukocyte   Literally "white cell." A general term formerly used to refer to any cell found in the blood that was not of the erythroid series. No longer particularly useful since the extensive functional and morphological categorization of white blood cells.

Leukopenia   A condition in which the number of circulating white blood cells is decreased below normal (ca. $5 \times 10^3/mm^3$ in humans).

Ligand   A substance that attaches to something else.

Local Immunity   Immunity that develops in a local site, relatively independently of the network of lymph glands and ducts throughout the body. Production of IgA antibodies to bacterial antigens in the gut is an example of local immunity.

Locus   Genetic term referring to a chromosomal segment containing a particular gene. Adjacent genes belong to separate loci if and only if they can be separated by a crossing over event.

LPC   Large pyrininophilic cell(s). Lymphoid cells in a blastoid state with abundant pyrinine-staining material (RNA) in the cytoplasm. A term used mostly to describe T cells activated in an MLC.

LPS   Lipopolysaccharide. A bacterial endotoxin, usually obtained from *E. coli,* capable of activating B cells in an antigen-independent fashion.

Lymph Fluid   The acellular serous exudate from capillaries picked up by the lymphatic drainage vessels and thus circulated throughout the lymphatic network.

Lymphoid   Having the characteristics of, and referring specifically to, cells of the lymphocytic series.

Lymphokine   Any of a number of substances produced and secreted by activated T lymphocytes, which affect other cell types.

Lymphoma   A general term that includes any tumor arising in lymphoid tissue.

Lymphopoiesis   Generation of the cellular elements of the spectrum of lymphocytes.

MAb   Monoclonal antibody.

Malignant   With regard to tumors, having the capacity to invade and disrupt surrounding normal tissues. Malignant tumors may be fast or slow growing; malignancy has nothing to do with growth rate. Cf. *Benign,* metastasis.

Mast Cell   A free-standing cell found almost exclusively in tissue compartments. It resembles blood basophils but is not derived from the granulocytic series. Mast cells release histamine on sensitization by antibody and antigen.

Medulla   The inner or central region of a defined anatomical structure.

Megakaryocyte   A white blood cell distinct from the lymphoid, monocytic, or granulocytic lines. Megakaryocytes produce *platelets* by a process of cytoplasmic budding.

Metastasis   With regard to tumors, the tendency of cells to break away from the primary tumor and migrate to secondary locations via the blood or lymph. Cf. malignant.

Memory   An altered immunological response to a given antigen resulting from exposure to that antigen.

MHC   Major histocompatibility complex. Originally defined as the genetic locus coding for those cell surface antigens presenting the major barrier to transplantation between allogeneic individuals. Now known to encode a wide range of genes coding for or controlling immunological functions.

Mitogen   Any substance capable of inducing a cell to begin DNA synthesis and cell division.

MLC   Mixed leukocyte (or lymphocyte) culture. Generally interpreted to include both proliferation and generation of cytotoxicity against allogeneic lymphocytes *in vitro*.

MLR   Mixed leukocyte (or lymphocyte) reaction. Often used in a more restricted sense than MLC (q.v.) to refer to just the proliferative phase of the reaction of T lymphocytes to allogeneic cells *in vitro*.

Monoclonal   Ultimately deriving from a single cell. Monoclonal antibodies are produced by populations of B lymphocytes that all derive from a single precursor hybridoma cell.

Multiparous   A female who has conceived more than once.

Multiple Myeloma   An oncologic disorder characterized by uncontrolled proliferation of myeloid cells, malignant lesions of bone, and the presence in the serum and urine of high levels of immunoglobulin-related proteins.

Multispecificity   The ability of a given immunoglobulin combining site to bind more than one type of antigen molecule. Multispecificity reduces the total number of combining sites needed to deal with the antigenic universe.

Murine   Of or pertaining to mice.

Myeloma Protein   A monoclonal immunoglobulin or immunoglobulin chain produced in an animal or a human with myeloma.

NK Cells   "Natural killer" cells. Cells present in the system that kill target cells, particularly tumor cells, without previous sensitization.

Necrosis   Disruption and atrophy of tissue through cell death.

Northern Blot   An experimental technique in which RNA species are separated on the basis of size by electrophoresis and then developed by hybridization with a highly radioactive nucleic acid probe. The location of RNA fragments hybridizing with the probe is determined by autoradiography of the dried electrophoresis gel.

Null Cells   White blood cells that are neither monocytes nor granulocytes, yet lack T- or B-lymphocyte surface markers. Null cell populations contain the effectors detected in ADCC and NKCC (q.v,).

Oncogenes   Altered forms of protooncogenes (q.v.) that promote or allow uncontrolled cellular proliferation.

Oncogenic   Capable of causing cancer.

Oncology   The study of tumors.

Ontogeny   The developmental history of an individual organism from conception to birth.

Opsonin   Any substance that enhances phagocytosis of a cell or particle. Antibodies and certain complement components are the major opsonins occurring normally in the body.

Opsonization   Usually involves coating a particle or cell with an antibody or complement, enabling it to adhere firmly to the surface of a phagocyte bearing appropriate receptors. The stable contact thus created enhances phagocytosis.

Ovine   Of or pertaining to sheep.

PAGE   *Polyacrylamide gel electrophoresis.*

Palliation   Relief of symptoms, as opposed to cure of the underlying problem or disease.

Parous Having given birth.

Pathogenic Capable of causing disease.

PBA Polyclonal B-cell activator. Most substances mitogenic for B cells, such as LPS (q.v.) are effective PBA.

PBL Peripheral blood lymphocytes (i.e., lymphocytes found in the blood circulation).

PHA Phytohemagglutinin, a plant lectin from kidney beans, which activates principally T lymphocytes.

Phagocytosis Literally, "eating of cells." The process by which certain cells, principally PMNs and macrophages, ingest cellular and particulate matter.

Phagosome Digestive vacuole within a phagocyte. Also called secondary granule.

Phylogeny The evolutionary history of a species.

Pinocytosis A generalized process by which a wide variety of cells ingest extracellular materials.

P-K Antibodies Prauznitz-Küstner antibodies. (Also called reaginic antibodies.) The antibodies in humans (now known to be IgE) responsible for atopic allergy.

Plasma Blood minus whole cells; includes the complete set of blood clotting factors.

Plasma Cells The terminally differentiated antibody producing and secreting progeny of activated B cells.

Platelet Small anuclear cell structure that derives from megalokaryocytes. Platelets (also called thrombocytes) are easily ruptured and release thrombin, which is important in blood clotting.

PMN Polymorphonuclear granulocyte; also called neutrophil.

Polyclonal Activator A substance that activates large numbers of different lymphocytes, independent of their antigenic specificity.

Porcine Of or pertaining to pigs.

PPD Purified protein derivative, prepared by $(NH_4)_2SO_4$ precipitation of the supernate of *M. tuberculosis* cultures.

Private Specificity A serologically defined antigenic specificity associated with a cell-surface protein coded for by the MHC. Private specificities are restricted to specific MHC haplotypes (cf. *Public specificity*).

Prophylaxis Preventive treatment—vaccination, for example.

Protooncogenes Genes involved in the induction, modulation, or suppression of proliferation of normal cells. When altered by translocation or recombination with viral nucleic acids, they may be transformed into oncogenes (q.v.).

Prozone Effect Failure of immune precipitation to occur in the presence of high antibody concentration.

Public Specificity An antigenic determinant, present on an MHC-coded protein, that is found in common among many different allelic forms (haplotypes) of the same protein.

Pyrininophilic Absorbing the stain pyrinine, which is specific for RNA.

Quiescent At rest; inactive.

Reaginic Antibody Antibody mediating release of vasoactive amines from appropriate storage cells (mast cells, basophils, etc.). In humans, IgE is the reaginic antibody.

Relapse In cancer, reappearance of clinically detectable disease after a period of remission (q.v.).

Remission   In cancer, a state of absence of clinically detectable tumor cells in the body. Should not be confused with cure.

RES   Reticuloendothelial system (q.v.).

Reticuloendothelial system   A collective term for cells of various origin, morphology, and residence active in phagocytosis. RES cells form much of the matrix of lymphoid organs.

RIA   Radioimmunoassay.

Sarcoma   Tumor originating in connective tissue.

SD determinants   Antigenic determinants on MHC gene products that are defined principally by their serological reactivity.

Serum   The noncellular elements of blood remaining after removal of clotting proteins.

Southern Blot   An experimental technique in which DNA fragments are separated on the basis of size by electrophoresis and then developed by hybridization with a highly radioactive nucleic acid probe. The location of DNA fragments hybridizing with the probe is determined by autoradiography of the dried electrophoresis gel.

Syngeneic   The genetic relationship between identical twins, or between two members of the same inbred strain (if they are the same sex).

T Cells   Lymphocytes that matured in, or were absolutely dependent for their differentiation on, the thymus.

Terpolymers   Polymers (usually linear) of three different amino acids in defined ratios.

Thrombocyte   See *Platelet.*

Thymocytes   Lymphoid cells resident in the thymus. Not to be confused with T cells (q.v.).

Titer   A term used to connote the relative strength of an antiserum. An antiserum is progressively diluted until some measurable property of the antiserum (agglutination, facilitation of complement-mediated lysis, etc.) is reduced by some predetermined amount. That dilution (i.e., 1:256) is then defined as the titer for that particular antiserum.

Tolerance   A natural or artificially induced state of nonresponsiveness to a specific antigen.

Toxoids   Toxins that have been modified in some way to reduce or eliminate their toxic effects while retaining their immunogenic and antigenic properties.

Trabeculum   A portion of an encapsulating connective tissue sheet that penetrates into (and often partially compartmentalizes) a gland or organ.

Tuberculin   Crude protein fraction isolated from the supernate of cultures of *M. tuberculosis.*

Tumor Antigens   Antigens found on tumor cells, but not on normal cells (including immature cell forms) of the tissue of origin.

Vasculitis   Inflammation of blood vessels.

Vasoactive   Affecting blood vessels.

Xenogeneic   Immunogeneic term defining the relationship between individuals belonging to different species.

Xenograft   Graft transplanted from one species to another.

Index